Immunologically Mediated
Pulmonary Diseases

Immunologically Mediated Pulmonary Diseases

Edited by

Joseph P. Lynch III, MD

Associate Professor of Internal Medicine
Division of Pulmonary and Critical Care Medicine
University of Michigan Medical School
University of Michigan Hospitals
Ann Arbor, Michigan

Richard A. DeRemee, MD

Professor of Medicine
Mayo Medical School
Consultant, Division of Thoracic Diseases
  and Internal Medicine
Mayo Clinic and Mayo Foundation
Rochester, Minnesota

With 31 additional contributors

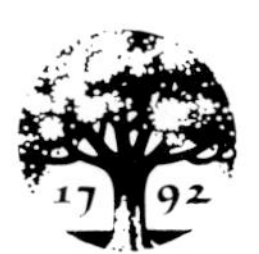

J.B. LIPPINCOTT COMPANY
Philadelphia   New York
London   Hagerstown

Acquisitions Editor: Charles McCormick, Jr.
Assistant Production Manager: Lori J. Bainbridge
Production Coordinator: Michael Bass & Associates
Compositor: Bookmasters
Printer/binder: Arcata Graphics/Halliday

6   5   4   3   2   1

Library of Congress Cataloging-in-Publication Data
Immunologically mediated pulmonary diseases/edited by Joseph P. Lynch III,
    Richard A. DeRemee with 31 additional contributors.
        p.   cm.
    Includes bibliographical references.
    Includes index.
    ISBN 0-397-51051-9
    1. Lungs—Diseases—Immunological aspects.   2. Lungs—
Pathophysiology.   3. Lungs—Diseases—Pathogenesis.   I. Lynch, Joseph P.
II. DeRemee, Richard A. (Richard Arthur), 1933–
    [DNLM: 1. Lung Diseases—immunology.   WF 600 I332]
RC756.I46   1991
616.2'4'079—dc20
DNLM/DLC
for Library of Congress   90-13691
                                        CIP

Contributors

Moira Chan-Yeung, MD, FRCPC
Professor of Medicine
University of British Columbia
Professor, Respiratory Division
Vancouver General Hospital
Vancouver, British Columbia, Canada

James H. Dauber, MD
Associate Professor of Medicine
University of Pittsburgh
Chief, Pulmonary Service
Veterans Administration Hospital
Pittsburgh, Pennsylvania

Gerald S. Davis, MD
Professor of Medicine
Director, Pulmonary Unit
University of Vermont Medical Center
Burlington, Vermont

Richard A. DeRemee, MD
Professor of Medicine
Mayo Medical School
Consultant, Division of Thoracic
  Diseases and Internal Medicine
Mayo Clinic and Mayo Foundation
Rochester, Minnesota

Paul Detjen, MD
Clinical Instructor of Medicine
Northwestern University Medical
  School
Fellow, Allergy and Immunology
Northwestern Memorial Hospital
Chicago, Illinois

Gary R. Epler, MD
Chairman, Department of Medicine
New England Baptist Hospital
Associate Clinical Professor
Boston University School of Medicine
Boston, Massachusetts

Joseph C. Fantone III, MD
Associate Professor of Pathology
University of Michigan Medical School
University of Michigan Hospitals
Ann Arbor, Michigan

Jordan N. Fink, MD
Professor of Medicine
Medical College of Wisconsin
Chief, Allergy-Immunology Division
Milwaukee County Medical Complex
Milwaukee, Wisconsin

Paul A. Greenberger, MD
Professor of Medicine
Division of Allergy-Immunology
Northwestern University Medical
  School
Attending Physician
Northwestern Memorial Hospital
Chicago, Illinois

Robert Hoffman, MD
Assistant Professor of Medicine
University of Pittsburgh School
  of Medicine
Director, Bronchoscopy Service
Presbyterian-University Hospital
Pittsburgh, Pennsylvania

Gary W. Hunninghake, MD
Professor of Medicine
University of Iowa College of Medicine
Director of Pulmonary/Critical Care
  Medicine
University of Iowa Hospitals and Clinics
Iowa City, Iowa

Elaine S. Jaffe, MD
Chief, Hematopathology Section
Deputy Chief, Laboratory of Pathology
National Cancer Institute
National Institutes of Health
Warren Grant Magnuson Clinical Center
Bethesda, Maryland

Talmadge E. King, Jr, MD
Associate Professor of Medicine
University of Colorado School of
  Medicine
Chairman, Clinical Affairs
National Jewish Center for Immunology
  and Respiratory Medicine
Denver, Colorado

James W. Leatherman, MD
Associate Professor of Medicine
University of Minnesota
Pulmonary Division
Department of Medicine
Hennepin County Medical Center
Minneapolis, Minnesota

Manuel Lopez, MD
Professor of Medicine
Tulane Medical School
Head, Clinical Immunology Laboratory
Tulane Medical Center
New Orleans, Louisiana

Joseph P. Lynch III MD
Associate Professor of Internal Medicine
Division of Pulmonary and Critical Care
  Medicine
University of Michigan Medical School
University of Michigan Hospitals
Ann Arbor, Michigan

Ralph J. Panos, MD
Instructor in Medicine
National Jewish Center for Immunology
  and Respiratory Medicine
University of Colorado Health Science
  Center
Denver, Colorado

Roy Patterson, MD
Professor of Medicine
Chief, Division of Allergy-Immunology
Northwestern University Medical
  School
Attending Physician
Northwestern Memorial Hospital
Chicago, Illinois

Udaya B. S. Prakash, MD, FRCP(C)
Consultant in Thoracic Diseases and
  Internal Medicine
Director of Bronchoscopy
Mayo Clinic and Mayo Medical Center
Professor of Medicine
Mayo Medical School
Rochester, Minnesota

Charles E. Reed, MD
Professor of Medicine
Mayo Medical School
Consultant in Allergy and Internal
  Medicine
Mayo Clinic
Rochester, Minnesota

Robert M. Rogers, MD
Professor of Medicine and
 Anesthesiology
Division of Pulmonary and Critical Care
 Medicine
Chief, Pulmonary Medicine
Presbyterian-University Hospital
Pittsburgh, Pennsylvania

Edward C. Rosenow III, MD
Arthur M. and Gladys D. Gray Professor
 of Medicine
Mayo Medical School
Rochester, Minnesota

Milton D. Rossman, MD
Associate Professor of Medicine
University of Pennsylvania School of
 Medicine
Hospital of the University of
 Pennsylvania
Philadelphia, Pennsylvania

John E. Salvaggio, MD
Henderson Professor of Medicine
Tulane Medical School
New Orleans, Louisiana

Robert M. Strieter, MD
Assistant Professor of Internal Medicine
Division of Pulmonary and Critical Care
 Medicine
University of Michigan Medical Center
Ann Arbor, Michigan

Paul E. Swanson, MD
Assistant Professor of Pathology
Washington University School of
 Medicine
St. Louis, Missouri

William D. Travis, MD
Staff Surgical Pathologist
Chief, Pulmonary and Postmortem
 Section
Laboratory of Pathology
National Cancer Institute
National Institutes of Health
Bethesda, Maryland

Mark R. Wick, MD
Professor of Pathology
Washington University School of
 Medicine
Associate Director of Anatomic
 Pathology
Barnes Hospital
St. Louis, Missouri

Robert A. Wise, MD
Associate Professor of Medicine
Johns Hopkins University School of
 Medicine
Johns Hopkins Hospital and
 Francis Scott Key Medical Center
Baltimore, Maryland

Craig A. Wolfe, MD
Fellow Associate
University of Iowa
University of Iowa Hospitals and Clinics
Iowa City, Iowa

Adriana Zeevi, PhD
Associate Professor of Pathology
University of Pittsburgh School of
 Medicine
Presbyterian-University Hospital
Pittsburgh, Pennsylvania

Preface

Rapid advances in cellular and molecular biologic techniques have led to significant insights into the pathogenesis of a variety of pulmonary disorders, particularly the interstitial lung disorders (such as sarcoidosis, idiopathic pulmonary fibrosis, and hypersensitivity pneumonitis). Bronchoalveolar lavage has allowed retrieval of inflammatory and immune effector cells from the lower respiratory tract and has provided a closer look into events leading to inflammation, fibrosis, and repair. Although the clinical relevance and application of bronchoalveolar lavage in the management of these disorders remain controversial, insights gleaned from the technique have brought us closer to unraveling the complex cellular interactions involved in the pathogenesis of some of these disorders. It is hoped that increased understanding of the mechanisms of inflammation, fibrosis, and repair will lead to novel and improved therapeutic strategies. Thus, the role of immunosuppressive and cytotoxic agents in the treatment of sarcoidosis, interstitial pneumonias, and vasculitis is addressed.

The development of new biologic tools at the cellular and molecular levels has led to more sensitive and more specific techniques (such as monoclonal antibodies and immunofluorescent and immunohistochemical stains) for the diagnosis of specific diseases (such as lymphoproliferative disorders and eosinophilic granuloma).

For the practicing clinician, the proliferation of new data may be confusing and the extrapolation to clinical medicine of many of these advances in immunology may be obscure. Although several textbooks have dealt with basic mechanisms of disease from the cellular or molecular level, an integrated approach that combines basic science and clinical insights is often lacking. In *Immunologically Mediated Pulmonary Diseases*, we present new insights into the pathogenesis of such disorders and we integrate advances made in the basic science arena with a clinical approach to the diagnosis and management of these heterogeneous disorders. The book is aimed at individuals who have a keen interest in immunology and pulmonology, such as pulmonologists, allergists, rheumatologists, and immunologists. It also represents an invaluable resource as a reference text for medical students, housestaff, and both practicing and academic physicians interested in immune-mediated pulmonary disorders.

Contributors were selected not only for their particular expertise but also for their ability to compile and present both new and historical data in a pragmatic and clinically relevant fashion. State-of-the-art discussion of both common diseases (such as asthma) and uncommon diseases (such as eosinophilic granuloma, chronic beryllium disease, lymphomatoid granulomatosis, and alveolar hemorrhage syndrome) is provided. Chest radiographs and histopathologic material highlight important points. The bibliographies are current and selectively comprehensive, and they allow the reader easy access to original and detailed investigations.

Many interstitial disorders (such as idiopathic pulmonary fibrosis, drug-induced or collagen-vascular–associated interstitial pneumonitis, and bronchiolitis obliterans) have overlapping features, but the salient characteristics of each have been elegantly addressed by individual authors. A detailed discussion of occupational disorders is beyond the scope of this text, but specific chapters on beryllium disease, occupational asthma, and silicosis/asbestosis are presented, recent advances in the understanding of these disorders having made them instructive in the broad category of immune-mediated disorders. The sections on vasculitis are subdivided into several chapters to allow sufficient individualized detail without losing coherence.

Certain disorders covered in *Immunologically Mediated Pulmonary Diseases* (such as pulmonary alveolar proteinosis, eosinophilic granuloma, and angiolympho-proliferative disorders) are of uncertain pathogenesis, and nonimmune mechanisms may be operative. Significant insights into these rare disorders have been gained within the past 5 years, however, and inclusion of these fascinating entities is warranted. A discussion of angiolymphoproliferative disorders in the context of pulmonary vasculitis (particularly lymphomatoid granulomatosis) presents new laboratory techniques (T-cell gene rearrangements, monoclonal antibodies) in this poorly understood group of disorders. The final chapter provides a comprehensive review of novel laboratory techniques that may be used in the management of disorders of uncertain pathogenesis.

As editors, we are delighted with the organization and coherence of *Immunologically Mediated Pulmonary Disorders* and are grateful to the authors for their skillful, comprehensive, and scholarly contributions.

Joseph P. Lynch III, MD
Richard A. DeRemee, MD

Contents

xii   Contents

1

Idiopathic Pulmonary Fibrosis

Ralph J. Panos
Talmadge E. King, Jr.

Idiopathic pulmonary fibrosis is one of the common forms of interstitial lung disease of unknown etiology. This disorder has been referred to as Hamman-Rich syndrome, idiopathic pulmonary fibrosis, cryptogenic fibrosing alveolitis, usual interstitial pneumonitis, desquamative interstitial pneumonitis, fibrosing alveolitis, diffuse alveolar fibrosis, and honeycomb or end-stage lung disease. Hamman-Rich syndrome, however, usually refers to a more fulminant disease, frequently associated with a connective tissue disease, especially rheumatoid arthritis.[1,2] Further, many of the cases originally described by Hamman and Rich,[1,2] and those subsequently reported under this designation, are now considered to be cases of organizing diffuse alveolar damage or cryptogenic organizing pneumonitis (idiopathic bronchiolitis obliterans with patchy organizing pneumonia).[3,4]

Although the cause and pathogenesis of idiopathic pulmonary fibrosis (IPF) are not known, the clinical, physiologic, radiographic, and pathologic findings in this disorder are well characterized. The diagnostic evaluation of a patient with suspected interstitial lung disease requires several sequential steps to differentiate the many possible causes and to stage adequately the extent and severity of the disease process. The initial approach should include a history, physical examination, posteroanterior and lateral chest radiographs, pulmonary function testing (specifically lung volumes, spirometry, diffusing capacity, and arterial blood gas measurements at rest). The most important step in this evaluation is a comprehensive clinical history to ascertain known causes of interstitial lung disease. Particular emphasis must be placed on occupational and environmental exposures of patient and spouse (especially the home and work environment, hobbies, pets, heating and cooling systems), previous illnesses (connective tissue diseases, cardiac or renal disorders), drug ingestion (prescribed, illicit, or

---

Supported in part by SCOR Grant no. HL 27353, National Heart, Lung and Blood Institute.

over-the-counter medicines, including health foods and vitamins), and family history of similar problems or other inherited diseases.

The prevalence of IPF is not known, but it is estimated to be 3 to 5 per 100,000 population.[5] The clinical course of IPF is variable with a mean survival following diagnosis of 3 to 5 years. Most patients with IPF are middle-aged and present with gradually increasing breathlessness on exertion that may be accompanied by a dry, nonproductive cough. Physical examination usually reveals bibasilar, dry, end-inspiratory rales. Signs of pulmonary hypertension and cor pulmonale develop as the disease progresses. Pulmonary function testing reveals reduced lung volumes and decreased diffusing capacity for carbon monoxide. Gas exchange is invariably abnormal either at rest or with exercise. The chest roentgenogram reveals a reticulonodular infiltrate that is more prominent in the lower lobes. Importantly, the diagnosis of IPF requires an open lung biopsy. The predominant histopathologic findings on open lung biopsy are an inflammatory alveolitis and derangement of the alveolar wall structures by fibrous tissue formation.

This chapter will review the current concepts of the pathogenesis of IPF. In addition, the clinical, radiographic, physiological, and histopathologic manifestations of idiopathic pulmonary fibrosis will be presented. Finally, the staging and monitoring of disease progression and available therapies will be discussed.

PATHOGENESIS

The factors that initiate the development of IPF are not known; however, genetic, viral, immune, and inflammatory processes are believed to play important roles in the sequence of events that culminates in the irreversible fibrotic derangements of the pulmonary parenchyma. An unknown inciting injury appears to activate immune and inflammatory processes in the lung that result in altered lung repair and fibrosis in susceptible individuals. Although the sequence of events in the pathogenesis of IPF is not fully known, many of the factors regulating immune, inflammatory, and fibrotic processes in the lung have been implicated in the development of IPF.

Genetic Factors

The hypothesis that there may be a genetic basis for the development of IPF is supported by several findings. This disorder may occur in genetically susceptible individuals who are unable to control the inflammatory, immune, and fibrotic processes in the lung after exposure to some unknown stimulus. The genetic factor may be a gene or group of genes associated with the regulation of pulmonary inflammatory or immune processes.[6] Because of the close association of diseases mediated by immune mechanisms and the HLA genes of the major histocompatibility system on chromosome 6, several studies have evaluated the phenotypic frequencies of the HLA antigens in patients with IPF.[7-10] Two studies found no significant association between HLA antigens and IPF.[11,12] Others reported conflicting evidence of an increased frequency of HLA-B12,[7] HLA-B15,[9] HLA-Dw6,[9] HLA-DR2,[10] and HLA-B8 (in patients with the onset of symptoms before the age of 50 and in women),[8] and a decreased incidence of HLA-

Dw3[9] among patients with IPF. Unfortunately, several problems exist with these studies: only one study evaluated all four HLA loci; different numbers of antigens, ranging from 24 to 65, were examined in each study; and the number of patients in each study was small, ranging from 20 to 50. Therefore, given the disparate results of these linkage studies, no definite association between an HLA locus and IPF has been established.

Evaluation of the alpha-1-antitrypsin locus on chromosome 14 in patients with IPF demonstrated a significant increase in non-MM phenotypes, especially MZ.[13] Another locus on chromosome 14, immunoglobulin gamma (Gm), has been associated with familial pulmonary fibrosis.[14] Further linkage studies of loci on chromosome 14 in individuals with sporadic and familial IPF are needed to determine the role that genetic elements on this chromosome might play in the development of pulmonary fibrosis.

Additional evidence of a genetic basis for IPF is suggested by the association of pulmonary fibrosis with inherited diseases such as Hermansky-Pudlak syndrome,[15,16] Gaucher's disease,[17,18] neurofibromatosis,[19–21] Niemann-Pick disease,[22] and tuberous sclerosis.[23–25]

Familial pulmonary fibrosis provides further evidence of a genetic basis for IPF. Familial pulmonary fibrosis was first described by Sandoz[26] in 1907, predating Hamman and Rich's[1,2] description of diffuse interstitial fibrosis (IPF). The clinical presentation, physical examination findings, and radiographic, physiological, and histopathologic abnormalities in familial pulmonary fibrosis are indistinguishable from findings described in sporadic cases of IPF.[27,28] Disease onset occurs from infancy to middle age and the disease duration is highly variable, ranging from months to many years.[29–37] Identical twins affected by familial pulmonary fibrosis often have a contemporaneous onset of illness and similar clinical presentation and disease course even if they are separated geographically.[32,38,39] Studies of several large kindreds affected by familial pulmonary fibrosis have determined that the pattern of inheritance is autosomal dominant with variable penetrance.[30,32–35] Genetic linkage studies of one family affected by familial pulmonary fibrosis suggest a possible association between the immunoglobulin haplotype Gm 1 on chromosome 14 and the development of familial pulmonary fibrosis.[14]

In an evaluation of 17 clinically unaffected family members of patients with familial pulmonary fibrosis, Bitterman and coworkers[40] found four individuals with positive gallium-67 lung scans and eight with increased numbers of neutrophils and activated macrophages in bronchoalveolar lavage fluid. However, no clinical evidence of pulmonary fibrosis appeared during a follow-up period of 2 to 4 years in these family members with evidence of "alveolar inflammation." Thus, "alveolar inflammation" is either an early development in the pathogenesis of familial pulmonary fibrosis and clinically overt pulmonary fibrosis will be detected in these family members during long-term follow-up or "alveolar inflammation" in these individuals is a mild form of familial pulmonary fibrosis that does not cause clinically apparent pulmonary fibrosis.

Viral Infection

A history of a prodromal flu-like illness[41–46] and the presence of intracellular inclusion bodies in alveolar epithelial cells in lung biopsy specimens from some patients with IPF suggest a viral etiology.[41,47,48] However, little additional evidence exists to support this hypothesis. Intranuclear inclusion bodies have been described by several investigators in patients with desquamative interstitial pneumonitis.[41,44,47] These nuclear inclusions were acidophilic and were separated by a clear halo from a deeply staining and sometimes nodular peripheral basophilic rim of nuclear material. Ultrastructural findings suggested that these intranuclear inclusions were laminated structures resembling myelin figures, and they were considered to be due to nuclear degeneration[41] or nucleoli altered by increased nucleoprotein synthesis in metabolically active alveolar epithelial cells[44] or intranuclear channel systems formed by tubular growth of the inner nuclear membrane in association with cellular growth and increased metabolic activity,[49] rather than viral particles. Not only were these inclusion bodies not viral particles, they were not specific for desquamative interstitial pneumonitis since they have been demonstrated in lung biopsy specimens from patients with tuberculosis, arc-welder's lung, eosinophilic granuloma of the lung, and asbestosis.[44] Furthermore, except for one study of a patient with Hamman-Rich syndrome examined by electron microscopy,[48] viral particles have not been found in other ultrastructural studies,[49–56] nor has a definite viral pathogen been cultured from pulmonary specimens.[53]

An association between Epstein-Barr virus infection and IPF has been suggested by viral serologic studies.[57] In a series of 13 patients, 10 had raised serum IgG against Epstein-Barr (EBV) viral capsid antigen (VCA), early antigen (EA), and nuclear antigen (NA); 3 had IgM against VCA; 13 had IgA against VCA; and 2 had IgA against EA. IgG against VCA was detected in the bronchoalveolar lavage fluid of 5 patients, 3 of whom had alveolar IgA against VCA. Serologic profiles for cytomegalovirus and herpes simplex virus were normal. These findings are intriguing but additional studies supporting these findings are lacking, and confirmation of EBV in pulmonary specimens from patients with IPF is required to determine the role EBV infection may play in the pathogenesis of IPF.

Immune Processes

Immunoglobulins and Autoantibodies

Approximately 20% of patients with pulmonary fibrosis that is indistinguishable from the histopathologic and physiological features of IPF have or develop a rheumatologic disorder, most often rheumatoid arthritis, progressive systemic sclerosis, polymyositis-dermatomyositis, or systemic lupus erythematosus.[46] Consequently, many of the immunologic abnormalities associated with these connective tissue disorders have been sought in patients with IPF.

Evidence of immunologic abnormalities is often present in the blood, bronchoalveolar lavage fluid, and lung tissue of patients with IPF. Hypergammaglobulinemia is present in 17% to 80% of patients with IPF.[46,58–60] The increase in gammaglobulin is due usually to a single class of immunoglobulin, most commonly IgG.[60] Cryoglobulins have been reported in 41% of patients with IPF[46] and the erythrocyte sedimentation rate is elevated in 60% to 94% of cases.[46,61] Serologic autoantibodies are common in these patients,[43,46,58,60–64] including elevated titers of antinuclear antibody (7–25%) and rheumatoid factors (14%) and decreased complement levels (6%).[47,64] Although these serologic abnormalities are common, their role in the pathogenesis of IPF is not known and they are considered to be epiphenomena.[5]

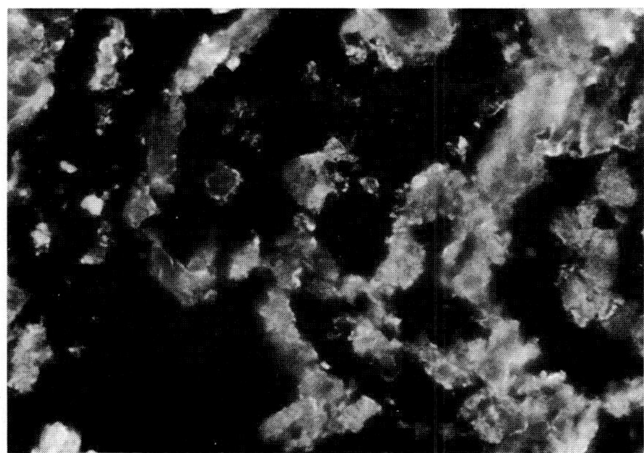

Figure 1-1. Immunofluorescent studies of lung tissue in IPF. This lung biopsy sample shows a cellular pattern of disease and demonstrates granular deposition of IgG along alveolar walls and capillaries. Several interstitial and intra-alveolar mononuclear cells are also positive.

Immune Complexes

Circulating soluble immune complexes are often present in patients with IPF.[65-67] Several investigators have found that elevated circulating immune complexes are associated with greater cellular inflammation in lung specimens[71,72] whereas others have not.[68] Increased IgG levels are found in the bronchoalveolar lavage fluid from patients with IPF,[69-71] and increases in IgG-secreting cells have been detected in lavage fluid from patients with active inflammation.[72] Immunohistochemical staining has detected immunoglobulins and complement lining alveolar walls and capillaries[73,74] (Fig. 1-1), but ultrastructural studies have not detected immune complexes[56,57,74] nor has a specific antigen or group of antigens been identified within the immune complexes. Walker and colleagues[75] have demonstrated immune deposits in about half of their patients with IPF by immunoelectron microscopy. These deposits were localized to the alveolar epithelial surface and/or to the luminal side of the capillary walls. No deposits were seen within the basement membrane. All cases positive for immune deposits by electron microscopy also had increased levels of circulating immune complexes and/or positive findings on light microscopic immunofluorescence. These data suggest that immune complexes are present in the pulmonary parenchyma and further support a role for these immune complexes in the initiation and maintenance of the immune and inflammatory processes that result in lung injury and fibrosis.

Immune Effector Cells

Production of a specific antibody response requires a number of cellular interactions beginning with antigen processing and presentation to T cells by accessory cells.[76] During activation, T cells interact with the antigen and with class II molecules of the major histocompatibility complex on the accessory cells. Class II molecules are expressed on alveolar capillary endothelial cells, alveolar epithelial cells, and alveolar macrophages in patients with IPF[77-83] and lymphocytes (predominantly OKT8+ T cells) are found in the interstitium.[78,80] Aberrant expression of class II molecules on epithelial cells with subsequent presentation of autoantigens to T lymphocytes may initiate autoimmune diseases such as thyroiditis and diabetic insulinitis[84]; therefore a similar mechanism may be present in IPF. In addition, alveolar macrophages may function as accessory cells for antigen presentation to lymphocytes and they are also capable of secreting lymphokines, including interleukin-1, that stimulate T lymphocyte proliferation.[85–89]

In addition, a fraction of the B cells recovered from bronchoalveolar lavage from patients with IPF secrete immunoglobulins that are directed against type I collagen and, further, circulating lymphocytes from these patients are activated when exposed to type I collagen.[90,91] Also, circulating antibodies to alveolar type II cells have been detected in patients with IPF.[92] Thus, although the expression of class II molecules on pulmonary epithelial cells in the proximity of T cells and the presence of lymphocytes that are sensitized to type I collagen in the circulation and bronchoalveolar lavage of patients with IPF suggest the presentation of autoantigens and the activation of an autoimmune process, it is not known if alveolar epithelial cells can present antigen to T lymphocytes functionally. Since class II molecules are expressed on alveolar epithelial cells in sarcoidosis and in pulmonary infections, their role in the pathogenesis of IPF remains uncertain.[81]

Thus, in IPF, immune complexes and complement are deposited along alveolar walls and capillaries, there are increased numbers of IgG-secreting B lymphocytes and activated macrophages in bronchoalveolar lavage fluid, and alveolar capillary endothelial cells, alveolar epithelial cells, and macrophages express class II molecules. These findings suggest immune activation within the lung. The stimulus for this activation and the processes that sustain it are not known, but immune activation appears to initiate alveolar inflammation.

Alveolar Inflammation

Studies of the bronchoalveolar lavage fluid from patients with IPF demonstrate a several-fold increase in the total cell number and changes in the composition of the cells within the alveolar space.[69,71,93] Most studies of bronchoalveolar lavage in groups of patients with IPF have found increases in the numbers of neutrophils and macrophages but some patients may have significant increases in the fraction of lymphocytes or eosinophils.[5,46,93–96] In contrast to the findings in lavage fluid, lymphocytes are the predominant immune effector cells in the interstitium,[61] and the differential cell counts of eosinophils and lymphocytes extracted from biopsy specimens do not correlate significantly with lavage differential cell counts.[93] The processes controlling the influx and efflux of inflammatory cells in the alveolar space are not well understood. In addition to changes in the total numbers and composition of inflammatory cells in the lungs of patients with IPF, many of these cells are activated and are releasing a variety of mediators, enzymes, and immunoglobulins that act to sustain the alveolar inflammation. Many of these factors may also cause derangements in the alveolar interstitium that result ultimately in fibrosis and loss of lung function.

Macrophages

Macrophages appear to play a central role in the pathogenesis of IPF. These pluripotent cells are found in increased numbers and in an activated state both within the alveolar space and within the alveolar interstitium in the lungs of patients with IPF. Whereas resting alveolar macrophages demonstrate little effector cell function, stimulated macrophages produce a variety of enzymes, complement components, cytokines, and other mediators of inflammatory and fibroblast cell function that could initiate or maintain the inflammatory and immune processes that precede and result in the fibrotic stage of this disease.[97] The stimulus for alveolar macrophage activation in IPF is not known but may be immune complexes.[98] Other factors that might activate macrophages include complement, microorganisms, and organic and inorganic particulates.[97,98]

Activated macrophages can release a variety of fibrogenic mediators that stimulate mesenchymal cell proliferation, including platelet-derived growth factor (PDGF), fibroblast growth factors, fibroblast activating factors, transforming growth factor beta, insulin-like growth factor, interleukin-1, and tumor necrosis factor.[97] An exaggerated spontaneous release of PDGF by cultured alveolar macrophages from patients with IPF has been reported.[99] Shaw and coworkers[100] have recently shown that alveolar macrophages from these patients have an increased relative abundance of PDGF(B) mRNA. Further, they demonstrated that interferon-gamma increased PDGF(B) mRNA production in these macrophages. These studies suggest an important role for PDGF gene activation in the chain of command linking lymphocytes, macrophages and fibroblasts in the pathogenesis of the fibrosis in these patients.

Extracellular matrix proteins such as fibronectin are also secreted by macrophages and may function as chemotaxins and growth factors for fibroblasts.[101–103] Activated macrophages may also modulate mesenchymal cell proliferation through decreased production of growth inhibitor factor.[104–107] Alveolar macrophages may affect the composition of the interstitial matrix components by secreting collagenase and lysosomal enzymes.[108,109] Finally, activated macrophages amplify the alveolar inflammatory process by recruiting neutrophils into the alveolar space through the release of chemotactic factors for circulating granulocytes.[98,110,111]

Neutrophils

Sustained neutrophil accumulation in the alveolar space and persistent neutrophil mediated injury and destruction of alveolar architecture are believed to be major factors that culminate in abnormal lung repair and interstitial fibrosis.[5] The processes that sustain neutrophil influx into the alveolar space are unclear but appear to be mediated in part by neutrophil chemotactic factors released by activated macrophages.[110,111] Neutrophils are capable of causing damage to the alveolar epithelial, parenchymal, and endothelial cells and to the extracellular matrix components of the alveolar wall by secreting proteases, hydrolases, and reactive oxidant species.[112] Neutrophil collagenases and other neutral proteases, as well as myeloperoxidase, are found in bronchoalveolar lavage fluid from patients with IPF.[113,114] Fibronectin, a cell surface protein and component of the pulmonary interstitium, is degraded by neutrophil proteases and is found in increased amounts in bronchoalveolar lavage fluid from these patients.[115,116]

Neutrophils isolated from lavage fluid injure lung parenchymal and epithelial cells in vitro by secreting oxygen radicals, and blood neutrophils stimulated by supernatant from cultured lavage macrophages are cytotoxic to lung fibroblasts.[112] The cytotoxicity of activated neutrophils is enhanced by a deficiency in glutathione, a scavenger of injurious oxidant species, in the alveolar lining fluid.[112] Thus, the number of neutrophils in bronchoalveolar lavage fluid from patients with IPF is increased and these neutrophils are capable of injuring lung cells and degrading interstitial matrix components by secreting proteases and oxidants, many of which are found in the bronchoalveolar lavage fluid of patients with IPF.

Lymphocytes

Whereas increased numbers of neutrophils are the striking finding in the bronchoalveolar lavage of patients with IPF, histopathologic examination of lung biopsy specimens demonstrates a predominance of mononuclear cells within the lung parenchyma.[78,80,93] T lymphocytes, predominantly OKT8+ T cells, are distributed throughout the interstitium whereas B lymphocytes are organized into follicles, occasionally with germinal center formation.[78–80] The OKT4+/OKT8+ ratio in the bronchoalveolar lavage fluid of patients with IPF is decreased when compared to the ratio in the peripheral blood.[117]

Lymphocyte migration into the alveolar interstitium is probably stimulated by macrophage- and/or lymphocyte-derived lymphocyte chemotactic factors.[118] Interstitial T cells are activated and express interleukin-2 receptors and class II antigens,[80] and intra-alveolar B cells are also actively secreting immunoglobulins.[72] Activated cytolytic lung lymphocytes, as determined by a lectin-dependent cell-mediated cytotoxicity assay that detects specific cytolytic cells and interleukin-2–activated killer cells but not natural killer cells, have been reported recently in a small number of patients with IPF.[119]

The factors that activate lymphocytes are not known but may be autoantigens presented by alveolar macrophages or pulmonary endothelial or epithelial cells.[81,82,85,88,89] One possible antigen is type I collagen, since circulating lymphocytes from patients with IPF are activated in the presence of type I collagen and some lavage B cells secrete immunoglobulins directed against type I collagen.[90,91]

Activated lymphocytes release a variety of mediators that can stimulate and sustain inflammation and fibrosis, including interleukin-2, interferons, transforming growth factor beta, and lymphocyte-derived chemotactic factor for fibroblasts.[106,107,120]

Other Cells

Eosinophils, basophils, and mast cells are also found in increased numbers in the bronchoalveolar lavage fluid and lung tissue of patients with IPF.[5,61,114] Potential roles for mast cells and eosinophils in alveolar inflammation are suggested by increased levels of histamine and eosinophil cationic protein, respectively, in lavage fluid.[114,121,122] Eosinophils are capable of injuring lung parenchymal cells and secrete a collagenase that cleaves type I and III collagen, two major constituents of lung extracellular matrix.[114,122] Since these cells compose a small fraction of the cells within the alveolar space and lung tissue, their role in alveolar injury remains speculative.

Mesenchymal Cells and the Interstitium

Irreversible fibrotic derangement of the alveolar parenchyma cause impairment in pulmonary gas exchange function and contribute to the clinical manifestations of IPF. The processes initiating and perpetuating the changes in the cellular and extracellular matrix components of the alveolar interstitium are not known but appear to be mediated in part by the inflammatory and immune effector cells that characterize the alveolar inflammation found in IPF.

IPF is characterized by changes both in the numbers and types of alveolar parenchymal cells and in the components of the extracellular matrix. The number of fibroblasts, the principal mesenchymal cells, is increased.[5,46,55] The increase in the number of fibroblasts appears to be caused both by the release of fibroblast chemoattractants that stimulate the migration of fibroblasts into the areas of alveolar inflammation and by cytokines released by inflammatory and immune effector cells that promote fibroblast proliferation.[97,120] Fibroblasts isolated from the lungs of patients with IPF proliferate significantly faster than fibroblasts from normal lungs cultured under the same conditions in vitro.[123] Nearly 15% of the clones from patients with IPF had growth rates twice that of normal fibroblasts.[123] Thus, within the population of fibroblasts inhabiting the interstitium in IPF are heterogeneous clones with different proliferative potentials. The factors that stimulate these growth patterns and regulate the proliferative characteristics of these different fibroblast subsets are not known.

Fibroblasts produce most of the extracellular matrix.[124] Although initial studies of the collagen content of lung biopsy specimens from patients with IPF found no changes in collagen content,[125] subsequent studies utilizing both biochemical and immunohistochemical methods found significant increases in the amount of collagen in fibrotic lungs compared to normal lungs.[126–130] The collagen concentration of autopsy specimens was greater than that of biopsy samples, suggesting continuing deposition of collagen during the course of IPF.[126] Studies of the rate of collagen synthesis suggest that the synthesis rate in IPF biopsy specimens is no different from the rate in normal lung specimens,[125,130] but in vivo studies of synthesis rates in animals after experimentally induced fibrosis demonstrate increased synthesis rates.[131,132] These differences may be due to the manner in which synthesis is expressed or to limitations of in vitro studies.[130] Cultured fibroblasts from normal and fibrotic human lung specimens synthesized similar amounts and proportions of type I, III, and V collagens.[133] Kuhn and colleagues[134] recently demonstrated that foci of active matrix deposition are present in the majority of biopsies in IPF, providing additional evidence of the progressive nature of the collagen deposition in this disease. Interestingly, these foci contained both collagen and fibronectin and were consistently localized outside remnants of basal lamina, therefore confirming that the fibrosis in this disease results primarily from the organization of exudate within airspaces.

The finding of increased levels of type III procollagen N-terminal peptides, a cleavage product released during secretion of type III collagen from cells, in the bronchoalveolar lavage fluid and serum of patients with IPF provides indirect evidence for an increased level of collagen synthesis in IPF.[135–138] Decreased collagen degradation may also contribute to the accumulation of collagen in the interstitium, and decreased collagenolytic activity and increased inhibitory collagenase activity has been demonstrated in lung biopsy specimens from patients with IPF.[130,139] Therefore, increased total collagen concentration may be due to increased numbers of collagen-secreting cells, decreased enzymatic degradation, and possibly increased rates of collagen synthesis.

Immunohistochemical studies of collagen types in fibrotic lung specimens have shown that in early active fibrosis there is an increased proportion of type III collagen.[127,135,140,141] Late fibrosis appears to be characterized by increased type I collagen.[129,142] The ratio of type III to type I collagen in lung biopsy specimens from patients with IPF was greater than the ratio in subsequent postmortem lung samples, and patients with a greater proportion of type III collagen had a better clinical course, further suggesting that type III collagen was increased in early IPF.[141] The concept that fibrotic collagen evolves in the lung over several months has been supported recently by Last and coworkers.[143] In this study, content of collagen crosslinks, hydroxylsinonorleucine (HLNL), dihydroxylysinonorleucine (DHLNL), and hydroxypyridinium (OHP) was determined in lung tissue from patients with interstitial lung disease, from patients with adult respiratory distress syndrome, and control subjects. Patients with IPF had increased lung OHP content compared to normals and patients with acute lung injury, whereas patients with ARDS had significant elevations of the DHLNL:HLNL ratio. These results are consistent with data obtained from animal models of fibrotic lung injury that suggest that an increase in the DHLNL:HLNL ratio serves as a marker of early fibrosis, whereas increased lung OHP content serves as a marker of chronic lung fibrosis.

The factors regulating the cellular processes that control the production of different collagen species are not well understood, but fibroblast cell density may influence the production of different types of collagen.[144] Fibroblasts from normal embryonic, adult, and fibrotic lung produced more type III collagen at confluency than at low plating densities in vitro.[144] Whether heterogeneous fibroblast subsets in IPF secrete different types of collagen species as well as exhibit different growth rates is not known.[123]

In addition to fibroblast proliferation, the numbers of other mesenchymal cells are also increased. Among these mesenchymal cells are contractile cells, including smooth muscle cells, contractile interstitial cells or myofibroblasts, and capillary pericytes.[145] Myofibroblasts, smooth muscle cells, and other contractile interstitial cells contain actin filaments and have the capability to contract.[145] The role these cells play in the functional impairments of IPF—especially decreases in lung compliance and lung volumes—is not certain, but similar cells appear to be responsible for scar contraction in granulation tissue.[146] There is no direct evidence for the production of extracellular matrix components by these cells but in the aorta myofibroblast-like cells produce elastin, collagen, and matrix material.[147]

HISTOPATHOLOGIC MANIFESTATIONS

The gross morphologic findings in IPF range from a normal appearance in early cases to diffuse honeycombing in the later stages of the disease process. Disease involvement is usually heterogeneous, and worse in the lower lobes. Areas of mildly involved or even normal pulmonary parenchyma may be interspersed throughout a background of extensive fibrosis and honeycombing. Consequently, an open lung biopsy is required if the diagnosis of IPF is to be established. Further, this approach decreases the sampling error found with transbronchial lung biopsy using the fiberoptic bronchoscope[148] and it also allows one to distinguish between active inflammation and end-stage fibrosis. This assessment of disease activity is important and aids in justifying the commitment to long-term, potentially toxic immunosuppressive or cytotoxic therapy.

Open lung biopsy is a relatively safe procedure with little morbidity and less than 0.5% mortality.[149,150] A limited thoracotomy is usually performed under general anesthesia. It is important that the surgeon obtain an adequate sample. Biopsies are taken from at least two sites, an upper lobe and a lower lobe site, and should include both abnormal and normal-appearing areas. Small subpleural samples, especially if pleuritis is present, and dependent segments of the right middle lobe and lingula may obfuscate histopathologic assessment. Atelectasis and hemorrhage into the tissue can be prevented by avoiding palpation and clamps and by delineating the wedge during full inflation. Sample processing, including inflating the tissue and immediate fixation, should be done immediately by the pathologist.[151] Multiple sections from all the biopsies should be stained with pentachrome, hematoxylin/eosin, iron, and toluidine blue (other special stains may be required). Not only is the routine diagnostic analysis and comment required but the pathologist should quantitate both the extent and the severity of the inflammatory/exudative and fibrotic/reparative lesions present. Although the major histopathologic abnormalities occur in the lung parenchyma, attention to the airways and vessels is also important. Communication between the clinician and the pathologist is vital if the correct diagnosis is to be obtained.

Three broad patterns of histopathologic findings have been described in IPF.[46,152,153] A cellular pattern characterized by the presence of increased numbers of macrophages and lymphocytes in the intra-alveolar space is a common finding, especially in early phases of the disease process (Fig.1-2A). This pattern has been inappropriately termed *desquamative interstitial pneumonia* (DIP) as a result of the incorrect identification of the intra-alveolar cells as alveolar type II cells.[47] The alveolar walls are lined by hyperplastic alveolar type II cells. "Desquamation," however, is not the mechanism by which these cells accumulate in the alveolar space. Lymphocytes and occasionally eosinophils infiltrate the alveolar septae and there may be a slight increase in the number of interstitial mesenchymal cells, but fibrosis and honeycombing are usually absent or only minimally present. Organizing diffuse alveolar damage or cryptogenic organizing pneumonitis (idiopathic bronchiolitis obliterans with patchy organizing pneumonia) should be considered when a cellular pattern is associated with extensive fibroblast proliferation, relatively little collagen deposition, and edema in a patient with a sudden onset and rapid course of respiratory failure.

Usual interstitial pneumonitis (UIP), a mixed cellular-fibrotic pattern, is characterized by intense interstitial inflammation composed of lymphocytes, eosinophils, monocytes, and plasma cells and thickening of the alveolar walls by increased numbers of mesenchymal cells (Fig. 1-2B, C).[152,153] The intra-alveolar space may contain proteinaceous debris and early honeycombing may be present in some areas. The mixed cellular-fibrotic pattern is characterized by a heterogeneous appearance in which areas of inflammation are intermixed with areas of fibrosis. The end-stage or honeycomb pattern is characterized by replacement of the pulmonary parenchyma by irregular cysts that are 1.0 to 2.5 mm in diameter.[152] The septae are thickened and lined by metaplastic alveolar epithelial cells (Fig. 1-2D). As with the mixed cellular-fibrotic pattern, the distribution of honeycombing is heterogeneous.

Although some researchers consider UIP and DIP to be distinct processes,[4,42,47,153] most authors consider these three patterns of histopathologic findings in IPF to be a spectrum of a single disease process.[5,154] The cellular pattern represents the earliest stage and is characterized by alveolar and interstitial inflammation. During the mixed cellular-fibrotic pattern, fibrotic changes within the alveolar wall begin to occur, and these derangements lead ultimately to the final histopathologic pattern, honeycomb lung.

Correlative studies have shown that the extent and severity of inflammation present on open lung biopsy correspond to disease stage, prognosis, and response to therapy.[93,96,153,154] Patients with a cellular pattern on open lung biopsy had a mean

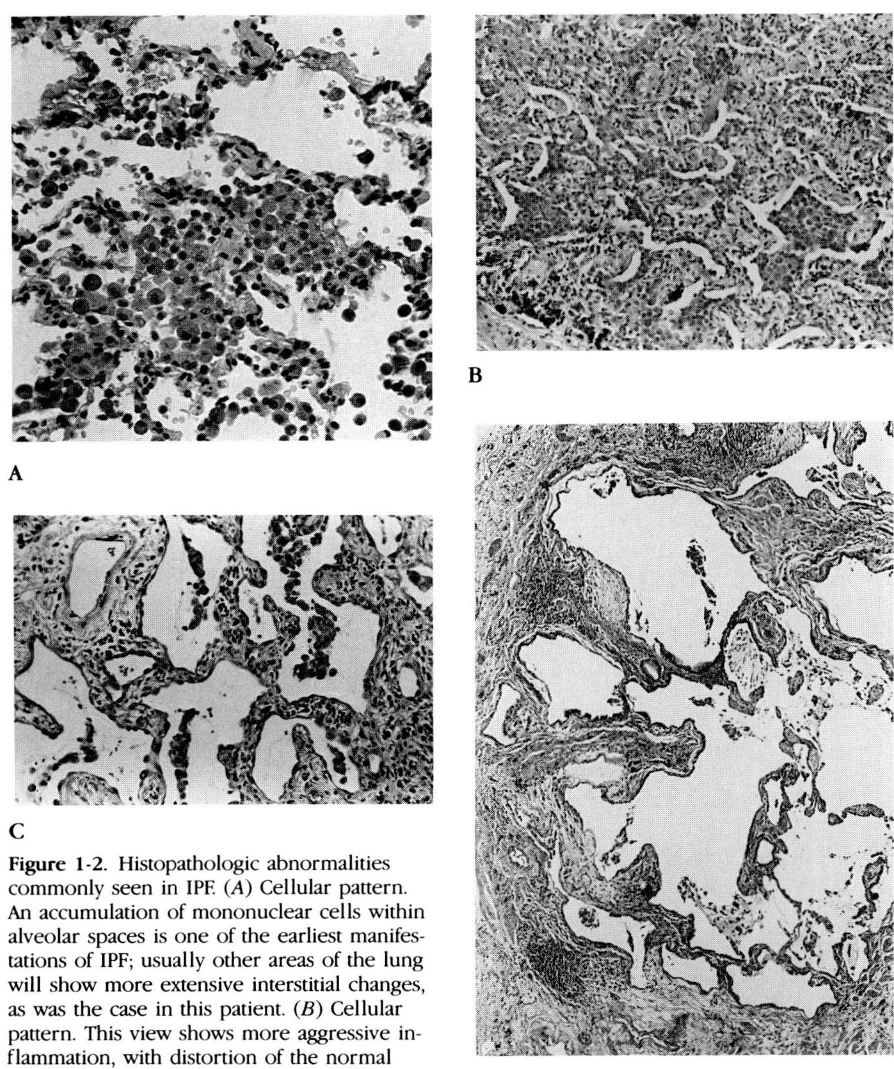

Figure 1-2. Histopathologic abnormalities commonly seen in IPF. (*A*) Cellular pattern. An accumulation of mononuclear cells within alveolar spaces is one of the earliest manifestations of IPF; usually other areas of the lung will show more extensive interstitial changes, as was the case in this patient. (*B*) Cellular pattern. This view shows more aggressive inflammation, with distortion of the normal lung architecture. There is a mild thickening of the alveolar walls and a marked accumulation of mononuclear cells (mostly alveolar macrophages) within the alveolar spaces. (*C*) Mixed cellular-fibrotic pattern of usual interstitial pneumonitis (UIP). There is active interstitial infiltration by mononuclear cells associated with interstitial widening and scarring. Hyperplastic type II cells line the alveolar walls. (*D*) End-stage honeycombed lung. The pulmonary architecture is destroyed and replaced by irregular cysts lined by metaplastic bronchiolar epithelium. Smooth muscle proliferation is also present, consistent with stromal metaplasia. Mucus, foamy macrophages, and other debris are in the airspaces.

survival of 12.2 years whereas those with a more fibrotic pattern had a mean survival of only 5.6 years.[153] A more cellular histopathologic pattern was also associated with a greater response to corticosteroid therapy.

CLINICAL MANIFESTATIONS

Patients with IPF are usually between 40 and 70 years of age, and men are affected slightly more frequently than women.[46,155] The initial symptom is usually breathlessness with exertion but some patients may present with a dry, nonproductive cough.[156,157] The onset of disease is occasionally associated with a flu-like illness and there have been several reports of a preceding mycoplasma or viral infection.[158–160] Although cough may be the initial symptom in some patients, all patients with IPF develop breathlessness with exercise as the disease progresses. Malaise and weight loss are common associated symptoms. Arthralgias, myalgias, and fever have been reported[46] but are rare manifestations of IPF in our experience and the presence of these symptoms should prompt a continued search for another diagnosis.

Physical examination may be normal at the onset of IPF. However, the most common physical examination finding is bibasilar end-inspiratory dry crackles ("Velcro" rales). Clubbing occurs commonly, usually late in the clinical course, whereas hypertrophic pulmonary osteoarthropathy is rare.[161,162] The cardiac examination may be normal early in the course of IPF but findings of pulmonary hypertension, cor pulmonale, and right-sided heart failure develop as the disease progresses. Cyanosis may be present in advanced IPF.

CHEST IMAGING STUDIES

Chest Roentgenogram

The chest roentgenogram may be normal in up to 14.8% of patients with IPF.[41,47,163,164] Epler and coworkers[163] described the roentgenographic and histopathologic findings in 115 patients with IPF. Of the 47 patients with a more cellular histopathologic pattern (desquamative interstitial pneumonitis), 12 (26%) had normal roentgenograms, whereas only 5 of 68 patients (7%) with a more fibrotic histopathologic pattern (usual interstitial pneumonitis) had normal roentgenograms. Serial chest roentgenograms may reveal a progression of roentgenographic abnormalities during the course of IPF,[46,155] but roentgenographic patterns correlate with lung histopathology only when honeycombing is present (Fig. 1-3).[154] Initially, the chest roentgenogram may show only a reduction in lung volume (usually only evident when previous films are available for comparison) or have a ground glass appearance—that is, a fine, homogeneous, hazy process. The most common radiographic findings are a reticular pattern, a lace-like network of curvilinear opacities that may be fine, medium, or coarse depending on their thickness, and a reticulonodular pattern, the superimposition of nodular densities on a network of curvilinear opacities. These patterns involve both lungs equally and are generally more prominent in the lower lobes. As IPF progresses, a

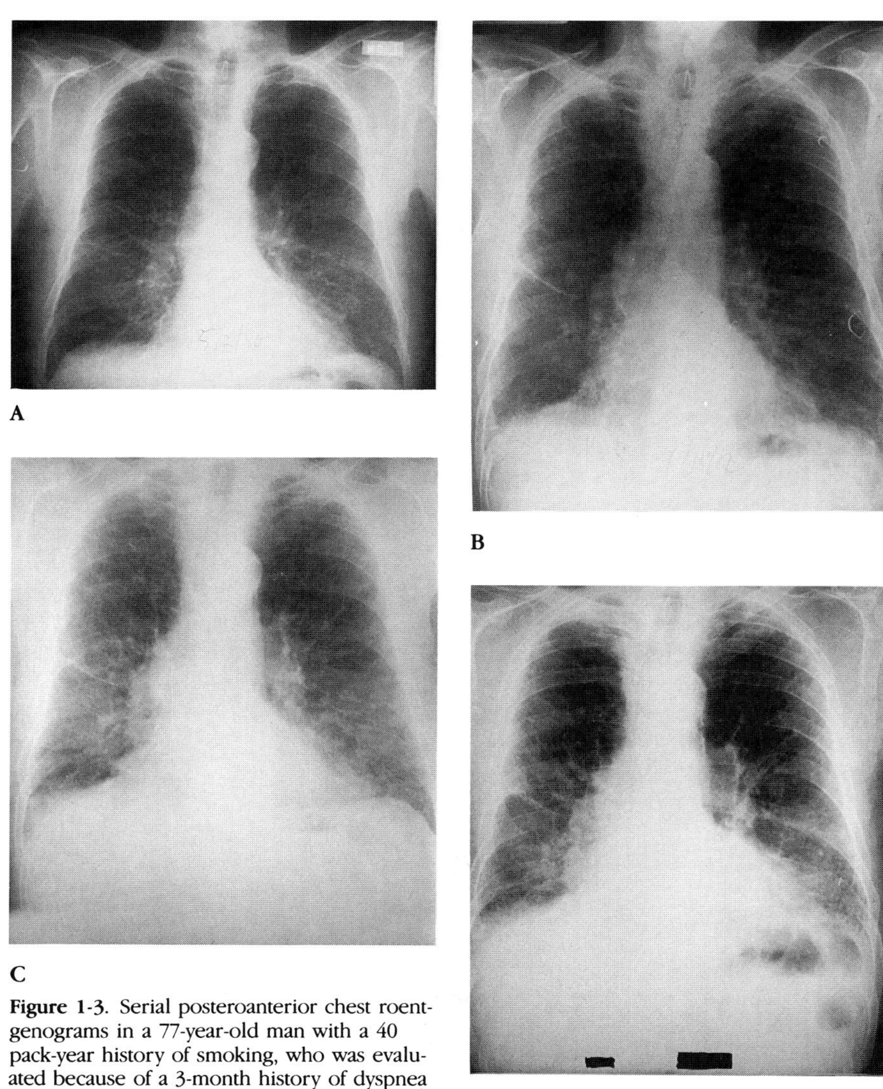

Figure 1-3. Serial posteroanterior chest roentgenograms in a 77-year-old man with a 40 pack-year history of smoking, who was evaluated because of a 3-month history of dyspnea with exertion. These roentgenograms illustrate two important points: (1) often radiographic abnormalities are present months to years before the onset (or recognition) of symptoms; and (2) there may be a marked disparity between the radiographic appearance and the physiological or pathologic abnormalities. (*A*) Roentgenogram taken 28 months prior to evaluation revealed a reticulonodular pattern most prominent in the lower lung zones, especially the left. Chest films taken 2 years earlier were essentially the same. (*B*) Roentgenogram taken at the time of evaluation revealed progression of the reticulonodular pattern with involvement in the mid- and upper lung zones. The lung volumes are maintained, presumably because of associated chronic obstructive lung disease. Physical examination revealed crackles (Velcro rales) at both bases. Results of pulmonary function studies were normal except for a reduction in the diffusing capacity (42% of predicted). The pressure-volume curve revealed an increase in elastic recoil: it was shifted slightly down and to the right, with a marked increase in the maximal

Text continued on p. 15

honeycomb pattern may develop: a coarse reticular pattern with translucencies or cysts measuring 0.5 to 1.0 cm in diameter.[165,166] Progressive loss of lung volume, deviation of the trachea to the right, and tracheomegaly are also typical roentgenographic findings in IPF.[167] Pleural involvement, adenopathy, or localized parenchymal densities are uncommon in IPF and suggest another interstitial process or a disease-associated complication such as an infectious process or neoplasm.

Computed Tomography

Computed tomography (CT), especially high-resolution, thin-section computed tomography (HRCT), may be useful in the differentiation of IPF from other interstitial lung diseases, determination of the extent and localization of disease activity, and detection of disease, especially in patients with normal or minimal change on chest roentgenograms (Fig. 1-4).[168–172] HRCT findings in IPF include a lower lung zone predominant, usually subpleural, reticular pattern with areas of haziness or airspace opacification. Honeycombing may also be present. HRCT may aid in the differentiation of IPF from silicosis, sarcoidosis, and lymphangitic carcinomatosis.[169] Airspace opacification on HRCT correlates with histopathologic findings of increased alveolar inflammation and with disease stabilization or improvement after corticosteroid therapy.[172] In a study of 23 patients with IPF, Staples and colleagues[168] demonstrated that CT assessment of disease extent by a visual score correlated significantly with severity of dyspnea, diffusing capacity, and total lung capacity. The use of HRCT in the assessment of disease extent and activity is still preliminary and is dependent on the expertise and experience of those who interpret the images. These initial studies are encouraging but require verification and more universal application of this technique.

Gallium-67 Scintillation Scanning

Nuclear scintigraphic scanning utilizing gallium-67 has been used to stage alveolar inflammation in patients with IPF.[46,173,174] Gallium-67 is a radionucleotide with a half-life of 78 hours. Within the lung, it is concentrated predominantly in activated macrophages and to a lesser extent in neutrophils. The gallium-67 index, a visual measure of the extent, intensity, and texture of gallium-67 uptake in the lung, correlates with interstitial

---

transpulmonary pressure (the coefficient of retraction was 12.2 cm H_2O/L). Arterial blood gases obtained while breathing room air (Denver, Colorado, elevation 5000 feet) were: pO_2, 46; pCO_2, 31; pH, 7.47; (A–a)O_2, 39. Bronchoalveolar lavage demonstrated an increase in total cells with an increase in neutrophils (10%) and eosinophils (4%). Open lung biopsies from the upper and lower lobes revealed an advanced stage of IPF with regions of normal lung surrounded by focal areas of cellularity, extensive regions of fibrosis, and subpleural honeycombing. (C) Roentgenogram taken 13 months later shows progression of the interstitial infiltrates, with evidence of honeycombing and pulmonary hypertension, despite aggressive treatment with corticosteroids and cytoxan and the institution of oxygen therapy. (D) Roentgenogram taken approximately 4 years after diagnosis demonstrates further progression with volume loss. He now reported breathlessness at rest. The patient died of respiratory failure 1 month after this film was taken.

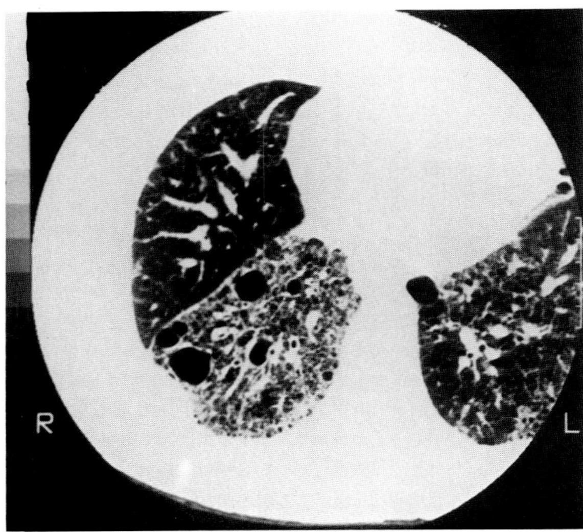

Figure 1-4. High-resolution, thin-section CT scan. The CT scan reveals extensive parenchymal involvement. Irregular fibrotic areas contain small honeycomb-like airspaces in the periphery of the lower lung zones. This scan reveals the inhomogenous distribution of the disease: changes are severe in the lower lobes and minimal in the upper lobes.

and alveolar cellularity in open lung biopsies and with the percentage of neutrophils but not lymphocytes, eosinophils, or macrophages in bronchoalveolar lavage cell counts.[173] Other studies have shown that the gallium-67 index usually correlates inversely with the severity of pulmonary fibrosis and does not correlate with a patient's clinical course (Fig. 1-5).[175,176]

A computer-assisted method of gallium-67 index calculation has been developed and greatly reduces the variability of the visual index.[177] However, no standardized method of interpretation of gallium-67 scans has been defined. In addition, gallium-67 scanning is expensive and may pose a moderate radiation hazard. Therefore, although gallium-67 is frequently concentrated in the lungs of patients with IPF, technical problems in the quantitative interpretation of the scans and lack of standardization limit the usefulness of this test in the evaluation of patients with IPF.

PHYSIOLOGICAL STUDIES

Pulmonary Function Testing

Pulmonary function tests in patients with IPF may yield normal results during early disease but usually reveal a reduced vital capacity and total lung capacity consistent with a restrictive process. As the disease progresses, pressure-volume studies demonstrate a reduction in lung compliance. The pressure-volume curve is shifted down and to the right by the stiff, noncompliant pulmonary parenchyma (Fig. 1-6). This decrease in pulmonary compliance causes a reduction in lung volumes. All lung volume components, total lung capacity, functional residual capacity, and residual volume, are reduced as the disease process progresses.

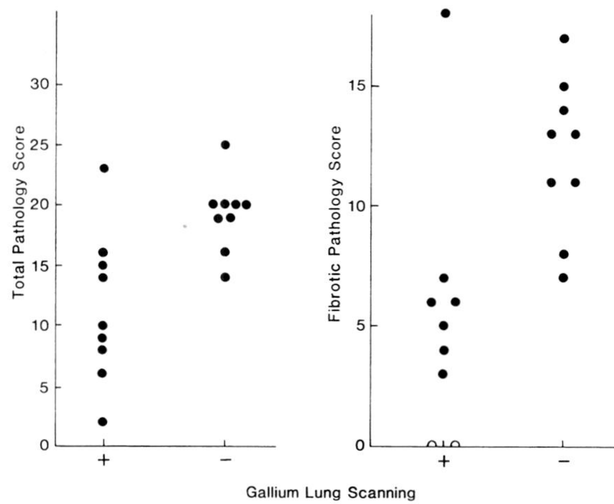

Figure 1-5. Correlation of gallium-67 index with histopathologic features in IPF. The gallium-67 scan index is a measure of gallium-67 uptake in the lung and was determined by a modification of the method of Line.[173] Gallium-67 uptake was classified as either increased (+; n = 9) or negative (−; n = 9). Open lung biopsies were evaluated using a pathologic scoring system that graded the extent and severity of 11 cellular and fibrotic histopathologic abnormalities.[96] The total pathology score measures the overall derangement of lung structure and is the sum of the fibrotic and cellular scores. The higher the score the more prominent the abnormality. (*Left panel*): Patients with more severe total pathologic derangement tended to have negative gallium-67 scans. (*Right panel*): Patients with negative scans had moderate-to-severe fibrosis and those with positive scans tended to have less fibrosis. No correlation was noted with the degree of cellularity found on the biopsies.

Spirometric measures of pulmonary function, forced expiratory volume in 1 second (FEV_1) and forced vital capacity (FVC), are usually reduced because of the reduction in lung volumes. The ratio of FEV_1 to FVC is usually normal or increased because airflow rates are elevated because of the increased static elastic recoil. The decreased lung compliance increases the work of breathing, and patients with IPF are frequently tachypneic and breathe with rapid, shallow breaths.[178,179] The stimulus for the increased respiratory rate and subsequent increase in minute ventilation is uncertain. Since the ventilatory response to hypercapnea is not increased in patients with IPF, the altered breathing pattern appears to be due to mechanoreceptors and vagal mechanisms rather than abnormal chemical ventilatory control.[180–182]

Gas Exchange

The diffusing capacity for carbon monoxide (DLCO) is usually reduced and may become abnormal early in the course of IPF.[183] Several common misconceptions exist regarding the usefulness of the DLCO in patients with IPF. First, the DLCO does not predict the extent or severity of the pathologic derangement—that is, neither the alveolitis nor the fibrosis is reflected by the level of DLCO (Fig. 1-7A).[184,185] Second, the initial DLCO or the change in DLCO over time does not accurately predict the clinical course or response to therapy.[186]

The resting arterial oxygen tension (PaO_2) is frequently normal at the onset of IPF. However, with exercise, the PaO_2 decreases and the alveolar-arterial oxygen gradient ($P(A-a)O_2$) widens.[46,185,187] With disease progression, resting hypoxemia is a universal finding (Fig. 1-7B). The major cause of resting hypoxemia in IPF is ventilation–perfusion

(*Text continued on page 20.*)

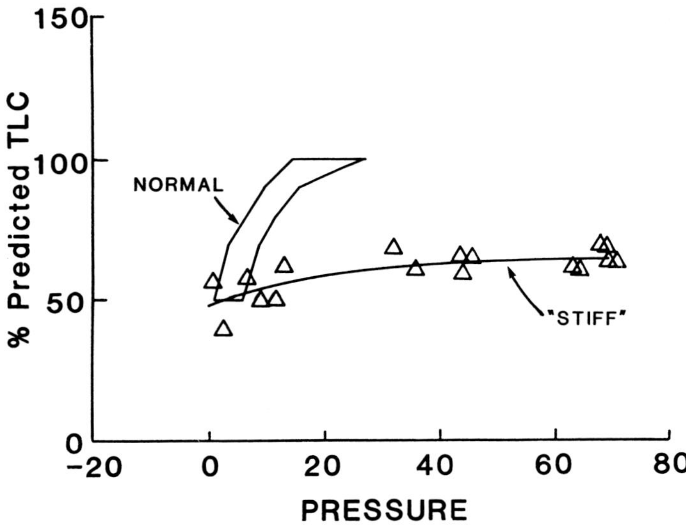

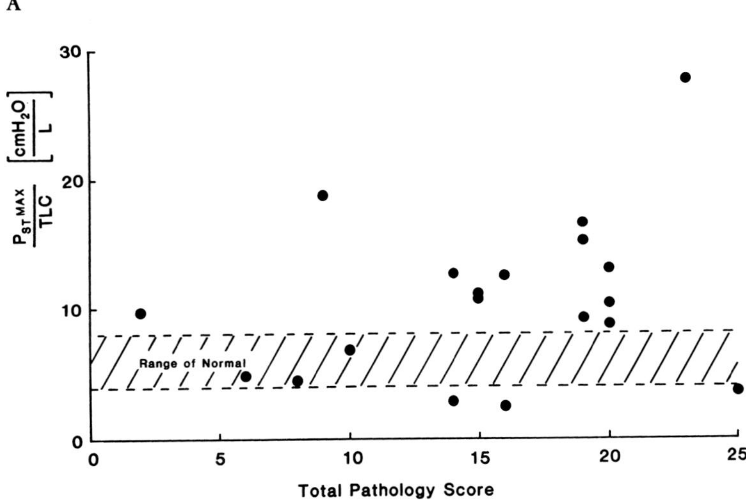

Figure 1-6. (*A*) Relationship of the static deflation volume and pressure in a patient with IPF. The percentage of predicted total lung capacity (TLC) is plotted against the static transpulmonary pressure (cm H_2O) for a patient with moderate-to-severe fibrosis and honeycombing. (*B*) Relationship of the coefficient of retraction, Pst max/TLC, and the total pathology score. In general, the compliance, maximum static transpulmonary pressure (Pst max) and the coefficient of retraction (the maximum transpulmonary pressure at TLC) tend to correlate with the extent of pathologic derangement, especially fibrosis, observed on open lung biopsy.

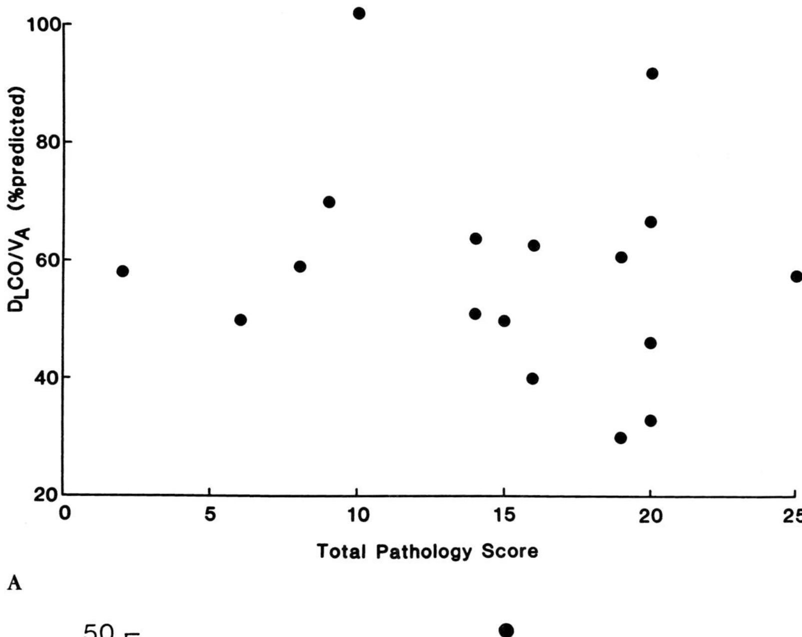

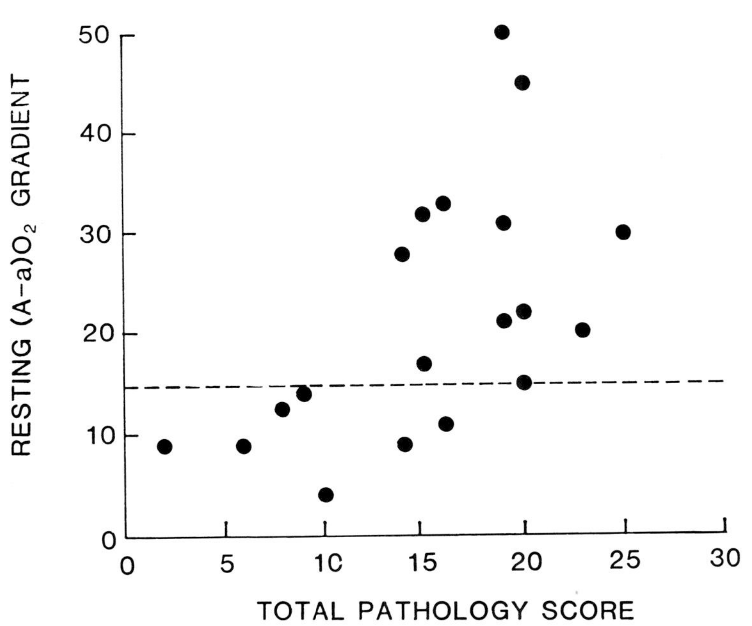

Figure 1-7. The relationship between gas exchange and histopathologic abnormalities in IPF. The total pathology score represents an approximation of the overall derangement of lung structure found on open lung biopsy and is the sum of the fibrotic and cellular abnormalities. (*A*) The initial diffusing capacity for carbon monoxide (D$_L$CO/V$_A$) and the total pathology score. There is no significant correlation between the estimation of the overall pathologic derangement and the D$_L$CO/V$_A$ (n = 17). (*B*) The initial resting alveolar-arterial oxygen gradient [(A–a)O$_2$] and the total pathology score. There is a significant correlation between the estimation of the overall pathologic derangement and the (A–a)O$_2$ gradient at rest (n = 19; Spearman's rank correlation coefficient = 0.40; p < 0.05). The dashed line represents the upper limit of normal.

mismatching.[46,187–189] However, approximately 20% of the widening in the $P(A-a)O_2$ that occurs during exercise may be due to an impairment of oxygen diffusion.[187] There is general agreement that gas exchange measurements [PaO_2 and $P(A-a)O_2$ with exercise] are the most sensitive functional tests of the overall process of IPF.[184,186]

DISEASE COURSE AND COMPLICATIONS

The natural and treated course of IPF varies from patient to patient. Some patients improve after treatment, a few patients have a relatively stable course, most, unfortunately, deteriorate and are unresponsive to therapy.[96,153] Although some patients may survive for more than 10 years, the mean duration of illness is 3 to 5 years. The causes and assessment of clinical deterioration in IPF have been reviewed recently.[190]

Respiratory failure due to pulmonary insufficiency accounts for nearly 40% of deaths. Approximately 25% of patients die from cardiovascular complications, including heart failure, myocardial infarction, and stroke. Bronchogenic carcinoma, pulmonary embolism, and infections are the other major causes of death. During the course of their illness most patients experience episodes of increased breathlessness, worsening hypoxemia, decreased exercise tolerance, or other declines in functional status. The most frequent cause of clinical deterioration is progression of the fibrotic process, and patients are disabled by hypoxemia and breathlessness. Cardiovascular disease affects nearly all patients with IPF. In advanced disease, approximately 70% of patients have clinical evidence of pulmonary hypertension that may progress to cor pulmonale and right heart failure.[46] Left ventricular heart failure is usually caused by atherosclerotic heart disease or systemic hypertension and may be exacerbated by hypoxemia, hypercapnea and acidosis, right heart failure, and right ventricular and septal hypertrophy.[190]

Patients with IPF have an increased incidence of bronchogenic carcinoma.[191–194] Squamous metaplasia, epithelial cell proliferation, and extension of cuboidal and columnar epithelial cells into the terminal bronchioles are potential predisposing factors for the development of bronchogenic carcinomas in IPF.[194] The distribution of histologic types of carcinomas found in IPF is not different from bronchogenic carcinomas not associated with pulmonary fibrosis.[191] If detected early, resectional surgery should be attempted. However, surgery is often not possible because of the degree of respiratory disability that would result.

Inactivity, heart failure, and bronchogenic carcinoma may predispose patients with IPF to pulmonary thromboembolism. Other than the rapidity of onset, pulmonary thromboembolism is often indistinguishable from disease progression because the symptoms of increased breathlessness, hypoxemia, tachycardia, and electrocardiographic findings of right ventricular strain are the same in both processes. Pulmonary angiography is usually required to diagnose pulmonary thromboembolism because ventilation–perfusion scans are often abnormal because of the pulmonary fibrosis.[188,189]

Spontaneous pneumothoraces are another cause of morbidity in patients with IPF.[34,155,195,196] Large cysts or blebs on chest roentgenograms may be a risk factor for pneumothoraces.[34,196] Because of the increased lung elastic recoil in IPF, tube thoracostomy is occasionally unsuccessful in achieving lung reexpansion and patients may require thoracotomy, bleb resection, and pleurectomy.

Pulmonary infection may worsen hypoxemia and breathlessness and precipitate respiratory decompensation. The incidence of pulmonary infections may be slightly increased in patients with pulmonary fibrosis, and therapy with corticosteroids and cytotoxic agents may further increase the risk of both pulmonary and systemic infections. A recent study, from an area where tuberculosis is more prevalent, has suggested that patients with interstitial lung disease may have an increased incidence of tuberculosis.[197] In our experience this is extremely rare, and common bacterial organisms are the most frequent pathogens. Importantly, despite the treatment with corticosteroids opportunistic infections are unusual complications in these patients.

STAGING AND MONITORING DISEASE ACTIVITY

The care of patients with IPF is complicated by the variable natural and treated course of this disorder. Some patients experience a rapid, inexorable deterioration, others may have a more stable course, and some may improve for variable periods after therapy.[153] Most patients experience declines in their functional level during the course of their illness. The most common cause of functional deterioration in IPF is disease progression but disease-associated complications such as heart failure, bronchogenic carcinoma, and adverse effects of therapy or acute processes such as pulmonary embolism, pneumothorax, and infection may intervene.[190] Because the manifestations of disease progression are multiple and nonspecific, a combination of diagnostic tests is often used to monitor the clinical course of patients with IPF. These diagnostic tests usually include chest roentgenograms, pulmonary function and exercise physiological testing, and bronchoalveolar lavage.

Chest Imaging Procedures

Chest roentgenography and gallium-67 lung scanning are the chest imaging procedures most commonly used to monitor the clinical course of patients with IPF. Since the chest roentgenogram may be normal when significant physiological abnormalities and histopathologic derangements are present, routine chest roentgenograms are poor indicators of the histopathologic extent and severity of disease and of its subsequent clinical course.[163] Honeycombing is the only radiographic pattern that correlates with lung histopathology.[154] Clinical and physiologic deterioration may occur with little or no change in the chest roentgenogram.

The usual quantitative interpretation of gallium-67 scanning, the gallium-67 index, does not correlate with the subsequent clinical course and correlates inversely with the severity of fibrosis that is present on histopathologic examination of lung biopsy specimens.[175,176,198] Therefore, neither the routine chest roentgenogram nor gallium scanning are sensitive indicators of the histopathologic extent and severity of disease and the subsequent clinical course in IPF.

Improved radiologic detection of disease extent and correlation with clinical course have been demonstrated in studies using high-resolution, thin-section computed tomography (HRCT).[170-172] It has been demonstrated that airspace opacification on HRCT correlates with a predominantly inflammatory pattern on lung biopsy and may predict disease stabilization or improvement after corticosteroid therapy.[171,199]

Other new technologies such as positron emission tomography (PET) and ^{99m}Tc-diethylenetriaminepentaacetate (^{99m}TcDTPA) have been used to determine disease activity and clinical course in IPF.[200,201] In preliminary studies, Pantin and coworkers[200] demonstrated that a glucose uptake that was normal or normalized after corticosteroid therapy, as measured by PET, correlated with a stable or improving clinical course whereas an elevated or increasing glucose uptake correlated with clinical deterioration. While these reports of noninvasive determination of disease activity and prediction of clinical course are encouraging, these techniques remain experimental and will require further validation and verification.

Pulmonary Function and Physiological Testing

Measurements of pulmonary function may correlate with the severity of pulmonary fibrosis but predict neither the degree of alveolar inflammation nor the subsequent clinical course.[46,184,185,202] A more fibrotic pattern on histopathologic examination of open lung biopsy specimens correlates with reduced vital capacity and compliance and increased coefficient of retraction (see Fig. 1-6*B*).[185,202] A marked reduction in vital capacity is associated with the presence of pulmonary hypertension and a reduced 2-year survival.[203]

Physiological assessments of gas exchange correlate well with the histopathologic abnormalities observed on open lung biopsy and with the clinical course of IPF.[185,202,204,205] Resting hypoxemia is correlated with the extent of fibrosis, the presence of pulmonary hypertension, and a poorer prognosis.[205] The D$_L$CO does not correlate with histopathologic derangements but a markedly reduced D$_L$CO (less than 50% of predicted) is associated with pulmonary hypertension and widened P($_A$–a)O$_2$ with exercise.[185,202,204]

Bronchoalveolar Lavage

Differential cell counts on bronchoalveolar lavage correlate with histopathologic changes on open lung biopsy and may predict responsiveness to therapy (Fig. 1-8).[93,96,206] Lymphocytosis correlates with alveolar septal inflammation and a relative absence of honeycombing whereas there is no correlation between any histopathologic abnormality and neutrophilia or eosinophilia.[96] An increase in the percentage of lymphocytes has been associated with a higher rate of response to corticosteroids.[93,96,206] Increases in neutrophils or eosinophils in lavage fluid have limited prognostic value, as increases in either or both cell types may be observed in both treatment responders and non-responders.[206,207] Neutrophilia or eosinophilia without lymphocytosis in lavage fluid was associated with a poor response to corticosteroids but a more favorable response to cyclophosphamide.[208] In one study of serial bronchoalveolar lavages in patients with IPF treated with prednisolone or with prednisolone and cyclophosphamide, abnormalities in lavage differential cell counts tended to normalize in patients who responded clinically.[208] However, abnormal lavage differential cell counts persisted in several patients who responded clinically. In another study comparing corticosteroids and cyclophosphamide, lavage neutrophilia persisted in the corticosteroid-treated group whereas the proportion of neutrophils decreased in the cyclophosphamide group.[209] The clinical response of the two groups was the same, however.

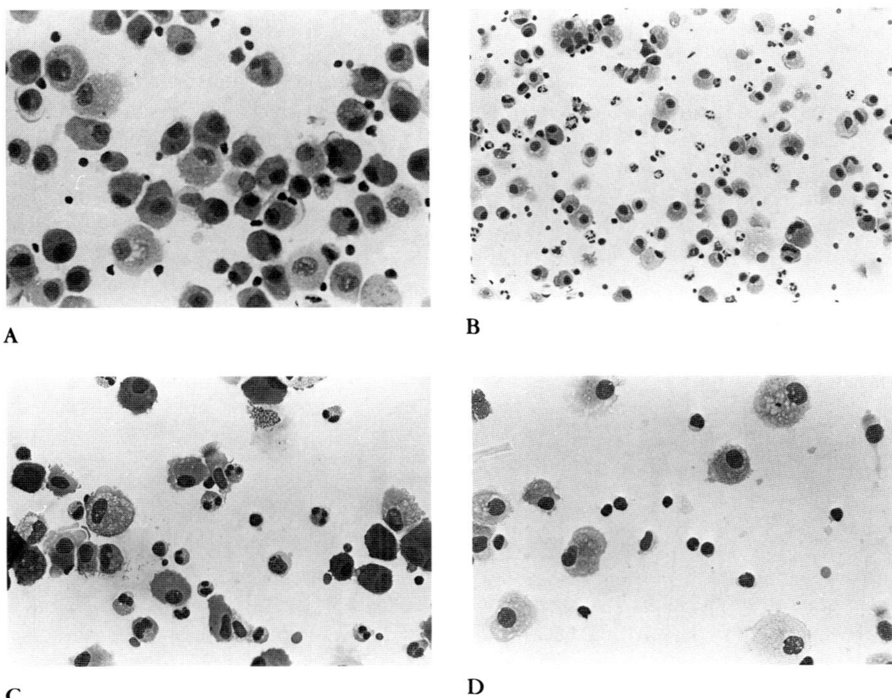

Figure 1-8. Bronchoalveolar lavage. (*A*) Cells recovered from a **normal** never-smoker (Diff Quik stain, ×40). The lavage technique, race, history of cigarette smoking, and age greatly influence the lavage cell composition. In a normal never-smoker, lavage reveals a predominance of macrophages (85 ± 2%) and lymphocytes (12 ± 1%); rarely are other cells seen (neutrophils 1.6 ± 0.7%; and eosinophils 0.2 ± 0.1%).[232] (*B*) A lavage specimen from a patient with active IPF shows a **neutrophilia** (Diff Quik stain, ×20). An increase in the total number of neutrophils is very common. Usually they compose 5–10% of the cells in patients with IPF and only rarely do they exceed 30%. (*C*) A lavage specimen from a patient with progressive IPF shows an **eosinophilia** (Diff Quik stain, ×40). Usually, eosinophils compose less than 5% of the cells in patients with IPF; rarely do they exceed 20%. (*D*) A lavage specimen from a patient with IPF shows a **lymphocytosis** (Diff Quik stain, ×40). An excessive number of lymphocytes is characteristic of IPF. However, lymphocytes rarely exceed 20% of the total because the number of macrophages is always increased as well.

In addition to changes in the bronchoalveolar lavage differential cell counts, abnormalities in the phospholipid components of pulmonary surfactant are present in IPF.[210–213] Honda and colleagues[213] described a decrease in the phospholipid content of bronchoalveolar lavage fluid from patients with IPF, a decrease in the phosphatidylglycerol to phosphatidylinositol ratio, and a relative decrease in the dipalmitoyl species of phosphatidylcholine. In addition, lipoprotein macroaggregates have been detected in lavage fluid from patients with IPF.[212] These abnormalities in surfactant components have been correlated with the clinical course of IPF. Hughes and Haslam[214] found that the proportion of phosphatidylglycerol (percentage of total phospholipid) did not predict response to prednisolone. However, in serial bronchoalveolar lavages in 14 patients treated with prednisolone, an early and sustained increase in phosphatidylglycerol was associated with clinical improvement. Robinson and coworkers[210] reported that a more normal phospholipid amount and composition in the lavage of patients with IPF correlated with a cellular pattern on open lung biopsy whereas less total recovered phospholipid and a more abnormal phospholipid composition were associated with a more fibrotic histopathologic pattern. Clinical improvement after corticosteroid therapy correlated with a more normal amount of total phospholipid but not with abnormalities in the phospholipid composition.

The role of bronchoalveolar lavage in monitoring disease course in patients with IPF requires further evaluation, but bronchoalveolar lavage differential cell counts do appear to predict responsiveness to corticosteroids (i.e., an increased proportion of lymphocytes correlates with better response) and analysis of surfactant phospholipids in lavage fluid may be useful in determining prognosis and monitoring disease course.

Multifarious Analysis

Although many different studies are used to evaluate and monitor patients with IPF, these histopathologic, radiographic, physiological, nuclear scintigraphic, and bronchoalveolar lavage parameters often change in discordant directions. Several investigators have devised multifarious scoring systems that combine several different studies into a single parameter that may be used to monitor disease progression.[96,202] Watters and colleagues[96] formulated the clinical, radiographic, and physiological (CRP) score from seven variables: dyspnea, chest roentgenogram, spirometry, lung volumes, diffusing capacity, resting alveolar–arterial oxygen difference, and exercise oxygen saturation. The CRP score correlated with the histopathologic abnormalities present on open lung biopsy better than any single component of the score.

A multifarious approach to monitoring patients with IPF necessitates a comprehensive assessment of a patient's functional status and provides a quantitative means of assessing therapeutic responsiveness and clinical course. While the CRP score is principally a research tool for the longitudinal assessment of patients with IPF and for determining response to various therapeutic interventions, a multifarious analysis of several clinical tests is required in clinical practice to monitor disease course in IPF because no single study adequately assesses clinical status and various studies may change discordantly. Furthermore, because disease progression and therapeutic responsiveness may be prolonged, a multifarious analysis is an objective quantitative assessment of the clinical course of patients with IPF.

THERAPY

Corticosteroids

Corticosteroids are the standard therapy for IPF. Approximately 40% to 70% of patients treated with corticosteroids report subjective improvement, whereas only 10% to 30% demonstrate subjective and objective improvement.[153,157,215,216] Patients responding to corticosteroids generally have earlier and less fibrotic disease and tend to survive longer.[153,157,206,216,217]

Corticosteroids are believed to suppress alveolar inflammation and decrease inflammation-mediated derangements in alveolar structure.[46,174] The mechanism of action of corticosteroids is not known but these agents can inhibit the migration of inflammatory cells into affected areas by decreasing neutrophil adherence to endothelial cells in areas of inflammation and suppressing production of migration inhibitory factors.[218] Corticosteroids also decrease the release of proteolytic enzymes by macrophages and impair the interactions between macrophages and lymphocytes, thereby altering lymphocyte function and proliferation.[97,219]

We believe that high-dose corticosteroid therapy should be initiated at the first sign of respiratory symptoms or physiological impairment. Frequently, treatment is delayed until the patient is significantly symptomatic (breathlessness impairing ability to work or severe coughing). This delay is inappropriate because invariably the patient will have severe, potentially irreversible, histopathologic changes by this time and is therefore much less likely to respond to treatment. If the 50% 5-year mortality for IPF is to be reduced,[153] we believe that therapy should be instituted as soon as the illness is recognized by clinical symptoms, chest roentgenogram, or physiological abnormality.

Although the optimal dosage and duration of corticosteroid therapy remain to be established, treatment is usually initiated with prednisone, 1 to 2 mg per kilogram per day (using ideal body weight) not to exceed a total daily dose of 100 mg per day. Prednisone is given as a single, oral dose in the morning. Alternate-day therapy or periodic injections of long-acting corticosteroids are not recommended since no data are available to suggest that these therapies are effective. The patient should be evaluated 2 to 3 weeks after starting therapy to ensure that he or she is tolerating the medication. The minimum length of the steroid trial is unknown, but 3 months is recommended because responsiveness to therapy is often delayed. A typical course we follow is to begin treatment with 1.5 mg to 2.0 mg per kilogram per day (usually 60–100 mg/day) for 6 weeks, followed by 1.0 mg per kilogram per day for the ensuing 6 weeks and then 0.5 mg per kilogram per day for the next 3 months. Approximately 3, 6, 12, and 24 months after initiating therapy, chest roentgenograms (insensitive parameter of change) and pulmonary physiological studies (most sensitive parameters of change, especially gas exchange at rest and particularly with exercise) should be obtained to assess the response to the treatment. If, after 3 to 6 months of therapy, stabilization or improvement is documented, then therapy should be tapered over several weeks until a maintenance dose of 0.25 mg per kilogram per day is reached. This dose is continued for an additional 3 to 6 months with the realization that the prednisone dose may have to be increased to previous "effective" dose levels (usually greater than 0.5mg/kg/day) to obviate further progression of the disease. We believe that treatment should be given for not less than 1 year. Most often, if effective, corticosteroids must be continued for even longer periods since the disease often flares several months after it appeared to stabilize. Many clinicians feel that lifelong treatment is required in the management of IPF. If the patient's pulmonary status (determined by objective measurements) is worse after 3 to 6 months of continuous treatment, then the therapy is discontinued or lowered (0.25 mg/kg/day) and another form of therapy, such as cyclophosphamide, is instituted.

Intermittent high-dose parenteral corticosteroid "pulse therapy" (intravenous methylprednisolone, 2 g once a week), plus low-dose oral prednisone (0.25 mg/kg/day) has been found to suppress the lavage neutrophilia and to reduce the uptake of gallium-67 in the lungs of patients with IPF (n = 5) compared to low-dose (0.25 mg/kg/day oral prednisone) oral therapy (n = 7) in patients treated for 6 months in a single-blind random trial.[220] However, the patients did not show a significant change in pulmonary function during the 6-month study period. Also, high-dose parenteral corticosteroid therapy has been recommended as the initial treatment in patients with aggressive severe disease. Methylprednisolone, 250 mg every 6 hours, has been utilized in an attempt to "control" the disease as soon as possible. No control trials exist to support any of these recommendations; however, our experience is that high-dose corticosteroids are more effective than the lower doses, although the incidence of complications may be higher. We hold strongly to the view that since the disease prognosis is extremely poor, an aggressive therapeutic approach is necessary to effect any change in the clinical course of these patients.

Although therapy with corticosteroids is usually well tolerated by patients, side effects are common. Peptic ulcer disease, posterior capsular cataracts, osteoporosis and vertebral compression fractures, psychologic effects including depression, hyperexcitability, or psychosis, and fluid and electrolyte abnormalities may occur.[219] Corticosteroid-induced myopathy may impair diaphragmatic and intercostal muscle strength and endurance and these changes may complicate the evaluation of the effectiveness of the therapy.[219]

Cytotoxic and Other Therapeutic Agents

Several cytotoxic agents including cyclophosphamide, azathioprine, chlorambucil, and vincristine have been used alone or in combination with corticosteroids in the treatment of IPF.[154,208,215,221–226] The most commonly used and best studied agents are azathioprine and cyclophosphamide. Winterbauer and coworkers showed that azathioprine appeared to have a beneficial effect on clinical function measured by vital capacity and gas exchange at rest and with exercise.[154] In an uncontrolled study, therapy with prednisone and azathioprine prolonged survival compared to treatment with prednisone alone.[215] In a study of serial bronchoalveolar lavages in patients with IPF, patients with increased neutrophils and eosinophils without lymphocytosis appeared to respond better to cyclophosphamide, whereas patients with lymphocytosis responded more frequently to prednisone.[208]

Cyclophosphamide is the most common second-line drug used as initial therapy in patients with contraindications to the use of corticosteroids or in those who failed or could not tolerate corticosteroid treatment. Cyclophosphamide is an alkylating agent of the nitrogen mustard group. It is absorbed orally and activated in the liver to several cytotoxic compounds. Its mode of action is the depletion of lymphocytes, thereby suppressing lymphocyte function. The usual dose for cyclophosphamide is 2 mg per kilogram (ideal body weight) as a single daily oral dose. Because of the increased incidence of gastrointestinal side effects at doses greater than 200 mg per day, we generally do not exceed this dose. Often, low-dose corticosteroids (0.25 mg/kg/day) are given concurrently with cyclophosphamide. In a randomized, controlled study, alternate-day prednisolone with an initial high-dose phase (60 mg daily for one month, then reduced by 5 mg a week to 20 mg on alternate days or to the minimum dose to maintain early improvement) was compared to cyclophosphamide plus alternate day low-dose prednisolone (100, 110, or 120 mg cyclophosphamide daily, depending on body weight,—i.e., 70 kg or more, 120 mg/day; 60–69 kg, 110 mg/day; less than 60 kg, 100 mg/day, plus 20 mg prednisolone on alternate days) in 43 patients with IPF.[226] The cyclophosphamide/prednisolone-treated group appeared to do better, in terms of the number who remained stable or improved and in terms of survival, over 3 years of follow-up compared to the prednisolone-only group. At 3 years, 10 of 22 patients in the prednisolone-only group had died, compared to 3 of 21 patients in the cyclophosphamide/prednisolone-treated group. This advantage was partially explained by better lung volumes in the cyclophosphamide/prednisolone-treated group at admission into the study. Importantly, it appears that cyclophosphamide has to be given for at least 3 months or longer before a positive effect can be demonstrated. Therefore, because of this data and from our own experience, we advocate at least 6 months of treatment with adequate doses of cyclophosphamide, prednisone, or both. Most patients should be treated for 1 year or longer. Further, failure to respond to one regimen should not discourage a trial of another, since a few patients will respond to the alternative therapy after failing the initial regimen.

Adverse effects of cyclophosphamide, including leukopenia, thrombocytopenia, hemorrhagic cystitis, and gastrointestinal disturbances, may necessitate adjustment of the dose. We generally aim to maintain the total white blood cell count at greater than 4000 per mm^3 or the neutrophil count greater than 1500 per mm^3. Increased fluid intake, 8 glasses of water or more per day, and frequent bladder emptying are recommended to prevent hemorrhagic cystitis. Bimonthly urinalysis is recommended to monitor for this potential complication.

The dose of azathioprine is usually 1 to 3 mg per kilogram per day. Side effects include drug fever, pancreatitis, and skin rashes. Both cyclophosphamide and azathioprine have been associated with interstitial lung disease and the development of hematologic malignancies.

Pencillamine has been used in small therapeutic trials but its usefulness has not been established.[215,224] Colchicine decreases alveolar macrophage release of fibronectin and alveolar macrophage-derived growth factor, two mediators that have been implicated in alveolar inflammation.[227] Whether colchicine has any therapeutic benefit in IPF has not yet been determined.

Other Management Issues

Although most therapeutic emphasis in IPF is directed against the underlying pulmonary process, other treatments for the nonpulmonary consequences of pulmonary fibrosis are often indicated. The most important therapy is oxygen for hypoxemia at rest and with exercise. Oxygen improves pulmonary hypertension caused by hypoxic pulmonary vasoconstriction and may modulate the development of cor pulmonale and right heart failure.[228] Higher oxygen flow rates than frequently used in the management of hypoxemic chronic obstructive lung disease may be required. Hydralazine improves the pulmonary hemodynamics of patients with IPF and cor pulmonale.[229] The effect of vasodilators on morbidity and mortality will determine the role of these agents in the treatment of patients with IPF.

Transplantation

Both unilateral lung and heart-lung transplantations have been performed successfully in patients with IPF.[230,231] Transplantation candidates are generally younger and do not have severe concomitant illnesses. Until more successful medical therapies are available for patients with progressive fibrosis that is not responsive to corticosteroids or cytotoxic agents, transplantation is the only therapy that offers the hope of long-term survival.

REFERENCES

1. Hamman L, Rich AR. Fulminating diffuse interstitial fibrosis of the lungs. Trans Am Clin Climatol Assoc 1935; 51:154–163.
2. Hamman L, Rich AR. Acute diffuse interstitial fibrosis of the lungs. Bull Johns Hopkins Hosp 1944; 74:177–212.
3. Colby TV, Churg AC. Patterns of pulmonary fibrosis. In: Sommers SC, Rosen PP, Fechner RE, eds. 1986 Pathology Annual. Part 2, Vol 21. Appleton-Century-Crofts, Norwalk, Conn, 1986; 277–309.
4. Katzenstein ALA, Myers JL, Mazur MT. Acute interstitial pneumonia: A clinicopathologic, ultrastructural, and cell kinetic study. Am J Surg Pathol 1986; 10:256–267.
5. Crystal RG, Bitterman PB, Rennard SI, Hance AJ, Keogh BA. Interstitial lung diseases of unknown cause: Disorders characterized by chronic inflammation of the lower respiratory tract. N Engl J Med 1984; 310:154–166.
6. Bitterman PB, Crystal RG. Is there a fibrotic gene? Chest 1980; 78:549–550.
7. Evans CC. HLA antigens in diffuse fibrosing alveolitis. Thorax 1976; 31:483. Abstract.
8. Turton CWG, Morris LM, Lawler SD, Turner-Warwick M. HLA in cryptogenic fibrosing alveolitis. Lancet 1978; i:507–508.
9. Varpela E, Tiilikainen A, Varpela M, Tukiainen P. High prevalences of HLA-B15 and HLA-Dw6 in patients with cryptogenic fibrosing alveolitis. Tissue Antigens 1979; 14:68–71.
10. Libby DM, Gibofsky A, Fotino M, Waters SJ, Smith JP. Immunogenetic and clinical findings in IPF association with the B-cell alloantigen HLA-DR2. Am Rev Respir Dis 1983; 127:618–622.
11. Strimlan CV, Taswell HF, DeRemee RA, Keuppers F. HLA antigens and fibrosing alveolitis. Am Rev Respir Dis 1977; 116:1120–1121. Letter.
12. Fulmer JD, Sposovska MS, von Gal ER, Crystal RG, Mittal KK. Distribution of HLA antigen in idiopathic pulmonary fibrosis. Am Rev Respir Dis 1978; 118:141–147.
13. Geddes DM, Brewerton DA, Webley M, Turton CW, Turner-Warwick M, Murphy AH, Ward AM. Alpha-1-antitrypsin phenotypes in fibrosing alveolitis and rheumatoid arthritis. Lancet 1977; ii:1049–1051.
14. Musk AW, Zilko PJ, Manners P, Kay PH, Kamboh MI. Genetic studies in familial fibrosing alveolitis: Possible linkage with immunoglobulin allotypes (Gm). Chest 1986; 89:206–210.
15. Garay SM, Gardella JE, Fazzini EP, Goldring RM. Hermansky-Pudlak syndrome: Pulmonary manifestations of a ceroid storage disorder. Am J Med 1979; 66:737–747.
16. Hoste P, Williams J, Devriendt J, Lamont H, vander Straeten M. Familial diffuse interstitial pulmonary fibrosis associated with oculocutaneous albinism: Report of two cases with a family study. Scand J Respir Dis 1979; 60:128–134.

17. Schneider EL, Epstein CJ, Kaback MJ, Brandes D. Severe pulmonary involvement in adult Gaucher's disease: Report of three cases and review of the literature. Am J Med 1977; 63:475–480.

18. Wolson AH. Pulmonary findings in Gaucher's disease. Am J Roentgenol 1975; 123:712–715.

19. Klatte EC, Franken EA, Smith JA. The radiographic spectrum in neurofibromatosis. Sem Roentgenol 1976; 11:17–33.

20. Massaro D, Katz S, Matthews MJ, Higgins G. Von Recklinghausen's neurofibromatosis associated with cystic lung disease. Am J Med 1965; 38:233–240.

21. Webb WR, Goodman PC. Fibrosing alveolitis in patients with neurofibromatosis. Radiology 1977; 122:289–293.

22. Lynn R, Terry RD. Lipid histochemistry and electron microscopy in adult Niemann-Pick disease. Am J Med 1964; 37:987–994.

23. Harris JO, Waltuck BL, Swenson EW. The pathophysiology of the lungs in tuberous sclerosis: A case report and literature review. Am Rev Respir Dis 1969; 100:379–387.

24. Dwyer JM, Hickie JB, Garvan J. Pulmonary tuberous sclerosis: Report of three patients and a review of the literature. Q J Med 1971; 40:115–125.

25. Medley BE, McLeod RA, Howser OW. Tuberous sclerosis. Sem Roentgenol 1976; 11:35–54.

26. Sandez E. Uber zwei Falle von fotaler bronchektasie Beitr Pathol Anat 1907; 41:495–516.

27. Rosenberg DM. Inherited forms of interstitial lung disease. Clin Chest Med 1982; 3:635–641.

28. Watters LC. Genetic aspects of idiopathic pulmonary fibrosis and hypersensitivity pneumonitis. Sem Respir Med 1986; 7:317–325.

29. MacMillan JM. Familial pulmonary fibrosis. Dis Chest 1951; 20:426–436.

30. Donohue WL, Laski B, Uchida I, Munn JD. Familial fibrocystic pulmonary dysplasia and its relation to the Hamman-Rich syndrome. Pediatrics 1959; 24:786–813.

31. Hughes EW. Familial interstitial fibrosis. Thorax 1964; 19:515–525.

32. Bonanni PP, Frymoyer JW, Jacox RF. A family study of idiopathic pulmonary fibrosis: A possible dysproteinemic and genetically determined disease. Am J Med 1965; 39:411–421.

33. Swaye P, Van Ordstrand HS, McCormack LJ, Wolpaw SE. Familial Hamman-Rich syndrome: Report of eight cases. Dis Chest 1969; 55:7–12.

34. Solliday NH, Williams JA, Gaensler EA, Coutu RE, Carrington CB. Familial chronic interstitial pneumonia. Am Rev Respir Dis 1973; 108:193–204.

35. Beaumont F, Jansen HM, Elema JD, Ten Kate LP, Sluiter HJ. Simultaneous occurrence of pulmonary interstitial fibrosis and alveolar cell carcinoma in one family. Thorax 1981; 36:252–258.

36. Murphy A, O'Sullivan BJ. Familial fibrosing alveolitis. Ir J Med Sci 1981; 150:204–209.

37. Tal A, Maor E, Bar-Ziv J, Gorodischer R. Fatal desquamative interstitial pneumonia in three infant siblings. J Pediatrics 1984; 104:873–876.

38. Peabody JW, Peabody JW Jr, Hayes EW, Hayes EW Jr. Idiopathic pulmonary fibrosis; its occurrence in identical twin sisters. Dis Chest 1950; 18:330–344.

39. Javaheri S, Lederer DH, Pella JA, Mark GJ, Levine BW. Idiopathic pulmonary fibrosis in monozygotic twins: The importance of genetic predisposition. Chest 1980; 78:591–594.

40. Bitterman PB, Rennard SI, Keogh BA, Wewers MD, Adelberg S, Crystal RG. Familial idiopathic pulmonary fibrosis: Evidence of lung inflammation in unaffected family members. N Engl J Med 1986; 314:1343–1347.

41. Gaensler EA, Goff AM, Prowse CM. Desquamative interstitial pneumonia. N Engl J Med 1966; 274:113–128.

42. Klocke RA, Augerson WS, Berman HH, Burgos FL, Rivera RA. Desquamative interstitial pneumonia: A disease with a wide clinical spectrum. Ann Intern Med 1967; 66:498–506.

43. Nagaya H, Elmore M, Ford CD. Idiopathic interstitial pulmonary fibrosis: An immune complex disease? Am Rev Respir Dis 1973; 107:826–830.

44. Patchefsky AS, Banner M, Freundlich IM. Desquamative interstitial pneumonia: Significance of intranuclear viral-like inclusion bodies. Ann Intern Med 1971; 74:322–327.
45. McNary WF Jr, Gaensler EA. Intranuclear inclusion bodies in desquamative interstitial pneumonia: Electron microscopic observations. Ann Intern Med 1971; 74:404–407.
46. Crystal RG, Fulmer JD, Roberts WC, Moss ML, Line BR, Reynolds HY. Idiopathic pulmonary fibrosis: Clinical, histologic, radiographic, physiologic, scintographic, cytologic, and biochemical aspects. Ann Intern Med 1976; 85:769–788.
47. Liebow AA, Steer A, Billingsley JG. Desquamative interstitial pneumonia. Am J Med 1965; 39:369–404.
48. O'Shea PA, Yardley JH. The Hamman-Rich syndrome in infancy: Report of a case with virus-like particles by electron microscopy. Johns Hopkins Med J 1970; 126:320–336.
49. Kawanami O, Ferrans VJ, Fulmer JD, Crystal RG. Nuclear inclusions in alveolar epithelium of patients with fibrotic lung disorders. Am J Pathol 1979; 94:301–312.
50. Brewer DB, Heath D, Asquith P. Electron microscopy of desquamative interstitial pneumonia. J Pathol 1969; 97:317–323.
51. Shortland JR, Darke CS, Crane WAJ. Electron microscopy of desquamative interstitial pneumonia. Thorax 1969; 24:192–208.
52. Farr GH, Harley RA, Henningar GR. Desquamative interstitial pneumonia: An electron microscopic study. Am J Pathol 1970; 60:347–370.
53. Tubbs RR, Benjamin SP, Osborne DG, Barenberg S. Surface and transmission ultrastructural characteristics of desquamative interstitial pneumonitis. Hum Pathol 1978; 9:693–703.
54. Sutinen S, Rainio P, Sutinen S, Huhti E, Pokela R. Ultrastructure of terminal respiratory epithelium and prognosis in chronic interstitial pneumonia. Eur J Respir Dis 1980; 61:325–336.
55. Coalson JJ. The ultrastructure of human fibrosing alveolitis. Virchows Arch [A] Pathol Anat 1982; 395:181–199.
56. Corrin B, Dewar A, Rodriquez-Roisin R, Turner-Warwick M. Fine structural changes in cryptogenic fibrosing alveolitis and asbestosis. J Pathol 1985; 147:107–119.
57. Vergnon JM, Vincent M, DeThe G, Mornex JF, Weynants P, Brune J. Cryptogenic fibrosing alveolitis and Epstein-Barr virus: An association? Lancet 1984; ii:768–771.
58. Gottlieb AJ, Spiera H, Teirstein AS, Siltzbach LE. Serologic factors in idiopathic diffuse interstitial pulmonary fibrosis. Am J Med 1965; 39:405–410.
59. Turner-Warwick M, Doniach D. Autoantibody studies in interstitial pulmonary fibrosis. Br Med J 1965; i:886–891.
60. Hobbs JR, Turner-Warwick M. Assay of circulating immunoglobulins in patients with fibrosing alveolitis. Clin Exp Immunol 1967; 2:645–654.
61. Turner-Warwick M, Haslam PL. The immunology of cryptogenic fibrosing alveolitis (idiopathic pulmonary fibrosis). In: Daniele RP, ed. Immunology and immunologic diseases of the lung. Boston: Blackwell Scientific Publications, 1988: 377–395.
62. Turner-Warwick M, Haslam P, Weeks J. Antibodies in some chronic fibrosing lung diseases: Part 2: Immunofluorescent studies. Clin Allergy 1971, 1:209–219.
63. Nagaya H, Sieker HO. Pathogenetic mechanisms of interstitial pulmonary fibrosis in patients with serum antinuclear factor: A histologic and clinical correlation. Am J Med 1972; 52:51–62.
64. Chapman JR, Charles PJ, Venables PJW, Thompson PJ, Haslam PL, Maini RN, Turner-Warwick MEH. Definition and clinical relevance of antibodies to nuclear ribonucleoprotein and other nuclear antigens in patients with cryptogenic fibrosing alveolitis. Am Rev Respir Dis 1984; 130:439–443.
65. Dreisin RB, Schwarz MI, Theofilopoulos AN, Stanford RE. Circulating immune complexes in the idiopathic interstitial pneumonias. N Engl J Med. 1978; 298:353–357.
66. Gelb AF, Dreisin RB, Epstein JD, Silverthorne JD, Bickel Y, Fields M, Border WA, Taylor CR. Immune complexes, gallium lung scans, and bronchoalveolar lavage in idiopathic interstitial pneumonitis-fibrosis: A structure-function clinical study. Chest 1983; 84:148–153.

67. Haslam PL, Thompson B, Mohammed I, Townsend PJ, Hodson ME, Holborow EJ, Turner-Warwick M. Circulating immune complexes in patients with cryptogenic fibrosing alveolitis. Clin Exp Immunol 1979; 37:381–390.
68. Mortenson RL, Schwarz MI, Cherniack RM, Harbeck RJ, Watters LC, Niccoli SA, McDermott TL, King TE Jr. The clinical role of circulating immune complexes in idiopathic pulmonary fibrosis. Am Rev Respir Dis 1989; 139:A192. Abstract.
69. Reynolds HY, Fulmer JD, Kazmierowski JA, Robert WC, Frank MM, Crystal RG. Analysis of cellular and protein content of bronchoalveolar lavage fluid from patients with idiopathic pulmonary fibrosis and chronic hypersensitivity penumonitis. J Clin Invest 1977; 59:165–175.
70. Hunninghake GW, Gadek JE, Kawanami O, Ferrans VJ, Crystal RG. Inflammatory and immune processes in the human lung in health and disease: Evaluation by bronchoalveolar lavage. Am J Pathol 1979; 97:149–206.
71. Weinberger SE, Kelman JA, Elson NA, Young RC, Reynolds HY, Fulmer JD, Crystal RG. Bronchoalveolar lavage in interstitial lung disease. Ann Intern Med 1978; 89:459–466.
72. Lawrence EC, Martin RR, Blaese RM, Teague RB, Awe RJ, Wilson RK, Deaton WJ, Bloom K, Greenberg SD, Stevens PM. Increased bronchoalveolar lgG-secreting cells in interstitial lung diseases. N Engl J Med 1980; 302:1186–1188.
73. Schwarz MI, Dreisin RB, Pratt DS, Stanford RE. Immunofluorescent patterns in the idiopathic interstitial pneumonias. J Lab Clin Med 1978; 91:929–938.
74. Eisenberg H, Simmons DH, Barnett EV. Diffuse pulmonary interstitial disease: An immunohistologic study. Chest 1979; 75:262–264.
75. Walker S, Schwarz MI, Harbeck R, Wallace ME, Willcox ML, Cherniack RM, King TE, Jr. Ultrastructural immune deposits are present in the lungs of patients with interstitial lung disease. Am Rev Respir Dis 1988; 137:347. Abstract.
76. Schwartz RH. T-lymphocyte recognition of antigen in association with gene products of the major histocompatibility complex. Ann Rev Immunol 1985; 3:237–261.
77. Razma AG, Lynch JP, Wilson BS, Ward PA, Kunkel SL. Expression of Ia-like (DR) antigen on human alveolar macrophages isolated by bronchoalveolar lavage. Am Rev Respir Dis 1984; 129:419–424.
78. Campbell DA, Poulter LW, Janossy G, DuBois RM. Immunohistological analysis of lung tissue from patients with cryptogenic fibrosing alveolitis suggesting local expression of immune hypersensitivity. Thorax 1985; 40:405–411.
79. Beaumont F, Schilizzi BM, Kallenberg CGM, de Ley L. Expression of class II-MHC antigens on alveolar and bronchiolar epithelial cells in fibrosing alveolitis. Chest 1986; 89:136S–137S.
80. Kradin RL, Divertie MB, Colvin RB, Ramirez J, Ryu J, Carpenter HA, Bhan AK. Usual interstitial pneumonitis is a T-cell alveolitis. Clin Immunol Immunopathol 1986; 40:224–235.
81. Kallenberg CGM, Schilizzi BM, Beaumont F, De Leij L, Poppema S, The TH. Expression of class II major histocompatibility complex antigens on alveolar epithelium in interstitial lung disease: Relevance to pathogenesis of idiopathic pulmonary fibrosis. J Clin Pathol 1987; 40:725–733.
82. Komatsu T, Yamamoto M, Shimokata K, Nagura H. Phenotypic characterization of alveolar capillary endothelial cells, alveolar epithelial cells and alveolar macrophages in patients with pulmonary fibrosis, with special reference to MHC class II antigens. Virchows Archiv [A] Pathol Anat 1989; 415:79–90.
83. Kallenberg CGM, Schilizzi BM, Beaumont F, Poppema S, DeLeij L, The TN. Expression of class II MHC antigens on alveolar epithelium in fibrosing alveolitis. Clin Exp Immunol 1987; 67:182–190.
84. Bottazzo GF, Pujol-Borrell R, Hanafusa T, Feldmann M. Role of aberrant HLA-DR expression and antigen presentation in induction of endocrine autoimmunity. Lancet 1983; ii:1115–1119.
85. Eden E, Turino GM. Interleukin 1 secretion from human alveolar macrophages in lung disease. J Clin Immunol 1986; 6:326–333.

86. Ettensohn DB, Roberts NJ Jr. Human alveolar macrophage support of lymphocyte responses to mitogens and antigens: Analysis and comparison with autologous peripheral blood-derived monocytes and macrophages. Am Rev Respir Dis 1983; 128:516–522.

87. Rosenthal, AS. Regulation of the immune response: Role of the macrophage. N Engl J Med 1980; 303:1153–1156.

88. Rossi GA, Zocchi E, Sacco O, Balbi B, Ravazzoni C, Damiani G. Alveolar macrophage stimulation of T-cell proliferation in autologous mixed lymphocyte reactions: Role of HLA-DR antigens. Am Rev Respir Dis 1986; 133:78–82.

89. Rich EA, Tweardy DJ, Fujiwara H, Ellner JJ. Spectrum of immunoregulatory functions and properties of human alveolar macrophages. Am Rev Respir Dis 1987; 136:258–265.

90. Kravis TC, Ahmed A, Brown TE, Fulmer JD, Crystal RG. Pathogenic mechanisms in pulmonary fibrosis: Collagen-induced migration inhibition factor production and cytotoxicity mediated by lymphocytes. J Clin Invest 1976; 58:1223–1232.

91. Hunninghake GW, Bedell GN. Interstitial lung disease: Concepts of pathogenesis. Sem Respir Med 1984; 6:31–39.

92. Baumgartner U, Schoelmerich J, Becher S, Costabel U. Detection of antibodies in serum of patients with idiopathic pulmonary fibrosis against isolated rat alveolar type II cells. Respiration 1987; 52:122–128.

93. Haslam PL, Turton CWG, Heard B, Lukoszek A, Collins JV, Salsbury AJ, Turner-Warwick M. Bronchoalveolar lavage in pulmonary fibrosis: Comparison of cells obtained with lung biopsy and clinical features. Thorax 1980; 35:9–18.

94. Davis GS, Brody AR, Craighead JE. Analysis of airspace and interstitial mononuclear cell populations in human diffuse interstitial lung disease. Am Rev Respir Dis 1978; 118:7–15.

95. Haslam PL, Turton CWG, Lukoszek A, Salsbury AJ, Dewar A, Collins JV, Turner-Warwick M. Bronchoalveolar lavage fluid cell counts in cryptogenic fibrosing alveolitis and their relation to therapy. Thorax 1980; 35:328–339.

96. Watters LC, Schwarz MI, Cherniack RM, Waldron JA, Dunn TL, Stanford RE, King TE. Idiopathic pulmonary fibrosis. Pretreatment bronchoalveolar lavage cellular constituents and their relationships with lung histopathology and clinical response to therapy. Am Rev Respir Dis 1987; 135:696–704.

97. Johnston RB. Monocytes and macrophages. N Engl J Med 1988; 318:747–752.

98. Hunninghake GW, Gadek JE, Lawley TJ, Crystal RG. Mechanisms of neutrophil accumulation in the lungs of patients with idiopathic pulmonary fibrosis. J Clin Invest 1981; 68:259–269.

99. Martinet Y, Rom WN, Grotendorst GR, Martin GR, Crystal RG. Exaggerated spontaneous release of platelet-derived growth factor by alveolar macrophages from patients with idiopathic pulmonary fibrosis. N Engl J Med 1987; 317:202–209.

100. Shaw RJ, Benedict SH, Clark RAF, King TE Jr. Pathogenesis of pulmonary fibrosis in interstitial lung disease: Alveolar macrophage PDGF(B) gene activation and up-regulation by interferon gamma. Am Rev Respir Dis; In press.

101. Rennard SI, Crystal RG. Fibronectin in human bronchopulmonary lavage fluid: Elevation in patients with interstitial lung disease. J Clin Invest 1981; 69:113–122.

102. Rennard SI, Hunninghake GW, Bitterman PB, Crystal RG. Production of fibronectin by the human alveolar macrophage: Mechanism for the recruitment of fibroblasts to sites of tissue injury in interstitial lung diseases. Proc Natl Acad Sci USA 1981; 78:7147–7151.

103. Bitterman PB, Rennard SI, Adelberg S, Crystal RG. Role of fibronectin as a growth factor for fibroblasts. J Cell Biol 1983; 97:1925–1932.

104. Clark JG, Kostal KM, Marino BA. Bleomycin-induced pulmonary fibrosis in hamsters: An alveolar macrophage product increases fibroblast prostaglandin E2 and cyclic adenosine monophosphate and suppresses fibroblast proliferation and collagen production. J Clin Invest 1983; 72:2082–2091.

105. Elias JA, Zurier RB, Schreiber AD, Leff JA, Daniele RP. Monocyte inhibition of lung fibroblast growth: Relationship to fibroblast prostaglandin production and density defined monocyte subpopulations. J Leukocyte Biol 1985; 37:15–28.
106. Elias JA, Rossman MD, Zurier RB, Daniele RP. Human alveolar macrophage inhibition of lung fibroblast growth: A prostaglandin dependent process. Am Rev Respir Dis 1985; 131:94–99.
107. Elias JA, Jimenez SA, Freundlich B. Recombinant gamma, alpha, and beta interferon regulation of human lung fibroblast proliferation. Am Rev Respir Dis 1987; 235:62–65.
108. Welgus HG, Campbell EJ, Bar-Shavit Z, Senior RM, Teitelbaum SL. Human alveolar macrophages produce a fibroblast-like collagenase and collagenase inhibitor. J Clin Invest 1985; 76:219–224.
109. duBois RM, Townsend PJ, Cole PJ. Alveolar macrophage lysosomal enzyme and C3b receptors in cryptogenic fibrosing alveolitis. Clin Exp Immunol 1980; 40:60–65.
110. Hunninghake GW, Gadek JE, Fales HM, Crystal RG. Human alveolar macrophage-derived chemotactic factor for neutrophils: Stimuli and partial characterization. J Clin Invest 1980; 66:473–483.
111. Merrill WW, Naegel GP, Matthay RA, Reynolds HY. Alveolar macrophage-derived chemotactic factor: Kinetics of *in vitro* production and partial characterization. J Clin Invest 1980; 65:268–276.
112. Cantin AM, North SL, Fells GA, Hubbard RC, Crystal RG. Oxidant-mediated epithelial cell injury in idiopathic pulmonary fibrosis. J Clin Invest 1987; 79:1665–1673.
113. Gadek JE, Kelman JA, Fells G, Weinberger SE, Horwitz AL, Reynolds HY, Fulmer JD, Crystal RG. Collagenase in the lower respiratory tract of patients with idiopathic pulmonary fibrosis. N Engl J Med 1979; 301:737–742.
114. Haellgren R, Bjermer L, Lundgren R, Venge P. The eosinophil component of the alveolitis in idiopathic pulmonary fibrosis: Signs of eosinophil activation in the lung are related to impaired lung function. Am Rev Respir Dis 1989; 139:373–377.
115. McDonald JA, Kelly DG. Degradation of fibronectin by human leukocyte elastase release of biologically active fragments. J Biol Chem 1980; 255:8848–8858.
116. Gadek JE, Hunninghake GW, Zimmerman RL, Crystal RG. Regulation of the release of alveolar macrophage-derived neutrophil chemotactic factor. Am Rev Respir Dis 1980; 121:723–733.
117. Ginns LC, Goldenheim PD, Burten RC, Colvin RB, Miller LG, Goldstein G, Hurwitz C, Kazemi H. T-lymphocyte subsets in peripheral blood and lung lavage in idiopathic pulmonary fibrosis and sarcoidosis: Analysis by monoclonal antibodies and flow cytometry. Clin Immunol Immunopathol 1982; 25:11–20.
118. Kaelin RM, Center DM, Bernardo J, Grant M, Snider GL. The role of macrophage-derived chemoattractant activities in the early inflammatory events of bleomycin-induced pulmonary injury. Am Rev Respir Dis 1983; 128:132–137.
119. Karpel JP, Norin AJ. Association of activated cytolytic lung lymphocytes with response to prednisone therapy in patients with idiopathic pulmonary fibrosis. Chest 1989; 96:794–798.
120. Kehrle JH, Wakefield LM, Roberts AB, Jakowlew S, Alverez-Mon M, Derynck R, Sporn MB, Fauci AS. Production of transforming growth factor beta by human T lymphocytes and its potential role in the regulation of T cell growth. J Exp Med 1986;163:1037–1050.
121. Haslam PL, Cromwell O, Dewar A, Turner-Warwick M. Evidence of increased histamine levels of lung lavage fluids from patients with cryptogenic fibrosing alveolitis. Clin Exp Immunol 1981; 44:587–593.
122. Haslam PL, Dewar A, Turner-Warwick M. Lung lavage eosinophils and histamine. In: Cumming G, Bonsignore R, eds. Cellular biology of the lung. New York: Plenum Press, 1982: 77–94.
123. Jordana M, Schulman J, McSharry C, Irving LB, Newhouse MT, Jordana G, Gauldie J. Heterogeneous proliferative characteristics of human adult lung fibroblast lines and clonally derived fibroblasts from control and fibrotic tissue. Am Rev Respir Dis 1988; 137:579–584.

124. Cantin A, Crystal RG. 'Interstitial pathology': An overview of the chronic interstitial lung disorders. Int Arch Allergy Appl Immunol 1985; 76(suppl 1):83–91.
125. Fulmer JD, Bienkowski RS, Cowan MJ, Breul SD, Bradley KM, Ferrans VJ, Roberts WC, Crystal RG. Collagen concentration and rates of synthesis in idiopathic pulmonary fibrosis. Am Rev Respir Dis 1980; 122:289–301.
126. Kirk JME, DaCosta PE, Turner-Warwick M, Littleton RJ, Laurent GJ. Biochemical evidence for an increased and progressive deposition of collagen in lungs of patients with pulmonary fibrosis. Clin Sci 1986; 70:39–45.
127. Bateman ED, Turner-Warwick M, Adelmann-Grill BC. Immunohistochemical study of collagen types in human foetal and fibrotic lung disease. Thorax 1981; 36:645–653.
128. Bateman ED, Turner-Warwick M, Haslam PL, Adelmann-Grill BC. Cryptogenic fibrosing alveolitis: Prediction of fibrogenic activity from immunohistochemical studies of collagen types in lung biopsy specimens. Thorax 1983; 38:93–101.
129. Madri JA, Furthmayr H. Collagen polymorphism in the lung: An immunochemical study of pulmonary fibrosis. Hum Pathol 1980; 11:353–366.
130. Selman M, Montano M, Ramos C, Chapela R. Concentration, biosynthesis and degradation of collagen in idiopathic pulmonary fibrosis. Thorax 1986; 41:355–359.
131. Clark JG, Overton JE, Marino BA, Vitto J, Starcher BC. Collagen biosynthesis in bleomycin-induced pulmonary fibrosis in hamsters. J Lab Clin Med 1980; 96:943–953.
132. Kehrer JP. Collagen production rates following acute lung damage induced by butylated hydroxytoluene. Biochem Pharmacol 1982; 31:2053–2058.
133. Raghu G, Masta S, Meyers D, Narayanan AS. Collagen synthesis by normal and fibrotic human lung fibroblasts and the effect of transforming growth factor beta. Am Review Respir Dis 1989; 140:95–100.
134. Kuhn C, III, Boldt J, King TE, Jr., Crouch E, Vartio T, McDonald JA. An immunohistochemical study of architectural remodeling and connective tissue synthesis in pulmonary fibrosis. Am Rev Respir Dis 1989; 140:1693–1703.
135. Kirk JME, Bateman ED, Haslam PL, Laurent GL, Turner-Warwick M. Serum type III procollagen peptide concentrations in cryptogenic fibrosing alveolitis and its clinical relevance. Thorax 1984; 39:726–732.
136. Low RB, Cutroneo KR, Davis GS, Giancola MS. Lavage type III procollagen N-terminal peptides in human pulmonary fibrosis and sarcoidosis. Lab Invest 1983; 48:755–759.
137. Bjermer L, Lundgren R, Haellgren R. Hyaluronan and type III procollagen peptide concentrations in bronchoalveolar lavage fluid in idiopathic pulmonary fibrosis. Thorax 1989; 44:126–131.
138. Cantin AM, Boileau R, Begin R. Increased procollagen III aminoterminal peptide-related antigens and fibroblast growth signals in the lung of patients with idiopathic pulmonary fibrosis. Am Rev Respir Dis 1988; 137:572–578.
139. Montano M, Ramos C, Gonzales G, Vadillo F, Pardo A, Selman M. Lung collagenase inhibitors and spontaneous and latent collagenase activity in idiopathic pulmonary fibrosis and hypersensitivity pneumonitis. Chest 1989;1115–1119.
140. Raghu G, Striker LJ, Hudson LD, Striker GE. Extracellular matrix in normal and fibrotic human lungs. Am Rev Respir Dis 1985; 131:281–289.
141. Kirk JME, Heard BE, Kerr I, Turner-Warwick M, Laurent GJ. Quantitation of types I and III collagen in biopsy lung samples from patients with cryptogenic fibrosing alveolitis. Collagen Rel Res 1984; 4:169–182.
142. Seyer JM, Hutcheson ET, Kang AH. Collagen polymorphism in idiopathic chronic pulmonary fibrosis. J Clin Invest 1976; 57:1498–1507.
143. Last JA, King TE Jr, Nerlich AM, Reiser KM. Collagen crosslinking in adult patients with acute and chronic fibrotic lung disease: Molecular markers for fibrotic collagen. Am Rev Respir Dis 1990; 141:307–313.

144. Trombley L, Absher M, Kelley J. Lung cell population density determines the ratio of type III to type I collagens. Am Rev Respir Dis 1981; 123:694–696.
145. Adler KB, Craighead JE, Vallyathan NV, Evans JN. Actin-containing cells in human pulmonary fibrosis. Am J Pathol 1981; 102:427–437.
146. Seemayer TA, Lagace R, Schurch W, Thelmo WL. The myofibroblast: Biologic, pathologic, and theoretical considerations. Pathol Annu 1980; 15:443.
147. Weissler JC. Idiopathic pulmonary fibrosis: Cellular and molecular pathogenesis. Am J Med Sci 1989; 297:91–104.
148. Fortoul T. Comparison of transbronchial and open lung biopsies in interstitial lung diseases. Arch Invest Med (Mex) 1988; 19:7–11.
149. Gaensler EA, Carrington CB. Open biopsy for chronic diffuse infiltrative lung disease: Clinical, roentgenographic, and physiological correlations in 502 patients. Ann Thorac Surg 1980; 30:411–426.
150. Ray JF, III, Lawton BR, Myers WO, Toyama WM, Reyes CN, Emanuel DA, Burns JL, Pederson DP, Dovenbarger WV, Wenzel FJ, Sautter RD. Open pulmonary biopsy: Nineteen-year experience with 416 consecutive operations. Chest 1976; 69:43–47.
151. Churg A. An inflation procedure for open lung biopsies. Am J Surg Pathol 1983; 7:69–71.
152. Colby TV, Carrington CB. Infiltrative lung disease. In: WM Thurlbeck, ed. Pathology of the lung. Thieme Medical Publishers, New York. 1988: 425–517.
153. Carrington CB, Gaensler EA, Coutu RE, Fitzgerald MX, Gupta RG. Natural history and treated course of usual and desquamative interstitial pneumonia. N Engl J Med 1978; 298:801–809.
154. Winterbauer RH, Hammar SP, Hallman KO, Hays JE, Pardee NE, Morgan EH, Allen JD, Moores KD, Bush W, Walker JH. Diffuse interstitial pneumonitis: Clinicopathologic correlations in 20 patients treated with prednizone/azathioprine. Am J Med 1978; 65:661–672.
155. Livingstone JL, Lewis JG, Reid L, Jefferson KE. Diffuse interstitial pulmonary fibrosis: A clinical, radiological, and pathological study based on 45 patients. Q J Med 1964; 33:71–103.
156. Scadding JG. Chronic diffuse interstitial fibrosis of the lungs. Br Med J 1960; 1:443–450.
157. Wright PH, Heard BE, Steel SJ, Turner-Warwick M. Cryptogenic fibrosing alveolitis: Assessment by graded trephine lung biopsy histology compared with clinical, radiographic, and physiological features. Br J Dis Chest 1981; 75:61–70.
158. Kaufman JM, Cuvelier CA, van der Straeten M. Mycoplasma pneumonia with fulminant evolution into diffuse interstitial fibrosis. Thorax 1980; 35:140–144.
159. Pinsker KL, Schneyer B, Beckner N, Kamholz SL. Usual interstitial pneumonia following Texas A$_2$ influenza infection. Chest 1987: 80:123–126.
160. Tablan OC, Reyes MP. Chronic interstitial pulmonary fibrosis following *Mycoplasma pneumoniae* pneumonia. Am J Med 1985; 79:268–270.
161. Galko B, Grossman RF, Day A, Tenebaum J, Kirsh J, Rebuck AS. Hypertrophic pulmonary osteoarthropathy in four patients with interstitial pulmonary disease. Chest 1985; 88:94–97.
162. Kupfer Y, Groopman JE, Lenora A, Tessler S. Pulmonary hypertrophic osteoarthropathy as the initial manifestation of interstitial fibrosis. NY State J Med 1989; 89:234–235.
163. Epler GR, McLoud TC, Gaensler EA, Mikus JP, Carrington CB. Normal chest roentgenograms in chronic diffuse infiltrative lung disease. N Engl J Med 1978; 298:934–939.
164. Sahn SA, Schwarz MI. Desquamative interstitial pneumonia with a normal chest radiograph. Br J Dis Chest 1974; 68:228–234.
165. Johnson TH. Radiology and honeycomb lung disease. Am J Roentgenol 1968; 104:810–821.
166. Genereux GP. The end-stage lung: Pathogenesis, pathology and radiology. Radiology 1975; 116:279–289.
167. Woodring JH, Barrett PA, Rehm SR, Nurenberg P. Acquired tracheomegaly in adults as a complication of diffuse pulmonary fibrosis. Am J Roentgenol 1989; 152:743–747.

168. Staples CA, Mueller NL, Vedal S, Abboud R, Ostrow D, Miller RR. Usual interstitial pneumonia: Correlation of CT with clinical, functional, and radiologic findings. Radiology 1987; 162:377–381.
169. Mathieson JR, Mayo JR, Staples CA, Mueller NL. Chronic diffuse infiltrative lung disease: Comparison of diagnostic accuracy of CT and chest radiography. Radiology 1989; 171:111–116.
170. Mueller NL, Guerry-Force ML, Staples CA, Wright JL, Wiggs B, Coppin C, Pare P, Hogg JC. Differential diagnosis of bronchiolitis obliterans with organizing pneumonia and usual interstitial pneumonia: Clinical, functional, and radiologic findings. Radiology 1987; 162:151–156.
171. Mueller NL, Miller RR, Webb WR, Evans KG, Ostrow DN. Fibrosing alveolitis: CT-pathologic correlation. Radiology 1986; 160:585–588.
172. Mueller NL, Staples CA, Miller RR, Vedal S, Thurlbeck WM, Ostrow DN. Disease activity in idiopathic pulmonary fibrosis: CT and pathologic correlation. Radiology 1987; 165:731–734.
173. Line BR, Fulmer JD, Reynolds HY, Roberts WC, Jones AE, Harris EK, Crystal RG. Gallium-67 citrate scanning in the staging of idiopathic pulmonary fibrosis: Correlation with physiologic and morphologic features and bronchoalveolar lavage. Am Rev Respir Dis 1978; 118:355–365.
174. Crystal RG, Gadek JE, Ferrans VJ, Fulmer JD, Line BR, Hunninghake GW. Interstitial lung diseases: Current concepts of pathogenesis, staging, and therapy. Am J Med 1981; 70:542–568.
175. Bogin RM, Buschman DS, Cherniack RM, Schwarz MI, McDermott TL, King TE Jr. The role of gallium lung scanning in the evaluation of idiopathic pulmonary fibrosis. Chest 1988; 94:73S. Abstract.
176. Bogin RM, Buschman DS, Cherniack RM, Schwarz MI, King TE Jr. Gallium-67 lung scanning is not helpful in predicting the clinical course of patients with idiopathic pulmonary fibrosis. Am Rev Respir Dis 1989; 139:A193.
177. Wesselius LJ, Witztum KF, Taylor AT, Hartman MT, Moser KM. Computer-assisted versus visual lung gallium-67 index in normal subjects and in patients with interstitial lung disorders. Am Rev Respir Dis 1983; 128:1084–1089.
178. Kornbluth RS, Turino GM. Respiratory control in diffuse interstitial lung disease and diseases of the pulmonary vasculature. Clin Chest Med 1980; 1:91–102.
179. Renzi G, Milic-Emili J, Grassino AE. The pattern of breathing in diffuse lung fibrosis. Bull Eur Physiopathol Respir 1982; 18:461–472.
180. Renzi G, Milic-Emili J, Grassino AE. Breathing pattern in sarcoidosis and idiopathic pulmonary fibrosis. Ann NY Acad Sci 1986; 465:482–490.
181. Dimarco AF, Kelsen SG, Cherniack NS, Gothe B. Occlusion pressure and breathing pattern in patients with interstitial lung disease. Am Rev Respir Dis 1983; 127:425–430.
182. Burdon JGW, Killian KJ, Jones NL. Pattern of breathing during exercise in patients with interstitial lung disease. Thorax 1983; 38:778–784.
183. Englert M, Yernault JC, deCoster A, Clumeek N. Diffusing properties and elastic properties in interstitial diseases of the lung. Prog Respir Res 1975; 8:177–185.
184. Keogh BA, Crystal RG. Clinical significance of pulmonary function tests: Pulmonary function testing in interstitial pulmonary disease: What does it tell us? Chest 1980; 78:856–865.
185. Fulmer JD, Roberts WC, von Gal ER, Crystal RG. Morphologic-physiologic correlates of the severity of fibrosis and degree of cellularity in idiopathic pulmonary fibrosis. J Clin Invest 1979; 63:665–676.
186. Watters LC, King TE, Schwarz MI, Waldron JA, Stanford RE, Cherniack RM: A clinical, radiographic, and physiologic scoring system for the longitudinal assessment of patients with idiopathic pulmonary fibrosis. Am Rev Respir Dis 1986; 133:97–103.
187. Jernudd-Wilhelmsson, Hoernblad Y, Hedenstierna G. Ventilation-perfusion relationships in interstitial lung disease. Eur J Respir Dis 1986; 68:39–49.
188. Wagner PD, Dantzker DR, Dueck R, dePolo JL, Wasserman K, West JB. Distribution of ventilation-perfusion ratios in patients with interstitial lung disease. Chest 1976; 69:256–257.

189. Eary JF, Fisher MC, Cerguira MD. Idiopathic pulmonary fibrosis: Another cause of ventilation/perfusion mismatch. Clin Nucl Med 1986; 11:396–399.
190. Panos RJ, Mortenson R, Niccoli SA, King TE Jr. Clinical deterioration in patients with idiopathic pulmonary fibrosis. Am J Med 1990; 88:396–404.
191. Turner-Warwick M, Lebowitz M, Burrows B, Johnson A. Cryptogenic fibrosing alveolitis and lung cancer. Thorax 1980; 35:496–499.
192. Jones AW. Alveolar cell carcinoma occurring in idiopathic interstitial pulmonary fibrosis. Br J Dis Chest 1970; 64:78-84.
193. Beaumont F, Jansen HM, Elema JD, Ten Kate LP, Sluiter HJ. Simultaneous occurrence of pulmonary interstitial fibrosis and alveolar cell carcinoma in one family. Thorax 1981; 36:252–258.
194. Haddad R, Massaro D. Idiopathic diffuse interstitial pulmonary fibrosis (fibrosing alveolitis), atypical epithelial proliferation and lung cancer. Am J Med 1968; 45:211–219.
195. Laros CD, Bergstein PGM. Relief of breathlessness in a case of progressive pulmonary fibrosis. Respiration 1982; 43:452–457.
196. Picado C, Gomez de Almeida R, Xaubet A, Montserrat J, Letang E, Sanchez-Lloret J. Spontaneous pneumothorax in cryptogenic fibrosing alveolitis. Respiration 1985; 48:77–80.
197. Sachor Y, Schindler D, Siegal A, Lieberman D, Mikulski Y, Bruderman I. Increased incidence of pulmonary tuberculosis in chronic interstitial lung disease. Thorax 1989; 44:151–153.
198. Vanderstappen M, Mornex JF, Lahneche B, Chauvot P, Bouvier JF, Wiesendanger T, Pages J, Webert P, Cordier JF, Brune S. Gallium-67 scanning in the staging of cryptogenic fibrosing alveolitis and hypersensitivity pneumonitis. Eur Respir J 1988; 1:517–522.
199. Vedal S, Welsh EV, Miller RR, Mueller NL. Desquamative interstitial pneumonia: Computed tomographic findings before and after treatment with corticosteroids. Chest 1988; 93:215–217.
200. Pantin CF, Valind SO, Sweatman M, Lawrence R, Rhodes CG, Brudin L, Britten A, Hughes JMB, Turner-Warwick M. Measures of the inflammatory response in cryptogenic fibrosing alveolitis. Am Rev Respir Dis 1988; 138:1234–1241.
201. Rinderknecht J, Shapiro L, Krauthammer M, Taplin G, Wasserman K, Uszler JM, Effros RM. Accelerated clearance of small solutes from the lungs in interstitial lung disease. Am Rev Respir Dis 1980; 121:105–117.
202. Gaensler EA, Carrington CB, Coutu RE, Fitzgerald MX. Radiographic-physiologic-pathologic correlations in interstitial pneumonias. Prog Respir Res 1975; 8:223–241.
203. Enson Y. Pulmonary heart disease: Relation of pulmonary hypertension to abnormal lung structure and function. Bull NY Acad Med 1977; 53:551–566.
204. Risk C, Epler GR, Gaensler EA. Exercise alveolar-arterial oxygen pressure difference in interstitial lung disease. Chest 1984; 85:69–74.
205. Green GM, Graham WGB, Hanson JJ, Gump DW, Phillips CA, Brody AR, Sylvester DW, Landis JN, Davis GS, Chraighead JE. Correlated studies of interstitial pulmonary disease. Chest 1976; 69:S263.
206. Rudd RM, Haslam PL, Turner-Warwick M. Cryptogenic fibrosing alveolitis: Relationships of pulmonary physiology and bronchoalveolar lavage to treatment and prognosis. Am Rev Respir Dis 1981; 124:1–8.
207. Peterson MW, Monick M, Hunninghake GW. Prognostic role of eosinophils in pulmonary fibrosis. Chest 1987; 92:51–56.
208. Turner-Warwick M, Haslam PL. The value of serial bronchoalveolar lavages in assessing the clinical progress of patients with cryptogenic fibrosing alveolitis. Am Rev Respir Dis 1987; 135:26–34.
209. O'Donnell K, Keogh B, Cantin A, Crystal RG. Pharmacologic suppression of the neutrophil component of the alveolitis in idiopathic pulmonary fibrosis. Am Rev Respir Dis 1987; 136:288–292.

210. Robinson PC, Watters LC, King TE, Mason RJ. Idiopathic pulmonary fibrosis: Abnormalities in bronchoalveolar lavage fluid phospholipids. Am Rev Respir Dis 1988; 137:585–591.

211. Hughes DA, Haslam PL. Changes in phosphatidylglycerol in bronchoalveolar lavage fluids from patients with cryptogenic fibrosing alveolitis. Chest 1989; 95:82–89.

212. Haslam PL, Hughes DA, Dewar A, Pantin CFA. Lipoprotein macroaggregates in bronchoalveolar lavage fluid from patients with diffuse interstitial lung disease: Comparison with idiopathic alveolar lipoproteinosis. Thorax 1988; 43:140–146.

213. Honda, Y, Tsunematsu K, Suzuki A, Akino T. Changes in phospholipids in bronchoalveolar lavage fluid of patients with interstitial lung diseases. Lung 1988; 166:293–301.

214. Hughes DA, Haslam PL. Phosphatidylglycerol levels in bronchoalveolar lavage fluid from patients with cryptogenic fibrosing alveolitis in relation to response to prednisolone. Am Rev Respir Dis 1987; 135:A30. Abstract.

215. Meier-Sydow J, Rust M, Kronenberger H, Thiel C, Amthor M, Riemann H. Long-term follow-up of lung function parameters in patients with idiopathic pulmonary fibrosis treated with prednisone and azathioprine or D-penicillamine. Prax Pneumol 1979; 33:680–688.

216. Turner-Warwick M. Bronchoalveolar lavage fluid cell counts in cryptogenic fibrosing alveolitis and their relation to therapy. Thorax 1980; 35:328–339.

217. Tukiainen P, Taskinen E, Holsti P, Korhola O, Valle M. Prognosis of cryptogenic fibrosing alveolitis. Thorax 1983; 38:349–355.

218. Parrillo JE, Fauci AS. Mechanisms of glucocorticoid action on immune processes. Ann Rev Pharmacol Toxicol 1979; 19:179–201.

219. Change S-W, King TE. Corticosteroids. In: Cherniack RM, ed. Drugs for the respiratory system. Orlando. Grune and Stratton, 1986; 77–138.

220. Keogh BA, Bernardo J, Hunninghake GW, Line BR, Price DL, Crystal RG. Effect of intermittent high dose parenteral corticosteroids on the alveolitis of idiopathic pulmonary fibrosis. Am Rev Respir Dis 1983; 127:18–22.

221. Weese WC, Levine BW, Kazemi H. Interstitial lung disease resistant to corticosteroid therapy: Report of three cases treated with azathioprine or cyclophosphamide. Chest 1975; 67:57–60.

222. Brown CH, Turner-Warwick M. The treatment of cryptogenic fibrosing alveolitis with immunosuppressant drugs. Q J Med 1971; 40:289–302.

223. Meuret G, Fueter R, Gloor F. Early stage of fulminant idiopathic pulmonary fibrosis cured by intense combination therapy using cyclophosphamide, vincristine, and prednisone. Respiration 1978; 36:228–233.

224. Cegla UH, Kroidl RF, Meier-Sydow J, Thiel C, Czamecki GV. Therapy of the idiopathic fibrosis of the lung: Experiences with three therapeutic principles: Corticosteroids in combination with azathioprine, D-penicillamine, and para-amino-benzoate. Pneumonologie 1975; 152:75–92.

225. Costabel U, Matthys H. Different therapies and factors influencing response to therapy in idiopathic diffuse fibrosing alveolitis. Respiration 1981; 42:141–149.

226. Johnson MA, Kwan S, Snell NJC, Nunn AJ, Darbyshire JH, Turner-Warwick M. Randomised controlled trial comparing prednisolone alone with cyclophosphamide and low dose prednisolone in combination in cryptogenic fibrosing alveolitis. Thorax 1989; 44:280–288.

227. Rennard SI, Bitterman PB, Ozaki T, Rom WN, Crystal RG. Colchicine suppresses the release of fibroblast growth factors from alveolar macrophages *in vitro*: The basis of a possible therapeutic approach to the fibrotic disorders. Am Rev Respir Dis 1988; 137:181–185.

228. Kennedy JI, Fulmer JD. Pulmonary hypertension in the interstitial lung diseases. Chest 1985; 87:558–560.

229. Lupi-Herrera E, Seoane M, Verdejo S, Gomez A, Sandoval J, Barrios R, Martinez W. Hemodynamic effect of hydralazine in interstitial lung disease patients with cor pulmonale: Immediate and short term evaluation at rest and during exercise. Chest 1985; 87:564–573.

230. Toronto Lung Transplant Group. Unilateral lung transplantation for pulmonary fibrosis. N Engl J Med 1986; 314:1140–1145.
231. Hakim M, Wallwork J. Heart-lung transplantation. Hosp Update 1985; 11:653–663.
232. BAL Cooperative Group. Bronchoalveolar lavage constituents in healthy individuals, idiopathic pulmonary fibrosis, and selected comparison groups. Am Rev Respir Dis 1990; 141: 5169–5202.

2

Pulmonary Complications in Collagen Vascular Disease

Robert A. Wise

The collagen vascular diseases are a group of diseases that are loosely connected by the presence of chronic inflammatory musculoskeletal involvement. Although these disorders are usually within the province of the rheumatologist, some patients with collagen vascular disease will present with primary lung manifestations. The purpose of this chapter is to review the spectrum of pulmonary involvement in this fascinating class of diseases. Several excellent reviews of pulmonary involvement in collagen diseases have appeared in the past.[1-6] This chapter will review the current state of knowledge regarding lung disease caused by systemic lupus erythematosus, rheumatoid arthritis, polymyositis-dermatomyositis, Sjögren's syndrome, ankylosing spondylitis, relapsing polychondritis, and mixed connective tissue disease.

SYSTEMIC LUPUS ERYTHEMATOSUS

General Features

Systemic lupus erythematosus (SLE) is one of the most common and polymorphic of the connective tissue diseases. It afflicts women ten times more frequently than men.[7] The disease usually begins during young adulthood, but approximately 15% of cases begin after age 50.[8-10] It is estimated that SLE has a prevalence of 50 cases per 100,000 population but is three times more prevalent in blacks than in whites.[11-15]

The survival rate among patients with SLE, once a dreaded disease, has improved dramatically in the 50 years since the introduction of corticosteroids. At Johns Hopkins, a series of 99 patients treated in the 1950s had a 62% 3-year survival rate. A series of 140 patients from the same hospital in 1975 showed a 94% 5-year survival.[16] Although the mortality from renal disease is decreasing, there appears to be an increased mortality from opportunistic infections.[17]

Criteria for the diagnosis of SLE have been proposed by the American Rheumatism Association.[18–20] These criteria are 96% sensitive and 96% specific when applied prospectively in a rheumatic disease clinic. Four or more of the following characteristics without other clear cause must be present during any period of observation.

1. Malar rash
2. Discoid rash
3. Photosensitivity
4. Oral ulcers
5. Arthritis
6. Serositis (pleuritis or pericarditis)
7. Renal disorder (persistent proteinuria or cellular urinary casts)
8. Neurologic disorder (seizures or psychosis)
9. Hematologic disorder (hemolytic anemia, leukopenia, lymphopenia, or thrombocytopenia)
10. Positive LE cell prep or Anti-DNA antibody or Anti-Sm antibody or false positive syphilis serology.
11. Antinuclear antibody

Antinuclear antibodies to mouse liver cells are present in 95% of patients with SLE.[21] Although most authorities would agree that SLE can occur in the absence of such antibodies, when they are absent the diagnosis should be considered tentative.[22] In some instances, subsequent tests will convert to a positive finding.[23] Other patients prove to have antibodies directed against cytoplasmic macromolecules such as Ro and La or against single-stranded DNA.[21,22,24]

The autoimmune etiology of SLE is well accepted, although the genesis of autoimmunity and the linkage between autoantibodies and disease expression still need to be better understood.[25,26] There is a clear genetic predisposition to the development of SLE. Ten percent of first-degree relatives and two-thirds of monozygotic twins of SLE patients will develop the disease.[27,28] SLE is associated with specific major histocompatibility locus (HLA) phenotypes, particularly HLA-DR3.[29] The presence of viral antibodies and virus-associated inclusion bodies in patients has led to the hypothesis that viral infection is involved in the pathogenesis of autoimmunity in SLE.[30–32] Ultraviolet light can exacerbate or induce SLE, possibly through the induction of cytokines.[28] More than 50 drugs have been implicated in the induction of an SLE syndrome in susceptible individuals. The most common drugs are anti-arrhythmic and antihypertensive drugs. Common agents include procainamide, quinidine, hydralazine, isoniazid, beta-adrenergic blockers, and diphenylhydantoin.[33–39] The drug-induced form of SLE usually spares the kidneys and central nervous system and predominantly manifests as a polyserositis involving the pleura, pericardium, peritoneum, and synovia.[40] Usually, drug-induced SLE occurs in individuals who acetylate the drugs slowly and are HLA-DR4 positive.[41] Drug-induced SLE probably has several different pathogenetic mechanisms, including modulation of suppressor lymphocytes or binding of complement, that prevent clearance of immune complexes.[42–44]

Thoracic Manifestations

Pulmonary involvement in SLE is common. Among reported thoracic complications of SLE are the following:

1. Pleurisy and pleural effusion
2. Shrinking lung syndrome
3. Diaphragmatic dysfunction
4. Acute lupus pneumonitis
5. Pulmonary vasculitis
6. Massive pulmonary hemorrhage
7. Pulmonary embolism
8. Interstitial pulmonary fibrosis
9. Bilateral hilar adenopathy
10. Pulmonary hypertension
11. Necrotizing pulmonary nodules
12. Pulmonary infection
13. Amyloidosis
14. Peripheral airway obstruction

Pleurisy

Clinically, pleurisy is present in 40% of patients.[7,11] One out of three SLE patients has pleurisy as a presenting sign of disease.[45] At autopsy, 35% to 100% of SLE patients show some evidence of pleural thickening, and 34% to 56% have active pleural effusions.[46–48] Immunoglobulin and complement have been found adherent to pleural mesothelial cells, and immune complexes have been found in the walls of parietal pleural capillaries in SLE patients, suggesting that the pleuritis is immune mediated.[49–51] Some pathologic studies, however, have attributed the majority of postmortem pleural effusions to terminal complicating conditions such as heart failure, infection, or uremia.[48] The distinction between pleural effusion from SLE and that due to other causes may be difficult. Distinguishing characteristics are that the pleurisy of SLE is often painful, whereas that of uremia and heart failure is painless.[52] In half the cases, the effusion is bilateral, and it may alternate from side to side. When the effusion is unilateral, however, it is most commonly on the left side, which can be a sign of pericardial involvement.[45,53] Effusions from SLE are usually small, and although large effusions have been reported, the presence of a large effusion requires that other causes be ruled out by appropriate diagnostic studies. In particular, it may be difficult to distinguish SLE pleural effusions from those caused by pulmonary thromboembolism.

The pleural fluid in an SLE effusion is exudative with a high protein concentration and a normal glucose concentration. LE cells, which are phagocytes that have ingested complexes of immunoglobulin and nucleoproteins, may be present in the pleural fluid, usually (but not always) in conjunction with LE cells in the peripheral blood.[54,55] Total hemolytic complement, C3, and C4 are often reduced in the pleural fluid. Because pleural fluid complement is reduced out of proportion to serum complement and immune complexes may be found in the pleural fluid in concentrations greater than in the serum,[51,56] it is believed that there is local immune activation within the pleural space.

Shrinking Lung Syndrome

One of the most interesting and controversial pulmonary manifestations of SLE is the "shrinking lung syndrome."[57-60] This clinical syndrome presents with dyspnea associated with a restrictive ventilatory defect but with small, clear lungs on the chest radiograph. Initially this syndrome was attributed to diffuse microatelectasis of the lung[57] or to pleural adhesions that prevented diaphragmatic descent.[61] There is little reason to believe, however, that small degrees of pleural fibrosis would have any significant effect on lung function, since conditions such as asbestos-related pleural thickening and therapeutic pleuridesis do not ordinarily have major effects on diaphragm function. In recent years, however, there has been mounting evidence that this disorder is a consequence of diaphragmatic dysfunction. From a sample of 33 subjects, Gibson studied 5 patients with SLE and small lung volumes and found evidence of marked reductions of maximum transdiaphragmatic pressure in 4.[62] Martens tested 26 consecutive SLE patients and found diaphragm weakness in 7.[63] Wilcox confirmed these findings in a series of 30 patients with SLE, among whom 9 had inspiratory muscle weakness. Phrenic nerve function appeared normal on direct nerve stimulation and no associated peripheral neuropathy or myopathy could be detected.[64] Steroid-induced myopathy, which can affect respiratory muscle strength, does not appear to be a common etiologic factor.[65] In some instances, diaphragm dysfunction can be elicited in dyspneic patients without significant reductions in lung volume.[66]

Although neuropathy and myopathy can occur in SLE, the diaphragmatic dysfunction seems to be unrelated to these disorders and improves or remains stable over time without specific treatment.[63,67,68] One theory holds that the mechanism for diaphragm dysfunction is neural reflex inhibition of diaphragm contraction as a consequence of the active pleuritis such as occurs after upper abdominal surgery.[69,70] One case report of SLE with diaphragm weakness has shown a dramatic improvement in lung function after treatment with beta-adrenergic drugs, suggesting that the diaphragm weakness may respond to pharmacologic agents.[71,72]

Although transdiaphragmatic pressure measurements are necessary for confirmation of diaphragm dysfunction in SLE, diaphragm weakness may be suspected by the finding of a 25% or greater reduction in vital capacity when the patient is recumbent, associated with a reduction in maximum inspiratory mouth pressure, two simple screening tests.[73]

Acute Lupus Pneumonitis

Acute lupus pneumonitis is an uncommon but dramatic complication of SLE. Often occurring during a generalized exacerbation of the disease, it represents a syndrome of diffuse lung injury similar to adult respiratory distress syndrome from other causes.[74-76] The syndrome consists of fever, dyspnea, hypoxemia that is unresponsive to high concentrations of inspired oxygen, and diffuse pulmonary infiltrates. Acute lupus pneumonitis can occur as the presenting syndrome of SLE.[77] Pathologic studies show diffuse nonspecific alveolar damage with interstitial and intra-alveolar edema, hyaline membranes, pulmonary hemorrhage, and polymorphonuclear or mononuclear cell infiltrates in the interstitium. Capillary deposition of immunoglobulins, immune complexes, and complement may be found in some, but not all cases, which suggests that local immune activation is sometimes a factor in the diffuse alveolar damage.[47,78-81] Small vessels may be involved with fibrin thrombi and infiltration by necrotic neutrophils.[82] Although some authors have emphasized the pulmonary hemorrhage found post mortem in this disorder, massive hemoptysis is usually not a prominent clinical component but can occur in severe, life-threatening cases.[83-87]

It is often difficult to distinguish acute lupus pneumonitis, a primary disorder, from infections that may induce or exaggerate lung injury. Opportunistic infections such as cytomegalovirus, *Legionella, Pneumocystis carinii,* and *Candida* pneumonia all have been reported to manifest as syndromes resembling acute lupus pneumonitis.[17,75,88,89] Differentiation may require bronchoalveolar lavage (BAL) or lung biopsy. In one series, only 3 out of 15 opportunistic lung infections in SLE patients was diagnosed prior to autopsy.[17] In cases where pulmonary hemorrhage is prominent, the syndrome may resemble Goodpasture's syndrome. A renal biopsy that fails to show either linear immunoglobulin deposition or anti-glomerular basement membrane antibodies and a compatible clinical syndrome are needed to establish the diagnosis of acute lupus pneumonitis.

Specific treatment is unknown, but large doses of corticosteroids or cytotoxic agents are used with some reported successes. The mortality of acute lupus pneumonitis is about 50%.[74,90,91]

Interstitial Pulmonary Fibrosis
Restrictive ventilatory defects associated with comparable reductions in carbon monoxide diffusing capacity and lung compliance are common in SLE but tend to be nonprogressive. It remains to be determined how often these defects are related to respiratory muscle dysfunction, interstitial lung disease, or the residua of acute lupus pneumonitis.[67,92-94]

Interstitial pulmonary fibrosis is common in other connective tissue diseases, such as rheumatoid arthritis, systemic sclerosis and dermatomyositis, but is much less prevalent in SLE. Autopsy series show evidence of interstitial fibrosis in about one in five SLE patients, but it is usually localized and is not an important clinical feature.[47,57] Haupt found a 4% prevalence of diffuse interstitial fibrosis in 120 autopsied patients, and Eisenberg collected 18 clinically documented cases.[48,95] However, when diffuse pulmonary fibrosis is present in a patient with SLE, one should question whether an overlap syndrome or other connective tissue disease is present.

Pulmonary Vascular Disease
A microangiitis involving the small vessels of the lung occurs in the setting of acute lupus pneumonitis and has been associated with fatal massive hemoptysis.[82] In some rare cases, particularly those that show some features of systemic sclerosis, plexiform lesions of the pulmonary vessels indistinguishable from primary pulmonary hypertension may occur.[96,97] In other cases, vasculitis has been demonstrated.[98] Simonson and colleagues studied 36 SLE patients using echo Doppler estimates of pulmonary artery pressure.[99] They found that 14% had elevated pulmonary artery pressures, defined as a

systolic pressure greater than 30 mm Hg.[99] None of the subjects had severe pulmonary hypertension, but there was an association of higher pulmonary artery pressures with Raynaud's phenomenon, which raises the question of a generalized vasospastic disorder.[100] In a collection of 46 case reports from the literature, it was found that three-quarters of the patients with severe pulmonary hypertension had Raynaud's phenomenon compared with 10% to 15% of SLE patients in general.[97] The presence of Raynaud's phenomenon in SLE patients with pulmonary hypertension may be prognostic of a beneficial response to pulmonary vasodilators.[101]

Pulmonary thromboembolism, as well as thrombotic events in the cerebral and coronary vessels, occurs with increased frequency in patients with SLE.[102,103] In some cases, this can lead to pulmonary hypertension and cor pulmonale.[104] In particular, this occurs in the group of patients who have anti-phospholipid antibodies that cross-react with blood coagulation factors. This syndrome is associated with anti-cardiolipin antibodies, lupus anti-coagulant, biologic false positive serologic tests for syphilis, acquired Protein C or Protein S deficiency, and thrombocytopenia. Following a thrombotic event, the levels of anti-phospholipid antibodies may transiently decline and therefore testing may need to be repeated at a future time.[105–109]

Other Pleuropulmonary Complications of SLE

A few cases of peripheral airway obstruction resembling bronchiolitis obliterans have been reported to occur in SLE. In some cases it is reversible with corticosteroid treatment.[110–112]

Cavitating pulmonary nodules similar to those that occur in rheumatoid arthritis have been reported to occur in SLE.[113] In most cases, however, cavitating nodules are the result of infection or pulmonary infarction.[114] Amyloidosis of the lung has been reported as a rare complication of SLE.[115,116] Hilar adenopathy that is radiographically indistinguishable from that of sarcoidosis can be present in SLE.[117,118]

RHEUMATOID ARTHRITIS

General Features

Rheumatoid arthritis (RA) is a systemic disease with prominent symmetric deforming inflammatory arthritis of the small joints. The 1987 Revised American Rheumatism Association criteria for a diagnosis of rheumatoid arthritis include the presence of four or more of the following criteria.[119]

1. Morning stiffness for 1 hour or more for 6 weeks or more
2. Swelling of three or more joints for 6 weeks or more
3. Swelling of wrist, metacarpophalangeal, or proximal interphalangeal joints for 6 or more weeks.
4. Symmetric joint swelling
5. Hand radiographic changes of joint erosions or decalcification
6. Rheumatoid nodules
7. Serum rheumatoid factor

Three out of four patients have extra-articular involvement that includes vasculitis, skin ulcers, lymphadenopathy, splenomegaly, neuropathy, episcleritis, pericarditis, or pulmonary involvement.[120,121] Rheumatoid arthritis occurs in women two to three times more commonly than in men, but the extra-articular manifestations are more severe in men.[120–123]

The pathogenesis of rheumatoid arthritis appears to involve both cell-mediated and humoral immune mechanisms. Many experts believe that joint destruction is mainly a result of lymphocyte- and macrophage-dependent reactions to synovial antigens.[124,125] Rheumatoid arthritis patients demonstrate cell-mediated immunity to collagen and collagen subunits.[126] The extra-articular reactions, and particularly the pleural reactions, are mediated by humoral immune mechanisms, as evidenced by their association with high levels of IgM rheumatoid factor and local deposition of immunoglobulins and immune complexes.[142]

The prevalence of thoracic complications of rheumatoid arthritis varies widely depending upon the definitions used, the selection of the study population, and the thoroughness of the evaluation.[92,127–129] Radiographic surveys find interstitial or pleural changes in 5% to 50% of patients with rheumatoid disease.[130–136] The major thoracic complications of rheumatoid arthritis are diffuse interstitial fibrosis, chronic airflow limitation, rheumatoid (necrobiotic) nodules in the lung, pleural effusion, and upper airway obstruction.[137]

Thoracic Manifestations of Rheumatoid Arthritis

Diffuse Interstitial Fibrosis

Although some early studies questioned whether rheumatoid arthritis was associated with an increased incidence of interstitial pulmonary fibrosis, more recent studies leave little doubt that interstitial inflammation and fibrosis are seen more often in association with rheumatoid disease than in a normal population.[128,138,139] Physiological and radiographic surveys of unselected samples of rheumatoid arthritis patients show that 1 in 6 have evidence of interstitial lung disease.[134] Open lung biopsies done on unselected volunteers with rheumatoid arthritis show histologic evidence of interstitial inflammation and fibrosis in 60%.[140]

Histopathologic changes in diffuse interstitial lung disease associated with rheumatoid arthritis are indistinguishable from those seen in the idiopathic variety. There is a mixed inflammatory interstitial infiltrate of lymphocytes, plasma cells, and macrophages. As the disease advances, fibrosis becomes more prominent.[141–143] Yousem and colleagues studied 40 open lung biopsies obtained for clinical evaluation and classified the interstitial processes to include usual interstitial pneumonia with fibrosis (UIP); bronchiolitis obliterans with organizing pneumonia (BOOP); lymphoid hyperplasia; and cellular interstitial pneumonia without fibrosis. Biopsy specimens often showed a mixed pattern but patients with more fibrosis had a worse prognosis.[143] Several patients have been reported with rheumatoid arthritis and eosinophilic interstitial pneumonia, but the relationship between these entities is not clear.[143–145] Immunofluorescent studies show deposition of rheumatoid factor immunoglobulin in alveolar walls and blood vessels but absence of complement deposition, so antibody-mediated reactions are of uncertain importance.[142] Many recent studies of bronchoalveolar lavage fluid in rheumatoid arthritis patients with active disease have shown elevated levels of angiotensin converting enzyme,[146] histamine, neutrophils, eosinophils,[147] fibrin degradation products,[148] activated alveolar macrophages producing neutrophil chemotactic factors and fibronectin,[149,150] Increased numbers of OKT4+ helper T-lymphocytes,[151] immunoreactive neutrophil elastase,[149] and biochemically active neutrophil collagenase. These findings suggest that the pathogenesis of fibrosis in rheumatoid arthritis is similar to the pathogenesis of UIP, where activation of alveolar macrophages induces neutrophilic infiltration into the interstitium of the lung and production of fibroblast growth factors.[153,154] The role of the lymphocyte in the development of interstitial fibrosis is not clear.[154] Some studies show increased numbers of BAL lymphocytes in patients with rheumatoid arthritis and interstitial lung disease,[155] while others do not.[150,156] Because alveolar macrophages produce cytokines that suppress lymphocyte production, some have postulated that the primary function of these cells is to modulate immune reactions in the lung, preventing lung injury.[157,158] Alveolar macrophages from rheumatoid arthritis patients with active disease are not as effective as normal alveolar macrophages in suppressing lymphocyte proliferation, which may promote chronic inflammatory responses in the lung or make rheumatoid arthritis patients prone to develop antibody responses to inhaled antigens.[159]

Interstitial lung disease is more common in male patients who smoke, who are older than 60 years, who have other extra-articular manifestations with higher levels of rheumatoid factor, and lower levels of complement, and who are HLA type B8, DR4, and Dw3 positive.[135,160–164] One study showed that alpha-1-antitrypsin variant phenotypes are predictive of development of interstitial fibrosis in rheumatoid arthritis patients. Only 1 of 30 patients with the normal M1–M1 phenotype developed interstitial lung disease, whereas 13 of 32 with variant phenotypes developed interstitial fibrosis.[165]

The prognosis for patients with diffuse interstitial fibrosis is poor. Typical cor pulmonale and digital clubbing occur in the late stages of the disease.[166] In one series, 3 of 5 biopsied patients died of lung disease within 13 months[143]; in another series, the 5-year survival rate was only 39% among patients with rheumatoid arthritis who were hospitalized for interstitial lung disease.[167]

Rheumatoid and Drug-Induced Interstitial Lung Disease. Distinguishing drug-induced interstitial lung disease from rheumatoid interstitial lung disease presents a difficult clinical problem. Many of the patients who develop pulmonary interstitial disease have severe active disease and are treated with gold salts, penicillamine, or methotrexate. All of these agents have been associated with the development of rapidly progressive pulmonary fibrosis, but the etiologic relationship is difficult to determine in many cases.[168–177] The diagnosis is usually based on the rapidity of onset and reversal of the disease with discontinuation of the therapy. In hypersensitivity reactions to gold salts, lymphocytes and a reversed helper/suppressor T-cell ratio may be present in some but not all cases. The mechanism of gold lung toxicity is thought to be either the binding of gold salts to collagen, which stimulates a delayed hypersensitivity reaction, or direct stimulation of collagen synthesis.[143,178] Two specific HLA phenotypes have been reported to occur in 93% of rheumatoid arthritis patients who develop pulmonary gold toxicity, suggesting a genetic basis for this process.[179]

Pulmonary gold toxicity is uncommon compared with toxicity related to penicillamine or methotrexate. One series of 110 patients followed prospectively with pulmonary function testing while on gold therapy failed to show any adverse effect on lung function.[180] In another series of 89 patients followed clinically while on gold therapy none of the subjects developed pulmonary toxicity.[181] In contrast, 3% of 133 patients treated with penicillamine[181] and 5% of 168 patients receiving methotrexate developed pulmonary toxicity.[172]

The primary treatment for drug-induced pulmonary toxicity is, of course, withdrawal of the offending agent. Corticosteroids have been used commonly, but their beneficial effect has yet to be determined.

Rheumatoid Nodules

Subcutaneous necrobiotic or rheumatoid nodules develop on the extensor surfaces of the joints in many rheumatoid arthritis patients with high titers of rheumatoid factor, who tend to develop extra-articular disease.[182] Histologically, the nodules have a necrotic center surrounded by palisades of epithelioid cells with an outer rim of fibroblasts and mononuclear inflammatory cells. The nodules vary in size from microscopic to several inches in diameter and may involve the serous membranes of many internal organs, including the dura and peritoneum.[143,183,184] Multiple small rheumatoid nodules can occur in the lung and can be indistinguishable from other reticulonodular interstitial diseases leading to respiratory failure.[191] At times, typical rheumatoid nodules in the lung may precede the development of the articular manifestations of rheumatoid arthritis.[184–186]

A radiographic survey of 309 rheumatoid arthritis patients found only one person with rheumatoid nodules.[135] When found in the lung in biopsy specimens, they are the only specific histologic finding for rheumatoid disease, but they have been reported to occur in other disorders and can be difficult to distinguish from necrotizing granulomas in some cases.[143,187–191] When solitary, they may be confused with malignant tumors radiographically.[192] Rheumatoid nodules can occur in endobronchial locations and must be distinguished by biopsy from carcinoma.[193] Several case reports of bronchogenic carcinoma in proximity to rheumatoid nodules suggest that they may be the focus for scar carcinoma in some cases.[194–196] Because needle biopsy may be misleading in these cases, radiographic observation or open biopsy is indicated.[197,198] Computed tomography may be helpful in the diagnosis when the nodules are located characteristically in the subpleural surface of the lower lung zones and are present in clusters.[185,199,200]

Nodules may cavitate and, if present in the upper lung zones, can mimic tuberculosis.[201,202] Other cases of cavitary fibroapical disease resemble the lesions found in ankylosing spondylitis without evidence of typical necrobiotic nodules.[203–206] Bacterial, mycobacterial, or fungal infections can occasionally infect a cavitating necrobiotic nodule.[207–210] Cavitation of a subpleural nodule can cause spontaneous pneumothorax.[211]

Caplan's syndrome was first described as the development of nodules, either single or multiple, in the lungs of Welsh coal miners with rheumatoid arthritis.[212] The lesions are histologically similar to necrobiotic nodules except that they have an abundance of dust-containing macrophages.[213,214] Similar lesions may occur in rheumatoid arthritis patients in other dust-exposed occupations.[214–221] Frequently background pneumoconiosis is absent or trivial. Most authorities believe that the nodules represent a nonspecific immunologic response to inhaled dust particles in this susceptible population.[222]

Pleural Effusion

Pleural effusion is common in rheumatoid arthritis, occurring in about 3% of clinical series.[223–226] The effusion is usually unilateral, but a few cases of bilateral effusions have been recorded.[223] Pleural effusion may occur at any time during the course of disease but usually occurs after many years of active disease. Like other extra-articular manifestations, it is more common in men than in women.[137,223,227,228] Specific HLA subtypes HLA-B8 and Dw3 are more common in patients with pleural effusions.[229]

The pleural fluid is a xanthochromic exudate with high protein and LDH contents.[226] Of particular note, three-quarters of the specimens have low levels of glucose and low pH, similar to an infectious or malignant process.[230–232] Because the pleural fluid glucose concentration does not rise with intravenous infusion of glucose, in contrast to tuberculous effusions, it has been suggested that the pleural surface has a selective block to glucose filtration. It seems unlikely, however, that the filtration characteristics of the pleural membrane could develop a greater concentration gradient for glucose than for larger protein molecules. Because one can follow the development of low pleural fluid glucose and high acid content over nearly a week, it seems more likely that the pleural space is the site of increased glucose metabolism.[233] The pleural fluid has levels of rheumatoid factor, anti-immunoglobulin IgM, that are comparable to serum levels, which is a nonspecific finding.[234,235] Occasionally, however, the fluid has low levels of complement and positive assays for immune complex-like material, raising the possibility of local humoral immune activation in these cases.[232,236] Cholesterol levels above 1000 mg/dl were present in four out of seven samples studied by Lillington, but this is a nonspecific finding in chronic effusions.[226,237] A case of chylous effusion associated with amyloidosis has been reported, but this is a rare complication.[238]

The cell counts in rheumatoid pleural effusions usually are predominately lymphocytic, but polymorphonuclear leukocytes and even frank pus can be found in the absence of bacterial infection.[232,239,240] One characteristic cell, a "rheumatoid cell" resembling those found in joint fluid, can be found in pleural fluid. This cell, a lipid-laden polymorphonuclear leukocyte, can be experimentally induced by antigen-antibody complex formation or nonspecific irritants in animals, and it may lack specificity.[241–244] Cytologic specimens show a characteristic amorphous granular debris adjacent to multinucleated giant cells.[239,240,245,246]

At thoracoscopy, the pleural surface has a typical granular appearance, studded with 0.5-mm nodules confined to the parietal pleura. Histologically, the nodules contain pseudostratified epithelial cells overlying a fibrous stroma that contains multinucleated giant cells. The visceral pleura typically shows only nonspecific inflammatory changes.[247,248] This has been described as an opened rheumatoid nodule and can involve the pericardium as well as the pleura.[225,249] Needle biopsy shows nonspecific inflammation and fibrosis, and is helpful only insofar as it can exclude tuberculous or malignant diseases, which have similar biochemical constituents.[247]

The effusions may remain chronically for months or years but usually resolve spontaneously without specific therapy. In rare cases the effusions may become large enough to require surgical decortication.[223,250] Infected as well as sterile empyemas may occur, requiring placement of chest tube drainage. Jones and Blodgett reported that 5 of 10 patients with rheumatoid effusions followed for 5 years developed empyema.[251]

Obstructive Airways Disease

Rheumatoid disease can involve the airways in the form of bronchiolitis obliterans with interstitial pneumonia (BIP), bronchiolitis obliterans with organizing pneumonia (BOOP), follicular bronchiolitis, or nonspecific chronic airflow limitation.

Bronchiolitis obliterans typically presents as rapidly progressive airflow obstruction in HLA-DR4–positive patients with severe nodular deforming disease.[112,145,204,252–260] It is associated with diffuse nodular or reticulonodular infiltrates on the chest radiograph and usually, but not always, with airflow obstruction on forced expiratory spirometry and elevated residual volume. Lung biopsy discloses mixed plasma cell and mononuclear inflammatory cell infiltration around bronchioles, which progresses to fibrosis and obliteration of the airways.[261] Immunochemical studies have shown linear deposition of IgG on alveolar walls, suggesting an immune etiology.[255] Most of the patients have Sjögren's syndrome if it is sought, and it has been suggested that the peribronchial lymphocytic infiltration is a manifestation of that disease.[254]

Bronchiolitis obliterans has been reported to occur in patients on penicillamine or gold therapy, but the causal relationship is difficult to prove.[262–266] In one series, not one of 89 patients taking gold, nor any of 380 patients taking neither gold nor penicillamine, developed respiratory complications, whereas 4 of 89 patients on penicillamine developed severe respiratory disease, including 2 cases of bronchiolitis obliterans.[267] In other large series of patients treated with penicillamine or gold, however, no significant pulmonary toxicity has been reported.[180,268] Cyclophosphamide and corticosteroids have been reported as successful therapy in selected cases.[269]

Bronchiolitis with organizing pneumonia is an increasingly frequently recognized disorder that shows radiographic evidence of localized pulmonary infiltration that is often responsive to corticosteroids.[143] The histopathology shows tongues of exudative granulation tissue that extend from the bronchioles into the alveolar duct regions in a patchy distribution. There may be fibrinous alveolar exudate in the regions of consolidation. In one series of seven patients with rheumatoid arthritis and BOOP, two had evidence of eosinophilic pneumonia,[143] an association also noted by others.[145]

Follicular bronchiolitis is an uncommon disease characterized by lymphoid hyperplasia with germinal centers surrounding the peripheral airways. The chest radiograph shows a fine reticulonodular pattern. Follicular bronchiolitis may occur in association with connective tissue diseases other than rheumatoid arthritis.[270,271]

Some authors have suggested that nonspecific chronic obstructive pulmonary disease is more prevalent in smokers with rheumatoid arthritis than in the general smoking population. Characteristics that distinguish those rheumatoid arthritis patients who develop airflow obstruction include Sjögren's syndrome, heterozygous alpha-1-antitrypsin phenotype (MS), and HLA phenotype DR4 and DQw1/DQw3 heterozygotes.[272–277]

Cricoarytenoid Arthritis

Rheumatoid arthritis affects predominantly the small joints of the hands and feet. A well-described complication of rheumatoid arthritis is the involvement of the small joints of the larynx, specifically the cricoarytenoid joints. The prevalence of this abnormality varies with the method of identifying the lesion: up to 88% in autopsy series[278] and as low as 26% in series based on physical examination alone.[279] CT scanning studies have shown abnormalities of the larynx in 54%.[280] In some circumstances, this lesion may lead to severe upper airway obstruction with stridor and require tracheostomy or lead to death.[281–284]

Upper airway obstruction may result from rheumatoid nodules developing on the vocal cords and from laryngeal nerve neuropathy attributed to vasculitis of the vasa nervorum.[285]

Other Pulmonary Complications of Rheumatoid Arthritis

Pulmonary hemosiderosis in association with rheumatoid arthritis has been reported in four cases but is a rare complication.[286,287]

Peripheral arteritis is a common complication of rheumatoid arthritis but arteritis of the pulmonary vessels with severe pulmonary hypertension is quite rare.[288–294] The characteristic histology shows fibrous intimal hyperplasia of the small vessels with mononuclear infiltration of the adventitia and disruption of the elastic lamina. Plexiform lesions are usually absent but have been demonstrated in one case.[294] Many of the earlier case reports may represent examples of what is now called mixed connective tissue disease or undifferentiated connective tissue disease.

SYSTEMIC SCLEROSIS

Clinical Characteristics

Reportedly, systemic sclerosis (SSc) was first described by Hippocrates (*History of Epidemics,* Book 5, Case 9), who described a patient who developed typical skin changes and cor pulmonale.[295] The most prominent clinical characteristic is inflammation and fibrosis of the skin and internal organs. Associated with this is a vasospastic tendency, which most commonly appears as Raynaud's phenomenon but which may also affect internal organs. The American Rheumatism Association criteria for the diagnosis of SSc include as the major criterion scleroderma proximal to the metacarpalphalangeal joints and as minor criteria sclerodactyly, digital pitting scars, and bibasilar pulmonary fibrosis. The conjunction of one major or two minor criteria was 97% sensitive and 98% specific in differentiating SSc from other connective tissue disorders.[296] CREST syndrome (*C*alcinosis, *R*aynaud's, *E*sophageal dysmotility, *S*clerodactyly, and *T*elangectasia) is a variant of SSc that is considered to be more benign.

The clinical features of SSc in one typical series as are follows: Raynaud's phenomenon in 98%, esophageal dysmotility in 72%, telangectasia in 83%, musculoskeletal involvement with myositis or arthritis in 17%, renal involvement in 11%, and cardiac involvement in 9% of cases. Clinically evident pulmonary disease is present in 68% of patients.[297]

SSc is an uncommon but not a rare disease, with a reported incidence of 6.3 to 18.7 new cases per million population per year.[298] The prevalence of the disease is estimated to be about 126 cases per million population,[299,300] although one recent population survey finds the prevalence to be as much as 20 times greater.[301] The disease affects women three times more frequently than men, with a peak age of onset in the fifth and sixth decades.[302] The cumulative mortality is about 33% during the first 5 years.[303]

The pathogenesis of SSc is not known, but theories have centered around two major hypotheses: primary vascular endothelial injury and autoimmune inflammatory reactions.[304–308] Recently Claman has proposed a unifying hypothesis that postulates an interaction of mast cells with endothelial cells and fibroblasts that is stimulated by T-lymphocytes, macrophages, and platelets and is mediated by heparin and heparin-binding growth factors.[309]

Thoracic Manifestations of Systemic Sclerosis

Recently, several excellent comprehensive reviews of the pleuropulmonary complications of SSc have appeared.[310–312] Early descriptions of SSc noted respiratory symptoms as a prominent feature of the advanced disease. It was considered that this was the result of thickening of the skin of the thoracic wall.[313] Studies showing normal compliance of the chest wall make this an unlikely cause of lung disease, although it may contribute to respiratory symptoms in some rare cases.[314–316] It is now generally recognized that the major pulmonary complications of SSc are interstitial pulmonary fibrosis and pulmonary hypertension.

Interstitial Pulmonary Fibrosis

At the time of diagnosis, chest radiographic evidence of interstitial fibrosis is present in about 20% of SSc cases.[317,318] In a collection of cross-sectional studies, 36% of 1620 cases showed radiographic pulmonary fibrosis.[311] In contrast, only about 1 in 5 patients with CREST syndrome have radiographic evidence of pulmonary interstitial fibrosis, leading some authors to speculate that this is a more benign form of the disease.[311] CREST patients who demonstrate the anticentromere autoantibody have less interstitial lung disease.[319,320] Patients with anti-Scl-70 antibodies are more likely to have both diffuse skin involvement and interstitial disease.[364] The chest radiograph typically shows bilateral lower lobe reticular infiltration, which can progress to cystic "honeycomb" lesions. In a few reported cases, pulmonary fibrosis can precede other manifestations of SSc.[321] Even in patients who have normal chest radiographs, however, thin section computed tomography demonstrates fibrosis in 44% of SSc patients. The earliest changes are increased radiodensity in the subpleural regions of the lower lobes.[322,323] SSc is more common in miners exposed to silica dust, which may present a problem in differentiating it from pneumoconiosis.[324] Acute syndromes resembling SSc with diffuse pulmonary infiltration may also occur after exposure to vinyl chloride, benzene, toluene, epoxy resins, adulterated cooking oils, silicon or paraffin breast augmentation, and cancer chemotherapy agents.[325–328]

Although traditionally SSc fibrosis of the lung was considered to be a noninflammatory process of increased collagen deposition, many studies of lung histology and BAL fluid have shown a prominent inflammatory component. Lavage effluent in SSc patients contains increased numbers of neutrophils, eosinophils, and, in some studies, lymphocytes.[322,329–336] Gallium scans are also positive in the majority of patients with interstitial lung disease, indicating alveolar inflammation, although some patients demonstrate normal scans in conjunction with alveolitis identified on lavage.[329,330,333,334,337] Gallium uptake by the lung is prominent in patients with Sjögren's syndrome who have lymphocytic inflammation in the lung periphery.[330]

Patients with persistent alveolitis and the greatest intensity of neutrophilic alveolitis tend to show the greatest abnormalities of carbon monoxide diffusing capacity.[312,332,333,338] In contrast, high lymphocyte counts on BAL tend to be associated with Sjögren's syndrome and an overall favorable prognosis[339,340] despite more pulmonary fibrosis on the chest radiograph and more restriction of vital capacity.[341] Alveolar macrophages like those found in idiopathic pulmonary fibrosis are activated, spontaneously releasing fibronectin and growth factors.[334,337]

The pathogenesis of pulmonary fibrosis in SSc has some parallels with idiopathic pulmonary fibrosis, including increased rate of collagen production, increased amounts of intracellular protocollagen, and increased numbers of fibroblasts.[312] The activated alveolar macrophages produce fibronectin as well as alveolar macrophage–derived growth factor (AMDGF) and possibly other substances that stimulate fibroblasts, such as interleukin-1 and transforming growth factor beta. Activated alveolar macrophages may also play a central role in the pathogenesis of SSc lung fibrosis by producing neutrophil chemotactic factors that can lead to lung damage through neutrophilic oxygen radical production or release of proteolytic enzymes. Evidence supporting immune activation of the alveolar macrophage includes the presence of immune complexes in BAL fluid in concentrations higher than in serum, serum antibodies to type I and type IV collagen, and elevated levels of BAL IgG, which are all associated with increased pulmonary fibrosis.[332,342,343]

Histologic evaluation of the lung in SSc has mainly been from autopsy series, which have emphasized the end-stage fibrosis with bronchiectasis and subpleural cysts. Alveolar septae are edematous and hypercellular in the early stages, progressing to lesions with hypocellularity, fibrosis, and hyalinization of the alveolar walls. Capillaries are reduced in number in regions of fibrosis, which are often patchy.[344–346] Arterioles show intimal proliferation of endothelial cells and either medial hypertrophy or myxomatous degeneration. The arteriolar changes are, however, not proximately related to the fibrotic changes and reflect a primary vasculopathy.[347]

Pulmonary function tests commonly show a restrictive ventilatory defect with reductions in lung volumes or an isolated defect in carbon monoxide diffusing capacity (DLCO).[314,320,337,348–360] In contrast to patients with idiopathic interstitial fibrosis, however, patients with SSc and interstitial fibrosis often have elevations of residual volume, a finding that has been attributed to small airway dysfunction from peribronchial fibrosis.[92,351,360] In one controlled study, though, other tests of small airway function were normal in nonsmoking SSc patients.[361] Nonetheless, frank airflow obstruction occurs in 17% of 287 patients reported in the literature and is not more prevalent among smokers with SSc.[311] The presence of airflow obstruction is associated with a poor prognosis. In one study, Peters-Golden found the case fatality rate was 100% for patients with combined airflow obstruction and a DLCO less than 70% of predicted.[353] A DLCO less than 40% of predicted is highly correlated with the development of pulmonary arterial hypertension and portends a 90% 5-year mortality.[353,362]

Longitudinal studies of lung function in SSc have found remarkable stability over long periods, suggesting that the disease process causes lung damage over a short period early in the course of disease.[349,356,358,363] Many patients, particularly those with isolated defects in DLCO, actually show improvement in lung function over time even in the absence of specific treatment, which makes evaluation of uncontrolled treatment regimens difficult.[354] Male patients with severe Raynaud's phenomenon who have digital ulceration or pitting tend to show the greatest declines in lung function over time.[354,364] The effect of smoking status is controversial. One study shows greater declines in nonsmokers,[358] another study shows greater declines in former smokers only,[354] and a third study shows greater declines in active smokers.[358] The role of gastroesophageal reflux with recurrent aspiration in the production of interstitial lung disease is not clear. Although it certainly is not the major cause of pulmonary fibrosis,[365] as some early clinicians thought, food particles are often found in the lung at autopsy,[311] and impairment of D$_L$CO is correlated with severity of acid reflux recorded by pH monitoring.[366]

Pulmonary Hypertension

Pulmonary hypertension occurs in 25% to 50% of patients with SSc depending upon the diagnostic methodology.[315,362,367] Among patients with CREST syndrome, about two-thirds will show pulmonary hypertension.[311] Though not all authors agree that CREST patients more frequently have pulmonary hypertension, when it does occur, in patients with CREST it is frequently not associated with pulmonary fibrosis.[358] The pathology of the pulmonary vessels resembles that of the peripheral arterioles: intimal proliferation, medial hypertrophy, and perivascular fibrosis, particularly in patients with the CREST syndrome and limited skin involvement.[344,347,368–371] Plexiform lesions and fibrinoid necrosis, which are seen in primary pulmonary hypertension, are uncommon even in cases of severe fatal pulmonary hypertension.[347,371] Occasionally multiple pulmonary emboli may lead to pulmonary hypertension.[372]

The cause of pulmonary hypertension in SSc is not known. Some authorities have implicated diffuse endothelial injury leading to fixed vascular disease, while others have stressed the primary vasoreactivity leading to fixed vascular defects. Diffuse endothelial injury appears to be an initial lesion in the development of toxic pulmonary hypertension[373] and has been postulated to be an early event in the development of SSc.[306,374–376]

Some authors have proposed that the pulmonary hypertension that occurs in SSc is similar to Raynaud's phenomenon of the lung, an increase in cold vasoreactivity. Cannon found that two-thirds of scleroderma deaths occurred in the winter months while Peters-Golden found that three-quarters of SSc deaths occurred during the cold months, compared with an expected mortality of 52%.[354,377] Naslund reported a striking case of a patient with cold-induced pulmonary hypertension.[378] Furst found that 5 of 9 SSc patients with very early disease developed reduced pulmonary blood flow on Krypton lung scans during hand immersion in ice water.[379] Several series, however, have not been able to demonstrate evidence of pulmonary hypertension induced by acute cold exposure in SSc patients.[380–384] The weight of evidence therefore suggests that most patients with SSc do not have active pulmonary vasoreactivity, but that such a state exists transiently in some patients, perhaps during the early phases of the disorder.

Carcinoma

Many case reports of association of SSc with carcinoma of the lung suggest an increased prevalence, similar to that seen with interstitial fibrosis of other types.[385] Although most of the case reports have emphasized an association with bronchoalveolar cell carcinoma, most of the pulmonary malignancies appear to be other cell types.[386–393] In the Peters-Golden series, the relative risk of lung cancer was 16.5.[387] In the study of Roumm, the relative risk of lung cancer was 4.4, without a clear relationship to smoking.[392] Case reports of rapid onset of SSc associated with either lung or breast cancer suggest that SSc may be a paraneoplastic syndrome in some cases.[394,395] Lung cancer in SSc is almost always associated with pulmonary fibrosis. Among the mechanisms that have been proposed for the relationship of SSc and interstitial fibrosis to pulmonary malignancy are impaired immune surveillance; impaired clearance of carcinogens; increased susceptibility to malignant transformation of hyperplastic epithelial cells; and secretion of inflammatory mediators that promote or initiate tumor cells.[387]

Other Thoracic Disorders in Systemic Sclerosis

Other pulmonary disorders uncommonly associated with SSc are diffuse pulmonary hemorrhage,[396] hemoptysis from intrabronchial telangectasia,[397] spontaneous pneumothorax,[398] and alveolar hypoventilation from respiratory muscle weakness.[316,399,400]

Treatment

There is no convincingly proven treatment for either the interstitial lung disease or the pulmonary vascular disease associated with SSc. There are, however, two retrospective series that show either improvement or stabilization of D_LCO in patients treated with d-penicillamine compared with untreated patients, and one series that demonstrates improvement in BAL lymphocytic inflammation.[341,401–403] There was no significant effect in any study on lung volumes, however, and spontaneous improvement in D_LCO is a common finding.[354] Immunosuppressive agents with plasmapheresis and combinations of cyclophosphamide and prednisone have also been reported to improve pulmonary function.[312,404] One retrospective report indicates that patients who are able to tolerate para-aminobenzoate treatment tend to show improvement in vital capacity.[405] In a prospective controlled randomized clinical trial, chlorambucil failed to be of use.[406]

Vasodilators have been used for pulmonary hypertension with variable success. Phentolamine, tolazoline, diazoxide, and prostaglandin E_1 have shown little benefit, whereas captopril, nifedipine, and hydralazine have been reported to be useful in some patients.[407–411] As with primary pulmonary hypertension, the pulmonary vasodilator drug selected is likely of less importance than the reactivity of the pulmonary vascular bed in the particular patient.[412] The failure to reverse pulmonary hypertension in SSc is consistent with the finding of a fixed pulmonary vascular bed.[384,413] Some have questioned the value of vasodilator therapy, although short-term controlled trials have shown some beneficial hemodynamic effects in patients with primary pulmonary hypertension.[414,415]

POLYMYOSITIS-DERMATOMYOSITIS

General Features

Polymyositis and dermatomyositis (PM-DM) are considered to be subcategories of the same disease complex because of identical inflammatory myopathies. PM-DM is a rare disease with an incidence of five cases per million.[416] It occurs twice as frequently in women as men in all age categories. The disease has two ages of peak onset: in the first decade of life and in the fifth and sixth decades.[417-419] Diagnostic criteria for the disease include proximal muscle weakness and tenderness; elevation of serum muscle enzymes creatine phosphokinase, aldolase, transaminases, and lactic dehydrogenase; patchy muscle necrosis with regeneration and inflammation on biopsy specimens; and an electromyogram with fibrillations and high-frequency repetitive discharges.[420] The etiology of the disease is not known but there may be a genetic predisposition because of the association with HLA phenotypes B8 and DR3.[421] Viral antigens or antibodies have been identified in some cases, but the etiologic relationship is not known.[422,423] An autoimmune process has been presumed because of the inflammatory nature of the muscle lesions and the presence of multiple autoantibodies in most patients.[424] Anti-muscle antibodies are not specific for PM-DM, but muscle homogenates cause lympho-cyte proliferation, and PM-DM lymphocytes are toxic to cultured muscle cells.[425-427] A vascular etiology has been implicated because of the presence of microvascular inflam-mation associated with complement deposition in the walls of blood vessels.[428]

The association of PM-DM with internal malignancy, particularly adenocarcinoma of the breast, lung, ovary, and stomach in older patients, although often cited, is con-troversial. Retrospective surveys have found a 6% to 26% concordance of adult PM-DM and malignant disease, but prospective studies have not always confirmed this association.[429-434]

Pulmonary Complications

The major pulmonary complications of PM-DM are interstitial pulmonary fibrosis, res-piratory muscle weakness, aspiration pneumonia due to pharyngeal muscle weakness, and toxicity from cytotoxic drugs. Pulmonary involvement in PM-DM has been exten-sively reviewed.[435]

Interstitial Pulmonary Fibrosis

Radiographic series vary widely in the prevalence of interstitial pulmonary disease. Ten out of a series of 213 PM-DM patients (5%) from the Mayo Clinic showed radiographic findings of interstitial lung disease.[436] Salmeron found a 9% prevalence in 109 patients.[437] Bohan did not find any cases out of 153 patients.[419] The prevalence in a small Japanese series, however, was an impressive 64%.[438] The chest radiographic find-ings are nonspecific, showing bibasilar symmetric reticular or reticulonodular shadows similar to those seen with idiopathic pulmonary fibrosis or the pulmonary fibrosis syn-dromes found in SSc or rheumatoid arthritis.[439-447] In some cases, the interstitial lung disease may precede the clinical evidence of myositis by several months.[447,448]

The histologic findings most commonly reported are interstitial fibrosis with vari-able degrees of mononuclear inflammatory cells.[439,441,445,447] More recently, the diver-sity of histologic findings has been emphasized, with many patients showing bronchiolitis obliterans and organizing pneumonia (BOOP) identical to that seen in rheumatoid arthritis.[448] Six cases in the literature show a pattern of acute lung injury or diffuse alveolar damage with interstitial edema and hyaline membranes.[448-450] Of concern is a recent series of lung biopsy studies in 15 patients, 3 of whom developed the adult respiratory distress syndrome (ARDS) following surgery.[448] This was postulated to be the result of release of toxic muscle metabolites from inflamed muscle and suggests the need for caution in performing open lung biopsy or other general anesthetic procedures. Less information is available on BAL in PM-DM than in other connective tissue diseases, but available studies show both neutrophilic and lymphocytic alveolitis in PM-DM patients.[339]

The prognosis for PM-DM patients who show evidence of lung disease is poor. The case fatality rate for patients with histologically proven interstitial fibrosis and myositis is 62% over a 2-year period.[451] Half of the deaths were the consequence of progressive lung disease. This is worse than another recent series of PM-DM patients, where the case fatality rate was only 14% over 4 years.[419] Patients with BOOP as a histologic finding appear to have a better prognosis than those with usual interstitial fibrosis, as do patients with rheumatoid arthritis.[143,448]

About 30% of polymyositis patients have Anti-JO-1 antibody, which is an autoantibody to the enzyme histidyl-tRNA synthetase.[430] This antibody is present only rarely in patients with dermatomyositis or polymyositis associated with malignancy. It is associated, though, with a high prevalence of interstitial pulmonary fibrosis.[452–458] Between 50%–70% of patients with PM who have interstitial fibrosis show anti-Jo-1 whereas only one in eight without pulmonary disease have this antibody.[455] It is not clear whether this antibody plays an etiologic role in the development of the lung disease, but its presence, along with the presence of other tRNA synthetase antibodies PL7 and PL12 in PM has suggested a viral etiology for the development of the autoimmune process.[459–461]

Respiratory Muscle Weakness

Proximal muscle weakness of the limbs is frequently the presenting sign of PM-DM. Respiratory muscle weakness severe enough to cause dyspnea, however, is uncommon, occurring in less than 7% of subjects.[462] Dyspnea from myopathic involvement of the diaphragm, however, may be masked by immobility and overshadowed by pulmonary fibrosis. The diaphragm is often found to be involved at autopsy or at the time of open lung biopsy.[463,464] Hypercapnia in association with restrictive lung disease suggests that the cause of respiratory failure is respiratory muscle weakness rather than interstitial lung disease, which usually causes chronic hypocapnia. Hypercapnic respiratory muscle failure is common when the vital capacity is less than 55% of the predicted value or when the maximum inspiratory force is less than 30% of predicted.[465] When respiratory muscle weakness is combined with interstitial lung disease, the transpulmonary pressure measurements with an esophageal balloon may help determine the etiology. If the predominant cause is weakness, the maximum static recoil pressure of the lung will be reduced, whereas if the lung is stiff, the maximum static recoil pressure will be normal or increased. Lung compliance may be reduced in muscle weakness due to microatelectasis. In far advanced cases of respiratory muscle weakness, ventilatory support, particularly at night, is helpful.[466–469]

Other Pulmonary Complications of Polymyositis-Dermatomyositis

One case has been reported of a patient with pulmonary hypertension and plexiform lesions similar to primary pulmonary hypertension, but this must be an uncommon association.[470] Small vessel vasculitis resembling that seen in the myocardium has been reported in the lung in some autopsy series.[462] Pulmonary alveolar proteinosis is also reported to occur in one case of dermatomyositis in a 9-year-old boy.[471]

Dysphagia due to pharyngeal muscle weakness is a major risk factor for death in patients with PM-DM, often predisposing to aspiration pneumonia.[462,472]

Treatment with corticosteroids or immunosuppressive drugs (methotrexate, azothiaprine, cyclophosphamide, and cyclosporine) is often effective in treatment of the myositis, but can lead to pulmonary complications, including opportunistic infections and hypersensitivity pneumonitis.[457,473–475] When pleural effusions occur in patients with PM-DM, they result from disease complications such as infection or heart failure rather than from the underlying disease.[476]

SJÖGREN'S SYNDROME

General Characteristics

Sjögren's syndrome is a generalized exocrine gland disorder associated with widespread lymphocytic tissue infiltration. The traditional triad included dry eyes, dry mouth, and rheumatoid arthritis, but the syndrome can exist as a primary disorder or be associated with another autoimmune disorder such as rheumatoid arthritis, SLE, PM-DM, SSc, or primary biliary cirrhosis.[477,478] Secondary Sjögren's syndrome occurs in about half of the reported cases.[479] The peak age of onset is in the fifth decade, and the male : female ratio is 1:9. The diagnosis is based on finding two of the following: (1) lymphocytic infiltrates in the salivary gland; (2) definite keratoconjunctivitis sicca; (3) an associated connective tissue or lymphoproliferative disorder.[477] Diagnosis, therefore, usually requires either a simple lip biopsy of superficial salivary glands or slit-lamp examination for Rose Bengal staining of the conjunctiva or cornea.

Female patients with primary Sjögren's syndrome are distinguished by an association with phenotype HLA-B8 and HLA-DR3 in half of the cases, whereas this is absent in patients with secondary Sjögren's syndrome.[480] In contrast, patients with Sjögren's syndrome and rheumatoid arthritis have a high prevalence of HLA-DR4. At times, however, it may be difficult to distinguish primary from secondary Sjögren's syndrome at the time of clinical presentation. The pathogenesis of Sjögren's syndrome is not known, but it is considered to be of autoimmune origin because of its association with other autoimmune diseases, the prevalence of anti-Ro/SSA and anti-La/SSB autoantibodies, and the similarity to chronic graft-versus-host disease. Recent evidence has suggested that the presence of gene interaction at the HLA-DQ region is associated with more severe disease.[276,481] It is postulated that heterozygotes can produce hybrid dimers of HLA-DQ antigens that promote the autoimmune process.

Others have postulated, however, that Sjögren's syndrome is caused by a primary defect in immunosurveillance with a low-grade lymphoproliferative disorder.[482] Involved organs show infiltration with large numbers of activated T-helper cells as well as smaller numbers of activated B cells producing monoclonal immunoglobulins. Natural killer cells that aid in the natural host defense against malignancies are either defective or absent.[483,484]

One in ten patients with Sjögren's syndrome has clinical evidence of pulmonary involvement.[486] The most common disorders are xerotrachea, interstitial lung disease due to lymphocytic or fibrotic infiltration, or obstructive lung disease.

Thoracic Involvement in Sjögren's Syndrome

Xerotrachea (Bronchitis Sicca)

Xerotrachea, although said to be the most common form of pulmonary involvement in Sjögren's syndrome, remains predominantly a clinical diagnosis. Patients have unremitting cough that is nonproductive or associated with scant, thick sputum. Biopsy of the trachea shows atrophy and lymphocytic infiltration of the bronchial mucus glands. The condition occurs in one out of five patients with primary Sjögren's syndrome. In the few patients who have been studied, tracheal mucus velocity is normal, and whole lung clearance of particles is increased.[485]

Obstructive Lung Disease

The relationship of Sjögren's syndrome to obstructive lung disease is controversial. Several large series of Sjögren's syndrome patients show a prevalence of obstructive lung disease no greater than comparison populations without the disease.[486–490] Other series, however, show about half of the subjects to have chronic airflow obstruction.[491–493] The prevalence of airflow obstruction appears to be related to the selection of patients. More patients who have Sjögren's syndrome associated with rheumatoid arthritis demonstrate an obstructive ventilatory defect.[277] In some cases the degree of airway obstruction, even in the absence of cigarette smoking, can be severe, but it is not related to an abnormal protease inhibitor phenotype.[260,494] Lung biopsy frequently shows peribronchial infiltration with lymphocytes, and it has been suggested that this could be the initial lesion in airflow obstruction associated with Sjögren's syndrome.[491] Functional studies have shown high prevalence of small airways dysfunction on spirometry,[487,488] but the prevalence does not seem to be increased when compared with age- and sex-matched controls.[489]

Interstitial Lung Disease

In most series, interstitial lung disease with reticular or reticulonodular infiltrates and reduction in D$_L$CO is the most common pulmonary abnormality in patients with Sjögren's syndrome.[486,488,495,496] Histologic examination shows two distinct patterns: lymphocytic interstitial pneumonia (LIP) and interstitial fibrosis. It has been suggested that the LIP pattern is the consequence of Sjögren's syndrome and that fibrosis is the result of associated collagen disease,[1] but this has not been supported either by recent biopsy series or by examination of cellular material from terminal airspaces.[497]

LIP is so frequently associated with Sjögren's syndrome that the authors who first classified the disorder have suggested that LIP is no more than a *forme fruste* of Sjögren's syndrome confined to the lung.[498] The lymphocytic infiltrate starts in the peribronchial regions and extends into the perivascular and interstitial regions. Tissue histiocytes and multinucleated giant cells may be present in variable numbers. Even with adequate biopsy material, it can be difficult to differentiate LIP from malignant lymphoma of the lung or lymphomatoid granulomatosis.[499] Immunohistochemical studies may be helpful in some cases.[500] In some cases, nodular lymphocytic collections and pulmonary amyloidosis are present.[501–503] When nodular lesions are present, pseudolymphoma, which consists of localized inflammatory infiltrates of mature lymphocytes with germinal centers, must be distinguished from malignant lymphoma, which is composed of immature lymphocytes without germinal centers.

The prevalence of non-Hodgkins lymphoma is increased forty-fold in Sjögren's syndrome patients. Primary lymphoma of the lung can be either T-cell or B-cell in origin and varies from low-grade to high-grade malignant potential. In most cases, however, immunophenotyping has shown B-cell lymphomas, either monoclonal or polyclonal.[504–508] Intratracheal lymphoma may lead to severe upper airway obstruction, which could be confused with peripheral airway obstruction.[509] The finding of monoclonal light change immunoglobulin fragments in the concentrated urine has been proposed as a helpful test to distinguish malignant lymphoma, but this is only of value in B-cell lymphoma.[510]

Although a viral etiology of the disease has been suspected in some cases for many years, recent evidence indicates that primary HIV virus infection can induce a syndrome similar to Sjögren's syndrome with keratoconjunctivitis sicca and lymphocytic interstitial pneumonia.[511]

Even when chest radiographs are normal, Sjögren's syndrome patients show evidence of active inflammatory disease in the chest. In one study, 10 out of 12 patients with normal chest films and primary Sjögren's syndrome had abnormally increased gallium uptake on lung scanning.[512] Most studies of BAL fluid find increased numbers of inflammatory cells in effluent from Sjögren's syndrome patients. Sjögren's syndrome patients fall into two categories: those with lymphocytic alveolitis and those with neutrophilic alveolitis. Breit and colleagues proposed that patients with primary Sjögren's syndrome had lymphocytic alveolitis whereas those with associated connective tissue disease had neutrophilic alveolitis.[330] Hatron and colleagues found that 55% of Sjögren's syndrome subjects with normal chest radiographs and normal lung function had alveolitis on BAL. Two-thirds of those with alveolitis have a lymphocytic type and one-third a neutrophilic.[513] Wallaert and colleagues analyzed lymphocyte subpopulations in patients with primary and secondary Sjögren's syndrome and found that both groups could have either type of inflammation. Patients with primary Sjögren's syndrome had expanded numbers of helper T4 cells in the lavage, whereas patients with secondary Sjögren's syndrome had expanded T8 cells in the lavage. The number of T8 cells tended to correlate with the degree of neutrophilic inflammation.[514] More recently, both peripheral blood and pulmonary lavage mononuclear cells have been shown to have deficient production of interleukin-2 (IL2). This defect in IL2 production occurs in both T4 and T8 cells but can be restored toward normal with indomethacin or depletion of macrophages.[515] This raises the possibility that the alveolar macrophage plays an important role in modulating both T4 and T8 lymphocyte populations through production of cyclooxygenase products. The exact role of these two classes of lymphocytic inflammation is unclear but may be correlated with the clinical course of disease. It is attractive to speculate that those patients with neutrophilic alveolitis will be more prone to develop interstitial fibrosis, whereas those with T4+ lymphocytic infiltration will develop LIP.

ANKYLOSING SPONDYLITIS

Ankylosing spondylitis, like Reiter's syndrome and psoriatic arthritis, is a disorder of the axial skeleton associated with the HLA phenotype HLA-B27. Ankylosing spondylitis, besides involving the spine and sacroiliac joints, also is associated with uveitis (25%), aortic valve incompetence, and cardiac conduction defects (3.5–10%).[516,517] HLA-B27 is present in 90% of ankylosing spondylitis patients. Other hereditary or environmental factors are important, however, since ankylosing spondylitis will develop in 2% of HLA-B27–positive people, but in 20% of HLA-B27–positive relatives of ankylosing spondylitis patients.[518] There is a strong male predominance in the disease, but it has been questioned whether this is a bias due to more severe disease in men; HLA-B27–positive females with ankylosing spondylitis often have less severe spinal deformity and more peripheral arthritis, leading to a diagnosis of seronegative rheumatoid arthritis.[519–521]

Rosenow reviewed 2080 cases of ankylosing spondylitis at the Mayo Clinic and found that only 1.3% of the cases had pleuropulmonary disease. The most common abnormality was fibrobullous disease of the apices of the lung radiographically indistinguishable from tuberculosis.[522,523] Several series of patients with apical fibrobullous disease have appeared, and there are about 160 reported cases.[524–526] Usually, the apical disease occurs late in the process, many years after the inflammatory arthropathy has become quiescent.[527] In a few instances, however, apical fibrobullous disease has been found on routine chest radiographs without other symptoms in people subsequently found to have HLA-B27 phenotypes.[528,529] The common infectious complication of apical fibrobullous disease is aspergilloma or atypical mycobacteria.[530,531] It has been postulated that the chest wall restriction impairs ventilation to the upper lobes, which predisposes to the upper lobe fibrotic lesions.[532] Radionuclide measurement of apical ventilation, however, is normal in cases where there is not yet fibrotic change.[533] Further, clearance of particles is also normal in the lung apices, so this does not seem to predispose to localized infection.[534] It is more likely that the apical lung disease represents an inflammatory facet of this disease since similar lung lesions occur in rheumatoid arthritis in the absence of thoracic immobility.

During the slow course of the disease, there is progressive immobilization of the costovertebral joints, leading to a "frozen thorax" in the later stages of the disease. Chest wall compliance is reduced to as low as 25% of normal in severe cases, but functional residual capacity and residual volumes tend to be normal or increased because the chest wall becomes fixed in a more expanded position.[535,536] Although there may be little expansion of the rib cage, the lung volumes in ankylosing spondylitis show little if any impairment without parenchymal lung disease. The mean vital capacity is slightly reduced to 60% to 90% of normal,[537–539] and exercise capacity is only moderately reduced without ventilatory limitation.[540] The D_LCO is normal in most cases or slightly reduced, consistent with the mild degree of restriction.[541] The rather minimal impact of the severe chest wall restriction on ventilation and lung volumes is because the thorax has two degrees of freedom. When the ribcage expansion is impaired then the thorax can expand in the abdominal pathway. For this reason, ankylosing spondylitis patients tend to show compensatory increases in abdominal wall motion with ventilation.[542,543]

RELAPSING POLYCHONDRITIS

Relapsing polychondritis is a rare disease.[544,545] The condition is chronic and characterized by recurrent acute painful and destructive inflammation of the cartilage of the ears (88%), nose (82%), peripheral joints (78–81%), and larynx and trachea (56–70%).[544,546] Aortic valve incompetence may result from dilatation of the aortic valve ring, and is seen in about one in ten cases.[547] One out of seven patients presents with respiratory signs or symptoms.[544] The prognosis is similar to that of polymyositis: 5-year survival is 74% and 10-year survival is 55%. Infectious and malignant neoplastic diseases are the most common causes of death. Older studies attributed half of the deaths to pulmonary disease, but a recent large series from the Mayo Clinic found that only 10% of deaths were attributable to upper airway obstruction.[548]

The cause of relapsing polychondritis is thought to be immunologic. One out of five patients has evidence of another autoimmune disease. Peripheral blood lymphocytes are activated by exposure to cartilage antigen in vitro; immunofluorescent staining reveals complement deposition on involved cartilage; and circulating antibody to type II collagen is present.[546,549–552] Histologically, involved cartilage shows replacement of normal cartilage with fibrous tissue, loss of glycosaminoglycans, and degeneration of elastin and collagen fibers. When the disease is active, a polymorphous cellular inflammatory infiltrate is present in the fibrous tissue surrounding the cartilage.[553,554]

The lung parenchyma is not involved in relapsing polychondritis unless there is an associated connective tissue disease. Tracheobronchial involvement leads to stricture of the larynx, trachea, or peripheral airways, which causes a reduction of inspiratory as well as expiratory flow on maximum flow volume tracings. There is no good correlation, however, between morphologic findings at bronchoscopy or tomography and the degree of physiological impairment.[555,556] In some cases there is dynamic inspiratory collapse of the upper airway, which may be due to impaired vocal cord abduction during forced inspiration.[555,557] Static pressure maximum expiratory flow studies show that peripheral airway narrowing may also contribute to airflow limitation in some cases.[555] There does not appear to be any reduction in static recoil pressure of the lung in nonsmokers in the few cases that have been studied.[555]

Treatment of the disease requires replacement of the aortic valve when indicated and short courses of high-dose corticosteroids for episodes of painful chondritis. Surgical management of upper airway obstruction is difficult because of the diffuse nature of the airway narrowing.

MIXED CONNECTIVE TISSUE DISEASE

General Features

Disease nosology is a favorite pastime of rheumatologists, and this is nowhere more evident than with respect to the clinical entity of mixed connective tissue disease (MCTD). This disorder was first proposed to be a distinct disorder by Sharp and colleagues,[559] who found a group of patients with antibody to extractable nuclear antigen (anti-ENA; now designated anti-RNP because of its reactivity with ribonucleoprotein units). The original syndrome consisted of an overlap syndrome with characteristics of SLE, systemic sclerosis, and rheumatoid arthritis, which had a relatively mild course, sparing renal involvement.[558,559] Subsequent studies of the originally described series, however, showed that most of the patients went on to differentiate into one of the better classified diseases, usually systemic sclerosis.[560,561] More recently, preliminary criteria have been defined for this disorder that may be useful prospectively, but it remains to be determined whether MCTD represents a specific clinical entity or rather is an early undifferentiated form of other diseases with some overlap features.[562,563] The five features that have been proposed for the diagnosis of this disorder are edema of the hands, synovitis, myositis, Raynaud's phenomenon, and acrosclerosis. In one study, these criteria correctly diagnosed all patients with MCTD, but were also fulfilled in 45% of patients with systemic sclerosis.[564]

Pulmonary Involvement in Mixed Connective Tissue Disease

Interstitial Disease

Pulmonary involvement is common in MCTD but is usually asymptomatic: Although 80% of patients have impaired pulmonary function, the impairment is symptomatic in only 10% of those patients.[560,565,566] The D_LCO is the most common abnormality, being reduced in three-quarters of the patients classified as having MCTD.[567] In 15% of patients interstitial changes are present at the lung bases on chest radiograph.[566,568] In some unusual cases, the interstitial fibrosis can be rapidly progressive and fatal.[569,570] Although cases of diaphragmatic dysfunction similar to that found in SLE have been reported, most patients tested prospectively have normal diaphragm function.[490,567,571] In MCTD, as in systemic sclerosis—and unlike SLE—there is no deposition of immunoglobulin and complement in alveolar walls.[570]

Pulmonary Hypertension

Severe fatal pulmonary hypertension like that seen with systemic sclerosis is an uncommon but reported complication of MCTD.[560,570,572–580] Histologic sections show medial and intimal hyperplasia with recanalization and plexiform lesions that resembles the hyperplasia seen in the CREST variant of systemic sclerosis or primary pulmonary hypertension. In some cases immunoglobulin deposits have been found in pulmonary vessel walls.[570] As is the case with SSc, pulmonary hypertension may be present without other parenchymal abnormality. In one series of 17 patients who were screened for cardiac disease with right heart catheterization, 11 (65%) were found to have elevated pulmonary vascular resistance, despite the absence of symptoms.[581] In a second series of 15 patients, 10 had elevated pulmonary vascular resistance and 10 had elevated pulmonary arterial pressure.[560]

Unusual reported pulmonary complications of MCTD include sterile purulent pleural effusions[582] and pulmonary hemorrhage associated with membranous glomerulonephritis.[583]

CONCLUSION

The collagen diseases are a heterogeneous group of disorders that can affect the lung almost as often as the joints and muscles. An increased understanding of the interstitial, obstructive airway, and pulmonary vascular involvement in these disorders may give us insight into other disorders in which the lung alone is the target organ, such as idiopathic pulmonary fibrosis, chronic obstructive lung disease, and primary pulmonary hypertension. The multisystemic nature of these diseases presents a challenge to the physician and the scientist alike.

REFERENCES

1. Hunninghake GW, Fauci AS. Pulmonary involvement in the collagen vascular diseases. Am Rev Respir Dis 1979; 119:471–503.
2. Wiedemann HP, Matthay RA. Pulmonary manifestations of the collagen vascular diseases. Clin Chest Med 1989; 10:677–722.
3. Harmon KR, Leatherman JW. Respiratory manifestations of connective tissue disease. Semin Respir Infect 1988; 3:258–273.
4. Turner-Warwick M. Connective tissue disorders and the lung. Aust NZ J Med 1986; 16:257–262.
5. Boulware DW, Weissman DN, Doll NJ. Pulmonary manifestations of the rheumatic diseases. Clin Rev Allergy 1985; 3:249–267.
6. Fraser RG, Pare JAP, Pare PD, Fraser RS, Genereux GP. Diseases of altered immunologic activity. In: Diagnosis of diseases of the chest. 3rd ed, vol 2. Philadelphia: WB Saunders, 1989, 1177–1326.
7. Estes D, Christian CL. The natural history of systemic lupus erythematosus by prospective analysis. Medicine 1971; 50:85.
8. Wallace DJ, Podell T, Weiner J, et al. Systemic lupus erythematosus—survival patterns: Experience with 609 patients. JAMA 1981; 245:934.
9. Catoggio LJ, Skinner RP, Smith G, et al. Systemic lupus erythematosus in the elderly: Clinical and serological characteristics. Rheumatology 1984; 11:175.
10. Baker SB, Rovira JR, Campion EW, et al. Late onset systemic lupus erythematosus. Am J Med 1979; 66:727.
11. Fessel WJ. Systemic lupus erythematosus in the community. Ann Intern Med 1974; 134:1027.
12. Wallace SL, Diamond H, Kaplan D. Recent advances in rheumatologic diseases. Ann Intern Med 1972; 77:455.
13. Jonsson H, Nived O, Sturfelt G. Outcome in systemic lupus erythematosus: A prospective study of patients from a defined population. Medicine 1989; 68:141–150.
14. Lawrence RC, Hochberg MC, Kelsey JL, McDuffie FC, et al. Estimates of the prevalence of selected arthritic and musculoskeletal diseases in the United States. J Rheumatol 1989; 16:427–441.
15. Fessel WJ. Epidemiology of systemic lupus erythematosus. Rheum Dis Clin North Am 1988; 14:15–23.
16. Urman JD, Rothfield NF. Corticosteroid treatment in systemic lupus erythematosus: Survival studies. JAMA 1977; 238:2272–2276.
17. Hellmann DB, Petri M, Whiting-O'Keefe Q. Fatal infections in systemic lupus erythematosus: The role of opportunistic organisms. Medicine 1987; 66:341–348.
18. Cohen AS, Reynolds WE, Franklin EC, et al. Preliminary criteria for the classification of systemic lupus erythematosus. Bull Rheum Dis 1971; 21:643.
19. Rabhan NB, Minkin W. Criteria for classification of systemic lupus erythematosus. JAMA 1973; 231:846.
20. Tan EM, Choen AS, Fries JF, Masi AT, McShane DJ, Rothfield NF, et al. The 1982 revised criteria for the classification of systemic lupus erythematosus (SLE). Arthritis Rheum 1982; 25:1271–1277.

21. Synkowski DR, Mogavero HS Jr, Provost TT. Lupus erythematosus: Laboratory testing and clinical subsets in the evaluation of patients. Med Clin North Am 1980; 64:921.
22. Maddison PJ, Provost TT, Reichlin M. Serological findings in patients with "ANA-negative" systemic lupus erythematosus. Medicine 1981; 60:87.
23. Ferreiro JE, Reiter WM, Saldana MJ. Systemic lupus erythematosus presenting as chronic serositis with no demonstrable antinuclear antibodies. Am J Med 1984; 76:1100.
24. Harley JB, Gaither KK. Autoantibodies. Rheum Dis Clin North Am 1988; 14:43–56.
25. Steinberg AD, Klinman DM. Pathogenesis of systemic lupus erythematosus. Rheum Dis Clin North Am 1988; 14:25–41.
26. Smiley JD, Moore SE Jr. Molecular mechanisms of autoimmunity. Am J Med Sci 1988; 295:478–496.
27. Decker JL, Steinberg AD, Reinertsen JL, et al. Systemic lupus erythematosus: Evolving concepts. Ann Intern Med 1979; 91:587.
28. Steinberg AD, Raveche ES, Laskin CA, et al. Systemic lupus erythematosus: Insights from animal models. Ann Intern Med 1984; 100:714.
29. Pandey JP, Fudenberg HH. Immunogenetic markers in autoimmune disease. Ann Intern Med 1984; 101:868.
30. Phillips PE, Christian CL. Myxovirus antibody increases in human connective tissue disease. Science 1970; 168:892.
31. Block SR, Christian CL. The pathogenesis of systemic lupus erythematosus. Am J Med 1975; 59:453.
32. Rich S. Human lupus inclusions and interferon. Science 1981; 213:772.
33. Hahn BH, Sharp GC, Irvin WS, et al. Immune responses to hydralazine and nuclear antigens in hydralazine-induced lupus erythematosus. Ann Intern Med 1972; 76:365.
34. Blomgren SE, Condemi JJ, Vaughan JH. Procainamide-induced lupus erythematosus: Clinical and laboratory observations. Am J Med 1972; 52:338.
35. Byrd RB, Schanzer B. Pulmonary sequelae in procainamide lupus-like syndrome. Dis Chest 1969; 55:170.
36. Auerbach RC, Snyder NE, Bragg DG. The chest roentgenographic manifestations of pronestyl-induced lupus erythematosus. Radiology 1973; 109:287.
37. Harrington TM, Davis DE. Systemic lupus-like syndrome induced by methyldopa therapy. Chest 1981; 79:696.
38. West SG, McMahon M, Protanova JP. Quinidine-induced lupus erythematosus. Ann Intern Med 1984; 100:840.
39. Miller KB, Salem D. Immune regulatory abnormalities produced by procainamide. Am J Med 1982; 73:487.
40. Solinger AM. Drug-related lupus: Clinical and etiologic considerations. Rheum Dis Clin North Am 1988; 14:187–202.
41. Batchelor JR, Welsh KI, Tinoco RM, et al. Hydralazine-induced systemic lupus erythematosus: Influence of HLA-DR and sex on susceptibility. Lancet 1980; i:1107.
42. Cush JJ, Goldings EA. Drug-induced lupus: Clinical spectrum and pathogenesis. Am J Med Sci 1985; 290:36–45.
43. Bigazzi PE. Autoimmunity induced by chemicals. J Toxicol Clin Toxicol 1988; 26:125–156.
44. Sim E. Drug-induced immune-complex disease. Complement Inflamm 1989; 6:119–126.
45. Winslow WA, Ploss LN, Loitman B. Pleuritis in systemic lupus erythematosus: Its importance as an early manifestation in diagnosis. Ann Intern Med 1958; 49:70.
46. Gross M, Esterly JR, Earle RH. Pulmonary alterations in systemic lupus erythematosus. Am Rev Respir Dis 1972; 105:572–577.
47. Miller LR, Greenberg SD, McLarty JW. Lupus lung. Chest 1985; 88:265–269.
48. Haupt HM, Moore GM, Hutchins GM. The lung in lupus erythematosus: Analysis of the pathological changes in 120 patients. Am J Med 1981; 71:791–798.

49. Pertchuk LP, Moccia LF, Rosen Y, Lyons H, Marino CM, Rashford AA, et al. Acute pulmonary complications in systemic lupus erythematosus. Am J Clin Pathol 1977; 68:553–557.

50. Turner-Warwick M. Immunological aspects of systemic diseases of the lungs. Proc R Soc Med 1974; 67:541–547.

51. Schocket AL, Lain D, Kohler PF, et al. Immune complex vasculitis as a cause of ascites and pleural effusions in systemic lupus erythematosus. J Rheumatol 1978; 5:33.

52. Levin DC. Proper interpretation of pulmonary roentgen changes in systemic lupus erythematosus. Am J Roentgenol 1971; 111:510.

53. Weiss JM, Spodick DH. Association of left pleural effusion with pericardial disease. N Engl J Med 1983; 308:696–697.

54. Good JT, King TE, Antony VB, et al. Lupus pleuritis: Clinical features and pleural fluid characteristics with special references to pleural fluid antinuclear antibodies. Chest 1983; 84:714.

55. Carel RS, Shapiro MS, Shoham D, Gutman A. Lupus erythematosus cells in pleural effusion. Chest 1977; 72:670–672.

56. Andrews BS, Arora NS, Shadforth MF, et al. The role of immune complexes in the pathogenesis of pleural effusions. Am Rev Respir Dis 1981; 124:115.

57. Hoffbrand BI, Beck ER. Unexplained dyspnea and shrinking lungs in systemic lupus erythematosus. Br Med J 1963; 1:1273–1277.

58. Rubin LA, Urowitz MB. Shrinking lung syndrome in SLE: A clinical pathological study. Rheumatology 1983; 10:973–976.

59. Harvey AM, Shulman LE, Tumulty PA, Conley CL, Schoenrich EH. Systemic lupus erythematosus: Review of the literature and clinical analysis of 138 cases. Medicine 1954; 33:291–437.

60. Eisenberg H. The interstitial lung diseases associated with collagen vascular disorders. Clin Chest Med 1982; 3:565–578.

61. Chick TW, DeHoratius RJ, Skipper BE, Messner RP. Pulmonary dysfunction in systemic lupus erythematosus without pulmonary symptoms. J Rheumatol 1972; 3:262–268.

62. Gibson GJ, Edmonds JP, Hughes GRV. Diaphragmatic function and lung involvement in systemic lupus erythematosus. Am J Med 1977; 63:926–932.

63. Martens J, Demedts M, Vanmeenen MT, Dequeker J. Respiratory muscle dysfunction in systemic lupus erythematosus. Chest 1984; 84:170–175.

64. Wilcox PG, Stein HB, Clarke SD, Pare P, Pardy RL. Phrenic nerve function in patients with diaphragmatic weakness and systemic lupus erythematosus. Chest 1988; 93:352–357.

65. Picado C, Fiz JA, Montserrat JM, Grau JM, Fernandez-Sola J, Luengo MT, Casademont J, Agusti-Vidal A. Respiratory and skeletal muscle function in steroid-dependent bronchial asthma. Am Rev Respir Dis 1990; 141:14–20.

66. Jacobelli S, Moreno R, Massardo L, Rivero S, Lisboa C. Inspiratory muscle dysfunction and unexplained dyspnea in systemic lupus erythematosus. Arthritis Rheum 1985; 28:781–788.

67. Eichacker PQ, Pinsker K, Epstein A, Schiffenbauer J, Grayzel A. Serial pulmonary function testing in patients with systemic lupus erythematosus. Chest 1988; 94:129–132.

68. Bernstein RM, Ino PW, Elkon KB, et al. Pulmonary function in SLE with a longitudinal study of the shrinking lungs syndrome. Arthritis Rheum 1982; 25:S7.

69. Dureuil B, Vires N, Cantineau JP, Aubier M, Desmonts JM. Diaphragmatic contractility after upper abdominal surgery. J Appl Physiol 1986; 61:1775–1780.

70. De Troyer A, Rosso J. Reflex inhibition of the diaphragm by esophageal afferents. Neurosci Lett 1982; 30:43–46.

71. Thompson PJ, Dhillon DP, Ledingham J, Turner-Warwick M. Shrinking lungs, diaphragmatic dysfunction and systemic lupus erythematosus. Am Rev Respir Dis 1985; 132:926–928.

72. Aubier M, Vilres N, Marciano D, et al. Effects and mechanism of action of terbutaline on diaphragmatic contractility and fatigue. J Appl Physiol 1984; 56:922–929.

73. Mier-Jedrzejowicz A, Brophy C, Moxham J, Green M. Assessment of diaphragm weakness. Am Rev Respir Dis 1988; 137:877–883.

74. Matthay RA, Schwartz MI, Petty TL, et al. Pulmonary manifestations of systemic lupus erythematosus: Review of twelve cases of acute lupus pneumonitis. Medicine 1975; 54:397.
75. Carette S, Macher AM, Nussbaum A, Plotz PH. Severe, acute pulmonary disease in patients with systemic lupus erythematosus: Ten years of experience at the National Institutes of Health. Semin Arthritis Rheum 1984; 14:52–59.
76. Asherson RA, Ridley M, Fletcher CD, Hughes GR. Systemic lupus erythematosus, pulmonary hypertension and adult respiratory distress syndrome (ARDS). Clin Exp Rheumatol 1988; 6:301–304.
77. Clinicopathologic conference: Anemia, abdominal pain, and death in a 19-year-old woman. Am J Med 1987; 83:93–100.
78. Churg A, Franklin W, Chan KL, et al. Pulmonary hemorrhage and immune-complex deposition in the lung: Complications in a patient with systemic lupus erythematosus. Arch Pathol Lab Med 1980; 104:388.
79. Marino CT, Pertchuk LP. Pulmonary hemorrhage in systemic lupus erythematosus. Arch Intern Med 1981; 141:201.
80. Eagen JW, Memoli VA, Roberts JL, et al. Pulmonary hemorrhage in systemic lupus erythematosus. Medicine 1978; 57:545.
81. Desnoyers MR, Bernstein S, Cooper AG, et al. Pulmonary hemorrhage in lupus erythematosus without evidence of an immunologic cause. Arch Inter Med 1984; 144:1398.
82. Myers JL, Katzenstein AA. Microangiitis in lupus-induced pulmonary hemorrhage. Am J Clin Pathol 1986; 84:552.
83. Mintz G, Galindo LF, Fernandez-Diez J, et al. Acute massive pulmonary hemorrhage in systemic lupus erythematosus. J Rheumatol 1978; 5:39.
84. Ramirez RE, Glasier C, Kirks D, et al. Pulmonary hemorrhage associated with systemic lupus erythematosus in children. Radiology 1984; 152:409.
85. Abud-Mendoza C, Diaz-Jouanen E, Alarcon-Segovia D. Fatal pulmonary hemorrhage in systemic lupus erythematosus: Occurrence without hemoptysis. J Rheumatol 1985; 12:558.
86. Leatherman JW. Immune alveolar hemorrhage. Chest 1987; 91:891–897.
87. Leatherman JW, Davies SF, Hoidal JR. Alveolar hemorrhage syndromes: Diffuse microvascular lung hemorrhage in immune and idiopathic disorders. Medicine 1984; 63:343–361.
88. Kwong YL, Wong KL, Kung IT, Chan PC, Lam WK. Concomitant alveolar hemorrhage and cytomegalovirus infection in a patient with systemic lupus erythematosus. Postgrad Med J 1988; 64:56–59.
89. Senecal JL, St-Antoine P, Beliveau C. *Legionella pneumophila* lung abscess in a patient with systemic lupus erythematosus. Am J Med Sci 1987; 83:93–100.
90. Isbister JP, Ralston M, Hayes JM. Fulminant lupus pneumonitis with acute renal failure and RBC aplasia: Successful management with plasmapheresis and immunosuppression. Arch Intern Med 1981; 141:1081.
91. Matthay RA, Petty TL. Treatment of acute lupus pneumonitis with azathioprine. Chest 1974; 66:219.
92. Huang CT, Lyons HA. Comparison of pulmonary function in patients with systemic lupus erythematosus, scleroderma, and rheumatoid arthritis. Am Rev Respir Dis 1966; 93:865.
93. Huang CT, Hennigar GR, Lyons HA. Pulmonary dysfunction in systemic lupus erythematosus. N Engl J Med 1965; 272:288.
94. Gold WM, Jennings DB. Pulmonary function in patients with lupus erythematosus. Am Rev Respir Dis 1966; 93:556.
95. Eisenberg H, Dubois EL, Sherwin RP, et al. Diffuse interstitial lung disease in systemic lupus erythematosus. Ann Intern Med 1973; 79:37.
96. Schwartzberg M, Lieberman DH, Getzoff B, Ehrlich GE. Systemic lupus erythematosus and pulmonary vascular hypertension. Arch Intern Med 1984; 144:605–607.

97. Editorial: Pulmonary hypertension and systemic lupus erythematosus. J Rheumatol 1986; 13:1.

98. Marchesoni A, Messina K, Carrieri P, Sinigaglia L, Tosi S. Pulmonary hypertension and systemic lupus erythematosus. Clin Exp Rheumatol 1983; 1:247–250.

99. Simonson JS, Schiller NB, Petri M, Hellmann DB. Pulmonary hypertension in systemic lupus erythematosus. J Rheumatol 1989; 16:918–925.

100. Manemoto N, Sato M, Moriuchi J, Ichikawa Y, Goto Y, Sasadaira H. An autopsied case of systemic lupus erythematosus with pulmonary hypertension: a case report. Angiology 1988; 39:187–192.

101. Fisher J, Mack RJ, Likier HM, Schiff AN, Borer JS. Nifedipine in pulmonary arterial hypertension: Importance of Raynaud's phenomenon. Chest 1987; 92:400–405.

102. Howe HS, Boey ML, Fong KY, Feng PH. Pulmonary haemorrhage, pulmonary infarction and the lupus anticoagulant. Ann Rheum Dis 1988; 47:869–872.

103. James TN. Thrombi in antrum atrii dextri of human heart as clinically important source for chronic microembolisation to lungs. Br Heart J 1983; 49:122–132.

104. Asherson RA, Oakley CM. Pulmonary hypertension in systemic lupus erythematosus. J Rheumatol 1986; 1:1–5.

105. Asherson RA, Khamashta MA, Ordi-Ros J, Derksen RH, Machin SJ, Barquinero J, Outt HH, Harris EN, Vilardell-Torres M, Hughes GR. The primary antiphospholipid syndrome: Major clinical and serological features. Medicine 1989; 68:366–374.

106. Alarcon-Segovia D, Deleze M, Oria CV, Sanchez-Guerrero J, Gomez-Pacheco L, Cabiedes J, Fernandez L, Ponce de Leon S. Antiphospholipid antibodies and the antiphospholipid syndrome in systemic lupus erythematosus. A prospective analysis of 500 consecutive patients. Medicine 1989; 68:353–365.

107. Levine SR, Welch KM. Antiphospholipid antibodies. Ann Neurol 1989; 26:386–389.

108. Moreb J, Kitchens CS. Acquired functional protein S deficiency, cerebral venous thrombosis, and coumarin skin necrosis in association with antiphospholipid syndrome: Report of two cases. Am J Med 1989; 87:207–210.

109. Matthey F, Walshe K, Mackie IJ, Machin SJ. Familial occurrence of the antiphospholipid syndrome. J Clin Pathol 1989; 42:495–497.

110. Kallenbach J, Zwi S, Goldman HI. Airway obstruction in a case of disseminated lupus erythematosus. Thorax 1978; 33:814.

111. Venizelos PC, Al-Baxar F. Pulmonary function abnormalities in systemic lupus erythematosus responsive to glucocorticoid therapy. Chest 1981; 79:702.

112. Geddes DM, Corrin B, Brewerton DA, et al. Progressive airway obliteration in adults and its association with rheumatoid disease. Q J Med 1977; 46:427.

113. Muren C, Strandberg O. Cavitary pulmonary nodules in atypical collagen disease and lupoid drug reaction: Report of two cases. Acta Radiol 1989; 30:281–284.

114. Webb WR, Gamsu G. Cavitary pulmonary nodules with systemic lupus erythematosus: Differential diagnosis. Am J Roentgenol 1981; 136:27.

115. Chan CN, Li E, Lae FM, Pang JA. An unusual case of systemic lupus erythematosus with isolated hypoglossal nerve palsy, fulminant acute pneumonitis, and pulmonary amyloidosis. Ann Rheum Dis 1989; 48:236–239.

116. Nomura S, Kumagai N, Kanoh T, Uchino H, Kurihara J. Pulmonary amyloidosis associated with systemic lupus erythematosus. Arthritis Rheum 1986; 29:680–682.

117. Nolop KB, Loyd JE, Snell JD. Hilar adenopathy. South Med J 1986; 49:461–465.

118. Kassan SS, Moss ML, Reddick R. Progressive hilar and mediastinal lymphadenopathy in systemic lupus erythematosus on corticosteroid therapy. N Engl J Med 1976; 294:1382–1383.

119. Arnett FC, Edworthy S, Block DA, et al. The 1987 revised ARA criteria for rheumatoid arthritis. Arthritis Rheum 1987; 39:S17.

120. Gordon DA, Stein JL, Broder I. The extra-articular features of rheumatoid arthritis: A systematic analysis of 127 cases. Am J Med 1973; 54:445.

121. Hurd E. Extra-articular manifestations of rheumatoid arthritis. Semin Arthritis Rheum 1979; 8:151.
122. Kohler PF, Vaughan J. The autoimmune diseases. JAMA 1982; 248:2646.
123. Brannan H, Good C, Divertie M, Baggenstoss A. Pulmonary disease associated with rheumatoid arthritis. JAMA 1964; 189:138.
124. Decker JL, Malone DG, Haraoui B, et al. Rheumatoid arthritis: Evolving concepts of pathogenesis and treatment. Ann Intern Med 1984; 101:810.
125. Krane SM, Simon LS. Rheumatoid arthritis: Clinical features and pathogenetic mechanisms. Med Clin North Am 1986; 70:263–284.
126. Stuart JM, Postlethwaite AE, Townes AS, et al. Cell-mediated immunity to collagen and collagen alpha-chains in rheumatoid arthritis and other rheumatoid diseases. Am J Med 1980; 69:13.
127. Fraser RG, Pare JAP, Pare PD, Fraser RS, Genereux GP. Diagnosis of diseases of the chest. 3rd ed, vol 2. Philadelphia: WB Saunders, 1989; 1198–1220.
128. Talbott JA, Calkins E. Pulmonary involvement in rheumatoid arthritis. JAMA 1964; 189:911.
129. Rubin EH. Pulmonary lesions in rheumatoid disease with remarks on diffuse interstitial pulmonary fibrosis. Am J Med 1955; 19:569.
130. Locke CB. Rheumatoid lung. Clin Radiol 1963; 14:43.
131. Aho A, Julkunen H, Kaipainen WJ. Pleuropulmonary x-ray findings in systemic lupus erythematosus and rheumatoid arthritis. Ann Med Intern Fenn 1959; 48 (suppl 28):16.
132. Horler AR, Thompson M. The pleural and pulmonary complications of rheumatoid arthritis. Ann Intern Med 1959; 51:1179.
133. Lodge T. Pulmonary fibrosis and the collagen diseases: Radiological aspects. Br J Radiol 1965; 29:645.
134. Popper MS, Bogdonoff ML, Hughes RL. Interstitial rheumatoid lung disease: A reassessment and review of the literature. Chest 1972; 62:243.
135. Jurik AG, Davidsen D, Graudal H. Prevalence of pulmonary involvement in rheumatoid arthritis and its relationship to some characteristics of the patients: A radiological and clinical study. Scand J Rheumatol 1982; 11:217–224.
136. Payne CR. Pulmonary manifestations of rheumatoid arthritis. Br J Hosp Med 1984; 32:192–197.
137. Petty T, Wilkins M. The five manifestations of rheumatoid lung. Dis Chest 1966; 49:75.
138. Ellman P, Ball RE. Rheumatoid disease with joint and pulmonary manifestations. Br Med J 1948; 2:816.
139. Aronoff A, Bywaters EGL, Fearnley GR. Lung lesions in chronic rheumatoid arthritis. Br Med J 1955; 2:228.
140. Cervantes-Perez P, Toro-Perez AH, Rodriguez-Jurado P. Pulmonary involvement in rheumatoid arthritis. JAMA 1980; 243:1715–1719.
141. Scadding JG. The lungs in rheumatoid arthritis. Proc R Soc Med 1969; 62:226.
142. DeHoratius RJ, Abruzzo JL, Williams RC. Immunofluorescent and immunologic studies of rheumatoid lung. Arch Intern Med 1972; 129:441.
143. Yousem SA, Colby TV, Carrington CB. Lung biopsy in rheumatoid arthritis. Am Rev Respir Dis 1985; 131:770–777.
144. Winchester R, Litwin S, Koffler D, Kunkel H. Observations on the eosinophilia of certain patients with rheumatoid arthritis. Arthritis Rheum 1971; 14:650.
145. Cooney T. Interrelationship of chronic eosinophilic pneumonia, bronchiolitis obliterans, and rheumatoid disease. J Clin Pathol 1981; 34:129.
146. Specks U, Martin WJ, Rohrbach MS. Bronchoalveolar lavage fluid angiotensin-converting enzyme in interstitial lung diseases. Am Rev Respir Dis 1990; 141:117–123.
147. Casale TB, Little MM, Furst D, Wood D, Hunninghake GW. Elevated BAL fluid histamine levels and parenchymal pulmonary disease in rheumatoid arthritis. Chest 1989; 96:1016–1021.

148. Idell S, Garcia JG, Gonzalez, McLarty Fair DS. Fibrinopeptide A reactive peptides and procoagulant activity in bronchoalveolar lavage: Relationship to rheumatoid interstitial lung disease. J Rheumatol 1989; 16:592–598.
149. Garcia JG, James HL, Zinkgraf S, Perlman MB, Keogh BA. Lower respiratory tract abnormalities in rheumatoid interstitial lung disease: Potential role of neutrophils in lung injury. Am Rev Respir Dis 1987; 136:811–817.
150. Perez T, Farre JM, Gosset P, Wallaert B, et al. Subclinical alveolar inflammation in rheumatoid arthritis: Superoxide anion, neutrophil chemotactic activity and fibronectin generation by alveolar macrophages. Eur Respir J 1989; 2:7–13.
151. Balbi B, Cosulich E, Risso A, Sacco O, et al. The interstitial lung disease associated with rheumatoid arthritis: Evidence for imbalance of helper T-lymphocyte subpopulations at sites of disease activity. Bull Eur Physiopathol Respir 1987; 23:241–247.
152. Weiland JE, Garcia JG, Davis WB, Gadek JE. Neutrophil collagenase in rheumatoid interstitial lung disease. J Appl Physiol: Respir Environ Exercise Physiol 1987; 62:628–633.
153. Crystal RG, Bitterman PB, Rennard SI, Keogh BA. Interstitial lung disease of unknown etiology: Disorders characterized by chronic inflammation of the lower respiratory tract. N Engl J Med 1984; 310:154–166, 235–244.
154. Snider GL. Interstitial pulmonary fibrosis: Which cell is the culprit? Am Rev Respir Dis 1983; 127:535–539.
155. Tishler M, Grief J, Fireman EM, et al. Bronchoalveolar lavage: A sensitive test for early diagnosis of pulmonary involvement in rheumatoid arthritis. J Rheumatol 1986; 13:547–550.
156. Herer B, De Castelbajac D, Israel-Biet D, Venet A, et al. Broncho-alveolar lavage in pulmonary involvement in rheumatoid arthritis. Ann Med Interne (Paris) 1988; 139:304–310.
157. Weissler JC, Lyons CR, Lipscomb MF, Toews GB. Human pulmonary macrophages: Functional comparison of cells obtained from whole lung and by bronchoalveolar lavage. Am Rev Respir Dis 1986; 133:473–477.
158. Rossi GA, Zocchi E, Sacco O, Balbi B, Ravazzoni, Damiani G. Alveolar macrophage stimulation of T-cell proliferation in autologous mixed lymphocyte reactions: Role of HLA-DR antigens. Am Rev Respir Dis 1986; 133:78–82.
159. Fireman EM, Ben Efraim S, Grief J, Kivity S, Topilsky MR. Suppressor cell activity of human alveolar macrophages in interstitial lung diseases. Clin Exp Immunol 1988; 73:111–116.
160. Walker W, Wright V. Pulmonary lesions and rheumatoid arthritis. Medicine 1964; 47:501.
161. Walker W, Wright V. Diffuse interstitial pulmonary fibrosis and rheumatoid arthritis. Ann Rheum Dis 1969; 28:252.
162. Hyland RH, Gordon DA, Broder I, Davies GM, et al. A systematic controlled study of pulmonary abnormalities in rheumatoid arthritis. J Rheumatol 1983; 10:395–405.
163. Gladman DD, Anhorn KA. HLA and disease manifestations in rheumatoid arthritis: A Canadian experience. J Rheumatol 1986; 13: 274–276.
164. Hakala M, Ruuska P, Hameenkorpi R, et al. Diffuse interstitial lung disease in rheumatoid arthritis: Views on immunological and HLA findings. Scand J Rheumatol 1986; 15:368.
165. Michalski JP, McCombs CC, Scopelitis E, Biundo JJ, Medsger TA. Alpha-1-antitrypsin phenotypes, including M subtypes, in pulmonary disease associated with rheumatoid arthritis and systemic sclerosis. Arthritis Rheum 1986; 29:586–591.
166. Patterson CD, Harville WE, Pierce JA. Rheumatoid lung disease. Ann Intern Med 1965; 62:685.
167. Hakala M. Poor prognosis in patients with rheumatoid arthritis hospitalized for interstitial lung fibrosis. Chest 1988; 93:114–118.
168. Smith W, Ball G. Lung injury due to gold treatment. Arthritis Rheum 1980; 23:351.
169. Scott D, Bradby G, Altman T, Zaphiropoulos G, Hawkins C. Relationship of gold and penicillamine therapy to diffuse interstitial lung disease. Ann Rheum Dis 1981; 40:136–141.
170. Geddes D, Brostoff J. Pulmonary fibrosis associated with hypersensitivity to gold salts. Br Med J 1976; 1:1444.

171. Agarwal R, Sharma SK, Malviya AN. Gold-induced hypersensitivity pneumonitis in a patient with rheumatoid arthritis. Clin Exp Rheumatol 1989; 7:89–90.

172. Carson CW, Cannon GW, Egger MJ, Ward JR, Clegg DO. Pulmonary disease during the treatment of rheumatoid arthritis with low dose pulse methotrexate. Semin Arthritis Rheum 1987; 16:186–195.

173. Lertratankul Y, Budiman-Mak E, Dietz AA, Jablokow VR, et al. Gold pneumonitis: A case report with electron-microscopy and electron probe analysis. Clin Exp Rheumatol 1986; 4:371–374.

174. Weinblatt ME. Toxicity of low dose methotrexate in rheumatoid arthritis. J Rheumatol 1985; 12 (Suppl 12):35–39.

175. Schapira D, Nahir M, Scharf Y. Pulmonary injury induced by gold salts treatment. Med Interne 1985; 23:259–263.

176. Noseworthy TW, Davey RS, Percy JS, King EG. Hypoxemic respiratory failure in rheumatoid arthritis: Gold related? Crit Care Med 1983; 11:761–762.

177. Cooke N, Bamji A. Gold lung. Rheumatol Rehabil 1981; 20:129–135.

178. Evans RB, Ettensohn DB, Fawaz-Estrup F, Lally EV, Kaplan SR. Gold lung: Recent developments in pathogenesis, diagnosis, and therapy. Semin Arthritis Rheum 1987; 16:196–205.

179. Partanen J, van Assendelft AHW, Koskinies S, Forsberg S, Hakala M, Ilonen J. Patients with rheumatoid arthritis and gold-induced pneumonitis express two high-risk major histocompatibility complex patterns. Chest 1987; 92:277–281.

180. Cooke NT, Bamji AN. Gold and pulmonary function in rheumatoid arthritis. Br J Rheumatol 1983; 22:18–21.

181. Wolfe F, Schurle DR, Lin JJ, Polland SM, et al. Upper and lower airway disease in penicillamine treated patients with rheumatoid arthritis. J Rheumatol 1983; 10:406–410.

182. Bennett JC. Rheumatoid arthritis: Clinical features. In: Schumacher HR, Klippel JH, Robinson DR, eds. Primer on the rheumatic diseases. 9th ed. Atlanta: Arthritis Foundation 1988; 87–92.

183. Ellman P, Cudkowicz L, Elwood JS. Widespread serous membrane involvement by rheumatoid nodules. J Clin Pathol 1954; 7:239.

184. Walters MN, Ojeda VJ. Pleuropulmonary necrobiotic rheumatoid nodules: A review and clinicopathological study of six patients. Med J Aust 1986; 144:648–651.

185. Nusslein HG, Rodl W, Giedel J, Missmahl M, Kalden JR. Multiple peripheral pulmonary nodules preceding rheumatoid arthritis. Rheumatol Int 1987; 7:89–91.

186. Hull S, Mathews JA. Pulmonary necrobiotic nodules as a presenting feature of rheumatoid arthritis. Ann Rheum Dis 1982; 41:21–24.

187. Beumer H, van Belle C. Pulmonary nodules in rheumatoid arthritis. Respiration 1972; 29:556.

188. Hahn BH, Yardley JH, Stevens MB. "Rheumatoid" nodules in systemic lupus erythematosus. Ann Intern Med 1970; 72:49.

189. Fallahi S, Collins RD, Miller RK, Halla JT. Coexistence of rheumatoid arthritis and sarcoidosis: Difficulties encountered in the differential diagnosis of common manifestations. J Rheumatol 1984; 11:526–529.

190. Berendsen HH, Hofstee N, Kapsenberg PD, Siewertsz van Reesma DR, Klein JJ. Bronchocentric granulomatosis associated with seropositive polyarthritis. Thorax 1985; 40:396–397.

191. Fellbaum C, Domej W, Popper H. Rheumatoid arthritis with extensive lung lesions. Thorax 1989; 44:70–71.

192. Burrows FG. Pulmonary nodules in rheumatoid disease: A report of two cases. Br J Radiol 1967; 40:256.

193. Johnson TS, White P, Weiss ST, et al. Endobronchial necrobiotic nodule antedating rheumatoid arthritis. Chest 1982; 82:199.

194. Shenberger KN, Schned AR, Taylor TH. Rheumatoid disease and bronchogenic carcinoma: Case report and review of the literature. J Rheumatol 1984; 11:226–228.

195. Stack BHR, Grant JWB. Rheumatoid interstitial lung disease. Br J Dis Chest 1965; 59:202–211.

196. Blodgett RC, Cera PJ, Jones FL. Alveolar cell carcinoma associated with rheumatoid nodule. Chest 1972: 62:625–627.

197. Baylor P, Buck J, Blenkinsopp E, McNair M, Gabriel R. Carcinoma of the colon presenting as rheumatoid lung. Br J Clin Pract 1980; 34:229.

198. Jolles H, Moseley PL, Peterson MW. Nodular pulmonary opacities in patients with rheumatoid arthritis: A diagnostic dilemma. Chest 1989; 96:1022–1025.

199. Sienewicz DJ, Martin JR, More S, et al. Rheumatoid nodules in the lung. J Can Assoc Radiol 1962; 13:73.

200. Steinberg DL, Webb WR. CT appearances of rheumatoid lung disease. J Comput Assist Tomogr 1984; 8:881–884.

201. Yue CC, Park CH, Kushner I. Apical fibrocavitary lesions of the lung in rheumatoid arthritis: Report of two cases and review of the literature. Am J Med 1986; 81:741–746.

202. Mutschlechner R, Godzinski M. A rare form of rheumatic lung disease. Wien Klin Wochenschr 1985; 97:912–914.

203. Strohl KP, Feldman NT, Ingram RH Jr. Apical fibrobullous disease with rheumatoid arthritis. Chest 1979; 75:739.

204. McCann BG, Hart GJ, Stokes TC, et al. Obliterative bronchiolitis and upper zone pulmonary consolidation in rheumatoid arthritis. Thorax 1983; 38:73.

205. Petrie GR, Bloomfield P, Grant IW, Crompton GK. Upper lobe fibrosis and cavitation in rheumatoid disease. Br J Dis Chest 1980; 74:263–267.

206. Macfarlane JD, Franken CK, van Leeuwen AW. Progressive cavitation pulmonary changes in rheumatoid arthritis: A case report. Ann Rheum Dis 1984; 43:98–101.

207. Pillemer SR, Webb D, Yocum DE. Legionnaire's disease in a patient with rheumatoid arthritis treated with cyclosporine. J Rheumatol 1989; 16:117–120.

208. Case Records of the Massachusetts General Hospital. Case 49-1984: A 64-year-old man with rheumatoid arthritis and cavitary pulmonary disease. N Engl J Med 1984; 311:1496–1505.

209. Watkin SW, Bucknall RC, Nisar M, Agnew RA. Atypical mycobacterial infection of the lung in rheumatoid arthritis. Ann Rheum Dis 1989; 48:336–338.

210. McConnochie K, O'Sullivan M, Khalil JF, Pritchard MH, Gibbs AR. Aspergillus colonization of pulmonary rheumatoid nodule. Respiratory Medicine 1989; 83:157–160.

211. Crisp AJ, Armstrong RD, Grahame R, Dussek JE. Rheumatoid lung disease, pneumothorax, and eosinophilia. Ann Rheum Dis 1982; 41:137–140.

212. Caplan A. Certain unusual radiological appearances in the chest of coal-miners suffering from rheumatoid arthritis. Thorax 1953; 8:29.

213. Gough J, Rivers D, Seal RME. Pathological studies of modified pneumoconiosis in coal-miners with rheumatoid arthritis (Caplan's syndrome). Thorax 1955; 10:9.

214. Caplan A, Cowen EDH, Gough J. Rheumatoid pneumoconiosis in a foundry worker. Thorax 1958; 13:181.

215. Chatigidakis CB, Theron CP. Rheumatoid pneumoconiosis (Caplan's syndrome): A discussion of the disease and a report of a case in a European Witwaterstrand gold miner. Arch Environ Health 1961; 2:397.

216. Campbell JA. A case of Caplan's syndrome in a boiler-scaler. Thorax 1958; 13:177.

217. Rickards AG, Barrett GM. Rheumatoid lung changes associated with asbestosis. Thorax 1958; 13:185.

218. Morgan WKC. Rheumatoid pneumoconiosis in association with asbestosis. Thorax 1964; 19:433.

219. Jordan JW. Pulmonary fibrosis in a worker using an aluminum powder. Br J Industr Med 1961; 18:21.

220. Antila S, Sutinen S, Paakko P. Rheumatoid pneumoconiosis in a dolomite worker: A light and electron microscopic and x-ray microanalytical study. Br J Dis Chest 1984; 78:195.

221. Greaves IA. Rheumatoid pneumoconiosis (Caplan's syndrome) in an asbestos worker: A 17-year follow-up. Thorax 1979; 34:404.
222. Benedek TGG. Rheumatoid pneumoconiosis: Documentation of onset and pathogenic considerations. Am J Med 1973; 55:515.
223. Walker WC, Wright V. Rheumatoid pleuritis. Ann Rheum Dis 1967; 26:467.
224. Campbell GD, Ferrington E. Rheumatoid pleuritis with effusion. Dis Chest 1968; 53:521.
225. Berger HW, Seckler SG. Pleural and pericardial effusions in rheumatoid disease. Ann Intern Med 1966; 64:1291.
226. Lillington GA, Carr DT, Mayne JG. Rheumatoid pleurisy with effusion. Arch Intern Med 1971; 128:764.
227. Ward R. Pleural effusion and rheumatoid disease. Lancet 1961; ii:1336.
228. Mays EE. Rheumatoid pleuritis: Observations in eight cases and suggestions for making the diagnosis in patients without the "typical findings." Dis Chest 1968; 53:202.
229. Hakala M, Tiilikainen A, Hameenkorpi R, et al. Rheumatoid arthritis with pleural effusion includes a subgroup with autoimmune features and HLA-B8, Dw3 association. Scand J Rheumatol 1986; 15:290.
230. Carr DT, Mayne JG. Pleurisy with effusion in rheumatoid arthritis, with reference to the low concentration of glucose in pleural fluid. Am Rev Respir Dis 1962; 85:345.
231. Dodson WH, Hollingsworth JW. Pleural effusion in rheumatoid arthritis: Impaired transport of glucose. N Engl J Med 1966; 273:1337.
232. Pettersson T, Klockars M, Hellstrom PE. Chemical and immunological features of pleural effusion: Comparison between rheumatoid arthritis and other diseases. Thorax 1982; 37:354–361.
233. Sahn SA, Kaplan RL, Maulitz RM, et al. Rheumatoid pleurisy: Observations on the development of low pleural fluid pH and glucose level. Arch Intern Med 1980; 140:1237.
234. Editorial: Pleurisy and rheumatoid arthritis. Br Med J 1968; 2:1.
235. Levine H, Santo M, Grieble HG, et al. Rheumatoid factor in non-rheumatoid pleural effusions. Ann Intern Med 1968; 69:487.
236. Hunder GG, McDuffie FC, Hepper NGG. Pleural fluid complement in systemic lupus erythematosus and rheumatoid arthritis. Ann Intern Med 1972; 76:357.
237. Coe JE, Atkawa JK. Cholesterol pleural effusion. Arch Intern Med 1961; 108:763–774.
238. Baim S, Samuelson CO, Ward JR. Rheumatoid arthritis, amyloidosis, and chylous effusions. Arthritis Rheum 1979; 22:182.
239. Boddington MM, Springs AI, Morton A, Mowat AG. Cytodiagnosis of rheumatoid pleural effusions. J Clin Pathol 1971; 24:95–106.
240. Nosanchuck JS, Naylor B. A unique cytologic picture in pleural fluid from patients with rheumatoid arthritis. Am J Clin Pathol 1968; 50:330–335.
241. Faarup P, Faurschou P. Rheumatoid arthritis cells in experimental pleuritis in mice. Acta Pathol Microbiol Immunol Scand 1986; 93:209.
242. Faurschou P. Decreased glucose in RA cell positive pleural effusion. Eur J Respir Dis 1985; 65:272–277.
243. Faurschou P, Faarup P. Granulocytes containing cytoplasmic inclusions in human tuberculous pleuritis. Scand J Respir Dis 1973; 54:341–346.
244. Faurschou P, Grunnet N, Winding O, Dirksen A, Faarup P. Rheumatoid arthritis cells and biochemical changes in turpentine-induced pleuritis in rabbits. APMIS 1989; 97:413–418.
245. Carmichael DS, Golding DN. Rheumatoid pleural effusion with "RA cells" in the pleural fluid. Br Med Jour 1967; 2:814.
246. Mandl MAJ, Watson JI, Henderson JAM, Wang NS. Pleural fluid in rheumatoid pleuritis. Arch Intern Med 1969; 124:373–376.
247. Faurshou P, Francis D, Faarup P. Thoracoscopic, histological, and clinical findings in nine cases of rheumatoid pleural effusion. Thorax 1985; 40:371–375.

248. Aru A, Engel U, Francis D. Characteristic and specific histological findings in rheumatoid pleurisy. Acta Pathol Microbiol Immunol Scand 1986; 94:57.
249. Champion GD, Robertson MR, Robinson RG. Rheumatoid pleurisy and pericarditis. Ann Rheum Dis 1968; 27:521–530.
250. Feagler JR, Sorenson GD, Rosenfeld MG, Osterland CK. Rheumatoid pleural effusion. Arch Pathol 1971; 92:257–266.
251. Jones FL Jr, Blodgett RC Jr. Empyema in rheumatic pleuropulmonary disease. Ann Intern Med 1971; 74:665.
252. Jacobs P, Bonnyns M, Depierreux M, et al. Rapidly fatal bronchiolitis obliterans with circulating antinuclear and rheumatoid factors. Eur J Resp Dis 1984; 65:384.
253. Price TML, Skelton MD. Rheumatoid arthritis with lung lesions. Thorax 1956; 11:234–240.
254. Begin R, Masse S, Cantin A, Menard HA, Bureau MA. Airway disease in a subset of nonsmoking rheumatoid patients: Characterization of the disease and evidence for an autoimmune pathogenesis. Am J Med. 1982; 72:743–750.
255. Herzog CA, Miller RR, Hoidal JR. Case reports. Bronchiolitis and rheumatoid arthritis. Am Rev Respir Dis 1981; 124:636–639.
256. Lahdensuo A, Mattila J, Vilppula A. Bronchiolitis in rheumatoid arthritis. Chest 1983; 85:705.
257. Jansen HM, Elema JD, Hylkema BS, van Leeuwen MA, et al. Progressive obliterative bronchiolitis in a patient with rheumatoid arthritis. Eur J Respir Dis (suppl) 1982; 121:43–52.
258. Thurlbeck WM. The pathology of small airways in chronic airflow limitation. Eur J Respir Dis (suppl) 1982; 121:9–18.
259. Sweatman MC, Markwick JR, Charles PJ, Jones SE, et al. Histocompatibility antigens in adult obliterative bronchiolitis with or without rheumatoid arthritis. Dis Markers 1986; 4:19–26.
260. Forman MB, Zwi S, Gear AJ, Kallenbach J, Wing J. Severe airway obstruction associated with rheumatoid arthritis and Sjögren's syndrome. A case report. S Afr Med J 1982; 61:674–676.
261. Gosink BB, Friedman PJ, Liebow AA. Bronchiolitis obliterans, roentgenologic-pathologic correlation. Am J Roentgenol Radium Ther Nucl Med 1973; 117:816–832.
262. Murphy KC, Atkins CJ, Offer RC, Hogg JC, Stein HB. Obliterative bronchiolitis in two rheumatoid arthritis patients treated with penicillamine. Arthritis Rheum 1981; 24:557–560.
263. Stein HC, Patterson AC, Offer RC, Atkins CJ, Teufel A, Robinson A. Adverse effects of d-penicillamine in rheumatoid arthritis. Ann Intern Med 1980; 29:24–29.
264. Epler GR, Snider GC, Gaensler EA, Cathcart ES, Fitzgerald MX, Carrington.CB Bronchiolitis and bronchitis in connective tissue disease: A possible relationship to the use of penicillamine. JAMA 1979; 242:528–532.
265. Lyle WH. D-penicillamine and fatal obliterative bronchiolitis. Lancet 1977; i:105.
266. Holness L, Tenenbaum J, Cooter NBE, et al. Fatal bronchiolitis obliterans associated with chrysotherapy. Ann Rheum Dis 1983; 42:593.
267. Wolfe F, Schurie DR, Lin JJ, Polland SM, et al. Upper and lower airway disease in penicillamine treated patients with rheumatoid arthritis. J Rheumatol 1983; 10:406–410.
268. Halla JT, Cassady J, Hardin JG. Sequential gold and penicillamine therapy in rheumatoid arthritis: Comparative study of effectiveness and toxicity and review of the literature. Am J Med 1982; 72:423.
269. Fort JG, Scovern H, Abruzzo JL. Intravenous cyclophosphamide and methylprednisolone for the treatment of bronchiolitis obliterans and interstitial fibrosis associated with chrysotherapy. J Rheumatol 1988; 15:850–854.
270. Yousem SA, Colby TV, Carrington CB. Follicular bronchitis/bronchiolitis. Hum Pathol 1985; 16:700.
271. Fortoul TI, Cano-Valle F, Oliva E, et al. Follicular bronchiolitis in association with connective tissue diseases. Lung 1985; 163:305.
272. Collins RL, Turner RA, Johnson AM, Whitley NO, McLean RL. Obstructive pulmonary disease in rheumatoid arthritis. Arthritis Rheum 1976; 19:623–628.

273. Mountz JD, Turner RA, Collins RL, Gallup KR, Semble EL. Rheumatoid arthritis and small airways function: Effects of disease activity, smoking, and alpha-1-antitrypsin deficiency. Arthritis Rheum 1984; 27:728–736.

274. Sassoon CS, McAlpine SW, Tashkin DP, Baydur A, Quismorio FG, Mongan ES. Small airways function in nonsmokers with rheumatoid arthritis. Arthritis Rheum 1984; 27:1218–1226.

275. Radoux V, Menard HA, Begin, Decary F, Koopman WJ. Airways disease in rheumatoid arthritis patients: One element of a general exocrine dysfunction. Arthritis Rheum 1987; 30:249–256.

276. Wise RA, Wigley FM, Scott TE, Hochberg MC. HLA-DQw alloantigens and pulmonary dysfunction in rheumatoid arthritis. Chest 1988; 94:609–614.

277. Scott TE, Wise RA, Hochberg MC, Wigley FM. HLA-DR4 and pulmonary dysfunction in rheumatoid arthritis. Am J Med 1987; 82:765–771.

278. Bienenstock H, Ehrlich GE, Freyberg RH. Rheumatoid arthritis of the cricoarytenoid joint: A clinicopathologic study. Arthritis Rheum 1963; 6:48–62.

279. Lofgren RH, Montgomery WW. Incidence of laryngeal involvement in rheumatoid arthritis. N Engl J Med 1962; 267:193–195.

280. Lawry GV, Finerman ML, Hanafee WN, Mancuso AA, Fan PT, Bluestone R. Laryngeal involvement in rheumatoid arthritis: A clinical, laryngoscopic, and computerized tomographic study. Arthritis Rheum 1984; 27:873–882.

281. Darke CS, Wolman L, Young A. Laryngeal stridor in rheumatoid arthritis. Br Med J 1958; 1:1279–1282.

282. Chalmers A, Traynor JA. Cricoarytenoid arthritis as a cause of acute upper airway obstruction. J Rheumatol 1979; 6:541–542.

283. Polisar IA, Burbank B, Levitt LM, Katz HM, Morrione TG. Bilateral midline fixation of cricoarytenoid joints as a serious medical emergency. JAMA 1960; 172:901–906.

284. Baker OA, Bywaters EGL. Laryngeal stridor in rheumatoid arthritis due to crico-arytenoid joint involvement. Br Med J 1957; 2:1400.

285. Wolman L, Darke CS, Young A. The larynx in rheumatoid arthritis. J Laryngol 1965; 79:403–434.

286. Lemley DE, Katz P. Rheumatoid-like arthritis presenting as idiopathic pulmonary hemosiderosis: A report and review of the literature. J Rheumatol 1986; 13:954–957.

287. O'Brodovich HM, Way RC, Andrew M, Dent PB. Noninvasive diagnosis of pulmonary hemorrhage in rheumatoid arthritis. Pediatrics 1983; 72:720–723.

288. Jordan JD, Snyder CH. Rheumatoid disease of the lung and cor pulmonale: Observations in a child. Am J Dis Child 1964; 108:174.

289. Gardner DL, Duthie JJ, MacLeod J, Allan WS. Pulmonary hypertension in rheumatoid arthritis: Report of a case with intimal sclerosis of the pulmonary and digital arteries. Scott Med J 1957; 2:183–186.

290. Kay JM, Banik S. Unexplained pulmonary hypertension with pulmonary arteritis in rheumatoid disease. Br J Dis Chest 1977; 71:63.

291. Baydur A, Mongan ES, Slager UT. Acute respiratory failure and pulmonary arteritis without parenchymal involvement: Demonstration in a patient with rheumatoid arthritis. Chest 1979; 75:518.

292. Onodera S, Hill JR. Pulmonary hypertension: Report of a case in association with rheumatoid arthritis. Ohio State Med J 1965; 61:141–144.

293. Armstrong JG, Steel RH. Localized pulmonary arteritis in rheumatoid disease. Thorax 1982; 37:313.

294. Morikawa J, Kitamura K, Habuchi Y, Tsujimura Y, Minamikawa T, Takamatsu T. Pulmonary hypertension in a patient with rheumatoid arthritis. Chest 1988; 93:876–878.

295. Sackner MA. The visceral manifestations of scleroderma. Arthritis Rheum 5:184–194.

296. Masi AT, Rodnan GP, Medsger TA, et al. Preliminary criteria for the classification of systemic sclerosis (scleroderma). Arthritis Rheum 1980; 23:561.

297. Livingston JZ, Scott TE, Wigley FM, Anhalt GJ, Bias WB, McLean RH, Hochberg MC. Systemic sclerosis (scleroderma): Clinical, genetic, and serologic subsets. J Rheumatol 1987; 14:512–518.

298. Steen VD, Medsger TA. Epidemiology and natural history of systemic sclerosis. Rheum Dis Clin North Am 1990; 16:1–10.

299. Medsger TA. Epidemiology of progressive systemic sclerosis. In: Black CM, Myers AR, eds. Systemic sclerosis (scleroderma). New York: Gower, 1985, 53–60.

300. Hochberg MC, Lopez-Acuna D, Gittelsohn AM. Mortality from systemic sclerosis (scleroderma) in the United States 1969–1977. In: Black CM, Myers AR, eds. Systemic sclerosis (scleroderma). New York: Gower, 1985, pp. 61–69.

301. Maricq HR, Weinrich MC, Keil JE, et al. Prevalence of scleroderma spectrum disorders in the general population of South Carolina. Arthritis Rheum 1989; 32:998–1006.

302. Medsger TA, Masi AT. Epidemiology of systemic sclerosis (scleroderma). Ann Intern Med 1971; 74:714.

303. Masi AT. Clinical-epidemiological perspective of systemic sclerosis (scleroderma). In: Jayson MIV, Black CM, eds. Systemic sclerosis: Scleroderma. New York: John Wiley & Sons, 1988, 7–31.

304. Campbell PM, LeRoy EC. Pathogenesis of systemic sclerosis: A vascular hypothesis. Semin Arthritis Rheum 1975; 4:351.

305. Fries JF. The microvascular pathogenesis of scleroderma: An hypothesis. Ann Intern Med 1979; 91:788.

306. Marks R, Czerniecki M, Andrews S, et al. The effects of scleroderma serum on human microvascular endothelial cells. Arthritis Rheum 1988; 31:1524.

307. Tan EM, Rodnan GP, Garcia I, et al. Diversity of antinuclear antibodies in progressive systemic sclerosis. Arthritis Rheum 1980; 23:617.

308. Inoshita T, Whiteside T, Rodnan G, Taylor F. Abnormalities of T-lymphocyte subsets in patients with progressive systemic sclerosis. J Lab Clin Med 1981; 97:264–277.

309. Claman HN. On scleroderma: Mast cells, endothelial cells and fibroblasts. JAMA 1989; 262:1208.

310. Owens GR, Follansbee WP. Cardiopulmonary manifestations of systemic sclerosis. Chest 1988; 91:118–127.

311. Alton E, Turner-Warwick M. Lung involvement in scleroderma. In: Jayson MIV, Black CM, eds. Systemic sclerosis: Scleroderma. New York: John Wiley, 1988.

312. Silver RM, Miller KS. Lung involvement in systemic sclerosis. Rheum Dis Clin North Am 1990; 16:199–216.

313. Day WDF. Cast of scleroderma or sclerema with the autopsy and remarks. Am J Med Sci 1870; 59:350–359.

314. Adhikari PK, Bianchi FA, Boushy SF, et al. Pulmonary function in scleroderma: Its relation to changes in the chest roentgenogram and in the skin of the thorax. Am Rev Respir Dis 1962; 86:823–831.

315. Sackner MA, Akgun N, Kimbel P, Lewis DH. The pathophysiology of scleroderma involving the heart and respiratory system. Ann Intern Med 1964; 60:611–630.

316. Russell DC, Maloney A, Muir AL. Progressive generalized scleroderma: Respiratory failure from primary chest wall involvement. Thorax 1981; 36:219–220.

317. Taormina VJ, Miller WT, Gefter WB, Epstein DM. Progressive systemic sclerosis subgroups: Variable pulmonary features. Am J Radiol 1981; 137:277–285.

318. Zarafonetis CJ, Dabich L, Devol EB, Skovronski JJ, et al. Retrospective studies in scleroderma: Pulmonary findings and effect of potassium p-aminobenzoate on vital capacity. Respiration 1989; 56:22–33.

319. Steen VD, Ziegler GL, Rodnan GP, et al. Clinical and laboratory associations of anticentromere antibody in patients with progressive systemic sclerosis. Arthritis Rheum 1984; 27:125.

320. Owens GR, Fino GJ, Herbert DL, Steen V, Medsger T, Pennock B. Pulmonary function in progressive systemic sclerosis: Comparison of CREST syndrome variant with diffuse scleroderma. Chest 1983; 84:546–550.

321. Lomeo RM, Cornella RJ, Schabel SI, Silver RM. Progressive systemic sclerosis sine scleroderma presenting as pulmonary interstitial fibrosis. Am J Med 1989; 87:525–527.

322. Harrison NK, Glanville AR, Strickland B, Haslam PL, et al. Pulmonary involvement in systemic sclerosis: The detection of early changes by thin section CT scan, bronchoalveolar lavage and ^{99m}Tc-DTPA clearance. Respir Med 1989; 83:403–414.

323. Strickland B, Strickland NH. The value of high definition, narrow section computed tomography in fibrosing alveolitis. Clin Radiol 1988; 39:589–594.

324. Rodnan GP. The association of progressive systemic sclerosis (scleroderma) with coal miners' pneumoconiosis and other forms of silicosis. Ann Intern Med 1967; 66:323–334.

325. Walder BK. Do solvents cause scleroderma? Int J Dermatol 1983; 22:157–158.

326. Alonso-Ruiz A, Zea-Mendoza AC, Salazar-Vallinas JM, Rocamore-Ripoli A. Toxic oil syndrome: A syndrome with features overlapping those of various forms of scleroderma. Semin Arthritis Rheum 1986; 15:200–212.

327. Finch WR, et al. Bleomycin induced scleroderma. J Rheumatol 1989; 7:651–659.

328. Vargas J, Schumacher R, Jimenez SA. Systemic sclerosis after augmentation mammoplasty with silicon implants. Ann Intern Med 1989; 111:377–383.

329. Miller KS, Smith EA, Kinsella M, Schabel SI, Silver RM. Lung disease associated with progressive systemic sclerosis: Assessment of interlobar variation by bronchoalveolar lavage and comparison with noninvasive evaluation of disease activity. Am Rev Respir Dis 1990; 141:301–306.

330. Breit SN, Cairns D, Szentirmay A, Callaghan T, et al. The presence of Sjögren's syndrome is a major determinant of the pattern of interstitial lung disease in scleroderma and other connective tissue diseases. J Rheumatol 1989; 16:1043–1049.

331. Pesci A, Bertorelli G, Manganelli P, Ambanelli U. Bronchoalveolar lavage analysis of interstitial lung disease in CREST syndrome. Clin Exp Rheumatol 1986; 4:121–124.

332. Silver RM, Metcalf JF, LeRoy EC. Interstitial lung disease in scleroderma: Immune complexes in sera and bronchoalveolar lavage fluid. Arthritis Rheum 1986; 29:525–531.

333. Owens GR, Paradis IL, Gryzan S, Medsger TA Jr, et al. Role of inflammation in the lung disease of systemic sclerosis: Comparison with idiopathic pulmonary fibrosis. J Lab Clin Med 1986; 107:253–260.

334. Rossi GA, Bitterman PB, Rennard SI, Ferrans VJ, Crystal RG. Evidence for chronic inflammation as a component of the interstitial lung disease associated with progressive systemic sclerosis. Am Rev Respir Dis 1985; 131:612–617.

335. Silver RM, Metcalf JF, Stanley JH, LeRoy EC. Interstitial lung disease in scleroderma: Analysis by bronchoalveolar lavage. Arthritis Rheum 1984; 27:1254–1262.

336. Konig G, Luderschmidt C, Hammer C, Adelmann-Grill BC, et al. Lung involvement in scleroderma. Chest 1984; 85:318–324.

337. Baron M, Feiglin D, Hyland R, Urowitz MB, Shiff B. [67]Gallium lung scans in progressive systemic sclerosis. Arthritis Rheum 1983; 26:969–974.

338. Kinsella MB, Smith EA, Miller KS, LeRoy EC, Silver RM. Spontaneous production of fibronectin by alveolar macrophages in patients with scleroderma. Arthritis Rheum 1989; 32:577–583.

339. Wallaert B, Hatron P, Grosbois J, Tonnel AB, Devulder B, Voisin C. Subclinical pulmonary involvement in collagen vascular diseases assessed by bronchoalveolar lavage: Relationship between alveolitis and subsequent changes in lung function. Am Rev Resp Dis 1986; 133:574–580.

340. Wallaert B, Bart F, Aerts C, Ouassi A, Hatron P, Tonnel AB, Voisin C. Activated alveolar macrophages in subclinical pulmonary inflammation in collagen vascular diseases. Thorax 1988; 43:24–30.
341. Edelson JD, Hyland RH, Ramsden N, Chamberlain DW. Lung inflammation in scleroderma: Clinical, radiographic, physiologic and cytopathological features. J Rheumatol 1985; 12:957–963.
342. Mackel AM, DeLustro F, Harper FE. Antibodies to collagen in scleroderma. Arthritis Rheum 1982; 25:522–531.
343. Seibold JR, Medsger TA, Winklestein A, et al. Immune complexes in progressive systemic sclerosis (scleroderma). Arthritis Rheum 1982; 25:1167–1173.
344. D'Angelo WA, Fries JF, Masi AT, et al. Pathologic observations in systemic sclerosis (scleroderma): A study of 58 autopsy cases and 58 matched controls. Am J Med 1969; 46:428–440.
345. Getzowa S. Cystic and compact pulmonary sclerosis in progressive scleroderma. Arch Pathol 1945; 40:99:106.
346. Spain DM, Thomas AG. The pulmonary manifestations of scleroderma: An anatomic-physiological correlation. Ann Intern Med 1950; 32:152–161.
347. Young RH, Mark GJ. Pulmonary vascular changes in scleroderma. Am J Med 1978; 64:998.
348. Ashba JK, Ghanem MH. The lungs in systemic sclerosis. Dis Chest 1965; 47:52–64.
349. Bagg LR, Hughes DT. Serial pulmonary function tests in progressive systemic sclerosis. Thorax 1979; 34:224–228.
350. Colp CR, Riker J, Williams MH. Serial changes in scleroderma and idiopathic interstitial lung disease. Arch Intern Med 1973; 132:506–515.
351. Fraser RG, Pare JAP, Pare PD, Fraser RS, Genereux GP. Diseases of altered immunologic activity. In: Diagnosis of diseases of the chest. 3rd ed, vol 2. Philadelphia: WB Saunders, 1989, 1177–1326.
352. Hughes DT, Lee FI. Lung function in patients with systemic sclerosis. Thorax 1963; 18:16–20.
353. Peters-Golden M, Wise RA, Hochberg MC, Stevens MB, Wigley FM. Carbon monoxide diffusing capacity as predictor of outcome in systemic sclerosis. Am J Med 1984; 77:1027–1034.
354. Peters-Golden M, Wise RA, Schneider P, Hochberg M, Stevens MB, Wigley F. Clinical and demographic predictors of loss of pulmonary function in systemic sclerosis. Medicine (Baltimore) 1984; 63:221–231.
355. Ritchie B. Pulmonary function in scleroderma. Thorax 1964; 19:28–36.
356. Schneider PD, Wise RA, Hochberg MC, Wigley FM. Serial pulmonary function in systemic sclerosis. Am J Med 1982; 73:384–394.
357. Steen VD, Owens GR, Redmond C, Rodnan GP, Medsger TA Jr. The effect of D-penicillamine on pulmonary findings in systemic sclerosis. Arthritis Rheum 1985; 28:882–888.
358. Steen VD, Owens GR, Fino GJ, Rodnan GP, Medsger TA Jr. Pulmonary involvement in systemic sclerosis (scleroderma). Arthritis Rheum 1985; 28:759–767.
359. Greenwald GI, Tashkin DP, Gong H, Simmons M, et al. Longitudinal changes in lung function and respiratory symptoms in progressive systemic sclerosis: Prospective study. Am J Med 1987; 83:83–92.
360. Wilson RJ, Rodnan GP, Robin ED. An early pulmonary physiologic abnormality in progressive systemic sclerosis (diffuse scleroderma). Am J Med 1964; 36:361–369.
361. Bjerke RD, Tashkin DP, Clements PJ, et al. Small airways in progressive systemic sclerosis (PSS). Am J Med 1979; 66:201–209.
362. Ungerer RG, Tashkin DP, Furst D, et al. Prevalence and clinical correlates of pulmonary arterial hypertension in progressive systemic sclerosis. Am J Med 1983; 75:65–74.
363. Colp CR, Riker J, Williams MH. Serial changes in scleroderma and idiopathic interstitial lung disease. Arch Intern Med 1973; 132:506–515.
364. Manoussakis MN, Constantopoulos SH, Gharavi AE, Moutsopoulos HM. Pulmonary involvement in systemic sclerosis: Association with anti-Scl 70 antibody and digital pitting. Chest 1987; 92:509–513.

365. Mahrer PR, Evans JA, Steinberg I. Scleroderma: Relation of pulmonary changes to esophageal disease. Ann Intern Med 1954; 40:92–110.
366. Johnson DA, Drane WE, Curran J, Cattau EL, Ciarleglio C, Khan A, Cotelingam J, Benjamin S. Pulmonary disease in progressive systemic sclerosis: A complication of gastroesophageal reflux and occult aspiration? Arch Intern Med 1989; 149:589–593.
367. Steckel RJ, Bein ME, Kelly PM. Pulmonary arterial hypertension in progressive systemic sclerosis. Am J Roentgen 1975; 124:461–465.
368. Salerni R, Rodnan GP, Leon DF, et al. Pulmonary hypertension in the CREST syndrome variant of progressive systemic sclerosis (scleroderma). Ann Intern Med 1977; 86:394–399.
369. Enson Y, Thomas HM, Bosken CH, et al. Pulmonary hypertension in interstitial lung disease: Relation of vascular resistance to abnormal lung structure. Trans Assoc Am Phys 1975; 88:248–255.
370. Stupi AM, Steen VD, Owens GR, et al. Pulmonary hypertension in the CREST syndrome variant of systemic sclerosis. Arthritis Rheum 1986; 29:515–524.
371. Al-Sabbagh MR, Steen VD, Zee BC, Nalesnik M, Trostle DC, Bedetti CD, Medsger TA. Pulmonary arterial histology and morphometry in systemic sclerosis: A case-control autopsy study. J Rheumatol 1989; 16:1038–1042.
372. Servi RJ, Albertini RE, Torretti D. Pulmonary hypertension, hypoxemia, and death in a patient with scleroderma. South Med J 1985; 78:739–741.
373. Rosenberg HC, Rabinovitch M. Endothelial injury and vascular reactivity in monocrotaline pulmonary hypertension. Am J Physiol 1988; 255:H1484–H1491.
374. Spitzer R, Kahaleh MB, Barland P. Cytotoxic factors specific for endothelial cells: Progressive systemic sclerosis without cutaneous involvement. NY State J Med 1981; 81:1081–1083.
375. Kahaleh MB, Sherer GK, LeRoy EC. Endothelial injury in scleroderma. J Exp Med 1979; 149:1326–1335.
376. Kahaleh MB, LeRoy EC. Endothelial injury in scleroderma: A protease mechanism. J Lab Clin Med 1983; 101:553–560.
377. Cannon PJ, Hassar M, Case DB, Casarella WJ, Somers SC, LeRoy EC. The relationship of hypertension and renal failure in scleroderma (progressive systemic sclerosis) to structural and functional abnormalities of renal cortical circulation. Medicine 1974; 53:1.
378. Naslund M, Pearson T, Ritter J. A documented episode of pulmonary vasoconstriction in systemic sclerosis. Johns Hopkins Med J 1981; 148:78–80.
379. Furst DE, Davis JA, Clements PJ, Sawtantra KC, Argyrios NT, Chia D. Abnormalities of pulmonary vascular dynamics and inflammation in early progressive systemic sclerosis. Arthritis Rheum 1981; 24:1403–1408.
380. Fahey P, Utell M, Condemi J, Breen R, Hyde R. Raynaud's phenomenon of the lung. Am J Med 1984; 76:263–269.
381. Altschule MD, Linenthal H, Zamcheck N. Lung volume and pulmonary dynamics in Raynaud's disease: Effect of exposure to cold. Proc Soc Exp Biol Med 1941; 48:503–505.
382. Miller MJ. Effect of the cold pressor test on diffusing capacity: Comparison of normal subjects and those with Raynaud's disease and progressive systemic sclerosis. Chest 1983; 84:264–266.
383. Shuck JW, Oetgen WJ, Tesar JT. Pulmonary vascular response during Raynaud's phenomenon in progressive systemic sclerosis. Am J Med 1985; 78:221–227.
384. Wise RA, Wigley F, Newball HH, Stevens MB. The effect of cold exposure on diffusing capacity in patients with Raynaud's phenomenon. Chest 1982; 81:695–698.
385. Turner-Warwick M, Lebowitz M, Burrows B, et al. Cryptogenic fibrosing alveolitis and lung cancer. Thorax 1980; 35:496–499.
386. Sarma DP, Weilbaecher TG. Systemic scleroderma and small cell carcinoma of the lung. J Surg Oncol 1985; 29:28–30.
387. Peters-Golden M, Wise RA, Hochberg M, Stevens MB, Wigley FM. Incidence of lung cancer in systemic sclerosis. J Rheumatol 1985; 12:1136–1139.

388. Salvant EE, Careter JM, Armstrong EM, Polk OD, Austin KI. CREST syndrome: A variant of progressive systemic sclerosis, associated with interstitial pulmonary fibrosis and malignancy. South Med J 1988; 81:1185–1187.

389. Winkelmann RK, Flach DB, Unni KK. Lung cancer and scleroderma. Arch Dermatol Res 1988; 280 (suppl): S15–S18.

390. Talbott JH, Barrocas M. Progressive systemic sclerosis (PSS) and malignancy, pulmonary and non-pulmonary. Medicine (Baltimore) 1979; 58:182–207.

391. Talbott JH, Barrocas M. Carcinoma of the lung in progressive systemic sclerosis: A tabular review of the literature and a detailed report of roentgenographic changes in two cases. Semin Arthritis Rheum 1980; 9:191–217.

392. Roumm AD, Medsger TA Jr. Cancer and systemic sclerosis: An epidemiologic study. Arthritis Rheum 1985; 28:1336–1340.

393. Medsger TA. Systemic sclerosis and malignancy: Are they related? (Editorial) J Rheumatol 1985; 12:1041–1042.

394. Enzenauer RJ, McKoy J, Riel M. Case report: Rapidly progressive systemic sclerosis associated with carcinoma of the lung. Milit Med 1989; 154:574–577.

395. Goodfield MJ, Millard LG. Systemic sclerosis in association with multiple primary pulmonary malignancy: A marker of internal malignancy? Postgrad Med J 1988; 64:866–868.

396. Kallenbach J, Prinsloo I, Zwi S. Progressive systemic sclerosis complicated by diffuse pulmonary hemorrhage. Thorax 1971; 32:767–770.

397. Kim JH, Follett JV, Rice JR, Hampson NB. Endobronchial telangiectasis and hemoptysis in scleroderma. Am J Med 1988; 84:173–174.

398. Edwards WG Jr, Dines DE. Recurrent spontaneous pneumothorax in diffuse scleroderma: Report of a case. Dis Chest 1966; 49:96–98.

399. Chausow AM, Kane T, Levinson D, Szidon JP. Reversible hypercapnic respiratory insufficiency in scleroderma caused by respiratory muscle weakness. Am Rev Respir Dis 1984; 130:143–144.

400. Iliffe GD, Pettigrew NM. Hypoventilatory respiratory failure in generalized scleroderma. Br Med J 1983; 286:337–338.

401. Medsger TA Jr. D-penicillamine treatment of lung involvement in patients with systemic sclerosis (scleroderma). Arthritis Rheum 1987; 30:832–834.

402. de Clerck LS, Dequeker J, Francx L, Demedts M. D-penicillamine therapy and interstitial lung disease in scleroderma: A long-term followup study. Arthritis Rheum 1987; 30:643–650.

403. Steen VD, Owens GR, Redmond C, Rodnan GP, Medsger TA Jr. The effect of D-penicillamine on pulmonary findings in systemic sclerosis. Arthritis Rheum 1985; 28:882–888.

404. Akesson A, Wollheim FA, Thysell H, Gustafson T, et al. Visceral improvement following combined plasmapheresis and immunosuppressive drug therapy in progressive systemic sclerosis. Scand J Rheumatol 1988; 17:313–323.

405. Zarafonetis CJ, Dabich L, Devol EB, Skovronski JJ, et al. Retrospective studies in scleroderma: Pulmonary findings and effect of potassium p-aminobenzoate on vital capacity. Respiration 1989; 56:22–33.

406. Furst DE, Clements PJ, Hillis S, et al. Immunosuppression with chlorambucil, versus placebo, for scleroderma: Results of a three-year parallel, randomized, double-blind study. Arthritis Rheum 1989; 32:584–593.

407. Baron M, Skrinskas G, Hyland R, Urowitz MB. Effects of prostaglandin E_1 and other vasodilator agents in pulmonary hypertension of scleroderma. Br Heart J 1983; 48:304–305.

408. Ocken S, Reinitz E, Strom J. Nifedipine treatment for pulmonary hypertension in a patient with systemic sclerosis. Arthritis Rheum 1983; 26:794–796.

409. Prouse PJ, Lahiri A, Gumpel JM. The CREST syndrome: Successful reduction of pulmonary hypertension by captopril. Postgraduate Med J 1984; 60:672–674.

410. Rozkovec A, Bernstein R, Asherson RA, Oakley CM. Vascular reactivity and pulmonary hypertension in systemic sclerosis. Arthritis Rheum 1983; 26:1037–1040.
411. Ohar J, Polatty C, Robichaud A, Fowler A, et al. The role of vasodilators in patients with progressive systemic sclerosis: Interstitial lung disease and pulmonary hypertension. Chest 1985; 88 (suppl):263S–265S.
412. Reeves JT, Grover RM, Turkevich D. The case for treatment of selected patients with primary pulmonary hypertension. Am Rev Respir Dis 1986; 134:342–346.
413. Ettinger WH, Wise RA, Stevens MB, Wigley FM. Absence of positional change in pulmonary diffusing capacity in systemic sclerosis. Am J Med 1983; 75:305–312.
414. Robin ED. The kingdom of the near dead: The shortened unnatural life history of primary pulmonary hypertension. Chest 1987; 92:330–334.
415. Rubin LJ, Mendoza J, Hood M, McGoon M, Barst R, Williams WB, Diehl JH, Crow J, Long W. Treatment of primary pulmonary hypertension with continuous intravenous prostacyclin infusion (epoprostenol): Results of a randomized trial. Ann Int Med 1990; 112:485–491.
416. Medsger TA, Dawson WN, Masi AT. The epidemiology of polymyositis. Am J Med 1970; 48:715–723.
417. Bohan A, Peter JB: Polymyositis and dermatomyositis (first of two parts). N Engl J Med 1975; 292:344.
418. Bohan A, Peter JB. Polymyositis and dermatomyositis (second of two parts). N Engl J Med 1975; 292:403.
419. Bohan A, Peter JB, Bowman RL, et al. A computer-assisted analysis of 153 patients with polymyositis and dermatomyositis. Medicine (Baltimore) 1977; 56:255–286.
420. Cronin ME, Miller FW, Plotz PH. Polymyositis and dermatomyositis. In: Schumacher HR, Klippel JH, Robinson DR, eds. Primer on the rheumatic diseases. 9th ed. Atlanta: Arthritis Foundation, 1988, 120–123.
421. Pachman LM, Maryjowski MC. Juvenile dermatomyositis and polymyositis. Clin Rheum Dis 1984; 10:95–115.
422. Mikol J, Felten-Papaiconomou A, Ferchal F, et al. Inclusion body myositis: Clinicopathological studies and isolation of adenovirus type 2 from muscle biopsy specimen. Ann Neurol 1982; 11:576–581.
423. Christensen ML, Pachman LM, Schneiderman R, et al. Prevalence of coxsackie B virus antibodies in patients with juvenile dermatomyositis. Arthritis Rheum 1986; 29:1365–1370.
424. Reichlin M, Arnett FC. Multiplicity of antibodies in myositis sera. Arthritis Rheum 1984; 27:1150–1156.
425. Dawkins RL, Eghtedari A, Holborow EJ. Antibodies to skeletal muscle demonstrated by immunofluorescence in experimental autoallergic myositis. Clin Exp Immunol 1971; 9:329–337.
426. Currie S, Saunders M, Knowles M, et al. Immunological aspects of polymyositis: The in-vitro activity of lymphocytes on incubation with muscle antigen and with muscle cultures. Q J Med 1971; 40:63.
427. Dawkins RL, Mastaglia FL. Cell mediated cytotoxicity to muscle in polymyositis: Effect of immunosuppression. N Engl J Med 1973; 288:434.
428. Kissel JT, Mendell JR, Rammohan KW. Microvascular deposition of complement membrane attack complex in dermatomyositis. N Engl J Med 1986; 314:329–334.
429. Winkelmann RK, Mulder DW, Lambert EH, et al. Course of dermatomyositis-polymyositis: Comparison of untreated and cortisone-treated patients. Mayo Clin Proc 1968; 43:545.
430. Hochberg MC, Feldman D, Stevens MB. Adult onset polymyositis/dermatomyositis: An analysis of clinical and laboratory features and survival in 76 patients with a review of the literature. Semin Arthritis Rheum 1986; 15:168–178.
431. Barnes BE. Dermatomyositis and malignancy. Ann Intern Med 1976; 84:68–76.
432. Callen JP, et al. The relationship of dermatomyositis and polymyositis to internal malignancy. Arch Dermatol 1980; 116:295–298.

433. Callen JP. Malignancy in polymyositis/dermatomyositis. Clin Dermatol 1988; 6:55–63.
434. Manchul LA, Jin A, Pritchard KI, et al. The frequency of malignant neoplasms in patients with polymyositis-dermatomyositis: A controlled study. Arch Intern Med 1985; 145:1835–1839.
435. Dickey BF, Myers AR. Pulmonary disease in polymyositis/dermatomyositis. Semin Arthritis Rheum 1984; 14:60–76.
436. Frazier AR, Miller RD. Interstitial pneumonitis in association with polymyositis and dermatomyositis. Chest 1974; 65:403–407.
437. Salmeron G, Greenberg SD, Lidsky MD. Polymyositis and diffuse interstitial lung disease: A review of the pulmonary histopathologic findings. Arch Intern Med 1981; 141:1005–1010.
438. Takizawa H, Shiga J, Moroi Y, Miyachi S, et al. Interstitial lung disease in dermatomyositis: Clinicopathological study. J Rheumatol 1987; 14:102–107.
439. Duncan PE, Griffin JP, Garcia A, et al. Fibrosing alveolitis in polymyositis: A review of histologically confirmed cases. Am J Med 1974; 37:621–626.
440. Webb DR, Currie GD. Pulmonary fibrosis masking polymyositis. JAMA 1972; 222:1146.
441. Olsen GN, Swenson EW. Polymyositis and interstitial lung disease. Am Rev Respir Dis 1972; 105:611.
442. Camp AV, Lane DJ, Mowat AG. Dermatomyositis with parenchymal lung involvement. Br Med J 1972; 1:155.
443. Songcharoen S, Raju SF, Penebaker JB. Interstitial lung disease in polymyositis and dermatomyositis. J Rheumatol 1980; 7:353–360.
444. Fergusson RJ, Davidson NM, Nuki G, Crompton GK. Dermatomyositis and rapidly progressive fibrosing alveolitis. Thorax 1983; 38:71–72.
445. Thompson PL, Mackay JR. Fibrosing alveolitis and polymyositis. Thorax 1970; 25:504–507.
446. Lakhanpal S, Lie JT, Con DL, Marti WJ. Pulmonary disease in polymyositis/dermatomyositis: A clinicopathological analysis of 65 cases. Ann Rheum Dis 1987; 46:23–29.
447. Schwartz MI, Matthay RA, Sahn SA, Stanford RE, Marmorstein BL, Scheinhorn DJ. Interstitial lung disease in polymyositis and dermatomyositis: Analysis of six cases and review of the literature. Medicine (Baltimore) 1976; 55:89–104.
448. Tazelaar HD, Viggiano RW, Pickersgill J, Colby TV. Interstitial lung disease in polymyositis and dermatomyositis. Clinical features and prognosis as correlated with histologic findings. Am Rev Respir Dis 1990; 141:727–733.
449. Sandbank M, Grunebaum M, Katzenellenbogen I. Dermatomyositis associated with subacute pulmonary fibrosis. Arch Dermatol 1966; 94:432–435.
450. Weaver AL, Brundage BH, Nelson RA, Bischoff MB. Pulmonary involvement in polymyositis: Report of a case with response to corticosteroid therapy. Arthritis Rheum 1968; 11:765–773.
451. Arsura EL, Greenberg AS. Adverse impact of interstitial pulmonary fibrosis on prognosis in polymyositis and dermatomyositis. Semin Arthritis Rheum 1988; 18:29–37.
452. Wasicek CA, Reichlin M, Montes M, et al. Polymyositis and interstitial lung disease in a patient with anti-Jo-1 prototype. Am J Med 1986; 76:538.
453. Arnett FC, et al. The Jo-1 antibody system in myositis: Relationships to clinical features and HLA. J Rheumatol 1981; 8:925–930.
454. Yoshida S, et al. The precipitating antibody to an acidic nuclear antigen, the Jo-1, in connective tissue diseases, a marker for a subset of polymyositis with interstitial pulmonary fibrosis. Arthritis Rheum 1983; 26:606–611.
455. Hochberg MC, Feldman D, Stevens MB, Arnett FC, Reichlin M. Antibody to Jo-1 in polymyositis/dermatomyositis: Association with interstitial pulmonary disease. J Rheum 1984; 11:663–665.
456. Bernstein RM, et al. Anti-Jo-1 antibody: A marker for myositis with interstitial lung disease. Br Med J 1984; 289:151–152.
457. al-Janadi M, Smith CD. Cyclophosphamide treatment of interstitial pulmonary fibrosis in polymyositis/dermatomyositis. J Rheumatol 1989; 16:1592–1596.

458. Phillips TJ, Leigh IM, Wright J. Dermatomyositis and pulmonary fibrosis associated with anti-Jo-1 antibody. J Am Acad Dermatol 1987; 17 (pt 2) :381–382.

459. Targoff IN, Arnett FC, Reichlin M. Antibody to threonyl-transfer RNA synthetase in myositis sera. Arthritis Rheum 1988; 31:515–524.

460. Plotz PH, Dalakas M, Leff RL, Love LA, et al. Current concepts in the idiopathic inflammatory myopathies: Polymyositis, dermatomyositis, and related disorders. Ann Intern Med 1989; 111:143–157.

461. Mathews MB, Bernstein RM. Myositis autoantibody inhibits histidyl-tRNA synthetase: A model for autoimmunity. Nature 1983; 304:177–179.

462. Roose AL, Walton JN. Polymyositis: A survey of 89 cases with particular reference to treatment and prognosis. Brain 1966; 89:747.

463. Lakhanpal S, Lie JT, Conn DL, Martin WJ II. Pulmonary disease in polymyositis/dermatomyositis: A clinicopathological analysis of 65 autopsy cases. Ann Rheum Dis 1987; 46:23–29.

464. Schiavi EA, Roncoroni AJ, Puy RJ. Isolated bilateral diaphragmatic paresis with interstitial lung disease: An unusual presentation of dermatomyositis. Am Rev Respir Dis 1984; 129:337–339.

465. Braun NM, Arora NS, Rochester DF. Respiratory muscle and pulmonary function in polymyositis and other proximal myopathies. Thorax 1983; 38:616–623.

466. Haskard DO. Successful treatment of dermatomyositis complicated by ventilatory failure. Ann Rheum Dis 1983; 42:460.

467. James JL, Park HWJ. Respiratory failure due to polymyositis treated by intermittent positive pressure respiration. Lancet 1961; ii:1281–1282.

468. Carroll N, Branthwaite MA. Control of nocturnal hypoventilation by nasal intermittent positive pressure ventilation. Thorax 1988; 43:349–353.

469. Kerby GR, Mayer LS, Pingleton SK. Nocturnal positive pressure ventilation via nasal mask. Am Rev Respir Dis 1987; 135:738–740.

470. Bunch TW, Tancredi RG, Lie JT. Pulmonary hypertension in polymyositis. Chest 1981; 79:105.

471. Samuels MP, Warner JO. Pulmonary alveolar lipoproteinosis complicating juvenile dermatomyositis. Thorax 1988; 43:939–940.

472. Benbassat J, Gefel D, Larholt K, Sukenik S, et al. Prognostic factors in polymyositis/dermatomyositis: A computer-assisted analysis of ninety-two cases. Arthritis Rheum 1985; 28:249–255.

473. Bookbinder SA, Espinoza LR, Fenske NA, Germain BF, Vasey FB. Methotrexate: Its use in the rheumatic diseases. Clin Exp Rheumatol 1984; 2:185–193.

474. Rowen AJ, Reichel J. Dermatomyositis with lung involvement, successfully treated with azathioprine. Respiration 1983; 44:143–146.

475. Chan JK, Tsang DN, Wong DK. *Penicillium marneffei* in bronchoalveolar lavage fluid. Acta Cytol 1989; 33:523–526.

476. Light RW. Pleural diseases. Philadelphia: Lea & Febiger, 1983, 170.

477. Talal N. Sjögren's syndrome. In: Schumacher HR, Klippel JH, Robinson DR, eds. Primer on the rheumatic diseases. 9th ed. Atlanta: Arthritis Foundation, 1988, 136–138.

478. Whaley K, Webb J, McEvoy BA, et al. Sjögren's syndrome. 2: Clinical associations and immunological phenomena. Q J Med 1973; 42:513.

479. Whaley K, Williamson J, Chisholm DK, et al. Sjögren's syndrome: Sicca components. Q J Med 1973; 42:279.

480. Manthorpe R, Frost-Larsen K, Isager H, et al. Sjögren's syndrome : A review with emphasis on immunological features. Allergy 1981; 36:129.

481. Harley JB, et al. Gene interaction at HLA-DQ enhances autoantibody production in primary Sjögren's syndrome. Science 1986; 232:1145–1147.

482. Kradin RL, Mark EJ. Benign lymphoid disorders of the lung, with a theory regarding their development. Hum Pathol 1983; 14:857–867.

483. Adamson TC, Fox RI, Frisman DM, Howell FV. Immunohistologic analysis of lymphoid infiltrates in primary Sjögren's syndrome. J Immunol 1983; 130:203–208.

484. Miyasaka N, et al. Natural killing activity in Sjögren's syndrome: An analysis of defective mechanisms. Arthritis Rheum 1983; 26:954–960.
485. Fairfax AJ, Haslam PL, Pavia D, Sheahan NF, et al. Pulmonary disorders associated with Sjögren's syndrome. Q J Med 1981; 50:279–295.
486. Strimlan VC, Rosenow ED III, Divertie MB, Harrison EG. Pulmonary manifestations of Sjögren's syndrome. Chest 1976; 70:354–361.
487. Bariffi F, Pesci A, Bertorelli G, Manganelli P, Ambanelli U. Pulmonary involvement in Sjögren's syndrome. Respiration 1984; 46:82–87.
488. Constantopoulos SH, Papadimitriou CS, Moutsopoulos HM. Respiratory manifestations in primary Sjögren's syndrome: A clinical, functional, and histologic study. Chest 1985, 88:226–229.
489. Papathanasiou MP, Constantopoulos SH, Tsampoulas C, Drosos AA, Moutsopoulos HM. Reappraisal of respiratory abnormalities in primary and secondary Sjögren's syndrome: A controlled study. Chest 1986; 90:370–374.
490. Vitali C, Viegi G, Tassoni S, Tavoni A, et al. Lung function abnormalities in different connective tissue diseases. Clin Rheumatol 1986; 5:181–188.
491. Newball HH, Brahim SA. Chronic obstructive airways disease in patients with Sjögren's syndrome. Am Rev Respir Dis 1977; 115:295–304.
492. Segal I, Fink G, Machtey I, Gura V, Spitzer SA. Pulmonary function abnormalities in Sjögren's syndrome and the sicca complex. Thorax 1981; 36:286–289.
493. Andonopoulos AP, Constantopoulos SH, Drosos AA, Moutsopoulos HM. Pulmonary function of nonsmoking patients with rheumatoid arthritis in the presence and absence of secondary Sjögren's syndrome: A controlled study. Respiration 1988; 53:251–258.
494. Karsh J, Moutsopoulos HM, Vergalla J, Jones EA. Protease inhibitor phenotypes and pulmonary disease in patients with Sjögren's syndrome. Respiration 1981; 41:60–65.
495. Constantopoulos SH, Drosos AA, Maddison PJ, Moutsopoulos HM. Xerotrachea and interstitial lung disease in primary Sjögren's syndrome. Respiration 1984; 46:310–314.
496. Oxholm P, Bundgaard A, Birk Madsen E, Manthorpe R, Vejl Rasmussen F. Pulmonary function in patients with primary Sjögren's syndrome. Rheumatol Int 1982; 2:179–181.
497. Constantopoulos SH, Moutsopoulos HM. The respiratory system in Sjögren's syndrome. In: Talal N, Moutsopoulos HM, Kassan SS, eds. Sjögren's syndrome: Clinical and immunological aspects. New York: Springer-Verlag, 1987, 83–88.
498. Liebow AA, Carrington CB. Diffuse pulmonary lymphoreticular infiltrations associated with dysproteinemias. Med Clin North Am 1973; 57:809–842.
499. Marchevsky A, Padilla M, Kaneko M, Kleinerman J. Localized lymphoid nodules of lung: A reappraisal of the lymphoma versus pseudolymphoma dilemma. Cancer 1983; 51:2070–2077.
500. Weis JW, Winter MW, Phyliky RL, et al. Peripheral T-cell lymphoma: Histologic immunohistologic, and clinical characteristics. Mayo Clin Proc 1986; 61:411.
501. Bonner H, Ennis RS, Geelhoed GW, Tarpley EM. Lymphoid infiltration and amyloidosis of lung in Sjögren's syndrome. Arch Pathol 1973; 95:42.
502. Kornfeld S. Clinicopathologic conference: Subcutaneous masses and adenopathy in a 77-year-old man with Sjögren's syndrome and amyloidosis. Am J Med 1989; 86:585–590.
503. Batra P, Collins JD, Magidson JG. Pulmonary nodular amyloidosis presenting as Sjögren's syndrome. J Natl Med Assoc 1983; 75:903–905.
504. Hansen LA, Prakash UB, Colby TV. Pulmonary lymphoma in Sjögren's syndrome. Mayo Clin Proc 1989; 64:920–931.
505. Schuurman HJ, Gooszen HC, Tan IW, Kluin PM, et al. Low-grade lymphoma of immature T-cell phenotype in a case of lymphocytic interstitial pneumonia and Sjögren's syndrome. Histopathology 1987; 11:1193–1204.
506. Walters MT, Stevenson FK, Herbert A, Cawley MI, Smith JL. Lymphoma in Sjögren's syndrome: Urinary monoclonal free light chains as a diagnostic aid and a means of tumour monitoring. Scand J Rheumatol 1986; 61(Suppl):114–117.

507. Asherson RA, Muncey F, Pambakian H, Brostoff J, Hughes GR. Sjögren's syndrome and fibrosing alveolitis complicated by pulmonary lymphoma. Ann Rheum Dis 1987; 46:701–705.
508. Herbert A, Walters MT, Cawley MI, Godfrey RC. Lymphocytic interstitial pneumonia identified as lymphoma of mucosa associated lymphoid tissue. J Pathol 1985; 146:129–138.
509. Kamholz S, Sher A, Barland P, Rosen N, et al. Sjögren's syndrome: Severe upper airways obstruction due to primary malignant tracheal lymphoma developing during successful treatment of lymphocytic interstitial pneumonitis. J Rheumatol 1987; 14:588–594.
510. Walters MT, Stevenson FK, Herbert A, Cawley MI, Smith JL. Urinary monoclonal free light chains in primary Sjögren's syndrome: An aid to the diagnosis of malignant lymphoma. Ann Rheum Dis 1986; 45:209–210.
511. Itescu S, Brancato LJ, Buxbaum J, Gregersen PK, et al. A diffuse infiltrative CD8 lymphocytosis syndrome in human immunodeficiency virus (HIV) infection: A host immune response associated with HLA-DR5. Ann Intern Med 1990; 112:3–10.
512. Collins RD Jr, Ball GV, Logic JR. Gallium-67 scanning in Sjögren's syndrome: Concise communication. J Nucl Med 1984; 25:299–302.
513. Hatron PY, Wallaert B, Gosset D, Tonnel AB, et al. Subclinical lung inflammation in primary Sjögren's syndrome: Relationship between bronchoalveolar lavage cellular analysis findings and characteristics of the disease. Arthritis Rheum 1987; 30:1226–1231.
514. Wallaert B, Prin L, Hatron PY, Ramon P, et al. Lymphocyte subpopulations in bronchoalveolar lavage in Sjögren's syndrome: Evidence for an expansion of cytotoxic/suppressor subset in patients with alveolar neutrophilia. Chest 1987; 92:1025–1031.
515. Miyasaka N, Murota N, Yamaoka K, Sato K, et al. Interleukin 2 defect in the peripheral blood and the lung in patients with Sjögren's syndrome. Clin Exp Immunol 1986; 65:497–505.
516. Moll JM, Haslock I, Macrae IF, Wright V. Associations between ankylosing spondylitis, psoriatic arthritis, Reiter's disease, intestinal arthropathies, and Behçet's syndrome. Medicine 1974; 53:343–364.
517. Nagyhegyi G, Nadas I, Banyai F, Luzsa G, et al. Cardiac and cardiopulmonary disorders in patients with ankylosing spondylitis and rheumatoid arthritis. Clin Exp Rheumatol 1988; 6:17–26.
518. van der Linden S, Valkenburg H, Cats A. The risk of developing ankylosing spondylitis in HLA-B27 positive individuals: A family and population study. Br J Rheum 1983; 22 (suppl2): 18–19.
519. Marks SH, Barnett M, Calin A. Ankylosing spondylitis in women and men: A case-control study. J Rheumatol 1983; 10:624–628.
520. Gran JT, Ostensen M, Husby G. A clinical comparison between males and females with ankylosing spondylitis. J Rheumatol 1985; 12:126–130.
521. Calin A. Ankylosing spondylitis and the spondyl-arthropathies. In: Schumacher HR, Klippel JH, Robinson DR, eds. Primer on the rheumatic diseases. 9th ed. Atlanta: Arthritis Foundation, 1988, 142–147.
522. Rosenow EC, Strimlan CV, Muhm JR, Ferguson RH. Pleuropulmonary manifestations of ankylosing spondylitis. Mayo Clin Proc 1977; 52:641–649.
523. Rumancik WM, Firooznia H, Davis MS Jr, Leitman BS, et al. Fibrobullous disease of the upper lobes: An extraskeletal manifestation of ankylosing spondylitis. J Comput Tomogr 1984; 8:225–229.
524. Davies D. Ankylosing spondylitis and lung fibrosis. Q J Med 1972; 41:395–417.
525. Vale JA, Pickering JG, Scott GW. Ankylosing spondylitis and upper lobe fibrosis and cavitation. Guy's Hosp Rep 1974; 123:97–119.
526. Hurwitz SS, Conlan AA, Krige LP. Fibrocavitating pulmonary lesions in ankylosing spondylitis. S Afr Med J 1982; 61:168–170.
527. Boushea DK, Sundstrom WR. The pleuropulmonary manifestations of ankylosing spondylitis. Semin Arthritis Rheum 1989; 18:277–281.

528. Hillerdal G. Ankylosing spondylitis lung disease: An underdiagnosed entity? Eur J Respir Dis 1983; 64:437–441.
529. Crompton GR, Cameron SJ, Langlands AO, et al. Pulmonary fibrosis, mimicking tuberculosis, presenting before joint symptoms in a female with ankylosing spondylitis. Tubercle 1973; 54:317–320.
530. Levy H, Hurwitz MD, Strimling M, Zwi S. Ankylosing spondylitis lung disease and *Mycobacterium scrofulaceum*. Br J Dis Chest 1988; 82:84–87.
531. Elliott JA, Milne LJ, Cumming D. Chronic necrotizing pulmonary aspergillosis treated with itraconazole. Thorax 1989; 44:820–821.
532. Stewart RM, Ridyard JB, Pearson JD. Regional lung function in ankylosing spondylitis. Thorax 1976; 31:433–437.
533. Parkin A, Robinson PJ, Hickling P. Regional lung ventilation in ankylosing spondylitis. Br J Radiol 1982, 55:833–836.
534. Farquhar DR, Chamberlain MJ, McCain GA, Morgan WK. Clearance of inhaled particles in ankylosing spondylitis. Ann Rheum Dis 1989; 48:974–977.
535. Sharp JT, Sweany SK, Henry JP, Pietras RJ, Meadows WR, Amarat E, Rubinstein HM. Lung and thoracic compliances in ankylosing spondylitis. J Lab Clin Med 1964; 63:254–263.
536. Travis DM, Cook CD, Julian DG, Crump CH, Helliesen P, Robin ED, Bayles TB, Burwell CS. The lungs in rheumatoid spondylitis. Am J Med 1960; 29:623–632.
537. Fetelius N, Hedenstrom H, Hillerdal G, and Hallgren R. Pulmonary involvement in ankylosing spondylitis. Ann Rheum Dis 1986; 45:736–740.
538. Vanderschueren D, Decramer M, Van den Daele P, Dequeker J. Pulmonary function and maximal transrespiratory pressures in ankylosing spondylitis. Ann Rheum Dis 1982; 48:632–635.
539. Franssen MJ, van Herwaarden CL, van de Putte LB, Gribnau FW. Lung function in patients with ankylosing spondylitis: A study of the influence of disease activity and treatment with nonsteroidal anti-inflammatory drugs. J Rheumatol 1986, 13:936–940.
540. Elliott CG, Hill TR, Adams TE, Crapo RO, et al. Exercise performance of subjects with ankylosing spondylitis and limited chest expansion. Bull Eur Physiopathol Respir 1985, 21:363–368.
541. Citrin BL, Bradley GW. Ventilatory function and transfer factor in ankylosing spondylitis. Scott Med J 1973; 18:109–113.
542. Grimby G, Fighl Meyer AR, Blomstrand A. Partitioning of the contributions of ribcage and abdomen to ventilation in ankylosing spondylitis. Thorax 1972; 29:1779–1784.
543. Josenhans WT, Wang CS, Josenhans G, et al. Diaphragmatic contribution to ventilation in patients with ankylosing spondylitis. Respiration 1971; 28:331–346.
544. McAdam LP, O'Hanlan MA, Bluestone R, et al. Relapsing polychondritis: Prospective study of 23 patients and a review of the literature. Medicine 1976; 55:193.
545. Pearson CM, Kline HM, Newcomber VD. Relapsing polychondritis. N Engl J Med 1960; 263:51.
546. Dolan DL, Lemmon GB, Teitelbaum SL. Relapsing polychondritis: Analytical literature review and studies on pathogenesis. Am J Med 1966; 41:285.
547. Chondritis of the left ear, orbital swelling and respiratory stridor. Case Records of the Massachusetts General Hospital (Case 51-1982) N Engl J Med 1982; 307:1631–1639.
548. Michet CJ, McKenna CH, Luthra HS, O'Fallon WM. Relapsing polychondritis: Survival and predictive role of early disease manifestations. Ann Intern Med 1986; 104:74–78.
549. Valenzuela R, Cooperrider PA, Gogate P, et al. Relapsing polychondritis: Immunomicroscopic findings in cartilage of ear biopsy specimens. Hum Pathol 1980; 11:19.
550. Homma S, Matsumoto T, Abe H, et al. Relapsing polychondritis: Pathological and immunological findings in an autopsy case. Acta Pathol Jpn 1984; 34:1137.
551. Herman JH, Dennis MV. Immunopathologic studies in relapsing polychondritis. J Clin Invest 1973; 52:549.

552. Ebringer R, et al. Autoantibodies to cartilage and type II collagen in relapsing polychondritis and other rheumatic diseases. Ann Rheum Dis 1981; 40:473–479.
553. Kindblom LG, Dalen P, Edmar G, et al. Relapsing polychondritis: A clinical, pathologic-anatomic and histochemical study of 2 cases. Acta Pathol Microbiol Scand 1977; 85:656.
554. Dryll A, Lansaman J, Meyer O, et al. Relapsing polychondritis: An ultrastructural study of elastic and collagen fibers degradation revealed by tannic acid. Virchows Arch 1981; 390:109.
555. Krell WS, Staats BA, Hyatt RE. Pulmonary function in relapsing polychondritis. Am Rev Respir Dis 1986; 133:1120–1123.
556. Mohsenifar Z, Tashkin DP, Carson SA, Bellamy PE. Pulmonary function in patients with relapsing polychondritis. Chest 1982; 81:711–727.
557. Gibson GJ, Davis P. Respiratory complications of relapsing polychondritis. Thorax 1974; 29:726–731.
558. Reichlin M, Mattioli M. Correlation of a precipitin reaction to an RNA protein antigen and a low prevalence nephritis in patients with systemic lupus erythematosus. N Engl J Med 1972; 286:908–911.
559. Sharp GC, Irvin WS, Tan EM, et al. Mixed connective tissue disease: An apparently distinct rheumatic disease syndrome associated with a specific antibody to an extractable nuclear antigen (ENA). Am J Med 1972; 52:148–159.
560. Nimelstein SH, Brody S, McShane D. Mixed connective tissue disease: A subsequent evaluation of the original 255 patients. Medicine (Baltimore) 1980; 59:239–248.
561. Sullivan WD, Hurst DJ, Harmon CE, et al. A prospective evaluation emphasizing pulmonary involvement in patients with mixed connective tissue disease. Medicine 1984; 63:92–107.
562. Lazaro MA, Maldonado Cocco JA, Catoggio LJ, Babini SM, Messina OD, Garcia Morteo O. Clinical and serologic characteristics of patients with overlap syndrome: Is mixed connective tissue disease a distinct clinical entity? Medicine (Baltimore) 1989; 68:58–65.
563. Raumussen EK, Ullman S, Hier-Madsen M, Sorensen SF, Halberg P. Clinical implications of ribonucleoprotein antibody. Arch Dermatol 1987; 123:601–605.
564. Alarcon-Segovia D, Cardiel MH. Comparison between three diagnostic criteria for mixed connective tissue disease: Study of 593 patients. J Rheumatol 1989; 16:328–334.
565. Harmon C, et al. Pulmonary involvement in mixed connective tissue disease (MCTD). Arthritis Rheum 1976; 19:801.
566. Prakash UB, Luthra HS, Divertie MB. Intrathoracic manifestations in mixed connective tissue disease. Mayo Clin Proc 1985; 60:813–821.
567. Derderian SS, Tellis CJ, Abbrecht PH, Welton RC, Rajagopal KR. Pulmonary involvement in mixed connective tissue disease. Chest 1985; 88:45–48.
568. Silver TM, Farber SJ, Bole GG, Martel W. Radiological features of mixed connective tissue disease and scleroderma: Systemic lupus erythematosus overlap. Radiology 1976; 120:269–275.
569. Wiener-Kronish JP, Solinger AM, Warnock ML, Churg A, et al. Severe pulmonary involvement in mixed connective tissue disease. Am Rev Respir Dis 1981; 124:499–503.
570. Clinicopathologic Conference: Mixed connective tissue disease. Am J Med 1978; 65:833.
571. Martens J, Demedts M. Diaphragm dysfunction in mixed connective tissue disease: A case report. Scand J Rheumatol 1982; 11:165–167.
572. Yazdy AM, Park MC, Supinski G. Restrictive ventilatory defect associated with pulmonary hypertension in mixed connective tissue disease (letter). J Rheumatol 1990; 17:121–123.
573. Hosoda Y, Suzuki Y, Takano M, Tojo T, Homma M. Mixed connective tissue disease with pulmonary hypertension: A clinical and pathological study. J Rheumatol 1987; 14:826–830.
574. Kitridou RC, Akmal M, Turkel SB, Ehresmann GR, et al. Renal involvement in mixed connective tissue disease: A longitudinal clinicopathologic study. Semin Arthritis Rheum 1986; 16:135–145.

575. Hainaut P, Lavenne E, Magy JM, Lebacq EG. Circulating lupus type anticoagulant and pulmonary hypertension associated with mixed connective tissue disease. Clin Rheumatol 1986; 5:96–101.

576. Guit GL, Shaw PC, Ehrlich J, Kroon HM, Oudkerk M. Mediastinal lymphadenopathy and pulmonary arterial hypertension in mixed connective tissue disease. Radiology 1985; 154:305–306.

577. Ueda N, Mimura K, Maeda H, Sugiyama T, et al. Mixed connective tissue disease with fatal pulmonary hypertension and a review of literature. Virchows Arch 1984; 404:335–340.

578. Graziano FM, Friedman LC, Grossman J. Pulmonary hypertension in a patient with mixed connective tissue disease: Clinical and pathologic findings, and review of literature. Clin Exp Rheumatol 1983; 1:251–255.

579. Kobayashi H, Sano T, Ii K, Hizawa K, et al. Mixed connective tissue disease with fatal pulmonary hypertension. Acta Pathol Jpn 1982; 32:1121–1129.

580. Jones MB, Osterholm RK, Wilson RB, et al. Fatal pulmonary hypertension and resolving immune-complex glomerulonephritis in mixed connective tissue disease (MCTD). Am J Med 1978; 65:855–863.

581. Alpert MA, Goldberg SH, Singsen BH, Durham JB, et al. Cardiovascular manifestations of mixed connective tissue disease in adults. Circulation 1983; 68:1182–1193.

582. Hoogsteden HC, van Dongen JJ, van der Kwast TH, Hooijkaas H, Hilvering C. Bilateral exudative pleuritis, an unusual pulmonary onset of mixed connective tissue disease. Respiration 1985; 48:164–167.

583. Germain MJ, Davidman M. Pulmonary hemorrhage and acute renal failure in a patient with mixed connective tissue disease. Am J Kidney Dis 1984; 3:420–424.

3

Drug-Induced Infiltrative Lung Diseases

Edward C. Rosenow III

The clinician must always be concerned that a drug a patient is ingesting could be responsible for the diffuse inflitrative lung disease seen on the chest roentgenogram. More than 50 drugs are known to produce a diffuse infiltrative pulmonary process, and occasionally dyspnea or cough may be the only symptom before the chest roentgenogram becomes abnormal. Yet these symptoms may represent the early stages of a progressive pulmonary process, and only by recognizing that a drug is responsible, stopping it, and possibly initiating corticosteroids will the process be reversed. Table 3-1 lists the drugs that will be reviewed in this chapter.[1-11] The patient may not volunteer that he or she is taking one of these medications, making it important for the clinician to inquire specifically about all medications that the patient is taking or has recently taken. Some of the chemotherapeutic agents cause a diffuse pulmonary process not clinically evident for days, weeks, or occasionally months after completion of a course of therapy.

In the absence of a national registry, little is known about the incidence of the adverse effects of drugs on the lungs. It is estimated that only a little over half of the physicians in the United States are aware of the Food and Drug Administration's reporting system, and fewer than 1% of physicians report adverse drug reactions![12] The estimated incidence of adverse reactions to nitrofurantoin ranges from 0.0005% to 0.2%.[13-15] The incidence of drug-induced pulmonary disease in patients receiving a chemotherapeutic agent probably ranges from 1% to 10% and may reach as high as 50% when other risk factors are added, such as when high-concentration inspired oxygen is administered to a patient receiving bleomycin. In many of these patients, the diagnosis is of a fatal pulmonary disease due to an opportunistic infection. The infection may also be present, but it may be masking the seriousness of the chemotherapy-induced reaction affecting the lung. Since there is no specific diagnostic blood test, chest radiographic pattern, or characteristic histology, it is very difficult to make a specific diagnosis of an adverse drug reaction in almost any organ, including the lung.

TABLE 3-1. Drugs Causing Infiltrative Lung Diseases

Chemotherapeutic	**Illicit**
Azathioprine	Ethvinyl chloride (Placidyl)
Bleomycin	Heroin
Busulfan	Propoxyphene HCl (Darvon)
Chlorambucil	Methadone HCl
Cyclophosphamide	Talc (magnesium silicate)
Cytosine arabinoside (Ara-C)	**Anti-inflammatory**
Melphalan	Acetylsalicylic acid
Methotrexate	Gold
Mitomycin-C	Penicillamine
Nitrosoureas	**Miscellaneous**
Procarbazine	Hydantoins
Vinblastine	Hydralazine HCl
Cardiovascular	Isoniazid
Amiodarone	Penicillamine
Tocainide	Procainamide HCl
Antibiotics	Tricyclics
Nitrofurantoin	
Sulfasalazine (azulfidine)	

The following criteria must be met before it can be concluded that a patient has had an adverse pulmonary reaction to a drug: (1) the patient is taking or has recently taken a drug known to induce pulmonary disease; (2) the histology, even though relatively nonspecific, is consistent with an adverse drug reaction; and (3) other causes have been excluded.

PATHOGENESIS

The mechanisms of drug-induced infiltrative lung disease are not well understood. Unfortunately, there are no good animal models, with the exception of bleomycin in rodents. Several mechanisms are becoming clear; more knowledge will no doubt lead to further clarifications.[7,16–20] The adverse reaction can be either direct through the drug itself or a metabolite of the drug, or indirect through the induction of immune-mediated or inflammatory mechanisms. However, as stated, animal models are few, and attempts to identify particular drugs as antigens with laboratory procedures have met with little success. When known, mechanisms are discussed in this chapter within specific drug groupings. It is hypothesized that the chemotherapeutic agents and chronically used nitrofurantoin cause oxidant injury through oxygen-derived substances such as hydroxyl radicals ($\cdot$OH), superoxide (O_2^-), hydrogen peroxide (H_2O_2), and singlet oxygen ($^1O_2$).[18,21] Oxidant radicals generate single-electron transfers that disrupt critical cell functions, producing death of the cell. This is one explanation of why an elevated $F_{I_{O_2}}$ in the patient who is receiving or has recently received bleomycin leads to a severe and potentially lethal pulmonary reaction.[22] Not all those receiving supplemental oxygen develop this reaction, however, nor is this reaction seen with most of the other chemotherapeutic agents. Some of these single-electron transfers are momentary reactions lasting less than a second, making it difficult to measure the metabolite or the reaction itself.

There are 30 drugs known to produce an amphophilic reaction in various tissues, including the lung, with the deposition of phospholipids within the cell. The most important is amiodarone.[17,23,24] It is unknown whether phospholipid deposition is a primary reaction that leads to lung injury or an incidental or secondary phenomenon unrelated to the diffuse pulmonary infiltrative reaction.

With some chemotherapeutic drug–induced pulmonary disease, the mechanism is probably a direct toxic reaction. This may be particularly evident with bleomycin in addition to its single-electron oxidant mechanism. Certain epidermal cells in the lung and skin contain lower levels of a specific inactivating enzyme, which allows the drug to accumulate within these cells, pass through the nuclear membrane, and produce damage by fragmentation of DNA.[25] The type I epithelial cell is the first cell to be affected; type II cells attempt to repair the type I cell defect and in the process are converted to type I cells in order to restore the normal air-blood barrier. The reactivity of the type II cell depends on the phase of the cell cycle it is in; if it is in the resting G_0 phase, the cell appears resistant to bleomycin injury, whereas if it is in the proliferative or transformation phases, significant cellular changes occur. Bleomycin has also been shown to stimulate fibroblasts directly to increase collagen synthesis. If the drug is given repeatedly, as is done with bleomycin, it will eventually be given at a time when the type II cells are in the proliferative or transformation phase and thus cellular changes will occur, leading to eventual pulmonary reaction. With bleomycin, unlike some other chemotherapeutic agents, there is a definite correlation with age and with dose.

Drug-induced systemic lupus erythematosus (SLE) is another drug-induced diffuse infiltrative lung disease in which there is some understanding of the mechanism.[26] There appear to be two groups of drugs associated with drug-induced SLE. The first group commonly elicits antinuclear antibody (ANA) formation in a large percentage of individuals taking the drug, but only a small proportion of these develop typical clinical symptoms of SLE. The second group consists of numerous drugs that have been reported to induce SLE rarely. In this group, the positive ANA reaction appears to correlate with the clinical syndrome of SLE. It is unknown how drugs incite antibodies to nuclear protein, since these drugs in themselves are nonimmunogenic. In drug-induced SLE, the antibodies are primarily against histones. This is in contrast to idiopathic SLE, where the antinuclear antibodies are more heterogeneous and consist of antibodies against native DNA nonhistone ribonuclear protein and histones as well as antibodies against extranuclear host components such as clotting factors.[26] One hypothesis is that the drug acts as an adjuvant or an immunostimulant, producing a disorder in the immune regulation system rather than inducing an abnormality in the effector cell. Autoimmunity then develops from the clonal expansion of cell-reacting lymphocytes, which are ordinarily held in check by a balance of helper and suppressor influences. Thus, the autoimmunity is not due to an alteration of self-constituents.

CLINICAL PRESENTATION

Chemotherapeutic drug–induced infiltrative lung disorders are among the more common and serious problems the pulmonologist and oncologist encounter. If the disorder goes unrecognized and the drug is not discontinued, the course is frequently fatal. Even when the drug is discontinued and corticosteroids are administered the process may progress to an irreversible subacute lung injury, resulting in respiratory failure and death. Chemotherapeutic agents are usually classified as antibiotics, alkylating agents, antimetabolites, nitrosoureas, and others. However, this classification has shed very little light on their pathogenetic potential and does little to help the clinician predict which patient will develop a significant pulmonary disease. Therefore, in this chapter each drug is discussed individually without any relationship to the category in which it belongs.

The clinical presentation and histology, however, do allow chemotherapeutic agents to be categorized as cytotoxic or noncytotoxic. Table 3-2 lists the drugs in each category. A cytotoxic reaction characteristically produces atypia in type II pneumocytes and other epithelial cells and is frequently fatal if the disorder goes unrecognized and the drug is not discontinued. The noncytotoxic reactions, however, with the exception of the reaction to cytosine arabinoside, are largely hypersensitivity phenomena in which eosinophilia is common, the onset is acute, and reversal is fairly rapid on discontinuing the drug. These are rarely fatal. They may be associated with granuloma formation, unlike cytotoxic reactions.

The clinical presentation of patients with cytotoxic drug–induced infiltrative lung disorder characteristically consists of dyspnea, nonproductive cough, and frequently fever. These symptoms may occur before any abnormalities appear on a chest roentgenogram. Fever is usually not associated with chills and may not be present daily, but the vast majority of patients, at some time in the course of an adverse chemotherapeutic drug reaction affecting the lungs, have associated fever. This presentation mimics opportunistic infection or recurring underlying lung disease such as those associated with the hematologic malignancies, making at all the more difficult to diagnose the exact etiology of the patient's pulmonary problem.

TABLE 3-2. Cytotoxic and Noncytotoxic Chemotherapeutic Agents

CYTOTOXIC	**NONCYTOTOXIC**
Azathioprine	Bleomycin
Bleomycin	Cytosine arabinoside (Ara-C)
Busulfan	Methotrexate
Chlorambucil	Procarbazine
Cyclophosphamide	
Melphalan	
Mitomycin-C	
Nitrosoureas	
Procarbazine	
Vinblastine	

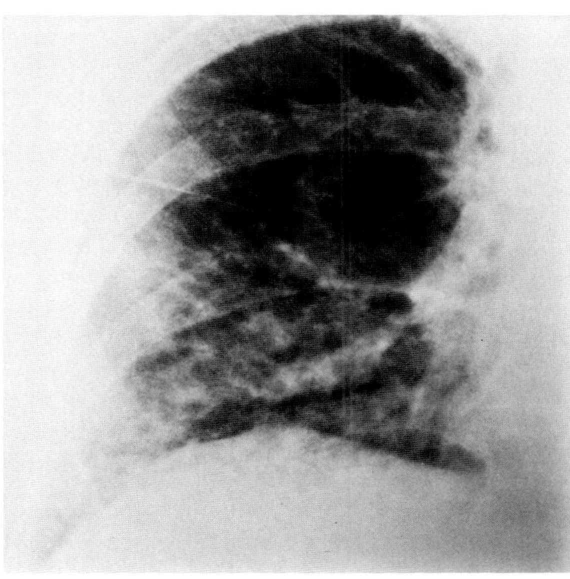

Figure 3-1. Cytotoxic lung. This enlarged view of a chest roentgenogram of cytotoxic lung shows predominantly interstitial changes with subtle intra-alveolar involvement. In this case, changes are greater at the bases, but involvement can be highly asymmetric.

Dyspnea, cough, and fever usually do not appear until at least a few weeks, and usually several weeks to a few months, after drug therapy is begun. In some situations, such as with busulfan (which is used over a period of years in some patients), symptoms may not begin for 6 to 12 months or more, and sometimes not for years. With cyclophosphamide there are several reports of the onset of the pulmonary process not beginning until months or even years after the discontinuation of therapy.

With the noncytotoxic drugs, particularly methotrexate and occasionally bleomycin and procarbazine, the onset of pulmonary symptoms and fever is more acute.

ASSESSMENT

A chest roentgenogram is usually the first test ordered in assessing new symptoms of cough and dyspnea; initially it may be unremarkable, but most commonly it shows an interstitial and occasionally an intra-alveolar process, sometimes before the patient is symptomatic (Figure 3-1). Initially it is very common for the infiltrates to be asymmetrical, sometimes apparently involving only one lung. The infiltrates do not migrate, even in hypersensitivity reactions involving eosinophilia. Pleural effusion occurs in fewer than 10% of these patients and is almost always a small amount. Hilar and mediastinal adenopathy is rare with the exception of methotrexate pneumonitis in children.

Pulmonary function tests invariably disclose abnormalities in individuals with diffuse infiltrative lung disease, particularly in comparison with pre-chemotherapeutic pulmonary function. If the patient is at risk because of limited respiratory reserve, then pulmonary function studies should be done and the risks of chemotherapy should be explained to the patient before the therapy is initiated. A decrease in the carbon monoxide diffusing capacity (DLCO) is usually the first abnormality seen, occurring before the onset of symptoms or chest roentgenographic abnormalities. DLCO monitoring may be an adequate test for following the patient at rest or with suspected early drug-induced infiltrative lung disorders. This parameter has been well studied with bleomycin; a decline greater than 15%, adjusted for hemoglobin, should be considered significant and the decision should be made as to whether to continue therapy or not.[27] It is possible that other "unrelated" disorders, such as congestive heart failure or pneumonia, also affect the DLCO. A fall in the DLCO is not as predictive of pneumonitis with methotrexate as it is with the cytotoxic agents.

CYTOTOXIC CHEMOTHERAPEUTIC AGENTS

Azathioprine.   **Azathioprine** has been associated with several well-documented instances of adverse interstitial lung disease, but considering that this drug is used in so many different disorders, including nonmalignant ones, the incidence of an adverse pulmonary reaction must be quite low.[28]

Bleomycin.   It is estimated that 10% of patients receiving **bleomycin** develop an adverse pulmonary reaction.[29–36] Of this group, in 10% (or 1% overall) the reaction is fatal. If supplemental oxygen or thoracic radiation is given within six months of bleomycin, the incidence of adverse reaction may be as high as 50%.[1,3,4,8,22,31,33,37–41] Also, if the total dose of bleomycin exceeds 450 units or if the patient is over age 70, the incidence increases significantly—a pattern that is unique to bleomycin and in contrast to that for other chemotherapeutic agents. In fact, bleomycin dosage is cumulative and the overall reaction does not necessarily relate to the current course of therapy.

As with other chemotherapeutic agents, the onset of dyspnea, nonproductive cough, and (almost always) fever is insidious. Chest roentgenograms show a diffuse interstitial process that is generally, but not always, greater at the bases and may be asymmetrical in its distribution, as stated earlier. In addition, bleomycin pneumonitis can produce a unique nodularity on chest roentgenogram and chest CT scan that mimics nodular metastasis.[42–47] It is important to recognize this possibility, because these nodules may be misinterpreted as malignancy, leading to further use of bleomycin with consequent further harm to the patient. Scharstain and colleagues state that the nodular radiologic findings are quite typical of bleomycin pneumonitis and, as such, biopsy to exclude metastatic disease may not be necessary. One group of authors reports granuloma formation within these nodules.[46]

Histologically, early endothelial damage is followed by destruction of type I and hyperplasia of type II pneumocytes. A "bizarre" atypia of type II pneumocytes is invariably present and is similar to that seen with all cytotoxic drug–induced interstitial pneumonitides (Fig. 3-2).

The association of supplemental oxygen and the onset of bleomycin pneumonitis cannot be stressed strongly enough, as many of these patients have been incorrectly diagnosed as having adult respiratory distress syndrome (ARDS). In many cases this course of events occurs during elective surgery, possibly for reasons unrelated to the

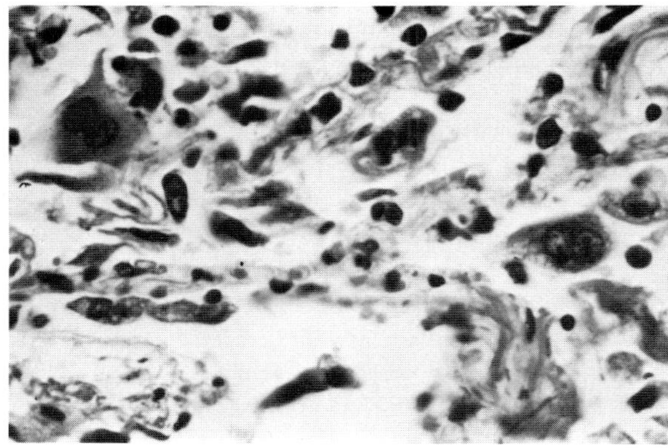

Figure 3-2. Cytotoxic lung. In this specimen there is marked atypia of almost all the cells, particularly the type II pneumocyte. Note that the nuclear:cytoplasmic ratio remains normal. In malignant cells, by contrast, the nuclear:cytoplasmic ratio is increased.

neoplastic process, the patient receiving supplemental oxygen during surgery and in the postoperative period as is routinely given. The anesthesiologist must be made aware that the patient has been receiving bleomycin, even as long ago as 1 year (? longer), and the $F_{I_{O_2}}$ must be kept below 0.25 if at all possible.[22] The intriguing question is why other chemotherapeutic agents with similar clinical, radiologic, and histologic findings do not show this supplemental oxygen–related toxicity.

Computed tomography of the chest may have some value in predicting bleomycin pulmonary toxicity.[43] Bleomycin produces its greatest effects radiologically in the posterior aspects of the lung. These changes may be seen on CT before becoming evident on the chest roentgenogram. The results of bronchoalveolar lavage have been reported in only four patients and show a wide range of abnormalities, including an increase in polymorphonuclear leukocytes (PMNs) and lymphocytosis.[48] Animal studies have shown that the type of cell increase depends on the stage of bleomycin toxicity: PMNs predominate early in the course of the disease while lymphocytes predominate after the third week.[49] It is not known whether supplemental oxygen or radiation influences the results of bronchoalveolar lavage. There is some indication that serum angiotensin converting enzyme can be used as a predictor of toxicity.[50] With toxicity the level recedes below normal.

Busulfan. **Busulfan** therapy for chronic hematologic disorders is unusual in that some patients may take this drug for 5 to 10 years or more before developing pulmonary toxicity. Masson and colleagues reviewed the literature, summarizing 56 cases, and estimated that 6% of patients receiving busulfan will develop an interstitial fibrosis and that 84% of these will die.[51] In at least two cases busulfan pneumonitis began within 6 weeks of initiation of therapy. The clinical, radiologic, and histologic presentations resemble those associated with other cytotoxic chemotherapeutic agents. Alveolar proteinosis is a very unusual complication of busulfan therapy; whether it is busulfan or an underlying chronic hematologic process that predisposes to this complication is unknown.[52,53] Vergnon and co-workers reported on bronchoalveolar lavage in three patients with busulfan pulmonary toxicity. A predominantly lymphocytic alveolitis indicated a more favorable prognosis than did a mixed alveolitis.[54]

Chlorambucil. Approximately a dozen well-documented cases of **chlorambucil** infiltrative lung disorder have been reported. The presentation and findings are similar to those associated with other cytotoxic agents.[55]

Cyclophosphamide. **Cyclophosphamide** may be one of the most underrated inducers of diffuse infiltrative lung disorders.[1,3–6,8,10,56–62] It has been well documented that the onset, progressing to a fatal pulmonary fibrosis, can occur after completion of therapy.[63,64] Cyclophosphamide interstitial pneumonitis and fibrosis does not appear to be age- or dose-related and the onset can occur at any time from less than 3 weeks to many years later. The incidence is probably under 1%; this drug has been available for many years and is used in a number of nonmalignant conditions, such as Wegener's granulomatosis and polyarteritis nodosa, for example. The clinical course and radiologic changes are similar to those associated with other cytotoxic agents.

Melphalan. There are 12 to 15 well-documented cases of **melphalan**-induced pulmonary toxicity. The clinical, radiologic, and histologic changes are similar to those already mentioned.[65,66]

Mitomycin-C. This is an unusual chemotherapeutic agent having three distinct types of adverse pulmonary reactions, which may overlap.[67–71] It is associated with the typical interstitial pneumonitis and fibrosis described with other cytotoxic agents, with a noncardiac pulmonary edema, and with a microangiopathic hemolytic anemia with renal insufficiency and pulmonary edema.

Noncardiac pulmonary edema has been reported to occur with a single dose of the drug, whereas in patients who develop microangiopathic hemolytic anemia and pulmonary edema the onset is usually delayed for 6 to 12 months. Most of those who develop microangiopathic hemolytic anemia and pulmonary edema have received either 5-fluorouracil (5-FU) or blood transfusions just before the onset of the adverse reaction. The treatment is supportive.

Nitrosoureas. All four **nitrosoureas** (BCNU, CCNU, methyl-CCNU, and DCNU) have been reported to produce pulmonary toxicity. The estimated incidence of adverse pulmonary effects ranges from 1% to 20%.[72–75]

Vinblastine. In addition to typical cytotoxic effects on the lungs, **vinblastine** can produce bronchospasm.[76–78] Even though it is one of the older chemotherapeutic agents, the adverse effects of vinblastine have been recognized only recently, probably because only in the last few years has it been used in combination with mitomycin-C, which may produce a synergistic pulmonary infiltrative disorder.

NONCYTOTOXIC CHEMOTHERAPEUTIC AGENTS

Bleomycin and Procarbazine. Both **bleomycin and procarbazine**, which produce predominant cytotoxic effects in the lung, have also been associated with a few cases each of a hypersensitivity type of pneumonitis, frequently associated with eosinophilia.[1,3,4] The pneumonitis has a rapid onset and regresses rapidly on discontinuing the drug. Sometimes the use of corticosteroids is required. No fatal case has been reported.

Cytosine Arabinoside.   Cytosine arabinoside (ARA-C) produces a most unusual adverse reaction in the lung, unlike that of any other drug-induced pulmonary disease—a noncardiac pulmonary edema with approximately 50% mortality.[79–82] Clinically, it presents as an adult respiratory distress syndrome (ARDS) and is frequently misdiagnosed as this entity. The treatment is unknown, but presumably an intensive trial of corticosteroids is worth considering in view of the highly fatal nature of this disorder.

Methotrexate.   Methotrexate is a unique drug with hundreds of case reports of a noncytotoxic effect that is frequently associated with eosinophilia.[1,3–6,8,10,83–85] In at least one-third of the cases, granulomas are evident on lung biopsy.

Methotrexate pneumonitis is most common in children being treated for acute lymphocytic leukemia, but an intriguing finding is that the leukemia is always in remission at the time of the onset and diagnosis of methotrexate pneumonitis. The pneumonitis can begin within a few days or after months of use of methotrexate. It is fairly rapid in onset, usually associated with fever, and rarely associated with adverse effects on other organs. Eosinophilia is seen in one-half of cases. The chest roentgenogram usually shows a uniform interstitial process and occasionally hilar lymphadenopathy. This is the only adverse drug effect on the lungs in which there is an associated adenopathy. Pleural effusion is seen in a small percentage of cases. Corticosteroids are the treatment of choice, although discontinuing the drug may be all that is necessary to bring about a resolution. An intriguing characteristic of methotrexate pneumonitis is that it may not recur after rechallenge with the drug. This is unexplained.

It is recognized that methotrexate pneumonitis occurs in about 5% of patients receiving this drug in low doses (averaging less than 15 mg/week), usually for rheumatoid arthritis.[2,3–6,9–11,86–88] The onset can occur from a few weeks to over a year after treatment is initiated. There have been a few fatal cases, but most patients respond to discontinuation of the drug and, if necessary, treatment with corticosteroids.[89] Granulomas are also seen histologically in this setting. An interesting association is a higher incidence of methotrexate pneumonitis in patients concomitantly using nitrofurantoin (Fig. 3-3).

Bronchoalveolar lavage in methotrexate pneumonitis shows a predominant lymphocyte alveolitis, mostly of the helper cell variety, suggesting a hypersensitivity pneumonitis.[83,90,91]

CARDIOVASCULAR DRUGS

Amiodarone.   Amiodarone pneumonitis is relatively common, affecting an estimated 6% of the patients receiving the drug. The adverse reaction is always in the form of an interstitial pneumonitis and fibrosis.[2,92,93] Over 90% of patients with an adverse reaction are receiving at least 400 mg amiodarone per day and have been on the medication for at least 2 months. In the majority, the onset is insidious, with dyspnea or

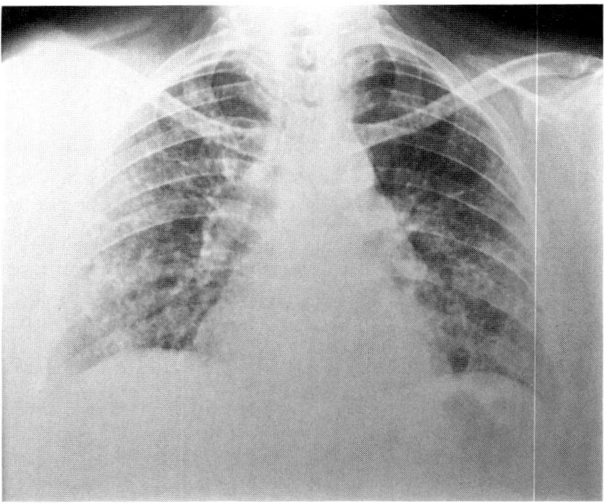

Figure 3-3. Methotrexate pneumonitis. This chest roentgenogram is from a 56-year-old patient with rheumatoid arthritis who received less than 15 mg of methotrexate per day. The pneumonitis was significantly reduced by stopping the drug and adding prednisone. Histology showed granulomas.

nonproductive cough being the first manifestations. A low-grade fever without chills can also occur. These symptoms usually precede chest roentgenographic findings, which consist of a diffuse interstitial or alveolar process (Fig. 3-4). Commonly these are initially asymmetric and occasionally they may mimic the peripheral infiltrative patterns seen in chronic eosinophilic pneumonitis. In a minority of the patients, the onset of symptoms is subacute to acute, mimicking pneumonitis, which is one of the major differential diagnoses in this setting. Pleuritic chest pain occurs in approximately 10% of patients. Pleural effusion has been reported in only a few cases. Clubbing has not been reported.

Because all of these patients have underlying heart disease, congestive heart failure is the usual major differential diagnosis in addition to an infectious pneumonia. An elevated sedimentation rate is very common and would help exclude congestive heart failure, but this is not sufficient alone to make the diagnosis. There is no eosinophilia and the antinuclear antibody test is usually negative. Pulmonary function tests disclose diminished total lung capacity and carbon monoxide diffusing capacity as well as hypoxemia, but these findings are also present with congestive heart failure and pneumonia.[92–94] A gallium-67 radionuclide lung scan will demonstrate increased uptake over the lungs with amiodarone pneumonitis whereas it would be negative in congestive heart failure. It may therefore be of some value in separating these two entities, as would the measurements of capillary wedge pressure.[95]

There is some evidence that prior amiodarone use with or without pulmonary toxicity predisposes to postoperative noncardiac pulmonary edema, possibly precipitated by supplemental oxygen.[96,97]

The results of bronchoalveolar lavage in amiodarone pneumonitis are variable.[23,92,98,99] All patients with amiodarone pneumonitis exhibit phospholipidosis of the alveolar macrophage; in fact, this is seen in the majority of patients on amiodarone for more than 2 months who die of nonpulmonary causes. Phospholipidosis of alveolar macrophages therefore cannot be used as a diagnostic feature; its absence, however, precludes a diagnosis of amiodarone pneumonitis and fibrosis. If the differ-

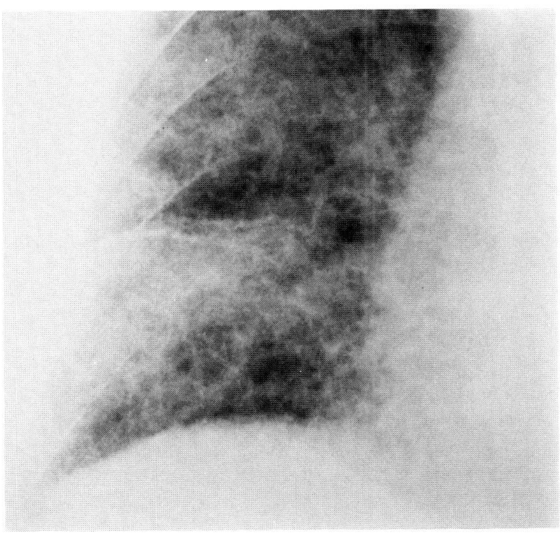

Figure 3-4. Advanced amiodarone pneumonitis and fibrosis. This is an enlarged view of the chest roentgenogram of a 76-year-old patient.

ential cell count of the bronchoalveolar lavage fluid is normal, the diagnosis of amiodarone pneumonitis cannot be made. If there are elevated levels of PMNs or lymphocytes and other causes have been excluded, then the diagnosis of amiodarone pneumonitis can be made.

Treatment consists of discontinuing the drug. In most cases this will be sufficient. Some patients will show no evidence of regression and will require the addition of corticosteroids. Approximately 10% of those affected will progress to diffuse pulmonary fibrosis and die. In some patients amiodarone is so critical for control of serious ventricular dysrhythmias that the cardiologist must maintain the drug. At this time, the dose is reduced to the lowest level to control the dysrhythmia and the patient is maintained on corticosteroids. The pulmonary process may progress in spite of such measures.

Lung biopsy is used primarily to exclude other disorders and is not usually done, the clinician relying on various features that have been mentioned above, such as high sedimentation rate, positive gallium-67 scan, and normal wedge pressure.

Tocainide. Tocainide has been available for only a few years, but there are at least a half-dozen case reports implicating it in the cause of acute interstitial pneumonitis beginning several months after initiation of therapy.[100] Discontinuing the medication is probably sufficient, but corticosteroids may be necessary.

ANTIBIOTICS

Nitrofurantoin, Acute Reaction. There have been over 500 documented case reports of acute nitrofurantoin pneumonitis.[2–6,9,10,14,101,102] However, it is likely that fewer than 2% of the patients receiving this drug develop an adverse reaction, either acute or chronic. The reaction is fatal in less than 1% of cases, with most fatalities occurring among the chronic nitrofurantoin pulmonary fibrosis group. The incidence of the chronic reaction varies from 1 in 550 to 1 in 5000 individuals.[14,15] The mechanism of the acute reaction is unknown, whereas the chronic reaction is possibly due to the induction of oxidant mechanisms. Yet supplemental oxygen has never been documented as a precipitating or additive factor, in contrast to bleomycin, which is also thought to cause an oxidant-mediated injury.[103] Interestingly, nearly 10% of the patients with an acute nitrofurantoin reaction have had a prior acute reaction to the drug.

With the acute reaction, there is, within a few hours to several days after initiation of therapy, the onset of dyspnea, fever, and nonproductive cough. The reaction does not appear to be dose-related. Other organ involvement is uncommon. Leukocytosis can occur and eosinophilia is seen in about one-third of cases. The chest roentgenogram shows an alveolar or interstitial process that may be quite asymmetric. Pleural effusion occurs in about 10% to 20% of the patients. Rales are heard in most patients. There are very few studies of the histology of acute nitrofurantoin pneumonitis. Although it is postulated to be a hypersensitivity phenomenon, this has not been documented. IgA-laden plasma cells have been demonstrated with immunofluorescence, but no other classes of immunoglobulins have been detected nor have antigen-antibody complexes been observed. The diagnosis is one of exclusion, as there is no confirmatory test. Rechallenging the patient to confirm the diagnosis is not recommended and is rarely needed with this particular class of antimicrobial as there are many substitutes.

Because nitrofurantoin is taken most commonly at the patient's discretion for a flare-up of symptoms related to urinary tract infection, the patient may neglect to mention that he or she is on nitrofurantoin. The clinician must therefore maintain a high index of suspicion in the patient who presents with recurring "pneumonia" that clears rapidly and is not associated with purulent sputum or positive sputum Gram stain or culture. Treatment consists of discontinuing the medication. There appears to be no indication for corticosteroids in the acute nitrofurantoin reaction.

Nitrofurantoin, Chronic Reaction.   Chronic nitrofurantoin pneumonitis and fibrosis is an entirely separate entity from the acute reaction and there appears to be no overlap.[14,101–104] The pathogenic mechanisms appear to be different, as do the clinical presentation, roentgenographic appearance, and probably histology (Figs. 3-5, 3-6). The patient has taken the medication more or less steadily for at least 6 months and frequently a few years before the insidious development of nonproductive cough and dyspnea without fever. Martin has shown with in vitro studies that parenchymal cells incubated with nitrofurantoin were injured through induction of oxygen radicals, which are thought to exert their effect by generating single-electron transfers within biologic systems; this is very similar to the mechanism of action of paraquat and possibly other drugs.[103] Bronchoalveolar lavage shows a lymphocytosis.[105]

The presentation, radiographic appearance, and histology are similar to those of idiopathic pulmonary fibrosis with the exception that clubbing has not been reported. Resolution after stopping the drug and treating with corticosteroids is much more frequently observed than with the idiopathic variety. The histologic pattern is similar to that of idiopathic pulmonary fibrosis, demonstrating a mild to moderate quantity of

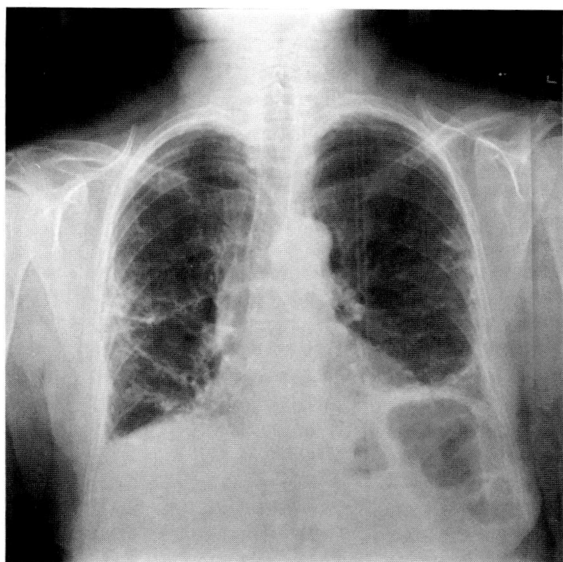

Figure 3-5. Chronic nitrofurantoin pulmonary fibrosis. This enlarged view of the chest roentgenogram of a 66-year-old woman shows a predominant interstitial pattern.

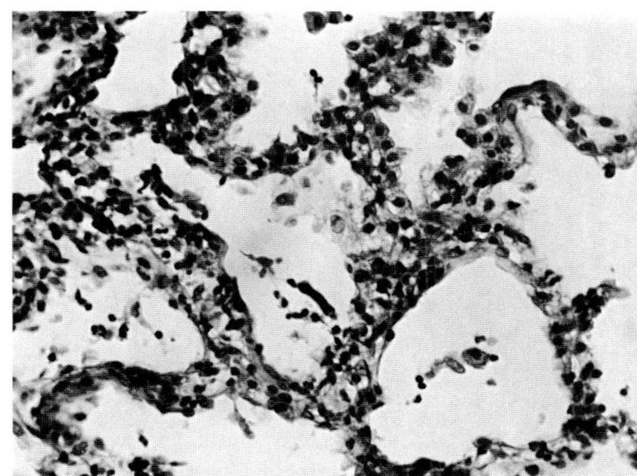

Figure 3-6. Chronic nitrofurantoin fibrosis. An infiltration of a mixture of inflammatory cells, includng polymorphonuclear leukocytes, lymphocytes, and plasma cells, is apparent.

inflammatory cells and eventually considerable fibrosis. However, as stated, this appears to be reversible in a fair percentage of the patients. The recommendation for treatment is to observe the patient for a few months after discontinuance of the drug. If there is no spontaneous resolution, then a trial of corticosteroids is indicated. Patients who are strongly symptomatic at the time of diagnosis should be considered for corticosteroid treatment immediately.

Sulfasalazine.   Sulfasalazine, or **azulfidine**, is an antimicrobial agent that has been used for many years in the treatment of chronic inflammatory bowel disease including chronic ulcerative colitis. The pulmonary reaction to sulfasalazine consists of cough, dyspnea, and, in approximately half the patients, fever beginning 1 to 8 months after initiation of therapy.[106–109] The chest roentgenogram shows a variable pattern of pulmonary infiltrates ranging from well-localized infiltrates to a diffuse interstitial process, sometimes mimicking that of chronic eosinophilic pneumonitis. In half the patients there is blood eosinophilia and bronchoalveolar lavage usually reveals a predominance of eosinophils.[108]

ILLICIT DRUGS

Heroin, propoxyphene hydrochloride (Darvon), methadone hydrochloride, ethvinyl chloride (Placidyl), and **talc** are all capable of producing a diffuse pulmonary infiltrate that is predominantly a noncardiac pulmonary edema.[2,3–5,7,110–115] However, there is also an infiltration of inflammatory cells into the interstitium. Several theories have been advanced to account for this: (1) an acute hypoxic effect on the alveolar capillary membrane with resultant increased permeability leads to an extravasation of fluid into the alveolar spaces; (2) neurogenic pulmonary edema occurs as a result of central nervous system irritation; (3) there is a direct toxic effect on the alveolar capillary membrane; and (4) there is a hypersensitivity reaction. Immunologic abnormalities have been reported, including depression of complement components and the deposition of immune complexes with immunoglobulins in the alveolar wall, but this finding has not been confirmed by others.[110] Somnolence and dyspnea begin within minutes to as long as an hour after intravenous injection of the drug or within an hour or two of ingesting the medication. Respiration is always depressed and the pupils are miotic. Noncardiac pulmonary edema is apparent on the chest roentgenogram. Hypoxia, hypercapnia, and acidosis are seen on arterial blood gas analysis. Treatment consists of assisted ventilation and, if necessary, intravenous naloxone to reverse respiratory depression. Aspiration pneumonia is common in this setting.

Talc in the form of **magnesium silicate** can produce a granulomatosis in the pulmonary bronchioles or arterioles.[116–119] It is used as a filler in oral preparations of amphetamines, methadone, propoxyphene hydrochloride, meperidine, and other drugs that are taken intravenously by drug addicts and should be considered in the evaluation of HIV-positive drug abusers.[117] With chronic abuse, a talc granulomatosis develops. The chest roentgenogram is normal in at least 50% of patients with subsequently proven talc granulomatosis. In the rest, a diffuse interstitial involvement is seen, sometimes with diffuse micronodular densities varying from 1 mm to 3 mm in size and mimicking alveolar microlithiasis, although the granulations are never as dense as in alveolar microlithiasis. Granulomatous changes can be seen in either the

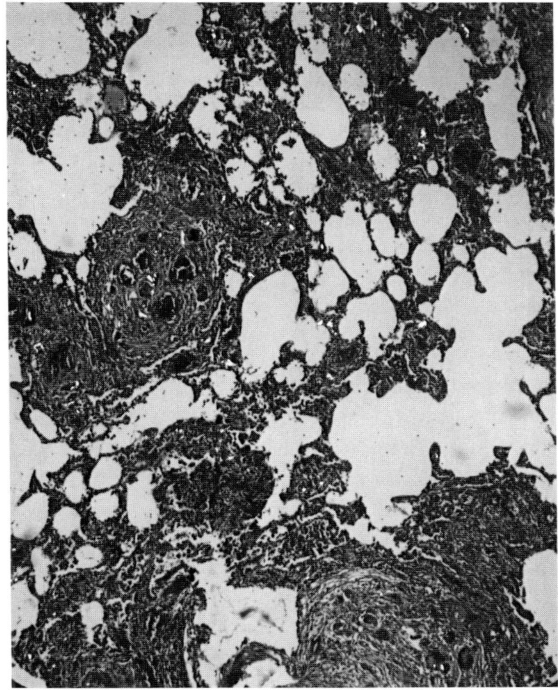

Figure 3-7. Talc granulomatosis. This H&E-stained preparation shows granulomas as well as birefringent particles (the small white dots scattered throughout the lung field).

bronchioles or the arterioles, and sometimes in both, along with an infiltration of multinucleated giant cells, lymphocytes, and other inflammatory cells. Eventually a peribronchial and/or periarteriolar fibrosis results. Birefringence is seen in the interstitium and the peribronchial and periarterial walls with the use of polarized light (Fig. 3-7). Bronchoalveolar lavage demonstrates an increased number of lymphocytes consistent with a granulomatous disease as well as free talc crystals.[120]

ANTI-INFLAMMATORY DRUGS

Acetylsalicylic Acid. **Aspirin** produces a noncardiac pulmonary edema in about a third of patients with a blood level greater than 40 mg per deciliter. The pulmonary edema occurs both in patients who have chronically ingested the medication for various inflammatory diseases and in those with acute ingestions as a suicide attempt. The mechanism is not known. The symptoms of cough and dyspnea begin within 1 to 2 hours of an acute overdose or insidiously hours and days after the salicylate level reaches 40 mg per deciliter. Rales are heard on auscultation of the lungs. Changes typical of noncardiac pulmonary edema are seen on the chest roentgenogram. The characteristic central nervous system stimulation seen with salicylate overdose causes hyperventilation, resulting in very low $PaCO_2$, sometimes below 15 mm Hg; of course, a low PaO_2 is also seen. Treatment requires supportive care, frequently intubation with ventilatory support, sometimes hemodialysis, and occasionally forced alkaline diuresis and hemodialysis. Bronchoalveolar lavage shows a predominance of PMNs.[124]

Gold.   Both forms of injectable **gold** have been reported to produce a diffuse interstitial pneumonitis and fibrosis. Thus far oral gold has not been reported to cause this.[125–127] Evans and co-workers have reviewed the world literature and include 60 cases in their report.[126] The reaction can mimic the interstitial pneumonitis and fibrosis seen with rheumatoid lung, but spontaneous resolution on discontinuing the gold clarifies the situation. Gold lung has been reported to occur in non-rheumatoid patients.[126] Symptoms of dyspnea and nonproductive cough begin several weeks to a few months after initiation of therapy. Peripheral eosinophilia has been seen in a few patients. An interstitial process is seen on the chest roentgenogram and in a few patients it has predominated in the upper lung fields. Histologically, lymphocytic and plasmacytic infiltration not unlike that of rheumatoid lung is seen. The mechanism is unknown, but one study demonstrated two major histocompatibility markers as predominant.[128] Bronchoalveolar lavage demonstrates a predominant lymphocytosis.[126–127] Treatment consists of discontinuing the drug and occasionally the addition of corticosteroids.

Penicillamine.   **Penicillamine** is unique in the three different disorders produced by it, including bronchiolitis obliterans, Goodpasture's syndrome, and drug-induced systemic lupus erythematosus.[129–132] A fourth entity that has been reported as "alveolitis or allergic pneumonitis" is probably drug-induced lupus. Bronchiolitis obliterans can have the appearance of an interstitial process on chest roentgenogram; however, in its purest form only endobronchial and peribronchial inflammation either with a normal chest roentgenogram or on hyperinflation are seen. There are now over a dozen case reports of penicillamine-induced Goodpasture's syndrome. The mechanism is unknown, but the features resemble those of the idiopathic variety of Goodpasture's syndrome. Therapy is the same, including hemodialysis, immunosuppressive agents, and occasionally plasmapheresis.

TRICYCLIC ANTIDEPRESSANTS

Tricyclic psychoactive drugs are now among the most common agents used in drug overdose.[136] The majority coming to an emergency room require intubation and assisted mechanical ventilation. The chest roentgenogram is abnormal in about 40% of patients and a third of these display a noncardiac pulmonary edema.

MISCELLANEOUS DRUG-RELATED DISORDERS

Drug-Induced Systemic Lupus Erythematosus.   Nearly 50 medications have been reported to induce systemic lupus erythematosus (SLE).[16,19,133–135] However, five of these produce over 90% of the reactions: procainamide hydrochloride, hydralazine hydrochloride, isoniazid, the hydantoins, and penicillamine. Many patients taking these medications for months or years develop antinuclear antibodies, particularly against histones, and a small percentage develop clinical symptoms of systemic lupus erythematosus. About half of this group demonstrate pleuropulmonary disease, including interstitial lung disease. The theory of the mechanism was discussed earlier in this chapter. The treatment consists of discontinuing the medication. In the majority, this is sufficient, and only a small number require the addition of corticosteroids to accelerate the resolution. The antinuclear antibody is positive in all patients with drug-induced SLE, with the anti-native (double-stranded) DNA being negative. Typical changes of SLE are seen on the chest roentgenogram, including interstitial infiltrates, apparent cardiomegaly from pericardial effusion, pleural effusion, and atelectasizing pneumonitis.

Drug-Induced Pulmonary Infiltrates and Eosinophilia   The pulmonary infiltration with blood eosinophilia (PIE) syndrome has been reported to be produced by over 30 drugs, but there is no single reference summarizing all of these.

REFERENCES

1. Cooper JAD Jr, White DA, Matthay RA. Drug-induced pulmonary disease: Part 1: Cytotoxic drugs. Am Rev Respir Dis 1986;133:321.
2. Cooper JAD Jr, White DA, Matthay RA: Drug-induced pulmonary disease: Part 2: Noncytotoxic drugs. Am Rev Respir Dis 1986;133:488.
3. Rosenow EC III. Chapter 371: Drug-induced lung diseases. In: Kelley WN, ed. Textbook of internal medicine. Vol. 2. Philadelphia: JB Lippincott, 1989:1939.
4. Rosenow EC III. Chapter 74: Drug-induced lung diseases. In: Murray JF, Nadel JA, eds. The textbook of respiratory medicine. Philadelphia: WB Saunders, 1988:1681.
5. Rosenow EC III, Martin WJ II. Chapter 8: Drug-induced interstitial lung disease. In: Schwarz MI, King TE Jr, eds. Interstitial lung disease. Philadelphia: BC Decker, 1988:123.
6. Treatment-induced respiratory disorders. In: Akoun GM, White JP, eds. Drug-induced disorders, Vol. 3. Amsterdam: Elsevier, 1989.
7. Rice KL. Pulmonary infiltrates associated with noncytotoxic drugs. Semin Respir Infect 1988;3:229.
8. Snyder LS, Hertz MI. Cytotoxic drug-induced lung injury. Semin Respir Infect 1988;3:217.
9. Rosenow EC III. Drug-induced bronchopulmonary pleural disease. J Allergy & Clin Immunol 1987;80:780.
10. Cooper JA Jr, Matthay RA. Drug-induced pulmonary disease. Dis Mon 1987; 33:61.
11. Rosenow EC III, Unni KK. Drug-induced pulmonary granulomas. In: Fanburg BL, ed. Sarcoidosis and other granulomatous diseases of the lung, Vol. 20. New York: Marcel Dekker, 1983:469.
12. Rogers AS, Israel E, Smith CR, et al. Physician knowledge, attitudes, and behavior related to reporting adverse drug events. Arch Intern Med 1988;148;1596.
13. Koch-Weser J, Sidel VW, Dexter M, Parish C, Finer DC, Kanarek P. Adverse reactions to sulfisoxazole, sulfamethoxazole, and nitrofurantoin. Arch Intern Med 1971;128:399.
14. Sovijärvi ARA, Lemola M, Stenius B, Idanpaan-Heikkila. Nitrofurantoin-induced acute, subacute, and chronic pulmonary reaction. Scand J Resp Dis 1977;58:41.
15. Jick SS, Jick H, Walker AM, Hunter JR. Hospitalizations for pulmonary reactions following nitrofurantoin use. Chest 1989;96:512.
16. Cooper JA Jr, Zitnik RJ, Matthay RA. Mechanisms of drug-induced pulmonary disease. Ann Rev Med 1988;39:395.
17. Reasor MJ. Phospholipidosis in the alveolar macrophage induced by cationic amphophilic drugs. Federation Proc 1984;43:2578.

18. Martin WJ II. Nitrofurantoin: Evidence for the oxidant injury of lung parenchymal cells. Am Rev Respir Dis 1983;127:482.

19. Lauterberg BH, Smith CV, Mitchell JR. Molecular mechanisms involved in drug-induced pulmonary injuries. Sem Resp Med 1980;2:45.

20. Daniel PT, Holzschuh J, Berg PA. Sulfadoxine specific lymphocyte transformation in a patient with eosinophilic pneumonia induced by sulfadoxine-pyrimethamine (Fansidar). Thorax 1989;44:307.

21. Chandler DB, Fulmer JD. The effect of deferoxamine on bleomycin-induced lung fibrosis in the hamster. Am Rev Respir Dis 1985;131:596.

22. Goldiner PL, Carlon GC, Cvitkovic E, Schweizer O, Howland WS. Factors influencing postoperative morbidity and mortality in patients treated with bleomycin. Br Med J 1978;1:1664.

23. Martin WJ II, Rosenow EC III. Amiodarone pulmonary toxicity. Recognition and pathogenesis (Part 2). Chest 1988;93:1242.

24. Martin WJ, Howard DM. Amiodarone-induced lung toxicity: In vitro evidence for the direct toxicity of the drug. Am J Pathol 1985;120:344.

25. Adamson IY. Drug-induced pulmonary fibrosis. Environ Health Perspect 1984;55:25.

26. Schoen RT, Trentham DE. Drug-induced lupus: An adjuvant disease? Am J Med 1981;71:5.

27. Bell MR, Meredith DJ, Gill PG. Role of carbon monoxide diffusing capacity in the early detection of major bleomycin-induced pulmonary toxicity. Aust NZ J Med 1985;15:235.

28. Krowka MJ, Breuer RI, Kehoe TJ. Azathioprine-associated pulmonary dysfunction. Chest 1983;83:696.

29. Quigley M, Brada M, Heron C, Horwich A. Severe lung toxicity with a weekly low dose chemotherapy regimen in patients with non-Hodgkin's lymphoma. Hematol Oncol 1988;6:319.

30. Van Barneveld PWC, Sleijfer DT, VanDerMark TW, et al. Natural course of bleomycin-induced pneumonitis: A follow-up study. Am Rev Respir Dis 1987;135:48.

31. White DA, Stover DE. Severe bleomycin-induced pneumonitis. Clinical features and response to corticosteroids. Chest 1984;86:723.

32. Van Barneveld PWC, VanDerMark TW, Sleijfer DT, et al. Predictive factors for bleomycin-induced pneumonitis. Am Rev Respir Dis 1984;130:1078.

33. Bauer KA, Skarin AT, Balikian JP, Garnick MB, Rosenthal DS, Canellos GP. Pulmonary complications associated with combination chemotherapy programs containing bleomycin. Am J Med 1983;74:557.

34. Samuels ML, Johnson DE, Holoye PY, Lanzotti VJ. Large-dose bleomycin therapy and pulmonary toxicity: A possible role of prior radiotherapy. JAMA 1976;235:1117.

35. Einhorn L, Krause M, Hornback N, Furnas B. Enhanced pulmonary toxicity with bleomycin and radiotherapy in oat cell lung cancer. Cancer 1976;37:2414.

36. Blum RH, Carter SK, Agre K. A clinical review of bleomycin: A new antineoplastic agent. Cancer 1973;31:903.

37. Goad ME, Tryka AF, Witschi HP. Acute respiratory failure induced by bleomycin and hyperoxia: Pulmonary edema, cell kinetics, and morphology. Toxicol Appl Pharmacol 1987;90:10.

38. Gilson AJ, Sahn SA. Reactivation of bleomycin lung toxicity following oxygen administration: A second response to corticosteroids. Chest 1985;88:304.

39. Cersosimo RJ, Matthews SJ, Hong WK. Bleomycin pneumonitis potentiated by oxygen administration. Drug Intell Clin Pharm 1985;19:921.

40. Matalon S, Harper WV, Goldinger JM, Nickerson PA, Olszowka J. Modification of pulmonary oxygen toxicity by bleomycin treatment. J Appl Physiol 1985;58:1802.

41. Tryka AF, Skornik WA, Godleski JJ, Brain JD. Potentiation of bleomycin-induced lung injury by exposure to 70% oxygen: Morphologic assessment. Am Rev Respir Dis 1982;126:1074.

42. Bellamy EA, Husband JE, Blaquiere RM, Law MR. Bleomycin-related lung damage: CT evidence. Radiology 1985;156:155.

43. Rimmer MJ, Dixon AK, Flower CD, Sikora K. Bleomycin lung: Computed tomographic observations. Br J Radiol 1985;58:1041.
44. Cohen MB, Austin JH, Smith-Vaniz A, Lutzky J, Grimes MM. Nodular bleomycin toxicity. Am J Clin Path 1989;92:101.
45. Santrach PJ, Askin FB, Wells RJ, Azizkhan RG, Merten DF. Nodular form of bleomycin-related pulmonary injury in patients with osteogenic sarcoma. Cancer 1989;64:806.
46. Scharstein R, Johnson JF, Cook BA, Stephenson SR. Bleomycin nodules mimicking metastatic osteogenic sarcoma. Am J Pediatr Hematol Oncol 1987;9:219.
47. Talcott JA, Garnick MB, Stomper PC, Godleski JJ, Richie JP. Cavitary lung nodules associated with combination chemotherapy containing bleomycin. J Urol 1987;138:619.
48. White DA, Kris MG, Stover DE. Bronchoalveolar lavage cell populations in bleomycin lung toxicity. Thorax 1987;42:551.
49. Giri SN, Hyde DM, Nakashima JM. Analysis of bronchoalveolar lavage fluid from bleomycin-induced pulmonary fibrosis in hamsters. Toxicol Pathol 1986;14:149.
50. Nussinovitch N, Peleg E, Yaron A, Ratt P, Rosenthal T. Angiotensin converting enzyme in bleomycin-treated patients. Int J Clin Pharmacol Ther Toxicol 1988;26:310.
51. Massin F, Fur A, Reybet-Degat O, Camus P, Jeannin L. Busulfan-induced pneumopathy. Rev Mal Respir 1987;4:3.
52. Bedrossian CWM, Luna MA, Conklin RH, MIller WC. Alveolar proteinosis as a consequence of immunosuppression: A hypothesis based on clinical and pathologic observations. Hum Pathol 1980;11:527.
53. Aymard JP, Gyger M, Lavallee R, Legresley LP, Desy M. A case of pulmonary alveolar proteinosis complicating chronic myelogenous leukemia: A peculiar pathologic aspect of busulfan lung? Cancer 1984;53:954.
54. Vergnon JM, Boucheron S, Riffat J, Guy C, Blanc P, Emonot A. Interstitial pneumopathies caused by busulfan: Histologic, developmental and bronchoalveolar lavage analysis of 3 cases. Rev Med Interne 1988;9:377.
55. Carr ME Jr. Chlorambucil induced pulmonary fibrosis: Report of a case and review. Vir Med 1986;113:677.
56. Kumar RK, Truscott JY, Rhodes GC, Lykke AW. Type 2 pneumocyte responses to cyclophosphamide-induced pulmonary injury: Functional and morphological correlation. Br J Exp Path 1988;69:69.
57. Quigley M, Brada M, Heron C, Horwich A. Severe lung toxicity with a weekly low dose chemotherapy regimen in patients with non-Hodgkin's lymphoma. Hematol Oncol 1988;6:319.
58. Stentoff J. Progressive pulmonary fibrosis complicating cyclophosphamide therapy. Acta Med Scand 1987;221:403.
59. Brooke BJ Jr, Seifter EJ, Walsh TE, et al. Pulmonary toxicity with combined modality therapy for limited stage small-cell lung cancer. J Clin Oncol 1986;4:200.
60. Cytoxan lung. CPC 16–1984. N Engl J Med 1984;310:1037.
61. Zimmerman MS, Ruckdeschel JC, Hussain M. Chemotherapy-induced interstitial pneumonitis during treatment of small cell anaplastic lung cancer. J Clin Oncol 1984;2:396.
62. Tsukamoto N, Matsukuma K, Matsuyama T, et al. Cyclophosphamide-induced interstitial pneumonitis in a patient with ovarian carcinoma. Gynecol Oncol 1984;17:41.
63. Hunt KK. Post-cyclophosphamide pneumonitis. N Engl J Med 1972;287:668.
64. Patel AR, Shah PC, Rhee HL, Sassoon H, Koduri PR. Cyclophosphamide therapy and interstitial pulmonary fibrosis. Cancer 1976;38:1542.
65. Goucher G, Rowland V, Hawkins J. Melphalan-induced pulmonary interstitial fibrosis. Chest 1980;77:805.
66. Westerfield BT, Michalski JP, McCombs C, Light RW. Reversible melphalan-induced lung damage. Am J Med 1980;68:767.

67. Verweij J, van Zanten T, Souren T, Golding R, Pinedo HM. Prospective study on the dose relationship of mitomycin C–induced interstitial pneumonitis. Cancer 1987;60:756.

68. Sheldon R, Slaughter D. A syndrome of microangiopathic hemolytic anemia, renal impairment, and pulmonary edema in chemotherapy-treated patients with adenocarcinoma. Cancer 1986;58:1428.

69. Doyle LA, Ihde DC, Carney DN, et al. Combination chemotherapy with doxorubicin and mitomycin C in non–small cell bronchogenic carcinoma. Severe pulmonary toxicity from q 3 weekly mitomycin C. Am J Clin Oncol 1984;7:719.

70. Cantrell JE Jr, Phillips TM, Schein PS. Carcinoma-associated hemolytic-uremic syndrome: A complication of mitomycin C chemotherapy. J Clin Oncol 1985;3:723.

71. McCarthy JT, Staats BA. Pulmonary hypertension, hemolytic anemia, and renal failure: A mitomycin-associated syndrome. Chest 1986;89:608.

72. Smith AC. The pulmonary toxicity of nitrosoureas. Pharmacol Ther 1989;41:443.

73. Weinstein AS, Diener-West M, Nelson DF, Pakuris E. Pulmonary toxicity of carmustine in patients treated for malignant glioma. Cancer Treat Rep 1986;70:943.

74. Mitsudo SM, Greenwald ES, Banerji B, Koss LG. BCNU (1,3-bis-(2-chloroethyl)-1-nitrosurea) lung: Drug-induced pulmonary changes. Cancer 1984;54:751.

75. Aronin PA, Mahaley MS Jr, Rudnick SA, et al. Prediction of BCNU pulmonary toxicity in patients with malignant gliomas: An assessment of risk factors. N Engl J Med 1980;303:183.

76. Hoelzer KL, Harrison BR, Luedke SW, Luedke DW. Vinblastine-associated pulmonary toxicity in patients receiving combination therapy with mitomycin and cisplatin. Drug Intell Clin Pharm 1986;20:287.

77. Konits PH, Aisner J, Sutherland JC, Wiernik PH. Possible pulmonary toxicity secondary to vinblastine. Cancer 1982;50:2771.

78. Rao SX, Ramaswamy G, Levin M, McCravey JW. Fatal acute respiratory failure after vinblastine-mitomycin therapy in lung carcinoma. Arch Intern Med 1985;145:1905.

79. Jehn U, Göldel N, Rienmüller R, Wilmanns W. Non-cardiogenic pulmonary edema complicating intermediate and high-dose Ara C treatment for relapsed acute leukemia. Med Oncol Tumor Pharmacother 1988;5:41.

80. Andersson BS, Cogan BM, Keating MJ, Estey EH, McCredie KB, Freireich EJ. Subacute pulmonary failure complicating therapy with high-dose Ara-C in acute leukemia. Cancer 1985;56:2181.

81. Kantarjian HM, Estey EH, Plunkett W, et al. Phase I-II clinical and pharmacologic studies of high-dose cytosine arabinoside in refractory leukemia. Am J Med 1986;81:387.

82. Haupt HM, Hutchins GM, Moore GW. Ara-C lung: Noncardiogenic pulmonary edema complicating cytosine arabinoside therapy of leukemia. Am J Med 1981;70:256.

83. White DA, Rankin JA, Stover DE, Gellene RA, Gupta S. Methotrexate pneumonitis: Bronchoalveolar lavage findings suggest an immunologic disorder. Am Rev Respir Dis 1989;139:18.

84. White DA, Orenstein M, Godwin TA, Stover DE. Chemotherapy-associated pulmonary toxic reactions during treatment for breast cancer. Arch Intern Med 1984;144:953.

85. Methotrexate pneumonitis. CPC 6–1985. N Engl J Med 1985;312:359.

86. Green L, Schattner A, Berkenstadt H. Severe reversible interstitial pneumonitis induced by low dose methotrexate: Report of a case and review of the literature. J Rheumatol 1988;15:110.

87. Carson CW, Cannon GW, Egger MJ, Ward JR, Clegg DO. Pulmonary disease during the treatment of rheumatoid arthritis with low dose pulse methotrexate. Sem Arthritis Rheum 1987;16:186.

88. McKendry RJR, Cyr M. Toxicity of methotrexate compared with azathioprine in the treatment of rheumatoid arthritis: A case-control study of 131 patients. Arch Intern Med 1989;149:685.

89. Newman ED, Harrington TM. Fatal methotrexate pneumonitis in rheumatoid arthritis (letter). Arthritis Rheum 1988;31:1585.

90. Akoun GM, Mayaud CM, Touboul JL, Denis MF, Milleron BJ, Perrot JY. Use of bronchoalveolar lavage in the evaluation of methotrexate lung disease. Thorax 1987;42:652.

91. White DA, Gellene R, Rankin JA, Gupta S, Cunningham-Rundles C, Stover DE. Methotrexate pneumonitis: Bronchoalveolar lavage findings suggest an immune mediated disorder. Am Rev Respir Dis 1984;129:A64.

92. Martin WJ II, Rosenow EC III. Amiodarone pulmonary toxicity: Recognition and pathogenesis (Part I). Chest 1988;93:1067.

93. Veltri EP, Reid PR. Amiodarone pulmonary toxicity: Early changes in pulmonary function tests during amiodarone rechallenge. J Am Coll Cardiol 1985;6:802.

94. Magro SA, Lawrence EC, Wheeler SH, Krafchek J, Lin HT, Wyndham CR. Amiodarone pulmonary toxicity: Prospective evaluation of serial pulmonary function tests. J Am Coll Cardiol 1988;12:781.

95. Zhu YY, Botvinick E, Dae M, Golden J, Hattern R, Scheinman M. Gallium lung scintigraphy in amiodarone pulmonary toxicity. Chest 1988;93:1126.

96. Kay GN, Epstein AE, Kirklin JK, Diethelm AG, Graybar G, Plumb VJ. Fatal postoperative amiodarone pulmonary toxicity. Am J Cardiol 1988;62:490.

97. Nalos PC, Kass RM, Gang ES, Fishbein MC, Mandel WJ, Peter T. Life-threatening postoperative pulmonary complications in patients with previous amiodarone pulmonary toxicity undergoing cardiothoracic operations. J Thorac Cardiovasc Surg 1987;93:904.

98. Israel-Biet D, Venet A, Caubarrere I, et al. Bronchoalveolar lavage in amiodarone pneumonitis: Cellular abnormalities and their relevance to pathogenesis. Chest 1987;91:214.

99. Akoun GM, Mayaud CM, Milleron BJ, Perrot JY. Drug-related pneumonitis and drug-induced hypersensitivity pneumonitis. Lancet 1984;1:1362.

100. Stein MG, Demarco T, Gamsu G, Finbeiner W, Golden JA. Computed tomography: Pathologic correlation in lung disease due to tocainide. Am Rev Respir Dis 1988;137:458.

101. Holmberg L, Boman G. Pulmonary reactions to nitrofurantoin: 447 cases reported to the Swedish Adverse Drug Reaction Committee 1966–1976. Eur J Respir Dis 1981;62:180.

102. Holmberg L, Boman G, Bottiger IE, Eriksson B, Spross R, Wessling A. Adverse reactions to nitrofurantoin: Analysis of 921 reports. Am J Med 1980;69:733.

103. Martin WJ II. Nitrofurantoin: Evidence for the oxidant injury of lung parenchymal cells. Am Rev Resp Dis 1983;127:482.

104. Robinson BWS. Nitrofurantoin-induced interstitial pulmonary fibrosis: Presentation and outcome. Med J Aust 1983;1:72.

105. Brutinel WM, Martin WJ II. Chronic nitrofurantoin reaction associated with T-lymphocyte alveolitis. Chest 1986;89:150.

106. Wang KK, Bowyer BA, Fleming CR, Schroeder KW. Pulmonary infiltrates and eosinophilia associated with sulfasalazine. Mayo Clin Proc 1984;59:343.

107. Williams T, Eidus L, Thomas P. Fibrosing alveolitis, bronchiolitis obliterans, and sulfasalazine therapy. Chest 1982;81:766.

108. Valcke Y, Pauwels R, Van Der Straeten M. Bronchoalveolar lavage in acute hypersensitivity pneumonitis caused by sulfasalazine. Chest 1987;92:572.

109. Steinfort CL, Wiggins J, Sheffield EA, Keal EE. Alveolitis associated with sulphamethoxypyridazine. Thorax 1989;44:310.

110. Brashear RE. Effects of heroin, morphine, methadone, and propoxyphene on the lung. Sem Resp Med 1980;2:59.

111. Tennant FS Jr. Complications of propoxyphene abuse. Arch Intern Med 1973;132:191.

112. Sarkar TK, Kumar RD, Cantacuzine D. Unilateral pulmonary edema following methadone ingestion (Roentgenogram of the Month). Chest 1975;68:723.

113. Conces DJ Jr, Kreipke DL, Tarver RD. Pulmonary edema induced by intravenous ethchlorvynol. Am J Emerg Med 1986;4:549.

114. Miller KS, Sahn SA. Bilateral exudative pleural effusions following intravenous ethchlorvynol administration. Chest 1989;95:464.
115. Miller KS, Harley RA, Sahn SA. Pleural effusions associated with ethchlorvynol lung injury result from visceral pleural leak. Am Rev Respir Dis 1989;140:764.
116. Radow SK, Nachamkin I, Morrow C, et al. Foreign body granulomatosis: Clinical and immunologic findings. Am Rev Respir Dis 1983;127:575.
117. Ben-Haim SA, Ben-Ami H, Edoute Y, Goldstien N, Barzilai D. Talcosis presenting as pulmonary infiltrates in an HIV-positive heroin addict. Chest 1988;94:656.
118. Crouch E, Churg A. Progressive massive fibrosis of the lung secondary to intravenous injection of talc: A pathologic and mineralogic analysis. Am J Clin Pathol 1983;80:520.
119. Schwartz IS, Bosken C. Pulmonary vascular talc granulomatosis. JAMA 1986;256:2584.
120. Farber HW, Fairman RP, Glauser FL. Talc granulomatosis: Laboratory findings similar to sarcoidosis. Am Rev Respir Dis 1982;125:258.
121. Heffner JE, Sahn SA. Salicylate-induced pulmonary edema: Clinical features and prognosis. Ann Intern Med 1981;95:405.
122. Thisted B, Krantz T, Strom J, Sorensen MB. Acute salicylate self-poisoning in 177 consecutive patients treated in ICU. Acta Anaesth Scan 1987;31:312.
123. McGuigan MA. A two-year review of salicylate deaths in Ontario. Arch Intern Med 1987;147:510.
124. Suarez M, Krieger BP. Bronchoalveolar lavage in recurrent aspirin-induced adult respiratory distress syndrome. Chest 1986;90:452.
125. McFadden RG, Fraher LJ, Thompson JM. Gold-naproxen pneumonitis: A toxic drug interaction? Chest 1989;96:216.
126. Evans RB, Ettensohn DB, Fawaz-Estrup F, Lally EV, Kaplan SR. Gold lung: Recent developments in pathogenesis, diagnosis, and therapy. Sem Arthritis Rheum 1987;16:196.
127. Ettensohn DB, Roberts NJ Jr, Condemi JJ. Bronchoalveolar lavage in gold lung. Chest 1984;85:569.
128. Partanen J, van Assendelft AH, Koskimies S, Forsberg S, Hakala M, Ilonen J. Patients with rheumatoid arthritis and gold-induced pneumonitis express two high-risk major histocompatibility complex patterns. Chest 1987;92:277.
129. Chalmers A, Thompson D, Stein HB, Reid G, Peterson AC. Systemic lupus erythematosus during penicillamine therapy for rheumatoid arthritis. Ann Intern Med 1982;97:659.
130. Murphy KC, Atkins CJ, Offer RC, Hogg JC, Stein HB. Obliterative bronchiolitis in two rheumatoid arthritis patients treated with penicillamine. Arthritis Rheum 1981;24:557.
131. Devogelaer JP, Pirson Y, Vandenbroucke JM, Cosyns JP, Brichard S, Nagant de Deuxchaisnes C. D-penicillamine induced crescentic glomerulonephritis: Report and review of the literature. J Rheumatol 1987;14:1036.
132. Peces R, Riera JR, Arboleya LR, Lopez-Larrea C, Alvarez J. Goodpasture's syndrome in a patient receiving penicillamine and carbimazole. Nephron 1987;45:316.
133. Totoritis MC, Rubin RL. Drug-induced lupus: Genetic, clinical, and laboratory features. Postgrad Med 1985;78:149.
134. Schoen RT, Trentham DE. Drug-induced lupus: An adjuvant disease? Am J Med 1981;71:5.
135. Ginsburg WW. Drug-induced systemic lupus erythematosus. Sem Resp Med 1980;2:51.
136. Roy TM, Ossorio MA, Cipolla LM, Fields CL, Snider HL, Anderson WH. Pulmonary complications after tricyclic antidepressant overdose. Chest 1989;96:852.

4

Immunologic Aspects of Pneumoconioses in Asbestosis and Silicosis

Gerald S. Davis

Diseases of the lungs caused by the inhalation of mineral dusts from the work place are among the oldest pulmonary disorders known. The distinctive diseases caused by silica and asbestos are the most severe, widespread, and intensively studied of the pneumoconioses. These diseases remain important public health problems throughout the world today, despite awareness of their causes and the availability of industrial hygiene measures to prevent them. Silicosis, and to a lesser extent asbestosis, remain common problems in developing economies, although their prevalence is decreasing in the more industrialized nations.

The importance of fundamental immunologic mechanisms in the pathogenesis of silicosis and asbestosis has become clear only recently. This is not to say that a specific immune response to the mineral as a traditional antigen is the cause of silicosis or asbestosis. Rather, it appears that many of the same cells, mediators, and mechanisms that control immunospecific responses are also the basis for the pulmonary reaction to these dusts. It is hoped that greater understanding of these mechanisms acquired through research with asbestosis and silicosis can then be applied to other idiopathic or autoimmune diseases where the causative agents are not known and cannot be traced in the lung through the course of the disease.

Many topics will not be discussed in detail that are important to an understanding of lung diseases caused by inhaled particles. This chapter will not present detailed information about mineralogy or geology, industrial hygiene, particle aerosol physics, particle deposition or clearance in the lung, pulmonary host defense mechanisms, or techniques for the analysis of minerals in lung tissue. Other sources should be sought for information about these topics. The focus of the presentation will lie with the clinical features of asbestosis and silicosis, some of the epidemiology related to them, and a detailed discussion of the cell biology believed to be responsible for their pathogenesis.

This chapter will focus on only two pneumoconioses among the many diseases caused by inhaled inorganic particles. Important diseases such as coal workers' pneumoconiosis, talcosis, or berylliosis will not be discussed. Silicosis and asbestosis will serve as examples of other pneumoconioses, but extension of findings from these two diseases to other conditions should be done with caution. These two conditions are more prevalent and have received much more research attention in human studies and animal models than any of the other mineral dust diseases. It is hoped that this review will provide substantial information about two important diseases and also will raise questions that suggest directions for future research.

ASBESTOSIS

Asbestos fibers produce a variety of chronic pulmonary diseases, including pulmonary fibrosis (asbestosis), fibrous thickening of the parietal pleura (plaques) and several other benign pleural reactions, a highly malignant cancer of pleural or peritoneal origin (mesothelioma), and an increased risk for carcinoma of the bronchus and other sites. In all of these diseases, the clinical signs of disease develop decades after asbestos exposure occurred or began, and the severity or likelihood of developing disease is proportional to the intensity of exposure.

Asbestos Minerals

Asbestos forms a group of naturally occurring minerals that are both crystalline in structure and fibrous in shape. Fibers are defined as having a length-to-width ratio (aspect ratio) of 3:1 or greater. The asbestos minerals are magnesium silicates, with additional elements (iron, calcium, sodium) present in various types of asbestos. There are six chemically distinct types of asbestos, grouped into two major physical forms, the serpentines and the amphiboles. The serpentines are long curly fibers, actually curled plates. The amphiboles are needle-like crystals composed of straight double chains. Chrysotile dominates commercial applications, and is the only serpentine of commercial use. The amphibole group of crocidolite, amosite, and anthophyllite have special properties that make them important for specific applications. The excessive health risks that may be associated with them have progressively curtailed their use. Two other amphiboles, tremolite and actinolite, have little direct commercial application but appear as contaminants in other minerals. For example, contamination of talc with tremolite will downgrade an ore from cosmetic to industrial uses. Asbestos rock is recovered from open pit mines (chrysotile) or tunnel mines (crocidolite). Asbestos is relatively abundant and easily retrieved in pure form, and thus inexpensive to produce. Chrysotile, mined in Quebec, Russia, Italy, South America, and China, accounts for most of the world production of asbestos, and is now the type used almost exclusively in the United States. Crocidolite is produced primarily in South Africa and Australia, while amosite from South Africa and anthophyllite from Finland are less important commercial sources of fiber. Naturally occurring exposed asbestos minerals, such as erionite in Turkey, are blamed for mesothelioma and other diseases in groups with intense environmental exposure.

The asbestos minerals are incredibly tough, and very stable even at high heat. These properties make them useful in manufactured products whenever friction or heat will be encountered, particularly for insulating and fire-retarding applications. The native minerals tend to shear length-wise under stress into progressively thinner long fibers, with some breakage of the strands into shorter fibers. The large rocks removed from mines are crushed and milled into a mass of dispersed fibers. The fibers may then be packed into a confined space, woven into cloth, mixed with a variety of binders for application as a paste, or mixed into other materials to add strength or fire-retarding properties to them. Aerosols of respirable asbestos fibers can be generated during mining, milling, fabrication of the asbestos products, or installation of them. Once these materials are in place in building structures, the asbestos product may deteriorate over time and liberate the fibers into the air of that site. Prolonged heating and cooling, combined with age, make asbestos friable, and small fibers may crumble from the surface of installed products.

The biologically hazardous forms of asbestos are the small fibers, which can be inhaled and deposited in the lower respiratory tract. Particles with aerodynamic diameter greater than 5 μm are largely deposited in the nose or large airways, while particles smaller than 0.1 μm to 0.5 μm remain suspended in the inhaled air and exhaled out of the lung. Notably, it is not the length of the asbestos fiber that limits inhalation, but rather its diameter. Fibers line up length-wise in an inhaled air stream, and follow kinetics of deposition that place their mass median aerodynamic diameter near their physical diameter rather than their length. Thus, very long, thin asbestos fibers can be deposited deep within the lung. These long fibers may have more biological activity, particularly in promoting cancer, than shorter fibers.[1] Asbestos fibers, some larger than could be inhaled, may be ingested in drinking water or swallowed after mucociliary clearance.

Commercial Applications of Asbestos

Asbestos was used widely in the past in many products and building construction materials. Awareness of the serious health hazards related to asbestos exposure has sharply reduced the use of this mineral. Stringent government regulations control the fabrication, installation, and removal of materials containing asbestos in the United States and in most industrialized nations. Asbestos is so well suited and economical for many of its uses that no good substitutes have been found. Many of the applications described below are no longer in use, but are important to the physician or epidemiologist because workers who received these exposures 30 years ago may present now with asbestos-related diseases.

Asbestos remains an important material for brake linings, friction bearings, and other applications where durability, heat resistance, and longevity of the product are paramount. Workers may be exposed to asbestos while manufacturing brake linings or friction pads. Mechanics, brakemen on railroads, and maintenance personnel may receive substantial asbestos exposure while servicing these parts, particularly when worn pads must be chipped or hammered for removal.

Insulation of pipes and buildings was the largest application for asbestos during the middle years of the 20th century. Steam pipes in commercial buildings, homes, boiler plants, and ships were usually insulated with asbestos; pipe fitters and insulation workers received high exposure. The construction and renovation of ships in the naval yards of World War II provided intense asbestos exposure for many workers. Walls, roofs, and other building structures were also commonly insulated with asbestos. Roof supports, girders, and other structural elements were sprayed with asbestos lagging (a paste mixture of asbestos, inert bulk agents, and binders) to prevent buckling in the heat of a fire. Health concerns have almost completely eliminated these insulating uses for asbestos, and replaced it with fibrous glass and other materials. Large amounts of asbestos insulation are still in place in buildings constructed between 1920 and 1960 or later. Workers can receive substantial exposure to asbestos in these buildings when the insulation is removed to service pipes or walls, the lagging crumbles and fibers fall into the air, or the site undergoes major renovation or demolition. Government regulations for asbestos construction and removal help control these exposures.

Asbestos is added to cement, floor tiles, asphalt roofing tiles, and other building materials during fabrication to provide strength and fire protection. Workers in plants where these products are made can receive substantial asbestos exposure, and develop asbestos-related diseases. Exposure during installation or renovation of the finished product is probably much less hazardous, since few fibers would be aerosolized. Cutting, drilling, or sawing materials that contain asbestos should be done with great caution. Asbestos has been used extensively for city water main pipes, and could expose citizens to fibers in their drinking water. The risk for cancer from asbestos in drinking water remains controversial.

Public concern remains high over asbestos materials in schools, homes, and public buildings. Some think that this installed asbestos represents a health hazard for children, office workers, or residents. Current scientific opinion favors the view that installed asbestos probably represents little or no public health risk, but with important reservations.[2] The installed asbestos must be contained, enclosed, and in good physical condition. Friable asbestos can generate potentially hazardous aerosols and should be removed or enclosed. Renovation, demolition, or asbestos abatement should be done only by trained personnel using approved techniques to protect themselves and bystanders from exposure. Maintenance workers who spend years cleaning and repairing structures that contain asbestos may be at much greater risk than the public passing through them. A reasonable balance in asbestos abatement is still being sought between needless cost and public safety.

Clinical Syndromes of Asbestos-Related Diseases

Asbestosis

The signs and symptoms of asbestosis are those of chronic diffuse interstitial lung disease in general, and closely parallel the clinical features of idiopathic pulmonary fibrosis (IPF). Symptoms usually are not apparent until 10 to 30 years after the asbestos exposure occurred or began. Gradually worsening shortness of breath with exertion is typically the first sign of asbestosis. Nonproductive cough may appear early as well. Both cough and exertional dyspnea gradually become more severe as the disease runs its course over several decades. Respiratory insufficiency may ultimately restrict patients to bed or chair and to continuous oxygen therapy. Cough may be quite disabling, with paroxysms interrupting conversation and exertion, but sputum production is usually minimal. Respiratory failure causes death for patients with severe asbestosis.

Physical examination reveals high-pitched end-inspiratory crackles (rales, crepitations) predominantly at the lung bases that become louder and more generalized as asbestosis progresses. Tachypnea with the use of accessory respiratory muscles and rapid expiration becomes apparent as the disease grows more severe. Digital clubbing without the associated findings or discomfort of hypertrophic pulmonary osteoarthropathy is a common finding in asbestosis, even early in the course of disease. Dependent edema, cardiomegaly, and elevated central venous pressure (cor pulmonale) complicate late asbestosis, as hypoxia and obliteration of the pulmonary capillary bed raise pulmonary artery pressure.

The pulmonary function abnormalities in asbestosis are typical of "restrictive" lung disease, and mimic those of IPF. Obliteration of airspaces and small vasculature with increased interstitial connective tissue produces characteristic derangements. Pulmonary compliance is reduced, airflow rates are rapid, and ventilation-perfusion matching is disturbed. The vital capacity is reduced. The total lung capacity and its subdivisions are decreased symmetrically. Quasi-static deflation pressure-volume curves are shifted down to the right, indicating decreased compliance. Airflow is rapid due to increased alveolar wall elastic recoil and well-tethered airways; thus the FEV_1/FVC ratio, $FEF_{25\%-75\%}$, and other measurements of airflow are normal or accelerated.

Gas exchange becomes increasingly abnormal as asbestosis progresses. The carbon monoxide diffusing capacity (DlCO) is reduced. Arterial blood gases obtained at rest may be normal early in asbestosis, then show hypoxemia with mild hypocarbia, and finally evidence hypercarbia as end-stage disease is reached. Arterial oxygen desaturation during exercise may occur quite early in asbestosis, and becomes more severe and constraining with progressive disease. The DlCO and exercise oxygen measurements may be abnormal before the vital capacity or resting arterial blood gases show much change, and therefore may be useful in the diagnosis and periodic evaluation of early asbestosis.

Radiology is an essential tool in the assessment of pulmonary disease caused by asbestos. The standard 72-inch posteroanterior chest radiograph is used to detect and follow the progress of patients with asbestosis. High-resolution computed tomography (CT) of the chest using standardized techniques has become a powerful adjunct for more sensitive or complete assessment of individual patients. As shown in the figures that illustrate this chapter, the CT scan clearly reveals parenchymal disease, honeycombing, pleural plaques, calcification, and other features that are seen with difficulty by plain radiograph.

A standardized scoring system has been developed by the International Labor Organization for the description and grading of chest radiographs in the pneumoconioses. The International Labor Organization, Union Internationale Contra Cancer (ILO-UICC) Classification System of radiographs of the pneumoconioses is the most current version of this scheme.[3,4] The ILO-UICC Classification System categorizes radiographic shadows in lung parenchyma as small or large opacities. The pattern of the small opacities is described as rounded (size *p, q, r*), such as might be seen in silicosis, or as irregular (size *s, t, u*), such as seen in asbestosis. The extent of small opacities is described as the profusion, referring to the number of small opacities per unit area. Profusion is scored on a 12-point scale as none (0/-, 0/0, 0/1), few but definite (1/0, 1/1, 1/2), moderate (lung markings visible; 2/1, 2/2, 2/3), or many (lung markings obscured;

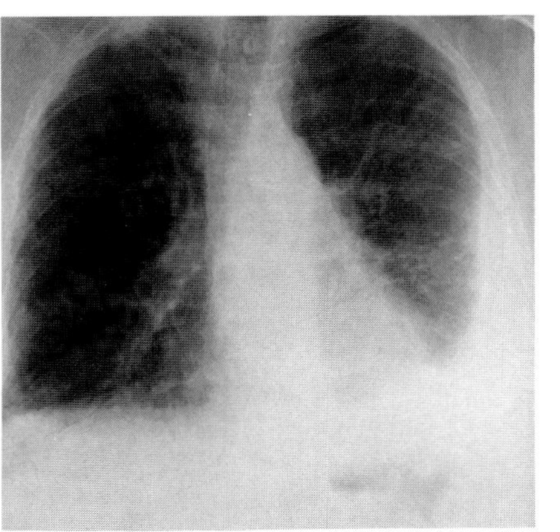
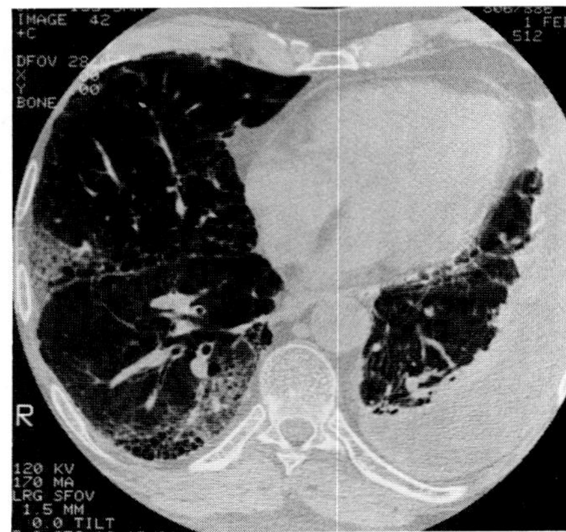

A   B

Figure 4-1. Asbestosis. (*A*) Plain chest radiograph reveals a pattern of small and medium irregular shadows in moderate profusion with somewhat of a lower zone predominance, and left pleural thickening with effusion. The patient was a 63-year-old man who had worked in a mill where 2 days per month he cut sheets of asbestos with a mechanical saw. (*B*) Computed tomogram reveals peripheral compartment interstitial fibrosis with honeycombing at pleural locations. A pleural-based mass with thickening and effusion is apparent on the left. Needle biopsy of the pleura recovered poorly differentiated carcinoma.

3/2, 3/3, 3/+). Large opacities are scored by size over 1 cm; a variety of pleural changes and other parenchymal findings can also be recorded. The system utilizes a set of standard reference films against which each worker's radiograph is compared. Readers who are specially trained in the use of this system record their findings on standardized forms. Interpretation of chest radiographs by a certified reader according to the ILO-UICC system is often required for legal compensation or to qualify for disability based on occupational lung disease.

The primary radiographic feature of asbestosis is a pattern of small irregular shadows with a lower lung zone predominance. In early or mild asbestosis, initial small irregular shadows, 1 mm to 5 mm in length and hairline thin, are scored as *s* opacities in low profusion, 1/0 or more, by the ILO-UICC classification scheme. As the disease progresses the opacities increase in size and become more extensive. Coarser shadows qualify for *t* or *u* designations and may be scored in higher profusions, up to 3/+. Dense small bands of fibrosis surrounding empty airspaces create a pattern of "honeycombing" in selected areas, particularly adjacent to pleural surfaces. Figure 4-1 illustrates the small irregular shadows of asbestosis on the plain radiograph and these opacities as well as honeycombing on the high-resolution CT scan. Evidence of other asbestos-related diseases, particularly pleural plaques, is commonly seen on the radiographs of patients with asbestosis. Cardiac enlargement due to cor pulmonale is a late feature of advanced disease. The chest radiograph in asbestosis is usually indistinguishable from that of a patient with idiopathic pulmonary fibrosis except for the pleural plaques that are sometimes seen, and for the history of asbestos exposure that the patient relates.

The pathology of asbestosis associates diffuse interstitial fibrosis with the presence of asbestos in the tissue.[5] On gross examination the lungs in advanced asbestosis are small and firm; the pleura is usually thickened, and parietal pleural plaques are usually present (see below). The cut surface of the lung is dark brown, with gray-white streaks of fibrous tissue that highlight septal planes. A firm reticular pattern of fibrosis is most apparent in the lower lung zones, and honeycombing may be seen. The central lymph nodes are usually normal in size, but may be discolored. In mild cases of asbestosis the lung may appear grossly normal.

The earliest or mildest lesions of asbestosis appear in the respiratory bronchioles. Alveolar duct bifurcations and respiratory bronchioles are the main sites of inhaled fiber deposition in animals exposed to asbestos[6] and the fibers penetrate the epithelium rapidly at these locations. Macrophages accumulate at sites of deposition and may promote both fiber transport and local tissue injury. Macrophages also accumulate in the airspaces of lungs affected by asbestosis. Interstitial cell accumulations are modest and primarily mononuclear. Neutrophils are usually few in number. Multinucleate giant cells are rare in most cases, but can be abundant in some instances. Granulomas do not occur in asbestosis, but collections of lymphocytes and plasma cells are found in some tissues. It is not yet clear whether these immune-inflammatory cell aggregates are part of the central pathogenesis of asbestosis or an incidental secondary response to the disease.

The walls of respiratory bronchioles are thickened by accumulations of connective tissue matrix with few cells, and the overlying epithelium may reveal cuboidalization and squamous metaplasia in human pathological specimens with asbestosis. Ultrastructural studies reveal epithelial and capillary injury and a pattern similar to idiopathic pulmonary fibrosis.[7] The first-order respiratory bronchioles of only occasional lobules are involved in the earliest disease. As asbestosis progresses, second- and third-order bronchioles and alveolar ducts become abnormal, and the process encompasses increasing numbers of lobules. Fibrosis appears to radiate out from the central unit along the septal planes. The process spreads outward in a centrifugal pattern that finally involves all parts of the lung. Extensive fibrosis finally engulfs and distorts the normal structures, and dense bands of collagen bordering cyst-like empty spaces create a honeycomb. Figure 4-2 illustrates asbestosis. Fibrosis is centered around small airways.

The lung reacts to asbestos fibers over time by coating some of them with biological materials. Asbestos bodies, or ferruginous bodies, are fibers coated with protein and iron deposits in a characteristic beaded pattern. Asbestos bodies form around long fibers and can be seen with the light microscope. Amphibole fibers generate asbestos bodies readily, whereas chrysotile produces them less frequently. The tendency of chrysotile to fragment into smaller fibers in lung tissue may contribute to its reduced tendency to form asbestos bodies. Thus, most asbestos bodies have amphibole cores. Figure 4-3 shows two asbestos bodies in lung tissue. A detailed discussion of asbestos bodies with illustrations of their many forms is included in a report from the College of American Pathologists by a panel chaired by Craighead.[5] Asbestos bodies in association with compatible histologic changes are required to establish a pathological diagnosis of asbestosis.[5] Detection of uncoated fibers by electron microscopy of tissue digestates is not sufficient to establish disease. Many workers have uncoated fibers and asbestos bodies in their lung tissues with no evidence of parenchymal disease or tissue reaction.

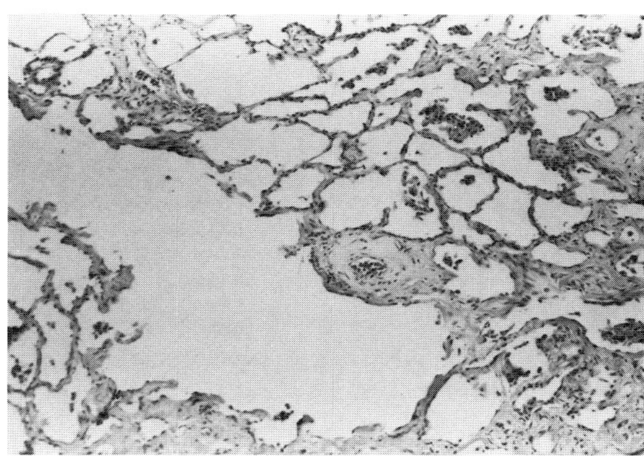

Figure 4-2. Asbestosis. Interstitial fibrosis and mild mononuclear cell inflammation are seen surrounding a terminal airway. Airspaces filled with macrophages are evident. The tissue was obtained from a 70-year-old retired surveyor of New York City subways and building sites who underwent thoracotomy for biopsy of an entrapping pleural lesion that proved to be a mesothelioma. Asbestos bodies and lesions typical of asbestosis were found in the lung parenchyma (see Fig. 4-3). (Original magnification × 25)

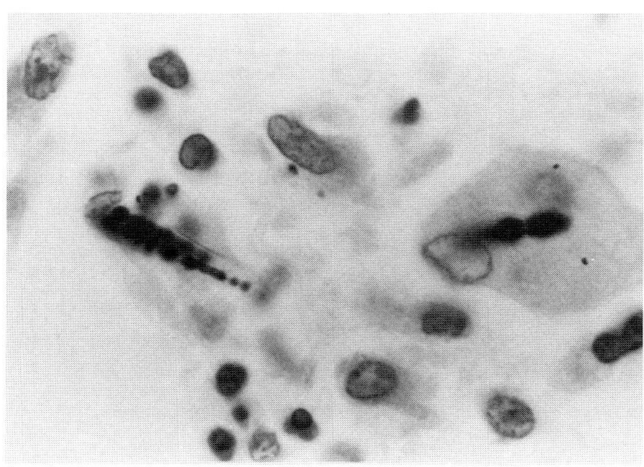

Figure 4-3. Asbestos bodies. Two ferruginous bodies are visualized with an iron stain in an area of interstitial fibrosis. The asbestos body on the left reveals a fibrous central core and the body on the right demonstrates a typical "dumbbell" shape. (Original magnification × 500)

Asbestosis usually runs its course over several decades or more after presentation. In general, the more intense the exposure and the greater the pulmonary fiber burden, the earlier asbestosis becomes apparent and the more rapidly it progresses. At least 10 years from initial exposure usually are required for clinical signs of disease, and 20 or 30 years often pass before symptoms are present. Another 5 to 30 years may pass before fibrosis becomes so severe as to cause respiratory failure. For example, a 20-year-old worker exposed to asbestos steam pipe insulation in the naval shipyards of World War II in 1940–1945 will typically not develop any signs of asbestosis until the 1960s or 1970s, and will not become substantially impaired until the 1970s or 1980s. Survival into the 21st century may be quite possible. Asbestosis patients with the most severe disease may succumb within 5 to 10 years of initial symptoms, and the course of their disease may be complicated by cancer or other asbestos-related problems.

Asbestosis can result from heavy exposure to any of the mineral forms of asbestos, although crocidolite and amosite are considered more fibrogenic than chrysotile. Quite heavy exposure is required to produce pulmonary fibrosis. The crocidolite asbestos mines and mills of South Africa, and asbestos cloth weaving mills of Britain, the asbestos cement plants of North America and Europe, and many other workplaces provided very high ambient fiber levels in the years between the late 19th century and the 1950s. Severe asbestosis with respiratory disability and death was an important industrial disease during and following those years of high exposure. The recognition of asbestos as the cause, and the imposition of industrial hygiene standards that reduce fiber levels a hundred-fold or more in the air of the workplace, has produced a dramatic reduction in the prevalence and severity of asbestosis.

Clinically significant pulmonary fibrosis due to asbestos will, in all likelihood, become rare or nonexistent in the industrialized nations over the next several decades. American workers presenting with asbestosis in the 1980s and 1990s received their initial fiber exposures in the 1940s, 1950s, and 1960s. Workplace conditions have changed substantially since that time. Industrial and environmental standards for airborne asbestos are now regulated vigorously in developed countries, and public awareness about asbestos hazards is high. The current Threshold Limit Values (TLV) for asbestos in workplace air (0.2 fibers/cc) appears to be a safe standard such that exposure at or below this level should not produce clinical asbestosis. It is to be hoped that asbestosis will soon become a disease of historical interest alone.

Pleural Plaques

Pleural plaques are patches of pleural thickening, sometimes with dystrophic central calcification, which occur on the parietal pleura in response to asbestos. These lesions cause no symptoms and are not a cause of disability, although they may be quite striking when seen in chest radiographs. Plaques appear typically on the lateral mid-chest parietal pleura and are seen frequently along the diaphragmatic and mediastinal pleural surfaces. Bilaterally symmetrical mid-chest pleural thickening with a line of central dystrophic calcification, or similar lesions on the surface of the diaphragm, are virtually diagnostic of asbestos-related pleural disease and thus of substantial asbestos exposure.

The pathology of pleural plaques is rather bland and does not usually reveal asbestos as the obvious cause of the lesions.[8] On gross examination, the plaques appear as glistening raised white islands with sharp borders arising from the parietal, or chest-wall, surface of the pleura, diaphragm, and mediastinum. Adhesions to the visceral pleura are not usually present. The plaques are usually multiple and bilateral, and vary in size from a few millimeters up to 5 cm to 10 cm in diameter and 1 mm to 15 mm in thickness. The pleural surface of the plaque is covered by normal mesothelium. The body of the plaque is composed of fibrous connective tissue, particularly fibrillar collagen. The chest wall surface of the plaque may reveal low-grade chronic inflammation. Dystrophic calcification is common in these plaques, with acicular apatite crystals aligned in parallel with the collagen fibers. Ferruginous bodies are generally not found in or adjacent to plaques, but small uncoated fibers may sometimes be found beneath the chest wall surface with special electron microscopic or digestion techniques.

The mechanisms by which plaques form is unclear. Asbestos fibers deposited deep in the lung parenchyma are transported centrifugally to subpleural locations as free

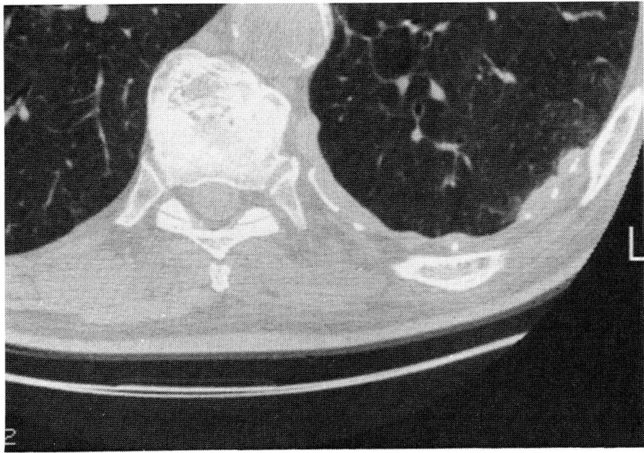

Figure 4-4. Asbestos-related pleural disease. Computed tomogram of the chest shows pleural thickening with linear calcification along the postero-lateral chest wall. The patient was a 64-year-old male smoker who had worked in an open pit asbestos mine in the 1950s. He was undergoing evaluation for a left lower lobe mass, which proved to be a small cell carcinoma.

fibers and by fiber-laden macrophages moving through interstitial lymphatics. Accumulations of fibers in subpleural locations can sometimes be found in tissues from animal models and human cases of asbestos exposure. The fibers are presumed to penetrate the visceral pleura, transit from the visceral pleura across the space to the parietal surface, penetrate, and produce an inflammatory and fibrotic response at the interface between the mesothelium and the underlying diaphragmatic or intercostal muscle. Mechanical trauma to the mesothelium does not appear to be an important pathogenetic mechanism in this response, since both the visceral and parietal pleura appear entirely normal. It is unknown why the inflammatory and fibrotic response does not occur beneath the visceral as well as the parietal pleura, or why deeper involvement of underlying chest wall structures is not seen.

Radiographically, pleural plaques appear as lines of pleural thickening along the mid-lateral chest wall, diaphragm, and/or mediastinum. Figure 4-4 illustrates the radiographic appearance of pleural plaques. Linear calcification can sometimes be seen within the thickening, particularly along the diaphragmatic pleura. The lesions appear as rounded or irregular densities when seen *en face.* Computed tomography (Fig. 4-4) shows plaques clearly, even when none are apparent by plain chest radiograph. The true plaques of asbestos-related disease must be read conservatively, and must be distinguished from unilateral pleural disease (with or without calcification), from other causes, from pleural reaction adjacent to rib injuries, and from subpleural fat in obese subjects.

The epidemiology of pleural plaques is related to exposure intensity and an appropriate lag time, as with pulmonary fibrosis (asbestosis). As many as 10% to 30% of men and 3% to 10% of women in urban areas evidence pleural plaques at autopsy, and 1% to 2% of chest radiographs of men show plaques.[9] Hillerdal[10] has estimated that only about 15% of subjects with plaques found by autopsy or incidental surgery will have plaques evident on chest radiograph. Most individuals with plaques give a history of exposure to asbestos, although it may be brief. A summer job in construction, a father or companion in the home who worked in asbestos, or living in an area near plants or mills using asbestos may be the only exposure identified. The latency time from initial asbestos exposure until plaques can be seen radiographically is usually 20 to 30 years.

The clinical importance of pleural plaques lies with these lesions as markers of asbestos exposure, and thus of other asbestos-related diseases. The plaques do not cause pain, irritate, or restrict ventilation. They may serve to substantiate asbestos exposure for individuals claiming compensation or disability for other asbestos-related diseases, but they are not in and of themselves a source of any disability.

Other Benign Pleural Lesions

Several other benign lesions of the pleura result from asbestos: benign effusion, pleuro-parenchymal strands ("crow's feet"), rounded atelectasis, and diffuse pleural thickening. Benign asbestos pleural effusion occurs during the first two decades following exposure, and thus usually is seen well before plaques or any other asbestos-related diseases (except possibly cancer) are evident. Effusion may occur later as well, but less commonly. The effusion is typically an exudate and may have great variability in cell composition, ranging from a few mononuclear cells to substantial blood. The mechanism of benign effusion is unclear, although immune-inflammatory mechanisms rather than mechanical ones appear to be implicated. Three criteria are required to establish the diagnosis: (1) exclusion of other causes (e.g., tuberculosis); (2) follow-up for 2 or more years to assure the effusion is benign; and (3) an identifiable exposure to asbestos.[10]

The lesion referred to as "crow's feet" on chest radiograph consists of several coarse linear shadows that converge on a pleural surface and extend from the visceral pleura into lung parenchyma. Areas of rounded atelectasis appear as dense, round masses several centimeters in diameter, with fine strands extending into the parenchyma. They occur just beneath the pleural surface. Rounded atelectasis is believed to be composed of a compressed portion of lung trapped in pleural-based strands of fibrous tissue; thus they resemble "crow's feet." Rounded atelectasis must be distinguished from carcinoma, a task that usually requires cytologic or tissue diagnosis unless the CT image is clearly distinctive.

Diffuse pleural thickening caused by asbestos is relatively rare but can produce significant entrapment and respiratory restriction.[8] This term does not apply just to a large plaque, but rather refers to thickening that surrounds most or all of the lung and that may cause substantial entrapment. The pleural fibrosis is often bumpy and varies in thickness at different sites. The thickening may extend over the pericardial surface and into the fissures of the lung, indicating involvement of visceral pleura as well as the parietal pleura, which is the primary site for plaques. These areas of thickening may demonstrate dystrophic calcification. Decortication surgery has been suggested to relieve the lung entrapment caused by diffuse pleural thickening, but overall results in comparison with patients managed more conservatively have not been reported. It may be very difficult to distinguish diffuse pleural thickening from mesothelioma without surgical exploration, except for the slow progression and calcification of the benign lesion.

Mesothelioma

Malignant mesothelioma arises from the mesothelial cells, or precursor cells, of the pleura and the peritoneum, or rarely from the pericardium or the tunica vaginalis testis. It is a terrible cancer, with virtually universal mortality, short survival after presentation, and no good treatment available. Mesothelioma is a rare cancer, with approximately 1500 to 2000 cases per year in America and about 600 per year in Britain.[11,12] Mesothelioma is very rare in the general population. Overall, approximately 80% of mesothelioma cases can be associated with some exposure to asbestos, with higher associations in geographic areas where asbestos work is common. The cumulative lifetime risk of developing mesothelioma may be as high as 10% among workers with heavy asbestos exposure.[13,14] Members of the households of asbestos workers and residents in the neighborhoods of asbestos mines, mills, and processing plants are also at increased risk of mesothelioma. There is a latency period of 20 to 30 years, often much longer, between initial asbestos exposure and the clinical presentation of mesothelioma. Very slight exposure to asbestos may produce increased risk for mesothelioma. There is a rough relation between a heavy asbestos exposure and the early development and increased incidence of mesothelioma, although this relationship is less complete than for other asbestos-related diseases. Tobacco smoking does not increase the risk of developing mesothelioma in humans, although bronchogenic carcinoma risk is enhanced (see below). Thus, asbestos is thought to be a complete carcinogen for mesothelioma, encompassing both initiator and promoter properties for inducing this cancer.[1,15]

Pleural mesotheliomas outnumber peritoneal tumors about 5:2 in most groups, although peritoneal mesotheliomas may predominate among very heavily exposed workers.[16] Asbestos fibers can cross the gastrointestinal epithelium as well as the pleura. Thus, peritoneal tumors could arise as a result of lymphatic transport of asbestos from the pleural space, swallowing fibers that were inhaled but cleared by mucociliary transport from the lung to the pharynx, or ingesting asbestos from water or other environmental sources.

Patients with mesothelioma typically present with symptoms of dyspnea related to lung entrapment or effusion, or with chest wall pain.[16,17] Most patients are 50 to 70 years of age at presentation, and men greatly outnumber women as a reflection of workplace exposures. Chest radiographs and CT scans reveal a "lumpy-bumpy" pattern of pleural thickening that is suggestive of the diagnosis, but certainly not unique for it. Most patients do not show asbestos pleural plaques or fibrosis on plain radiographs, although the majority reveal plaques and lines of dystrophic calcification by CT scan.

Mesothelioma is usually unilateral and spreads by local invasion to entrap the lung, central thoracic vessels, esophagus, heart, or abdominal structures, producing signs and symptoms related to specific organ involvement. Mesothelioma sometimes spreads to local or hilar lymph nodes, but only very rarely metastasizes outside of the chest or abdomen. Local extension along needle tracks and incision lines often complicates biopsy procedures. Pain in the chest wall, abdomen, and deep organs can be incapacitating. Large and recurrent collections of pleural or ascites fluid complicate direct tumor invasion.

Mesotheliomas are categorized histologically as epithelial, sarcomatous, or mixed cell types.[5] The major difficulty in pathological diagnosis is distinguishing mesothelioma from other cancers that may have metastasized to the pleural space, particularly adenocarcinoma of lung origin. Specialized histochemical or immunohistochemical staining may assist with the definitive identification of mesothelioma.[5,12] Asbestos bodies are not found in mesothelioma tissue, but fibers and asbestos bodies can be identified in many cases in the lung parenchyma, confirming an associated asbestos exposure.

The course and prognosis of mesothelioma are grim, and no satisfactory curative or palliative measures are available. Survival from diagnosis averages 18 months, with slightly better outlook for patients with epithelial and mixed cell types, and worse survival for patients with sarcomatous histology.[11,12] Initial management with frequent thoracentesis or paracentesis, decortication and debulking surgery, and aggressive chemotherapy or radiotherapy may help maintain functional status longer but probably do not extend survival substantially.[12] General supportive measures, with oxygen, nutrition, and pain control, are the main contributions to the treatment of mesothelioma.

The risk of mesothelioma depends greatly on the asbestos fiber type. The risk for mesothelioma from amphibole asbestos fibers is generally agreed, while the risk from chrysotile is still debated. The association between mesothelioma and asbestos was first reported among South African crocidolite workers[18] and has since been observed in many other worker groups exposed to amphibole. Endemic areas of mesothelioma have been found in the eastern mediterranean, where environmental exposures to the zeolite fiber erionite[19] and the amphibole tremolite[20] are implicated. A clear association between exposure to chrysotile alone and mesothelioma has not been proven. These cancers occur with slightly increased frequency among the chrysotile mine and mill workers of Quebec, but the neoplasms have been attributed to the amphibole tremolite that contaminates the primary serpentine fiber.[21] In the past, workers in many trades received exposure to a variety of different asbestos types, thus complicating risk assessment. Workers and others exposed exclusively to pure chrysotile after milling may have no increased risk of mesothelioma above the rare occurrence in the general population.[22]

The position that pure chrysotile does not confer an increased risk of mesothelioma has tremendous implications for public health and public policy. Most of the asbestos insulation and construction materials installed in buildings in the United States contain only chrysotile. Concerns have been raised that friable asbestos flaking off from these sources becomes airborne in schools and other buildings, and that children and others may be exposed to low doses of asbestos. These exposures are agreed to be well below levels that might cause pulmonary fibrosis or even benign pleural reactions, but theoretically they could enhance the risk of cancer. If chrysotile does not induce mesothelioma, then these construction materials provide little or no risk for the general (nonsmoking) public, and may not require special removal unless they are seriously deteriorated. The savings in time, disruption, and cost from not undertaking extensive asbestos abatement could be enormous. Many scientists now hold that mesothelioma is a disease caused only by amphibole asbestos fibers[22] and that the hazards of chrysotile exposure for the general public have been overrated.[2]

Bronchogenic Carcinoma

Asbestos exposure increases the risk of bronchogenic carcinoma in tobacco smokers in a dose-related manner. Asbestos appears to act as a "promoter" for lung cancer rather than as a complete carcinogen, with smoke acting as an "inducer." The effect of smoking is multiplicative, with a many-fold higher incidence of cancer among smoking asbestos workers than in any other groups. Individuals exposed to asbestos who do not smoke have a risk of bronchogenic carcinoma that is slightly[23] or not at all[24] increased compared to the general population. Asbestos workers who smoke have a risk of cancer that can be as high as 50-fold that of smokers without fiber exposure.[11,14,23,24] Lung cancer in smokers appears after a latency period of 10 to 30 years after initial asbestos exposure, but earlier than among nonexposed smokers.[5]

Greatly increased risk of lung cancer has been recorded among smokers who have worked with crocidolite and other amphibole asbestos fibers.[18] Cancer risk increases directly with the intensity and duration of asbestos exposure (fiber burden) and with cumulative smoking behavior (pack-years). Cancer risks may be increased slightly even for smokers whose asbestos exposure is too small to cause asbestosis or pleural plaques. Recent surveys among workers with modern exposure levels, hundreds of times less than those experienced in the past, do not support an increased risk of lung cancer, but these studies are limited by relatively short follow-up times since first exposure.[25,26] Cancer risk is increased, but to a lessor degree, among smokers who have worked with chrysotile asbestos only.[27] Since most asbestos workers who were exposed in previous decades were also heavy smokers, the assessment of lung cancer risks for nonsmokers has been difficult. Definitive proof that chrysotile fiber does not cause an increased risk for lung cancer in nonsmokers has not yet been provided, but awaits a large-scale study that would detect infrequent events reliably. Accurate assessment of the cancer risk caused by chrysotile for nonsmokers is of great importance, however, because of its public health implications related to asbestos abatement.

The signs and symptoms, radiographic findings, management, course, and prognosis for lung cancer in asbestos-exposed smokers are similar to those for lung cancer in the general population. Pleural plaques, and sometimes pulmonary fibrosis, can be identified on the chest radiographs and CT scans of many of these cancer patients, although the tumor may precede the other findings of asbestos-related disease. The cell types of lung cancer seen in association with asbestos are the same as for tobacco smokers in general. An increased frequency of adenocarcinoma, with decreased frequency of squamous cell cancer, has been observed in some series. Figures 4-1 and 4-4 illustrate examples of small cell undifferentiated and large cell undifferentiated carcinomas occurring in association with various manifestations of other asbestos-related diseases.

Disability or personal injury compensation has become an important issue for lung cancer patients with asbestos exposure; the risk of lung cancer is considered an important factor in compensating workers with evidence of other asbestos-related diseases. In several developed countries the cancer is determined to be caused by asbestos if radiographic or histopathologic evidence of asbestos-related diseases is found.[1] In the United States similar precedents for compensation have been established.

Current exposure to asbestos can be reduced through proper occupational and environmental hygiene measures. Previous exposure and lung asbestos fiber burdens cannot be changed. Thus, smoking cessation must receive the highest possible priority for individuals with past, or current, asbestos exposure. Aggressive, repeated measures to identify smokers and help them stop smoking are essential for reducing their cancer risks. Former smokers with asbestos exposure should receive ongoing close surveillance for lung cancer.

Bronchoalveolar Lavage Findings
in Asbestos-Related Disease

The profile of cells recovered by bronchoalveolar lavage from workers exposed to asbestos and from patients with overt asbestosis have been reported by authors from around the world. Table 4-1 summarizes results from several recent studies. Published reports describe most patients with clinical and radiographic asbestosis as evidencing increased proportions and total numbers of neutrophils, modestly increased eosinophils, and an increase in the proportion and number of lymphocytes.[28–36] The total number of macrophages is often increased, although the percentage is reduced by the influx of other inflammatory cell types. Among the subjects in each series, however, there appear always to be some patients who have relatively normal bronchoalveolar lavage (BAL) cell profiles despite asbestosis. Within the published reports there is considerable variation in results from workers who have been exposed to asbestos but who have no evidence of disease or who only have pleural plaques. The BAL cell populations for these exposed subjects vary from normal to mild changes similar to those found in asbestosis. Because of this variability, these results will not be reviewed in detail.

The proportions of T-lymphocyte surface antigen phenotypes in BAL fluid and in venous blood from the same subjects have been reported in two series,[31,36] as summarized in Table 4-2. The reports differ in that one studied workers with exposure alone whereas the other studied patients with asbestosis, they used different methods for enumerating T-cell phenotypes, and they obtained somewhat different values for normal subjects in blood and BAL fluid. Nonetheless, within each series the proportions of CD4+ T-cells, CD8+ T-cells, and the CD4+:CD8+ ratios in peripheral blood were similar between the controls and the asbestos-exposed workers. In these reports the percentage of T-cells expressing the CD4+ phenotype and the CD4+:CD8+ ratio were increased significantly in BAL fluid from asbestos-exposed subjects.

The recovery of asbestos fibers and ferruginous bodies in BAL fluid has generated considerable interest. Analysis of BAL fluid gives hope of establishing asbestos exposure in the potentially exposed subject and possibly quantitating the extent of that exposure. Standard methods have been proposed for digesting the cellular material in BAL fluid with sodium hypochlorite, trapping asbestos bodies and fibers on filters, and examining them by light microscopy to enumerate ferruginous bodies or by transmission electron microscopy to count small and large fibers.[21,37,38] Asbestos bodies are only rarely found in BAL specimens from nonexposed subjects but are abundant in fluid from workers with asbestos exposure.[28,34,36,38–40] Fewer than 1 asbestos body per ml of BAL fluid are found by light microscopy in samples from subjects with no workplace or environmental exposure to asbestos. Workers with mild exposure may have 2 to 20 asbestos bodies per ml, and workers with heavy exposure may demonstrate thousands of bodies per ml of fluid. The asbestos body counts in BAL fluid appear to correlate approximately with the presence and extent of parenchymal asbestosis, perhaps because both are a reflection of very heavy exposure. An important aspect of these reports is the finding that asbestos in BAL fluid does not represent recent exposure only; many subjects who have had no asbestos contact for 20 years or more still

TABLE 4-1. Bronchoalveolar Lavage Findings in Asbestos-Related Disease

Author	Begin	Rom	Costabel	Robinson	Hayes	Garcia	Cantin	Wallace
Year	1985	1987	1987	1988	1989	1989	1989	1989
Reference number	29	30	31	32	33	34	35	36
Location	Quebec	N I H	Germany	Australia	Australia	Texas	Quebec	California
Status	Asbestosis	Asbestosis	Asbestosis	Asbestosis	Asbestosis	Asbestosis	Asbestosis	Exposed
No. of subjects	17	18	7	26	15	12	10	15
BAL Volume (ml)	150	100	100	250	300	200	150	300
Recovery (%)	59.0		51.0	54.0		60.5		83.7
Total cells	37.2		30.0	39.0		22.7		42.7
AM %	88.0	76.0	71.0	83.0	84.2	82.9	89.7	80.0
LYS %	5.5	21.0	28.0	10.0	10.8	5.5	7.5	19.1
PMN %	5.0	3.0	2.0	5.4	3.2	8.0	3.1	.8
EOS %	1.0	.0		2.5	1.8	3.6	1.5	
Status	Control	Control	Control	Control		Control	Control	Control
No. of subjects	18	8	11	18		10	10	10
BAL Volume (ml)	150		100	250		200	150	300
Recovery (%)	61.0		54.0	51.0		54.5		60.0
Total cells	16.5		7.2	39.0		5.3		27.0
AM %	92.0	83.0	92.0	92.0		93.0	74.5	89.9
LYS %	7.6	15.0	7.0	8.0		5.0	24.5	9.7
PMN %	.4	2.0	1.0	2.0		1.3	.7	.5
EOS %	.1	.0		.2		.7	.3	

Total Cells shown $\times 10^{-6}$

AM % = % alveolar macrophages; LYS % = % lymphocytes; PMN % = % neutrophils; EOS % = % eosinophils

TABLE 4-2. T-Lymphocyte Surface Antigen Phenotypes from Asbestos-Exposed Workers

	NOMENCLATURE	**PERIPHERAL BLOOD**				**BAL FLUID**			
Author		Costabel		Wallace		Costabel		Wallace	
Year		1987		1989		1987		1989	
Reference number		31		36		31		36	
Methods used		IPS/LM		FS/FC		IPS/LM		FS/FC	
Location		Germany		California		Germany		California	
Status		Asbestosis	Control	Exposed	Control	Asbestosis	Control	Exposed	Control
No. of subjects		7	11	15	10	7	11	15	10
CD4+ %	Helper/Inducer	44.4%	43.7%	34.0%	34.5%	72.0%	55.0%	55.1%	48.9%
CD8+ %	Suppressor/Cytolytic	25.7%	25.8%	33.9%	34.0%	19.0%	31.0%	27.3%	27.8%
CD4+:CD8+	Helper:Suppres Ratio	2.00	1.80	1.07	1.05	4.50	1.90	2.88	1.99

The clusters of differentiation (CD) numerical designation is shown in the first column and the putative function of lymphocytes carrying that surface antigen is shown in the second column.

Methods used: IPS/LM = Immunoperoxidase-linked antibody stain/light microscopy
FS/FC = Fluorescein-linked antibody stain/flow cytometry

have numerous asbestos bodies in BAL fluid. It must be emphasized that the presence of asbestos fibers or bodies in BAL fluid only proves exposure to asbestos at some time in the past; it does not prove that any asbestos-related disease has occurred.

The results obtained to date provide a reasonable expectation that BAL will prove useful in the evaluation of selected patients with asbestos exposure. It should be particularly useful in research about the mechanisms of asbestosis, providing a closer look at events within the lung than peripheral blood samples. There is a continuum of changes in BAL cell types and T-lymphocyte phenotypes between normal subjects and patients with overt asbestosis, with substantial overlap and no clear dividing line between these groups. The findings in workers with exposure but no disease are even more variable. The confounding effects of smoking, age, extent of exposure, asbestos mineral type, and genetic variability among subjects have not been studied in detail. The data available do not permit interpretation of BAL cell type profiles for clinical diagnosis or management of patients with asbestos-related diseases. There appears to be a clear dichotomy between the numbers of asbestos bodies recovered from workers with significant exposure and from subjects with no asbestos exposure. Thus, analysis of BAL in search of asbestos may be useful in confirming asbestos exposure for patients with compatible clinical findings and an equivocal occupational history.

Immune Responses in Asbestos-Exposed Workers

The ways in which asbestos interacts with the immune system have generated considerable interest. In theory, an aberrant immunologic response to asbestos as a chronic "antigen," or to native proteins altered by asbestos to create neo-antigens, could be part of the pathogenetic mechanism of asbestos-related diseases. Alternatively, depression of immune surveillance as a secondary result of evolving asbestos-induced disease could permit other diseases to develop more readily, particularly cancer. Asbestos exposure has not been associated with increased susceptibility to infections in general or to any particular infectious agent, such as the link between silicosis and chronic tuberculosis. Investigators have surveyed asbestos-exposed workers, asbestosis patients, and animal models of asbestosis in an attempt to find evidence to support one or both of these hypotheses. Unfortunately, this has proved to be a difficult area with few simple or consistent answers. The literature is confusing.

Early epidemiologic studies of immunologic function in asbestos-exposed workers or patients with asbestosis provided somewhat contradictory results, and many of the reports were limited by small numbers of subjects and poorly matched control groups (see review by Morris and associates[41]). The most consistent finding that emerged from these studies was an elevation of serum immunoglobulins IgG, IgA, and IgM, but there was no apparent correlation between the degree of elevation and other exposure or disease parameters. In contrast, Israeli asbestos cement workers had normal serum immunoglobulin levels but other changes in cellular immune responses.[42] The appearance of auto-antibodies (rheumatoid factor, anti-nuclear antibodies) has provided conflicting results among various studies.[41] A case-control study of patients with multiple myeloma that sought associations with potential causative agents identified exposure to asbestos and exposure to petroleum products as the occupational factors increasing the odds ratio for this malignant plasma cell dyscrasia.[43] In aggregate, these reports suggest that polyclonal stimulation of B-lymphocyte or plasma cell function is a feature of selected phases of asbestos-related disease and is probably a secondary effect rather than a primary cause.

Studies of lymphocyte number and type and of cell-mediated immune function have produced confusing results. A group of asymptomatic asbestos cement workers with normal or near-normal chest radiographs were selected for further immunologic evaluation because of serum hypergammaglobulinemia.[44] These workers demonstrated reduced peripheral blood lymphocyte counts, decreased numbers of CD4+ (helper/ inducer) lymphocytes, and a diminished response to stimulation with phytohemagglu-tinin in vitro. U.S. asbestos insulation workers, 80% with radiographic disease, demonstrated an increased proportion of CD8+ (T-suppressor/cytolytic) lymphocytes, and a decreased CD4+:CD8+ (helper: suppressor) ratio, when compared to industrial controls without asbestos exposure.[45] Whereas most of the insulation workers showed normal lymphocyte natural killer (NK) cell activity, a fraction of workers evidenced increased NK activity, and another subset had depressed NK activity. Demographic or asbestos disease parameters did not correlate with NK activity. Asbestos-exposed iron and machinery workers evidenced an increased proportion of T-suppressor (CD8+) lymphocytes and a decreased CD4+:CD8+ (helper: suppressor) ratio.[46] The decreased CD4+:CD8+ ratio was associated with depressed lymphocyte NK cell activity and an increased proportion of a Leu 2+ Leu 8− subset proposed as effector suppressor T cells. The changes in the proportions of lymphocyte phenotypes were correlated with radiographic evidence of asbestos-related disease but not with age, smoking, or the extent of asbestos exposure. In a study from Australia, lymphocytes from patients with asbestosis evidenced normal NK activity.[47] The addition of subtoxic amounts of asbes-tos to normal blood and BAL lymphocytes in vitro suppressed NK cell activity equally in lymphocytes from normal subjects and from the asbestosis patients. Profiles of lym-phocytes recovered by BAL from asbestos-exposed workers are normal or show in-creased percentages of lymphocytes (see Table 4-1). The limited evidence available suggests that BAL T-lymphocyte surface antigen phenotypes demonstrate the reverse of that seen in peripheral blood, with an increase in the proportion of CD4+ cells, and an increase in the CD4+:CD8+ ratio, as discussed above (see Table 4-2).

Several laboratories have examined the proliferative responses of blood lympho-cytes challenged with common mitogens. U.S. West Coast shipyard workers with radio-graphic evidence of asbestos-related disease had an increased lymphocyte proliferative response to pokeweed mitogen stimulation, compared with shipyard workers with low asbestos exposure and normal radiographic appearance and with a pool of Red Cross blood donors.[48] Shipyard workers with and without radiographically evident disease had increased serum IgG and IgA levels, increased suppressor T-cell numbers, and a reduced T-helper to T-suppressor ratio when they were compared to the Red Cross donors. It is not clear whether the differences in serum immunoglobulins and lympho-cyte surface antigen phenotype proportions in this study were due to exposure to as-bestos or to other unidentified confounding differences between the blood donors and the shipyard workers. Conversely, Israeli cement plant workers demonstrated normal lymphocyte responses to pokeweed and conconavalin A (con A) mitogens, but aug-mented T-cell division in autologous mixed lymphocyte culture.[42] These cement work-ers had elevated T-cell suppressor activity, but normal peripheral blood counts, percentages and ratios of lymphocyte phenotype subgroups, and lymphocyte NK cell activity when compared with a similar group of transport workers. American asbestos cement workers showed a diminished response to stimulation with phytohemagglutinin in vitro.[44] Lymphocytes recovered by BAL from sheep chronically exposed to asbestos responded to pokeweed and con A mitogens with increased stimulation, as compared with cells from sham-control sheep.[49]

The majority of surveys indicate that asbestos-exposed individuals manifest a slight to moderate decrease in the proportion of CD8+ (T-suppressor/cytolytic) lymphocytes in peripheral blood, a normal percentage of CD4+ (T-helper/inducer) lymphocytes, and a decreased CD4+:CD8+ (T_h/T_s) ratio.[45,46] In BAL fluid, the percentage of lymphocytes may be increased, and the proportion of CD4+ cells and the CD4+:CD-8+ ratio are elevated.[31,36] Lymphocyte NK cell activity appears to be normal,[32,42] depressed,[45,46] or increased[45] in various subsets of asbestos-exposed workers. These reports also suggest, but do not confirm, that asbestos exposure or clinically evident asbestos-related disease sometimes is associated with "priming" peripheral blood lymphocytes for an augmented proliferative response to pokeweed mitogen,[48] con A,[49] and autologous mixed lymphocyte culture,[42] and possibly a decreased response to phytohemagglutinin.[44]

No clear picture of the effects of asbestos on humoral or cell-mediated immune responses has emerged from the many studies that have been reported. It appears that this may be largely a statistical problem created by a number of confounding factors. Genetic variation in the intensity of immune responses among workers is likely to produce subgroups that respond differently to the same stimulus. Immunologic responses that augment the pathogenetic processes of asbestos-caused disease may be confused or compounded by secondary reactions. Both the intensity and duration of asbestos exposure could influence immune responses. Subjects with full-blown asbestosis may have quite different immune reactions than workers with low-dose exposure and no manifestations of any disease. Lastly, most reports have focused on peripheral blood, whereas, the lung and pleural surface are the site of disease. Much more work is required to understand the role of immune responses in the pathogenesis of asbestosis and the impact of asbestos on immunocompetence.

Mechanisms of Asbestos-Related Diseases

We are beginning to understand the mechanisms by which asbestos fibers produce the various diseases associated with them. Many aspects of the pathogenesis of asbestos-related diseases remain obscure, however. Most observations related to mechanisms of disease have been derived from animal models or from in vitro cell culture systems, and extension to the realities of human disease requires substantial confirmation.

Recruitment of Inflammatory Cells

Asbestos fibers deposit preferentially at alveolar duct bifurcations in rats exposed to a chrysotile aerosol.[6] Within 24 hours macrophages have been recruited to these sites, many of the fibers have been ingested, and a substantial portion of the fiber burden has been translocated out of the lung by mucociliary clearance or into the interstitium. Asbestos can activate the chemotactic fifth component (C5a) from complement proteins, and complement activation in bronchoalveolar epithelial lining fluid is hypothesized as the mechanism for this early attraction of phagocytes where inhaled fibers land in the lung.[50,51]

Animal models of inhalation exposure of rats to asbestos,[52,53] intratracheal instillation in hamsters,[54] and an extensively documented model of repeated endobronchial instillation in sheep[55] have consistently demonstrated increased numbers of neutrophils and macrophages in the BAL fluids and lung tissues of animals developing asbestosis. As detailed above, BAL fluids from human cases of asbestosis evidence increased proportions of neutrophils. The macrophages recovered by BAL from human asbestosis patients secrete increased amounts of the potent neutrophils chemotactic leukotriene B_4 (LTB_4).[34] Alveolar macrophages from rats exposed to asbestos release a protein chemotactin for macrophages.[56] Chemotactic activity for neutrophils is released by alveolar macrophages recovered from various animal species after asbestos exposure,[54,57,58] and exposure of control alveolar macrophages to asbestos in vitro produces similar activity.

These data suggest that asbestos fibers can promote an inflammatory cell response of macrophages and neutrophils by triggering the release of potent chemotactins from macrophages that have ingested the fibers. Asbestos may also generate chemotactins for inflammatory cells in the extracellular milieu. For practical purposes these effects have been studied primarily utilizing free airspace cells and secretions, but a similar sequence of events is hypothesized to occur in the interstitium. Inflammation within the lumen and surrounding interstitium of terminal airways is the earliest/simplest pathological finding in asbestosis, and it could be explained by these mechanisms.

Injury to Lung Tissues

Investigation along several lines highlights the importance of reactive oxygen species as mediators of tissue injury, and possibly other effects, in diseases caused by asbestos. Macrophages, neutrophils, mesenchymal or epithelial target cells, and possibly the surface of the asbestos fiber itself, may generate high energy reactive forms of oxygen: superoxide (O_2^-), hydrogen peroxide (H_2O_2), hydroxyl radical ($\cdot OH$).

Alveolar macrophages recovered by BAL from human asbestosis patients spontaneously release increased amounts of O_2^- and H_2O_2.[30] BAL macrophages from sheep with experimental asbestosis release increased O_2^- with PMA stimulation but not spontaneously.[59] Cells exposed to asbestos in vitro also release reactive oxygen species. Tracheal epithelial cells and fibroblasts are killed by exposure to asbestos in vitro, and the damage can be blocked by antioxidant enzymes (superoxide dismutase, catalase), by $\cdot OH$ scavengers and by iron chelating agents.[60,61] Iron appears to play a key role in the generation of these reactive oxygen species, acting as a Fenton reagent to catalyze the production of $\cdot OH$ from H_2O_2 and O_2^- (see review by Mossman and March[62]). The addition of desferoxamine, an iron chelator, blocks asbestos toxicity in many systems.

The generation of O_2^- from alveolar macrophages appears to be partially dependent on the fibrous nature of a mineral, since a variety of fibers trigger O_2^- release, whereas nonfibrous but chemically identical particles do not enhance oxidant production.[62] The surface of silicates in the form of both fibers and nonfibrous particles can serve as Fenton catalysts in cell-free systems. Minerals that are fibrogenic (asbestos, silica, kaolin) are more potent O_2^- generators than minerals that cause little or no human pulmonary fibrosis (fiberglass, wollastonite).[63]

The reactive oxygen species generated in response to asbestos or on the fiber surface could injure cells by peroxidation of membranes and by DNA strand breakage.[62] Injury to genetic material could be particularly important as a mechanism of inducing or promoting neoplastic transformation of cells. The combination of cigarette smoke and asbestos, but not either one alone, caused breaks in strands of *E. coli* DNA in vitro,[64] and the addition of iron chelators or catalase reduced this effect. This growing body of evidence from human studies, animal models, and cell culture research all point to reactive oxygen species as important intermediates in both fibrosis and cancer caused by asbestos, and suggests that anti-oxidants and iron chelators could provide a means of altering these processes.

Fibrosis

Asbestos may promote fibrosis through a variety of mechanisms that lead to fibroblast proliferation and the deposition of excess connective tissue matrix material. Cytokines and other mediators released from pulmonary macrophages appear to be key elements in this process. The many interlocking pathways of cytokines and cell interactions in the lung have been reviewed in detail[65] and are also discussed in this chapter in relation to silicosis. Less comprehensive information has been assembled about asbestosis, but many of the final pathways appear to be similar.

Alveolar macrophages from asbestosis patients, and in some instances from workers exposed to asbestos who do not have disease, release increased amounts of fibronectin and somatomedin (insulin-like growth factor) activity,[30] increased interferon-gamma,[32] and increased plasminogen activator. Alveolar macrophages from sheep exposed to chrysotile asbestos by repeated endobronchial instillation also secrete increased growth-promoting activity for fibroblasts[66] and increased plasminogen activator.[35] BAL fluid from these animals contains fibronectin and plasminogen activator activity in excess amounts.[67] Increased thymidine incorporation, implying proliferation or DNA repair, is observed in epithelial and interstitial cells in the bronchiolar-alveolar regions of rats soon after asbestos inhalation.[68–70] It is not clear whether this effect is caused directly by asbestos or is mediated by cytokines released from other cells.

The mechanisms by which asbestos induces lung tissue injury, recruits inflammatory cells, stimulates fibrosis, and causes cancer require much more research before a real understanding is achieved. The limited, often disconnected, information summarized above provides many clues and several important directions for future investigation. These and many future findings must be drawn together in order to understand why asbestos produces its distinctive patterns of histopathologic response and why it takes so very long for these diseases to develop after asbestos exposure begins.

SILICOSIS

Silicosis is caused by the inhalation of dust containing crystalline free silica, SiO_2. Silicosis is a chronic disease that requires prolonged exposure to mineral dust and develops decades after exposure has begun. Acute silicoproteinosis, an acute alveolar epithelial injury associated with massive silica exposure, is discussed briefly below. Chronic silicosis is characterized by the progressive development of nodules and fibrosis in lung tissue, with gradual impairment of lung function and enhanced susceptibility to tuberculosis. In some workers with advanced silicosis the small individual pulmonary nodules coalesce to form large, conglomerate masses; this condition is then referred to as progressive massive fibrosis. The diagnosis is established by the combination of compatible chest radiographic changes and an appropriate history of occupational exposure, and lung biopsy is rarely required.

Silicosis is of great historical interest as one of the earliest occupational lung diseases whose cause and course were recognized.[71] The association between dust exposure and disease in miners has been noted since the time of Hippocrates. Complete descriptions of the signs, symptoms, and gross pathology of silicosis had appeared by the 16th century. A great deal of the epidemiology and the role of dust control measures were known by the late 18th and early 19th centuries. The prevalence and severity of silicosis increased in the late 19th and early 20th centuries: mechanized mining techniques and air-powered carving chisels generated much greater dust aerosols than hand-held tools. Although the important concepts were apparent a century earlier, substantial improvements in workplace safety did not occur until the union labor and public health movements of the early and mid-20th century drew attention to silicosis. Modern dust control measures are effective in preventing silicosis, but it remains an important industrial health problem in less developed countries and in workplaces where proper safety practices are ignored.

Mineralogy

Approximately 25% of the earth's crust is silicon, and this element is widely distributed in nature. Silicosis is caused by crystalline silica, occurring either in pure form or mixed with other minerals. The term "crystalline free silica" indicates a compound with a chemical formula SiO_2 in crystal matrix, rather than an amorphous form. Alpha-quartz is the most important mineral form of silica in human disease, and accounts for the bulk of clinical silicosis. Other crystalline forms, the polymorphs cristobalite and tridymite, are less widespread. A crystalline structure is important for toxicity, and noncrystalline forms of silica (diatomaceous earth, natural glass, etc.) are relatively innocuous. High temperature can convert noncrystalline materials into crystalline forms. Heating occurs in the mining and processing of diatomaceous earth and may convert this amorphous silicate into crystalline cristobalite.

Quartz is mixed with other minerals in many rocks. Conglomerates, such as granite, contain mixtures of quartz with feldspar, mica, and other silicates. Sandstones may consist of nearly 100% silica, while some shales contain only 10%. Workers in a variety of trades who blast, grind, drill, or crush these stones may be exposed to aerosols that include quartz, and thus may be at risk for silicosis.

The mixed silicates, which contain silicon and oxygen in combination with sodium, potassium, calcium, aluminum, magnesium, or other cations, are not "free silica." These mixed silicates are very common minerals geologically, but are much less fibrogenic than quartz. The mixed silicates are believed to be responsible for little or no lung disease unless exposure is massive and prolonged. Diseases due to mixed siliceous dusts, such as kaolin or mica, will not be discussed in this chapter.

Occupational Exposures to Silica

Many work environments that generate dust and aerosols containing silica provide a risk for silicosis. Underground mining, milling, stone crushing, tunnel construction, foundry work, sandblasting, and granite carving in stone sheds have historically been important sources of silicosis. The preparation and secondary use of finely divided silica additives (silica flour) for paints, plastics, and other minerals are newer industrial settings where silicosis may occur.

Virtually all mining operations that involve tunneling—"hard rock mining"—generate silica aerosols when the bedrock is drilled away to expose and follow veins of ore. For this reason, silicosis has been an important problem in the diamond and gold mines of South Africa, the tin mines of Britain, and the coal mines of Germany and America, and remains a major cause of disease and disability in miners in South America, China, and other developing areas. Tunnels beneath rivers or cities for subway trains can produce very high ambient dust levels and can cause rapidly progressive, early silicosis in exposed workers.

Foundries that cast ferrous and nonferrous metals use molds of sand and clay. Residues of sand from the mold or core can remain adherent to the castings, and removal often requires mechanical means that aerosolize silica. The high temperatures endured by the molds may convert other forms of silica to the more toxic polymorph cristobalite.

Sandblasting is a well-recognized cause of silicosis. Abrasive cleaning using sand is on the decline in the United States and has been prohibited in Great Britain and Europe. However, if the target of abrasive cleaning is siliceous, even steel shot or other blasting media may be associated with a risk of silicosis. Glassmaking may expose workers to aerosols of finely divided glass sand (quartz), and several polymorphs of silica can be generated as a result of the high temperatures involved in the manufacturing process. Workers who manufacture products from powdered silica or add it to other substances to lend bulk or texture are at risk for silicosis. Refractory brick workers produce silica-rich products for use in high-temperature furnaces employed in the steel and iron industries. These refractories often use crushed sandstone as a raw material, and therefore an increased risk of silicosis may result. Silica flour (finely ground silica) is used as a filler in the manufacture of paints, cosmetics, and plastics, and as an abrasive; millers who crush stone into powder or workers who add powder to mixtures of other materials may inhale silica aerosols.

The development of silicosis demonstrates a dose-response relationship with exposure to silica dust. The proportion of the dust represented by silica (free quartz), the percentage of particles of a size suitable for inhalation (respirable fraction), the concentration of the dust in the air (number of particles or weight per unit volume), and the duration of exposure (work years) all interact to determine the prevalence and rapidity of silicosis. Very high levels of exposure to silica, such as may occur in uncontrolled mine tunnels or granite sheds with pneumatic machinery, can produce radiographic evidence of disease within 5 years. More moderate exposure levels, those typical of most industries before dust controls were instituted, result in radiographic silicosis after several decades of exposure. Severe clinical impairment or death due to respiratory failure usually requires 20 to 40 years from first exposure to silica, but intense exposure can result in death from acute silicoproteinosis within 5 years.[72]

The intensity of exposure in the workplace can be quantitated using samples of air recovered with a stationary collector at a central location or with personal dust samplers that collect air from the zone near the wearer's face. The ambient dust is usually fractionated as it is collected, so that only the smaller respirable particles are measured. The number of respirable particles per volume of air sampled (millions of particles per cubic foot; mppcf) or the weight of dust per volume of air (milligrams per cubic meter; mg/m^3) are determined. Since dust concentrations will usually vary from site to site and from time to time within a workplace, a time-weighted average exposure is usually calculated. The collected dust can be analyzed to determine the percentage of quartz (free silica) it contains.

Modern industrialized nations have imposed standards of air quality for the workplace that specify a threshold limit value (TLV) or permissible exposure limit (PEL) for silica designed to provide a safe exposure level. These standards are usually specified for the amount of free quartz and the concentration of dust in the air and are weighted for time of exposure over the work week. Slightly different methods of measuring and computing standards are used by agencies responsible for underground mines (Mine Safety and Health Administration; MSHA) and for other industries (Occupational Safety and Health Administration; OSHA). The current PEL for respirable free silica, measured as a fraction mixed with other dusts and adjusted for time of exposure, is approximately 1.0 mg/m^3 in the United States.[73] In 1974 the National Institute of Occupational Safety and Health (NIOSH) recommended a 10-hour time-weighted average level for free silica or 0.05 mg/m^3 as the limit needed to prevent silicosis,[74] but this standard has not been adopted.

Dust control measures in the workplace can reduce dramatically the levels of airborne silica particles. Efficient fans and air exchange systems provide fresh air and remove dust-laden air. Applying water during cutting, drilling, milling, and grinding operations greatly reduces the dust generated. Personal respirator masks and positive pressure air hoods with independent air supplies protect workers from airborne dust. Obviously, these measures are effective only when the air cleansing machinery is working properly or when workmen wear the respirators provided for them. Compliance appears to be a much greater problem than the availability of adequate technology.

The Prevalence of Silicosis: the Safety of the Workplace

The prevalence of silicosis has dropped sharply since the widespread institution of dust control measures and safety regulations in the industrialized nations. Death certificate statistics derived by NIOSH, which probably underestimate the prevalence of the disease substantially, recorded 2152 deaths due to silicosis in the United States from 1975 to 1986.[75] Other national statistics report 250 individuals per year with a new diagnosis of silicosis.[76]

Costello and Graham[77] examined the frequency of death due to silicosis in a cohort mortality study of 5414 workers employed between 1950 and 1982 in the Barre, Vermont, granite industry. Workers employed before 1940 were exposed to high dust levels, exceeding 40 mppcf. Workers employed after the institution of dust controls in 1940 were exposed to levels below the current PEL, less than 10 mppcf. Deaths due to silicosis and tuberculosis were common among workers hired before 1940, with standardized mortality ratios 5 to 10 times those expected for the U.S. population. Virtually no deaths due to silicosis were observed among workers who had exposure to the granite industry after dust control measures were instituted. Previous surveys of this industry documented minimal or no loss of pulmonary function attributable to silica exposure among modern workers.[78–81]

Silicosis remains a major industrial health problem in less industrialized countries. Cases of silicosis and complicating tuberculosis are still common in China but appear primarily in workers exposed before the institution of effective dust controls in many mines in about 1960.[82,83] Reliable statistics are not always available, but recent estimates suggest ongoing problems in South Africa,[84] Chile,[85] and other countries with large mining efforts.

Exposures in selected industries remain higher than is desired. Recent surveys of silica flour mills in the United States revealed that one-third to one-half of the personal air samples in 28 plants exceeded the PEL, with occasional measurements 10 times the accepted standard.[75] Valiante and Rosenman[86] reported the findings of a silicosis registry developed for the New Jersey Department of Health. They utilized hospital discharge records, death certificates, and other sources to identify 401 individuals in the years 1979 to 1987 who had radiographic or other clear evidence of silicosis and an appropriate work history. Approximately two-thirds of the workers had moderate to severe silicosis by radiographic criteria. The investigators examined the mines, mills, and plants where many of the cases had originated, and there they documented excessive dust exposure levels and inadequate personal safety protection in most instances. Thus, hazardous exposures were continuing for other workers at these sites. These epidemiologists extrapolated their survey statistics to the United States as a whole, and projected 1500 new cases of silicosis per year, six times the federal register incidence.

The modern epidemiology of silicosis suggests several conclusions. Silicosis is now a rare disease in the United States and in other industrialized nations, although a large number of workers are employed in diverse industries where a potentially hazardous silica exposure could exist. Dust control measures can dramatically reduce the silica levels in workplace air. Industries in which dust control measures have been applied and maintained rigorously, such as the granite industry, have effectively eliminated silicosis as a health hazard. At least in this instance, the current federal standards appear to provide adequate safety. Problems with silicosis continue in many industries, however. In almost all instances these problems can be attributed to inadequate dust control measures, improper use or maintenance of available equipment, and ambient dust levels substantially in excess of regulated standards. The tremendous problem posed by silicosis in less industrialized nations, where dust control measures are not common, highlights the importance of this strategy. Silicosis is preventable without abandoning the industries in which silica exposure could occur. Rather than revision of the existing PEL, emphasis should be placed on thorough application of available technology for dust control and vigorous enforcement of existing standards. With these efforts silicosis will become even less common in the future.

Clinical Features of Silicosis

Dyspnea with exertion is the most common presenting symptom of silicosis. Usually onset and progression are very gradual. Cough and sputum production are also common, and many workers have associated bronchitis. Since most workers exposed to silica also smoke tobacco, it may be difficult to distinguish the symptoms of silicosis from those of chronic obstructive pulmonary disease. Rales and scattered wheezes may be found on physical examination of the chest, but often auscultation is normal despite relatively advanced silicosis. Digital clubbing is rare. The course of the disease is often insidious, and progression occurs in the absence of continued exposure to silica. Simple nodular silicosis is diagnosed by historical and radiographic criteria, and affected individuals are generally asymptomatic unless there is associated chronic bronchitis. At the other extreme, shortness of breath may become disabling if progressive massive fibrosis develops. Cor pulmonale is not common but may occasionally be found as an end-stage feature.

Pulmonary function is usually normal in simple nodular silicosis; a mixed pattern of obstruction and reduction in lung volumes appears in workers with more advanced disease. Progressive massive fibrosis produces severe restriction, loss of pulmonary compliance, and hypoxemia and may be associated with cor pulmonale. In general, the pulmonary physiologic abnormalities of silicosis are those typical of restrictive, chronic, interstitial lung disease, but with a substantial component of associated airflow limitation.

Simple silicosis is manifest on chest radiograph as diffuse rounded opacities (Fig. 4-5). A modest predominance of shadows in the upper lung zones is usually seen, but without complete sparing of lower zones. Eggshell calcification of the hilar nodes is characteristic of silicosis when it is present, but it is an uncommon finding (Fig. 4-6B). Simple nodular silicosis may calcify as well, but infrequently. The discrete rounded opacities may coalesce and fuse in advanced disease to form large irregular masses, as shown in Figure 4-6A, thus qualifying for the label of "progressive massive fibrosis." The pleural surface is relatively spared in silicosis, and pleural thickening or calcification, when present, is usually the result of tuberculosis rather than silicosis.

The ILO Classification system,[3] described above, includes a pattern for rounded opacities that are characteristic of silicosis. These are scored as small (p-type), medium (q-type), or large (r-type), and the profusion of the predominant pattern is quantitated using the 12-point scale (0/- to 3/+). The large conglomerate masses, lymph node enlargement, and calcification are also recorded in this system.

Pathology

The pathology of silicosis has been reviewed recently by a committee formed by NIOSH, and their definitive report explains and illustrates the histopathology in detail.[87] Collections of dust-laden macrophages mixed with loose, intermingled reticulin fibers form the earliest or smallest lesion of silicosis. These lesions gradually expand and mature to form the classic lesion of silicosis, the silicotic nodule or islet. The typical early silicotic nodule occurs adjacent to respiratory bronchioles and small blood vessels and in subpleural locations. It has a distinct architecture composed of whorled collagen and reticulin in the center, with macrophages, fibroblasts, and

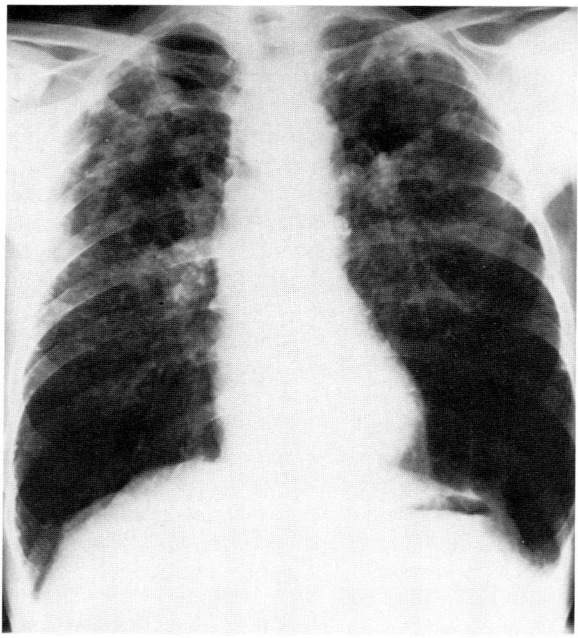

Figure 4-5. Moderate silicosis. This radiograph of a Vermont granite worker exposed to silica before the institution of dust controls in 1940 illustrates classic features of silicosis. A moderate profusion of small and medium rounded opacities is seen in an upper lung zone distribution, with some upward hilar retraction and hyperinflation of the lower lung zones. Calcification in hilar lymph nodes is apparent bilaterally.

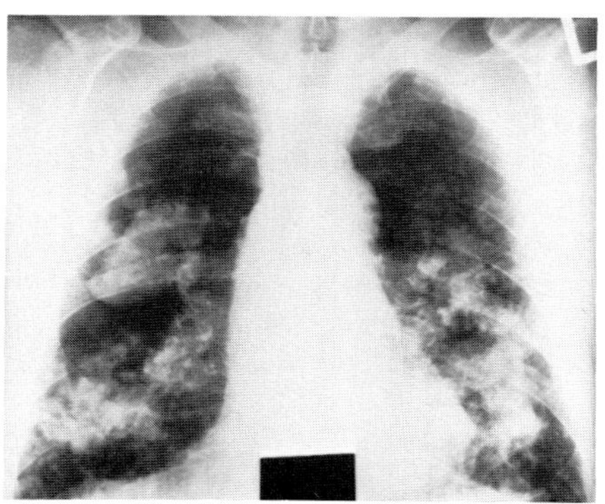

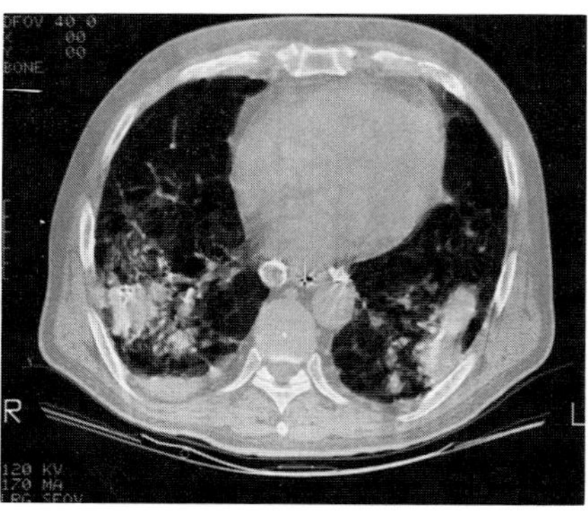

A   B

Figure 4-6. Advanced silicosis. (*A*) Advanced silicosis with large conglomerate masses is evident in the chest radiograph of a man who worked in an upstate New York tunnel iron mine from 1923 until 1940. Despite the extensive radiographic disease, he had few pulmonary symptoms and at age 79 his vital capacity measured 80% of the predicted value. (*B*) Computed tomogram of same patient reveals conglomerate masses with dense strands of fibrosis extending into the lung parenchyma. Extensive calcification is evident in these masses and in central lymph nodes. A large node in the right paraesophageal groove demonstrates a typical eggshell rim of calcification.

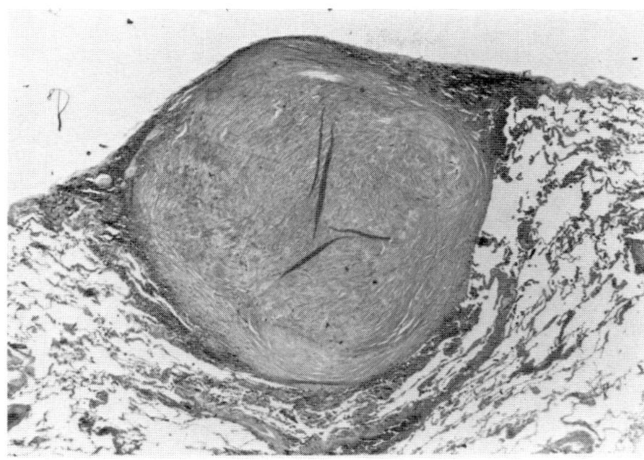

Figure 4-7. Silicotic nodule. A large subpleural silicotic nodule illustrates central whorled connective tissue with a thin rim of surrounding inflammatory cells. The nodule appears as a discrete lesion within relatively normal lung parenchyma. Birefringent particles were evident by polarized light microscopy. The tissue was obtained from a 68-year-old man who underwent left upper lobe resection for a mass lesion, which proved to a mixed adenosquamous carcinoma. (Original magnification ×33)

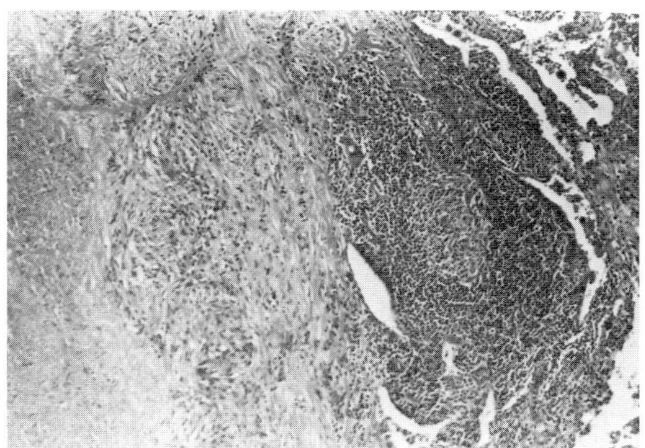

Figure 4-8. Silicosis. The architecture of a typical silicotic nodule reveals a central zone of whorled connective tissue and fibrosis *(left)*, an intermediate zone of cellular inflammation in which macrophages predominate *(center)*, and a peripheral zone of mononuclear cell inflammation in which lymphocytes predominate *(right)*. A smaller secondary nodule is forming within the zone of lymphocytes, and the process is extending outward into the interstitium of the lung. (Original magnification ×25)

lymphocytes surrounding this connective tissue matrix core. Epithelioid giant cells are a variable feature. Immunoglobulins have been demonstrated in silicotic nodules as well. The dust is initially centered within the earliest collections of macrophages and then moves out with the rim of mononuclear cells as the center of the lesion becomes a whorled, acellular mass of mature collagen. When examined with appropriate ultrastructural analytical techniques, very small particles of silica can be found in the center of these lesions, while the larger particles of mixed silicates predominate peripherally.[87] Silicotic nodules may be seen with the naked eye beneath the pleural surface of the lung and in tissue sections. In simple silicosis these nodules vary from barely visible pinpoint marks up to distinct round or stellate lesions several millimeters in diameter. Figures 4-7 and 4-8 illustrate typical silicotic nodules. The pathologic localization of the earliest silicotic lesions may be the result of the anatomy of dust deposition. Brody has shown that initial deposition of dust in animal models is concentrated at alveolar duct bifurcations, sites anatomically close to the respiratory bronchioles.[88]

The nodules in simple silicosis are isolated, less than 1 cm in diameter, and often appear to punctuate otherwise relatively normal alveolar architecture. This pathologic stage corresponds to radiographs with small nodules in low profusion, little pulmonary physiologic derangement, and minimal or no symptoms. These lesions can also be found in silica-exposed workers with normal chest radiographs who die of other causes.[89] Conglomerate silicosis develops as small nodules merge and interstitial fibrosis extends into the alveolar septal planes surrounding the nodular lesions. Nearby airways and pulmonary blood vessels can become distorted, narrowed, and obliterated by this process. Contracture and extensive fibrosis of involved areas progress as disease advances. Localized emphysema often develops in areas adjacent to these lesions, both from tissue destruction and from traction with overdistention. Perinodular emphysematous regions may coalesce to form macroscopic blebs. If these blebs develop in a subpleural location, they may rupture into the pleural space and cause pneumothorax. This stage of silicosis is associated with the typical radiographic, physiological, and clinical findings of classic silicosis.

Progressive massive fibrosis (PMF) is uncommon but may develop in severe silicosis as the individual silicotic nodules coalesce to form conglomerate masses 2 cm or greater in size. In contrast to PMF lesions in coal workers, silicosis PMF masses rarely or never cavitate by ischemic necrosis, and tuberculosis should be sought if cavitation is found.[87] Upper lung zone predominance of PMF lesions with surrounding scarring and contraction shrinks the size of the upper lobes dramatically in advanced silicosis.

The visceral pleural surface overlying parenchymal nodules is often involved with focal fibrosis in advanced silicosis. Calcification is rare and suggests tuberculosis. In contrast to asbestos-related disease, the parietal pleura is not involved in silicosis. The lymph nodes of the hilum and mediastinum enlarge in silicosis and are replaced by isolated or conglomerate silicotic nodules. Dust is abundant in these lesions. These nodes may exhibit layers of peripheral calcification, giving them the characteristic "eggshell" appearance on chest radiograph.

Tuberculosis

A clear association between silicosis and increased susceptibility to tuberculosis (TB) has been established in hard rock miners, coal miners, granite workers, and other industrial groups.[90,91] Workers with established silicosis appear to be more susceptible than the general population to developing active TB when exposed and evidence a more chronic persistent form of TB once infected. It has not yet been resolved whether low-level exposure to silica, without the development of overt silicosis, also predisposes to TB.

The reasons for enhanced susceptibility to TB in silicosis are not known. Silica added to macrophage cultures in vitro potentiates growth of *M. tuberculosis* in these cells,[92] but the organism also grows in such cultures without the addition of dust. As noted below, macrophages recovered from human workers exposed to silica and from animal models of silicosis demonstrate normal phagocytosis and killing of pyogenic bacteria. It is possible that the immune-inflammatory response that characterizes silicosis, as detailed below, creates favored locations in which cells aggregate that are particularly susceptible to infection by mycobacteria.

The diagnosis of TB may be difficult in patients with silicosis. The radiographic changes are similar in both diseases, and thus progression of densities and infiltrates in upper lung zones becomes nonspecific. TB in silicosis is often indolent and may progress slowly. Few organisms may be shed, and positive sputum smears or cultures may be difficult to obtain. Silicosis predisposes to infection with atypical mycobacteria as well as *M. tuberculosis*. If mycobacteria are recovered, the species and drug sensitivity must be confirmed. Silico-tuberculosis patients usually respond well to conventional antituberculous therapy in regard to clinical improvement and radiographic stabilization, but complete eradication of organisms may be impossible. It is hypothesized that organisms can be sequestered within the fibrotic lesions of silicosis and remain viable despite effective chemotherapy. Reactivation following an apparent cure is common in silico-tuberculosis. For this reason many experts follow multidrug treatment of silico-tuberculosis patients with isoniazide treatment for the rest of their lives.[90]

Acute Silicoproteinosis

An acute form of silicosis can develop shortly after intense exposure to finely divided silica in high doses. The clinical features of this disease resemble pulmonary alveolar proteinosis much more than silicosis, and thus the compound name for this syndrome. Animals develop a similar disease if exposed to high doses of silica.

The histopathology of silicoproteinosis (silicotic alveolar proteinosis, acute silicosis) is characterized by evidence of extensive injury to airspace epithelium with hyperplasia and regrowth of type II pneumocytes.[87] The airspaces are filled with a proteinaceous lipid-rich exudate. It appears to be the result of tremendous overproduction (and/or deficient removal) of surfactant lipids and apoproteins. An interstitial reaction is usually seen as well, and loose aggregates of mononuclear inflammatory cells are seen in lesions resembling early silicotic nodules. Patients report the rather rapidly progressive development of shortness of breath and nonproductive cough. Restriction of lung volumes and hypoxia are evident. Silicoproteinosis presents on chest radiograph as a diffuse ground glass infiltrate with a peripheral distribution in all lung zones.

Silicoproteinosis develops within months to a few years after an intense, high-dose exposure to finely divided silica. Tunnel workers, sand blasters, and workers manufacturing silica flour have been at particular risk, usually in circumstances where they did not realize their risk or proper respiratory protection was not utilized.[72,93] The disease progresses rapidly, and death usually occurs within a year of presentation. Therapeutic whole-lung bronchoalveolar lavage is effective in spontaneous pulmonary alveolar proteinosis, but it is not known whether this treatment alters the course of silicoproteinosis. Modern industrial hygiene measures and proper education of workers who could be exposed to finely divided silica should prevent future cases of this devastating disease.

Therapy of Silicosis

There is no accepted effective therapy for silicosis. The course of the disease is usually very slow, and respiratory failure or cor pulmonale are late consequences. Many patients outlive their silicosis to die of other causes. The symptoms are often less severe than the chest radiographs would suggest (see Fig. 4-6). Careful evaluation for TB, and prolonged treatment of that infection if found, are essential parts of the management of silicosis. Continuous oxygen therapy, diuretics, treatment of secondary infection, and other general supportive measures would be indicated by the same criteria used in other lung diseases.

Treatment of silicosis with agents designed to interrupt the inflammatory sequence of events leading to fibrosis has received very little attention in human studies or animal models. Corticosteroids are described as ineffective but have not received a well-controlled prospective evaluation. Recent studies of silicosis in the sheep model have focused on inhalation of aluminum salts as a means of reducing the toxicity of silica.[94] The early results appear promising, but it is not clear whether the aluminum is accelerating clearance of silica from the lung, and thus reducing the effective dose, or ameliorating the toxicity of the silica that remains in the lung. More study is needed to provide better and more specific treatment for workers with silicosis.

Mechanisms of Inflammation and Fibrosis in Silicosis

The pathogenetic mechanisms that induce silicosis are being clarified by ongoing research into basic immune-inflammatory responses. The section that follows provides a somewhat selective review of the existing evidence and puts forward cellular mechanisms for this disease that are still somewhat speculative.

Many of the same interactions between macrophages, lymphocytes, neutrophils, and fibroblasts that occur in chronic autoimmune or other idiopathic chronic inflammatory diseases also appear to be operative in silicosis. The unique aspects of silicosis relate to the presence of a persisting etiologic agent, silica particles, and the highly localized architectural response to it. The silicotic nodule represents both the fundamental building block of the histopathology of silicosis and a paradigm for the pathogenetic mechanisms of the disease. The interactions between various cells, and between cells and mineral particles, within the nodule should serve to explain the basic mechanisms of disease.

Most of the mechanisms that are believed to be responsible for the pathogenesis of silicosis have been observed in animal models or cell culture systems and then inferred for human disease. Several qualifications must be placed on this transfer of information from animals to man. Silicosis develops slowly in humans exposed to silica even at high concentrations. Although silicoproteinosis may develop rapidly under extreme exposure conditions (see above), classical silicosis requires years or decades to achieve full expression. Interactions between cells, conceived as due to the release of and responses to cytokines, are usually measured in hours or days. It is not at all clear why silicosis develops so slowly in humans and laboratory animals. Perhaps processes with much longer time scales than cytokine release are operative as well, such as clonal or phenotypic changes in cell populations.

A second problem area for extrapolation from cell and animal studies is the localized nature of silicosis. Silicosis appears as discrete foci of inflammation and fibrosis.

Until the most advanced stages of the disease, the lung tissue between these foci remains relatively normal. The inflammatory-fibrotic response is strictly limited to locations where mineral particles are also present. These observations imply that either the mediators that promote inflammation and fibrosis in silicosis must be very localized in activity or additional mechanisms that inhibit inflammation and down-regulate fibrosis predominate beyond the silicotic nodule. The mechanisms of localization, down-regulation, or damage control have received little attention.

The experimental evidence for the hypothetical mechanisms that are responsible for silicosis has been reviewed in detail,[95] and will be summarized below. Recent progress has added support to this proposed scheme and has suggested several additions.

Macrophage Interactions with Silica Particles

Alveolar macrophages (AM) containing refractile birefringent silica particles can be observed in the lungs of experimental animals several hours after inhalation of a silica aerosol.[88] Within several days of exposure, most of the inhaled dust is contained within the cells recovered by BAL, rather than free in the fluid. AM recovered by BAL from granite workers contain silica, and a substantial fraction of the cells retain the dust decades after workplace exposure ended. Almost all of the silica found in lung tissue sections, silicotic nodules, and lymph nodes is located within macrophages in animal models and in human cases of silicosis. Thus, pulmonary macrophages phagocytose silica readily and sequester the particles for long periods. These observations have focused attention on the macrophage as the primary interface between the mineral particles and the lung, and thus as the primary intermediate mechanism by which silicosis develops. It appears that the response of the macrophage to silica is manifested by the activation of this cell and the consequent release of a variety of mediators that then influence other cells to express the pathologic pattern we know as silicosis.

Early attempts to model silicosis centered on macrophages exposed to silica and other particles in vitro.[96] The investigators quickly observed that most macrophages died immediately after ingesting silica particles, whereas other particulates (diamond dust, latex) had little effect. They concluded that silica cytotoxicity was an important mechanism of the disease. Further studies have demonstrated that silica cytotoxicity for macrophages must play only a very minor role in silicosis. The macrophages recovered from rats immediately and at time points up to 1 year after silica exposure have normal viability and normal or enhanced cell function,[88,97] although initially 40% and later 5% of the cells contain particles. The AM recovered from granite workers also contain abundant particles and exhibit normal viability and normal cell function.[98] The particle burden of silica per cell observed in specimens recovered from humans or animals exposed in vivo is much less than the dose applied in vitro in many experiments, and thus dose alone may explain some of the cytotoxic effects seen in early studies. Furthermore, particles deposited in alveoli are immediately immersed and coated with alveolar lining material. The surfactant lipids and proteins can substantially reduce the cytotoxicity of silica particles for macrophages in vitro.[99] Although some macrophages in the lung may die prematurely after silica ingestion, it appears that most of the pathogenetic mechanisms of this disease are due to other alterations in macrophage function induced by these particulates.

Macrophages recovered from animals exposed to silica exhibit increased cell surface ruffling and spreading, increased oxygen consumption, enhanced phagocytosis of inert particles and bacteria,[97] increased release of superoxide anion after stimulation,[59] increased expression of class II major histocompatibility antigens,[100] and enhanced secretion of cytokines. These are the features of stimulated or activated macrophages. Some of these alterations can be reproduced in vitro, implying a direct effect by silica on the macrophage. Other effects have not been observed with in vitro exposure alone and imply a requirement for participation by lymphocytes or other cells, as discussed below. The macrophages within the lung interstitium, and possibly within lymph nodes, may be more important in these processes than the airspace cells, which are more easily recovered for research.[101] There is now a large body of evidence supporting the concept that the macrophage is activated in silicosis and that these activated cells promote inflammation and fibrosis through their effects on other cell types.

Macrophages aggregate promptly at alveolar duct bifurcations where silica particles impact.[88] Expansion of the airspace macrophage population accompanies silicosis in animal models and human patients. These observations suggest that silica, either alone or through its effects on macrophages that have ingested it, promotes recruitment of macrophages to sites where the mineral is located. Active complement fragments generated from complement proteins in alveolar lining material and chemotactins secreted by macrophages are likely candidates to explain these effects, as is discussed for neutrophils below. Macrophage aggregating, attracting, and immobilizing factors released by lymphocytes may also be important as disease progresses. Recruitment and possibly local proliferation greatly expand the population of macrophages in the lung in silicosis. This enlarged population then becomes available for quantitatively as well as qualitatively increased effects on other lung cells and on the lung connective matrix.

Macrophage Interactions with Lymphocytes

Lymphocytes accumulate within the evolving lesions of silicosis, and increased numbers of lymphocytes are recovered by BAL from the lungs of animals exposed to silica (see review by Davis[95]). Absher and associates observed an influx of CD4+ (putative helper/inducer) T lymphocytes into the lungs of rats exposed to an aerosol of silica (cristobalite), with an accompanying but less intense increase in CD8+ (putative suppressor/cytolytic) lymphocytes.[102] Struhar and colleagues made similar observations after intratracheal instillation of quartz.[103] In virtually all the animal studies, the increase in lymphocytes is a relatively late event that follows a transient increase in neutrophils and an initial increase in macrophages. Human patients with silicosis[30] and asymptomatic granite workers[98] evidence a slight increase in the proportion of lymphocytes recovered by BAL.

Macrophages could interact with lymphocytes to promote nodule formation through direct cell contact and by means of secreted cytokines. Macrophages treated with silica in vitro[104–107] and AM recovered from silica-exposed animals[100,108] secrete increased amounts of interleukin-1 (IL-1). This polypeptide cytokine can stimulate T-lymphocyte activation and proliferation and promote fibroblast proliferation.[65] An expanded population of T lymphocytes, activated through the influence of IL-1, might then in turn release interferon-gamma and other macrophage-activating substances. Current evidence suggests that secreted IL1 (probably IL-1β) may be elaborated in silicosis. Macrophage membrane IL1 (probably IL1α) could also be important through direct contact with the lymphocyte cell surface, but has not been studied in detail. Through this postulated loop, macrophages that contain silica might stimulate T cells that serve to amplify the signal and then indirectly stimulate additional macrophages that have not had direct contact with the mineral.

Human cases of silicosis provide evidence of polyclonal B-lymphocyte stimulation. It is not clear whether these manifestations of increased immunoglobulin synthesis are important mechanisms in the pathogenesis of silicosis or represent nonspecific secondary effects. Case series of workers with silicosis report increased prevalence of rheumatoid factor, antinuclear antibodies, and circulating immune complexes, as well as generalized increases in serum concentrations of immunoglobulins.[109] BAL fluid from silica-exposed granite workers contains increased concentrations of IgG, IgA, and IgM.[110] Increased levels of immunoglobulins have also been observed in animals exposed to silica, although B-lymphocyte function has been studied relatively little in animal models of silicosis.

Macrophage Interactions with Neutrophils

Neutrophils are abundant in the BAL fluid of animals soon after exposure to silica, particularly when doses are high or the route of exposure is by intratracheal instillation rather than inhalation. In this setting the neutrophils could be a reflection of acute injury rather an integral part of chronic silicosis. However, neutrophils are found in the BAL fluid of rats many months after exposure by aerosol to modest doses of quartz or cristobalite.[97,102] Several mutually supportive mechanisms could recruit neutrophils to sites of silica-induced inflammation. Silica particles could activate complement in alveolar lining material to generate C5a fragments, a potent chemotactin for macrophages and neutrophils.[50,51] Macrophages exposed to silica in vitro secrete a chemotactic activity for neutrophils into the cell culture medium.[111] Potentially, silica could stimulate macrophages to produce leukotriene B_4 (LTB_4) or to secrete a polypeptide chemotactic factor (IL-8), but these effects remain to be fully evaluated in silicosis.

Human patients with silicosis,[30] asymptomatic granite workers,[98] and patients with mixed dust pneumoconiosis[31] do not evidence any increase in the proportions of neutrophils recovered by BAL. Neutrophils are not a prominent feature of the tissue pathology of silicosis. These observations suggest that neutrophils may be less important than other mononuclear inflammatory cell types in the pathogenesis of silicosis.

Macrophage Interactions with Fibroblasts

Excessive connective tissue matrix material located at inappropriate sites within lung parenchyma is the hallmark of pulmonary fibrosis in general, and specific patterns of deposition characterize silicosis. Fibroblasts are increased in absolute number and extend to abnormal locations, such as alveolar spaces, where excess connective tissue matrix is deposited extracellularly. It is not yet clear whether these fibroblasts are altered in phenotype, produce increased amounts of collagen, or synthesize abnormal proportions of the different collagen types. The increase in tissue collagen could be the result of normal protein synthesis by an abnormally expanded number of cells or a result of altered synthesis by these cells.

The activated macrophage in silicosis is hypothesized to be the driving force behind fibroblast proliferation and possibly fibroblast migration and altered collagen synthesis as well. A substantial literature supports this idea (see review by Davis[95]). Mesenchymal cells continue accelerated collagen production when lung parenchyma from animal models of silicosis is placed in tissue culture.[112] Growth-promoting activity for fibroblasts is increased in the supernatant medium of cultured macrophages recovered from animals with silicosis.[102,113] Macrophages appear to be required to produce fibrosis with silica in subcutaneous chamber systems.[114] A protein of 16 kDa that stimulated collagen production by granulation-tissue cells was isolated from the lungs of rats with silicosis.[115]

Macrophages have the ability to secrete a variety of cytokines that can promote growth of fibroblasts. Platelet-derived growth factor (PDGF), transforming growth factor beta (TGFβ), IL-1, tumor necrosis factor alpha (TNFα), and insulin-like growth factor (IGF1) can be synthesized and secreted by pulmonary macrophages, and these cytokines have potent mitogenic effects on fibroblasts and other mesenchymal cells.[65] Macrophages exposed to silica in vitro secrete Il-1,[104–107] and alveolar macrophages recovered from animals with silicosis secrete increased IL-1.[100,108] Silica added to normal macrophages in vitro provokes enhanced secretion of TNFα,[116] and macrophages from rats with silicosis are primed for increased TNFα secretion following secondary stimulation with small amounts of endotoxin.[117] In silicosis, it is not yet clear exactly which of these growth promoters are most important or precisely how they interact with one another to produce the particular pattern of nodular and interstitial fibrosis that characterizes the disease.

Alterations in Lung Structural Elements

Injury to lung tissue is an important aspect of silicosis. The macrophages and neutrophils that are recruited to the silicotic nodule and surrounding tissues carry collagenolytic and elastolytic proteases, oxidant-generating systems, and potent enzymes with broad potential for destruction of parenchymal cells and connective tissue matrix components. The type II alveolar epithelial cell appears to be a particularly susceptible target for direct or secondary injury in silicosis. High-dose exposure to silica causes type II cell injury and proliferation, and excessive accumulation of surfactant lipids and proteins, both in human cases of silicoproteinosis[72] and in animal models of acute silicosis.[118] Tissue injury in silicosis has received less attention than the mechanisms of inflammation and fibrosis.

Mechanisms of Nodule Formation and Fibrosis

The primary lesion of silicosis is the silicotic nodule, described above as a rather spherical collection of macrophages, lymphocytes, fibroblasts, collagen, and dust particles in a distinctive architectural arrangement. Figure 4-8 depicts the architectural arrangement of the silicotic nodule. This lesion resembles a granuloma, and the factors that regulate granuloma formation may also be responsible for the formation of the silicotic nodule. The importance of macrophages in granuloma formation has been emphasized,[119] and the role of IL-1 and TNFα have been highlighted by several experiments. Kasahara and colleagues produced granulomatous lesions in the lungs of mice when agarose beads coupled with IL-1 or with TNFα were injected intratracheally, while beads coated with interferon-gamma or with IL-2 caused little effect.[120] The development of BCG-induced granulomas in the livers of mice was blocked by antibody against TNFα.[121] The authors postulated an autoamplification loop in which macrophage activation and TNFα secretion were perpetuated by TNFα released from the same or nearby macrophages. Thus, IL-1 and TNFα could play critical roles in silicosis through localized effects that (a) perpetuate macrophage activation, (b) promote silicotic nodule formation, (c) stimulate T-lymphocyte proliferation and activation, and (d) cause fibroblasts to replicate.

More research is required in order to understand in silicosis the timing, sequence, and precise roles of macrophages, neutrophils, lymphocytes, fibroblasts, and other cell types, and of the many cytokines and other signalling substances that they produce. Research utilizing silicosis provides a system in which the etiologic agent is known, the dose and timing of exposure can be manipulated precisely, and the amount and location of the causative agent can be tracked in lung tissue throughout the disease. Thus, silicosis may serve as a useful model for other immune/inflammatory/fibrotic diseases in which the inciting agents or events are not yet known.

Silicosis and Lung Cancer

Epidemiologic studies reveal an increased risk of bronchogenic carcinoma in workers with heavy silica exposure who smoke tobacco. Recent retrospective analyses of the causes of mortality in workers in Italy, Finland, Sweden, Canada, and the United States have shown excess prevalence of lung cancer among workers with occupational exposure to silica. In most of these studies, the worker groups were identified from state registries because of compensation for silicosis, and then their mortality rates and causes of death were determined from death certificate files and other sources.

Zambon and colleagues[122] examined 878 deaths among a cohort of 1313 workers in northern Italy compensated for silicosis between 1959 and 1963 and compared causes of mortality with age-matched national and regional mortality rates. They reported an increase in deaths due to lung cancer, with a mortality ratio approximately twice that expected. Among those for whom information on smoking status was available, 86.9% of the workers were current or former smokers, and only 13.1% had never smoked. Almost all of the lung cancers occurred in smokers; four occurred in non-smokers. The researchers concluded that tobacco smoking was the dominant environmental influence in causing lung cancer in this cohort but that silicosis produced a further two- or threefold increase in cancer death rates.

Finkelstein and associates[123] determined the lung cancer mortality among 1190 miners and 289 surface industry workers compensated for silicosis in Ontario, Canada, between 1940 and 1985 and compared death rates with those for the population of the province. They observed increased rates of lung cancer (about twofold) in both underground and surface worker groups after correction for age. Although only 13% of the workers had never smoked, about half the provincial frequency, these authors concluded that smoking habit alone was unlikely to account for the increased risk of lung cancer they observed.

Another recent study of Canadian workers was reported by Infante-Rivard and co-workers[124] describing lung cancer mortality in Quebec workers compensated for silicosis between 1938 and 1985. The causes of 565 deaths among 1062 registrants were reviewed; miners represented about 28% of the cohort, with surface industry silica exposure contributing the remainder. They observed 83 lung cancers, versus 24 expected, for a specific mortality ratio of 3.47:1. No cases of lung cancer occurred among nonsmokers, but only 7.1% of the workers had never smoked. The investigators concluded that there is a more than threefold increased risk of death from lung cancer in men who received compensation for silicosis in Quebec.

Mastrangelo and associates[125] compared the frequency of silica exposure and silicosis in 309 lung cancer patients and 309 age-matched case-referent controls admitted to a general hospital in Northern Italy during 1973–1980. Overt silicosis, determined by workman's compensation, increased the relative risk of lung cancer significantly by a factor of two or more. Only six cases of lung cancer occurred in nonsmokers among the 309 subjects. No increased risk for cancer was associated with silica exposure in the nonsmokers, but the validity of the analysis was limited by the small number of cases. The authors concluded that in smokers silicosis increases the risk of lung cancer but that exposure to silica without silicosis does not increase risk.

A cohort mortality study of 5414 Vermont granite industry workers employed from 1950 to 1982 was reported by Costello and Graham.[77] They analyzed causes of death from certificates of 1527 of the 1643 workers who died and obtained data about the men from a variety of other community sources. The deaths involved 1284 granite shed workers and 359 workers employed in quarries—a much less dusty environment. A dramatic reduction in the dust levels of the granite sheds took place in 1940 with the introduction of widespread dust control measures. Thus, workers hired before 1940 experienced high levels of silica exposure whereas those hired after 1940 did not. Silicosis was the cause for 37 among 931 deaths in workers hired before 1940, whereas no bona fide silicosis was found in any workers after 1940. Lung cancer mortality was increased in shed workers hired before 1940 but not in those hired later or in quarry workers. Chest radiographs were available for review on 62 workers hired before 1940 who died of respiratory cancer, and radiographic silicosis was evident in 33 (53%). All workers dying of lung cancer were smokers. The investigators concluded that high levels of silica exposure and tobacco smoking combined to produce increased risk of respiratory cancer for granite workers. They also noted that current levels of workplace dust exposure, below the threshold limit value, did not appear to increase the risk of lung cancer in the granite industry.

All these epidemiologic studies appear to generate comparable and mutually supportive conclusions, despite the differences in their methods and nations of origin. Exposure to high levels of silica dust (level and duration enough to cause overt silicosis in some workers) produces a two- to fourfold increased risk for lung cancer in tobacco smokers. This risk obtains for surface industry workers in granite sheds, foundries, and mills, as well as for underground miners, thus implicating a true effect of the mineral dust rather than an effect produced by radon daughters, trace elements, or other confounding carcinogens in the mine environment. Low levels of silica dust exposure, obtainable in modern industry, appear not to increase cancer risk. Silica exposure apparently does not produce an increased cancer risk for workers who do not smoke tobacco, but this conclusion requires more cases for greater statistical certainty. The effects of silica appear to parallel those of asbestos as a cause of increased lung cancer risk among smokers, with the important differences of less risk enhancement at all silica doses and an apparent threshold of low doses without increased cancer risk.

Larger, possibly prospective, studies will be needed to determine with confidence whether silica exposure within regulated safe levels causes a significantly increased lung cancer risk.

The mechanisms remain speculative by which silica potentiates tobacco smoke as a cause of cancer. Hypothetically, the mineral could act as a co-carcinogen inducing cancer, a cancer promoter stimulating growth of transformed cells, or a passive means of carrying tobacco carcinogens into the lung or impairing their clearance, or it could alter immune surveillance mechanisms resulting in a failure to eliminate malignant cells when they arise. More research is needed to assess which one or several of these possibilities is actually important.

CONCLUSIONS

The pneumoconioses are becoming diseases of historical interest in the industrialized world, targets of successful public health and industrial hygiene measures to reduce airborne dust in the work environment. Modern techniques for dust control are moderate in cost and effective in protecting workers. These methods have permitted continuing operations such as granite carving and sandblasting and continuing use of products such as silica flour. Application of these methods could provide safety for workers in tunnel mines, quarries, and dusty industries throughout the world. Asbestos presents a special problem because of its cancer-promoting properties with very low exposure and because asbestos products can remain hazardous throughout their life. Asbestos has been dealt with by limiting its use, removing it or encasing it where it is installed, and providing maximum protection for workers who must contact it. Other natural mineral and synthetic materials—safer, it is hoped, than asbestos—have been found to substitute for it. In all instances, prevention of pneumoconiosis by limiting exposure to airborne particles and fibers is the proper means of controlling these diseases.

The mechanisms of injury, inflammation, fibrosis, and tissue remodeling that occur in asbestosis and silicosis are of great interest even if prevention is the best way to control disease. Understanding these processes may provide insight into fundamental mechanisms of lung injury and repair and provide opportunities for intervention in patients who have received substantial dust exposure or who suffer from other lung diseases of unknown cause. Asbestosis and silicosis still stand as paradigms of occupational lung disease and still provide important opportunities for future research.

ACKNOWLEDGMENTS

The author thanks Peter A. Dietrich, M.D., Department of Radiology, for assistance with the radiographs, and Kevin E. Leslie, M.D., Department of Pathology, for help with the figures illustrating histopathology, and Jason Kelley, M.D., Department of Medicine, for his helpful comments on this manuscript. This work was supported in part by the Vermont Pulmonary Special Center of Research, HL-14212 (SCOR).

REFERENCES

1. Mossman BT, Gee JB. Asbestos-related diseases. N Engl J Med 1989; 320:1721–1730.
2. Mossman BT, Bignon J, Corn M, Seaton A, Gee JBL. Asbestos: Scientific developments and implications for public policy. Science 1990; 247:294–301.
3. Radiographs of the pneumoconioses—1980. The International Labor Office, 1750 New York Avenue, N.W., Washington, DC.
4. Classification of radiographs of the pneumoconioses. Med Radiogr Photogr 1981; 57:1–17.
5. Craighead JE, Abraham JL, Churg A, Green FHY, Kleinerman J, Pratt PC, Seemayer TA, Vallyathan V, Weill H. The pathology of asbestos-associated diseases of the lungs and pleural cavities: Diagnostic criteria and proposed grading schema. Arch Pathol Lab Med 1982; 106:540–597.
6. Brody AR, Hill LH, Adkins B Jr, O'Connor RW. Chrysotile asbestos inhalation in rats: Deposition pattern and reaction of alveolar epithelium and pulmonary macrophages. Am Rev Respir Dis 1981; 123:670–679.
7. Corrin B, Dewar A, Rodriguez Roisin R, Turner Warwick M. Fine structural changes in cryptogenic fibrosing alveolitis and asbestosis. J Pathol 1985; 147:107–119.
8. Wright PF, Hansson A, Kreel L, et al. Respiratory function changes after asbestos pleurisy. Thorax 1980; 35:31–36.
9. Hillerdal G, Lindgren A. Pleural plaques: Correlation of autopsy findings to radiographic findings and occupational history. Eur J Respir Dis 1980; 61:315–319.
10. Hillerdal G. Nonmalignant pleural disease related to asbestos exposure. Clin Chest Med 1985; 6:141–152.
11. Hughes JM, Weill H, Hammad YY. Mortality of workers employed in two asbestos cement manufacturing plants. Br J Ind Med 1987; 44:161–174.
12. Rudd R. Malignant mesothelioma. J R Soc Med 1989; 82:126–129.
13. Newhouse M. Epidemiology of asbestos-related tumors. Semin Oncol 1981; 8:250–257.
14. Selikoff IJ, Churg J, Hammond EC. Asbestos exposure and neoplasia. JAMA 1964; 188:142–146.
15. Barrett JC, Lamb PW, Wiseman RW. Multiple mechanisms for the carcinogenic effects of asbestos and other mineral fibers. Environ Health Perspect 1989; 81:81–89.
16. Antman KH, Corson JM. Benign and malignant pleural mesothelioma. Clin Chest Med 1985; 6:127–140.
17. Antman KH. Natural history and staging of malignant mesothelioma. Chest 1989; 96(1):93s–95s.
18. Wagner JC, Sleggs EA, Marchand P. Diffuse pleural mesothelioma and asbestos exposure in the North Western Cape Province. Br J Ind Med 1960; 17:260–271.
19. Baris YI, Sahin AA, Ozemi M, et al. An outbreak of pleural mesothelioma and chronic fibrosing pleurisy in the village of Karain/Urgup in Anatolia. Thorax 1978; 33:181–192.
20. McConnochie K, Simonato L, Mavrides P, Christophides P, Pooley FD, Wagner JC. Mesothelioma in Cyprus: The role of tremolite. Thorax 1987; 42:342–347.
21. Churg A, Warnock ML. Analysis of the cores of asbestos bodies from members of the general population: Patients with probably low-degree exposure to asbestos. Am Rev Respir Dis 1979; 120:781–786.
22. Craighead JE. The epidemiology and pathogenesis of malignant mesothelioma. Chest 1989; 96(1):92s–93s.
23. Saracci R. Asbestos and lung cancer: An analysis of the epidemiological evidence on the asbestos-smoking interaction. Int J Cancer 1977; 20:323–331.
24. Berry G, Newhouse ML, Antonis P. Combined effects of asbestos and smoking on mortality from lung cancer and mesothelioma in factory workers. Br J Ind Med 1985; 42:12–18.
25. Gardner MJ, Winter PD, Pannett B, Powell CA. Follow up study of workers manufacturing chrystotile asbestos cement products. Br J Ind Med 1986; 43:726–732.

26. Ohlson CG, Hogstedt C. Lung cancer among asbestos cement workers: A Swedish cohort study and a review. Br J Ind Med 1985; 42:397–402.

27. McDonald JC, Liddell FDK, Gibbs GW, et al. Dust exposure and mortality in chrysotile mining, 1910–1975. Br J Ind Med 1980; 37:11–24.

28. Jaurand MC, Gaudichet A, Atassi K, Sebastien P, Bignon J. Relationship between the number of asbestos fibers and the cellular and enzymatic content of bronchoalveolar fluid in asbestos exposed subjects. Bull Europ Physiopath Resp 1980; 16:595–606.

29. Begin R, Cantin A, Berthiaume Y, Boileau R, Bisson G, Lamoureux G, Rola-Pleszczynski M, Drapeau G, Masse S, Boctor M, Breault J, Peloquin S, Dalle D. Clinical features to stage alveolitis in asbestos workers. Am J Ind Med 1985; 8:521–536.

30. Rom WN, Bitterman PB, Rennard SI, Cantin A, Crystal RG. Characterization of the lower respiratory tract inflammation of nonsmoking individuals with interstitial lung disease associated with chronic inhalation of inorganic dusts. Am Rev Respir Dis 1987; 136:1429–1434.

31. Costabel U, Bross KJ, Huck E, Guzman J, Matthys H. Lung and blood lymphocyte subsets in asbestosis and in mixed dust pneumoconiosis. Chest 1987; 91:110–112.

32. Robinson BW, Rose AH, Hayes A, Musk AW. Increased pulmonary gamma interferon production in asbestosis. Am Rev Respir Dis 1988; 138:278–283.

33. Hayes AA, Mullan B, Lovegrove FT, Rose AH, Musk AW, Robinson BW. Gallium lung scanning and bronchoalveolar lavage in crocidolite-exposed workers. Chest 1989; 96:22–26.

34. Garcia JG, Griffith DE, Cohen AB, Callahan KS. Alveolar macrophages from patients with asbestos exposure release increased levels of leukotriene B_4. Am Rev Respir Dis 1989; 139:1494–1501.

35. Cantin A, Allard C, Begin R. Increased alveolar plasminogen activator in early asbestosis. Am Rev Respir Dis 1989; 139:604–609.

36. Wallace JM, Oishi JS, Barbers RG, Batra P, Aberle DR. Bronchoalveolar lavage cell and lymphocyte phenotype profiles in healthy asbestos-exposed shipyard workers. Am Rev Respir Dis 1989; 139:33–38.

37. Roggli VL, Piantadosi CA, Bell DY. Asbestos bodies in bronchoalveolar lavage fluid: A study of 20 asbestos-exposed individuals and comparison to patients with other chronic interstitial lung diseases. Acta Cytol 1986; 30:470–476.

38. de Vuyst P, Jedwab J, Dumortier P, Vandermoten G, Vande Weyer R, Yernault JC. Asbestos bodies in bronchoalveolar lavage. Am Rev Respir Dis 1982; 126:972–976.

39. Sebastien P. [Current possibilities of the biometrology of dust in specimens of bronchoalveolar lavage fluid]. Ann Biol Clin (Paris) 1982; 40:279–293.

40. Gellert AR, Kitajewska JY, Uthayakumar S, Kirkham JB, Rudd RM. Asbestos fibres in bronchoalveolar lavage fluid from asbestos workers: Examination by electron microscopy. Br J Ind Med 1986; 43:170–176.

41. Morris DL, Greenberg SD, Lawrence EC. Immune responses in asbestos-exposed individuals [editorial]. Chest 1985; 87:278–280.

42. Lahat N, Sobel E, Djerassi L, Kaufman G, Horenstein L, Gruener N. Immunological profile of chest X-ray–negative asymptomatic asbestos workers. Am J Ind Med 1988; 13:473–482.

43. Linet MS, Harlow SD, McLaughlin JK. A case-control study of multiple myeloma in whites: Chronic antigenic stimulation, occupation, and drug use. Cancer Res 1987; 47:2978–2981.

44. deShazo RD, Nordberg J, Baser Y, Bozelka B, Weill H, Salvaggio J. Analysis of depressed cell-mediated immunity in asbestos workers. J Allergy Clin Immunol 1983; 71:418–424.

45. Lew F, Tsang P, Holland JF, Warner N, Selikoff IJ, Bekesi JG. High frequency of immune dysfunctions in asbestos workers and in patients with malignant mesothelioma. J Clin Immunol 1986; 6:225–233.

46. Tsang PH, Chu FN, Fischbein A, Bekesi JG. Impairments in functional subsets of T-suppressor (CD8) lymphocytes, monocytes, and natural killer cells among asbestos-exposed workers. Clin Immunol Immunopathol 1988; 47:323–332.

47. Robinson BW. Asbestos and cancer: Human natural killer cell activity is suppressed by asbestos fibers but can be restored by recombinant interleukin-2. Am Rev Respir Dis 1989; 139:897–901.

48. Anton Culver H, Culver BD, Kurosaki T. Immune response in shipyard workers with x-ray abnormalities consistent with asbestos exposure. Br J Ind Med 1988; 45:464–468.

49. Rola-Pleszczynski M, Masse S, Sirois P, Lemaire I, Begin R. Early effects of low-dose exposure to asbestos on local cellular immune responses in the lung. J Immunol 1981; 127:2535–2538.

50. Warheit DB, George G, Hill LH, Snyderman R, Brody AR. Inhaled asbestos activates a complement-dependent chemoattractant for macrophages. Lab Invest 1985; 52:505–514.

51. Warheit DB, Hill LH, George G, Brody AR. Time course of chemotactic factor generation and the corresponding macrophage response to asbestos inhalation. Am Rev Respir Dis 1986; 134:128–133.

52. Kagan E, Oghiso Y, Hartmann DP. The effects of chrysotile and crocidolite asbestos on the lower respiratory tract: Analysis of bronchoalveolar lavage constituents. Environ Res 1983; 32:382–397.

53. Warheit DB, Chang LY, Hill LH, Hook GE, Crapo JD, Brody AR. Pulmonary macrophage accumulation and asbestos-induced lesions at sites of fiber deposition. Am Rev Respir Dis 1984; 129:301–310.

54. Glassroth JL, Bernardo J, Lucey EC, Center DM, Jung-Legg Y, Snider GL. Interstitial pulmonary fibrosis induced in hamsters by intratracheally administered chrysotile asbestos. Am Rev Respir Dis 1984; 130:242–248.

55. Begin R, Rola-Pleszczynski M, Masse S, Nadeau D, Drapeau G. Assessment of progression of asbestosis in the sheep model by bronchoalveolar lavage and pulmonary function tests. Thorax 1983; 38:449–457.

56. Kagan E, Oghiso Y, Hartmann DP. Enhanced release of a chemoattractant for alveolar macrophages after asbestos inhalation. Am Rev Respir Dis 1983; 128:680–687.

57. Schoenberger CI, Hunninghake GW, Kawanami O, Ferrans VJ, Crystal RG. Role of alveolar macrophages in asbestosis: Modulation of neutrophil migration to the lung after acute asbestos exposure. Thorax 1982; 37:803–809.

58. Rola-Pleszczynski M, Gouin S, Begin R. Asbestos-induced lung inflammation: Role of local macrophage-derived chemotactic factors in accumulation of neutrophils in the lungs. Inflammation 1984; 8:53–62.

59. Cantin A, Dubois F, Begin R. Lung exposure to mineral dusts enhances the capacity of lung inflammatory cells to release superoxide. J Leukocyte Biol 1988; 43:299–303.

60. Mossman BT, Marsh JP, Shatos MA. Alteration of superoxide dismutase activity in tracheal epithelial cells by asbestos and inhibition of cytotoxicity by antioxidants. Lab Invest 1986; 54:204–212.

61. Shatos MA, Doherty JM, Marsh JP, Mossman BT. Prevention of asbestos-induced cell death in rat lung fibroblasts by inhibitors of active oxygen species. Environ Res 1987; 44:103–116.

62. Mossman BT, Marsh JP. Evidence supporting a role for active oxygen species in asbestos-induced toxicity and lung disease. Environ Health Perspect 1989; 81:91–94.

63. Kennedy TP, Dodson R, Rao NV, Ky H, Hopkins C, Baser M, Tolley E, Hoidal JR. Dusts causing pneumoconiosis generate ·OH and produce hemolysis by acting as Fenton catalysts. Arch Biochem Biophys 1989; 269:359–364.

64. Jackson JH, Schraufstatter IU, Hyslop PA, Vosbeck K, Sauerheber R, Weitzman SA, Cochrane CG. Role of oxidants in DNA damage: Hydroxyl radical mediates the synergistic DNA damaging effects of asbestos and cigarette smoke. J Clin Invest 1987; 80:1090–1095.

65. Kelley J. Cytokines of the lung: State of the art. Am Rev Respir Dis 1990; 141:765–788.

66. Lemaire I, Rola-Pleszczynski M, Begin R. Asbestos exposure enhances the release of fibroblast growth factor by sheep alveolar macrophages. J Reticuloendothel Soc 1983; 33:275–285.

67. Begin R, Bisson G, Lambert R, Cote Y, Fabi D, Martel M, Lamoureux G, Rola-Pleszczynski M, Boctor M, Dalle D, Masse S. Gallium-67 uptake in the lung of asbestos exposed sheep: Early association with enhanced macrophage-derived fibronectin accumulation. J Nucl Med 1986; 27:538–544.

68. Brody AR, McGavran PD, Overby LH. Brief inhalation of chrysotile asbestos induces rapid proliferation of bronchiolar-alveolar epithelial and interstitial cells. IARC Sci Publ 1989; 93–99.

69. Brody AR, Overby LH. Incorporation of tritiated thymidine by epithelial and interstitial cells in bronchiolar-alveolar regions of asbestos-exposed rats. Am J Pathol 1989; 134:133–140.

70. McGavran PD, Brody AR. Chrysotile asbestos inhalation induces tritiated thymidine incorporation by epithelial cells of distal bronchioles. Am J Respir Cell Mol Biol 1989; 1:231–235.

71. Corn JK. Historical aspects of industrial hygiene, II: Silicosis. Am Ind Hyg Assoc J 1980; 41:125–133.

72. Suratt PM, Winn WC Jr, Brody AR, Bolton WK, Giles RD. Acute silicosis in tombstone sandblasters. Am Rev Respir Dis 1977; 115:521–529.

73. Office of the Federal Register. Code of federal regulations: Mineral resources—exposure limits for airborne contaminants (30 CFR 56.5001). Washington, DC: Office of the Federal Register, National Archives and Records Administration, 1988.

74. Centers for Disease Control. Criteria for a recommended standard: Occupational exposure to crystalline silica (NIOSH 75–120). Cincinnati, OH: US Dept of Health, Education, and Welfare; Health Services and Mental Health Administration, 1974.

75. Current trends: Exposure trends in silica flour plants—United States, 1975–1986. MMWR 1989; 39:380–383.

76. US Dept of Labor Supplementary Data System. Publication PB86-129830. Washington, DC: National Technical Information Service, 1983.

77. Costello J, Graham WG. Vermont granite workers' mortality study. Am J Ind Med 1988; 13:483–497.

78. Graham WGB, O'Grady RV, Dubuc B. Pulmonary function loss in Vermont granite workers: A long-term follow-up and critical reappraisal. Am Rev Respir Dis 1981; 123:26–28.

79. Theriault GP, Burgess WA, DeBeradinis LJ, Peters JM. Dust exposure in the Vermont granite sheds. Arch Environ Health 1974; 28:12–17.

80. Theriault GP, Peters JM, Fine LJ. Pulmonary function in granite shed workers of Vermont. Arch Environ Health 1974; 28:18–22.

81. Theriault GP, Peters JM, Fine LJ. Pulmonary function and roentgenographic changes in granite dust exposure. Arch Environ Health 1974; 28:23–27.

82. Lou JZ, Zhou C. The prevention of silicosis and prediction of its future prevalence in China. Am J Public Health 1989; 79:1613–1616.

83. Wegman DH, Wegman ME. Lessons from silicosis control in China [editorial]. Am J Public Health 1989; 79:1599–1600.

84. Cowie RL, van Schalkwyk MG. The prevalence of silicosis in Orange Free State gold miners. J Occup Med 1987; 29:44–46.

85. Prenafeta J. [Pneumoconiosis in Chile]. Rev Med Chil 1984; 112:511–515.

86. Valiante DJ, Rosenman KD. Does silicosis still occur. JAMA 1989; 262:3003–3007.

87. Craighead JE, Kleinerman J, Abraham JL, Gibbs AR, Green FHY, Harley RA, Ruettner JR, Vallyathan NV, Juliano EB. Diseases associated with exposure to silica and nonfibrous silicate minerals. Silicosis and Silicate Disease Committee. Arch Pathol Lab Med 1988; 112:673–720.

88. Brody AR, Roe MW, Evans JN, Davis GS. Deposition and translocation of inhaled silica in rats: Quantification of particle distribution, macrophage participation, and function. Lab Invest 1982; 47:533–542.

89. Craighead JE, Vallyathan V. Cryptic pulmonary lesions in workers occupationally exposed to dust containing silica. JAMA 1980; 244:1939–1941.

90. Snider DE. The relationship between tuberculosis and silicosis. Am Rev Respir Dis 1978; 118:455–460.

91. Westerholm P, Ahlmark A, Maasing R, Segelberg I. Silicosis and risk of lung cancer or lung tuberculosis: A cohort study. Environ Res 1986; 41:339–350.

92. Allison AC, D'Arcy Hart P. Potentiation by silica of the growth of *Mycobacterium* tuberculosis in macrophage cultures. Br J Exp Pathol 1968; 49:465–476.

93. Banks DE, Morring KL, Boehlecke BA, et al. Silicosis in silica flour workers. Am Rev Respir Dis 1981; 124:445–450.

94. Dubois F, Bégin R, Cantin A, Massé S, Martel M, Bilodeau G, Dufresne A, Perreault G, Sébastien P. Aluminum inhalation reduces silicosis in a sheep model. Am Rev Respir Dis 1988; 137:1172–1179.

95. Davis GS. Pathogenesis of silicosis: Current concepts and hypotheses. Lung 1986; 164:139–154.

96. Allison AC, Harington JS, Birbeck M. An examination of the cytotoxic effects of silica on macrophages. J Exp Med 1966; 124:141–154.

97. Davis GS, Hemenway DR, Evans JN, Lapenas DJ, Brody AR. Alveolar macrophage stimulation and population changes in silica-exposed rats. Chest 1981; 80:8–10.

98. Christman JW, Emerson RJ, Graham WG, Davis GS. Mineral dust and cell recovery from the bronchoalveolar lavage of healthy Vermont granite workers. Am Rev Respir Dis 1985; 132:393–399.

99. Emerson RJ, Davis GS. Effect of alveolar lining material–coated silica on rat alveolar macrophages. Environ Health Perspect 1983; 51:81–84.

100. Struhar DJ, Harbeck RJ, Gegen N, Kawada H, Mason RJ. Increased expression of class II antigens of the major histocompatibility complex on alveolar macrophages and alveolar type II cells and interleukin-1 (IL1) secretion from alveolar macrophages in an animal model of silicosis. Clin Exp Immunol 1989; 77:281–284.

101. Bowden DH, Hedgecock C, Adamson IYR. Silica-induced pulmonary fibrosis involves the reaction of particles with interstitial rather than alveolar macrophages. J Pathol 1989; 158:73–80.

102. Absher MP, Trombley L, Hemenway DR, Mickey RM, Leslie KO. Biphasic cellular and tissue response of rat lungs after eight-day aerosol exposure to the silicon dioxide cristobalite. Am J Pathol 1989; 134:1243–1251.

103. Struhar D, Harbeck RJ, Mason RJ. Lymphocyte populations in lung tissue, bronchoalveolar lavage fluid, and peripheral blood in rats at various times during the development of silicosis. Am Rev Respir Dis 1989; 139:28–32.

104. Schmidt JA, Oliver CN, Lepe Zuniga JL, Green I, Gery I. Silica-stimulated monocytes release fibroblast proliferation factors identical to interleukin 1: A potential role for interleukin 1 in the pathogenesis of silicosis. J Clin Invest 1984; 73:1462–1472.

105. Kampschmidt RF, Worthington ML 3d, Mesecher MI. Release of interleukin-1 (IL1) and IL1-like factors from rabbit macrophages with silica. J Leukocyte Biol 1986; 39:123–132.

106. Oghiso Y, Kubota Y. Interleukin 1 production and accessory cell function of rat alveolar macrophages exposed to mineral dust particles. Microbiol Immunol 1987; 31:275–287.

107. Hurme M, Seppala IJ. Differential induction of membrane-associated interleukin 1 (IL1) expression and IL1 alpha and IL1 beta secretion by lipopolysaccharide and silica in human monocytes. Scand J Immunol 1988; 27:725–730.

108. Oghiso Y, Kubota Y. Enhanced interleukin 1 production by alveolar macrophages and increase in Ia-positive lung cells in silica-exposed rats. Microbiol Immunol 1986; 30:1189–1198.

109. Doll NJ, Stankus RP, Hughes J, Weill H, Gupta R, Rodriguez M, Jones RN, Alspauge MA, Salvaggio JE. Immune complexes and autoantibodies in silicosis. J Allergy Clin Immunol 1981; 68:281–285.

110. Calhoun WJ, Christman JW, Ershler WB, Graham WG, Davis GS. Raised immunoglobulin concentrations in bronchoalveolar lavage fluid of healthy granite workers. Thorax 1986; 41:266–273.

111. Lugano EM, Dauber JH, Daniele RP. Silica stimulation of chemotactic factor release by guinea pig alveolar macrophages. J Reticuloendothel Soc 1981; 30:381–390.
112. Dauber JH, Rossman MD, Pietra GG, Jimenez SA, Daniele RP. Experimental silicosis: Morphologic and biochemical abnormalities produced by intratracheal instillation of quartz into guinea pig lungs. Am J Pathol 1980; 101:595–612.
113. Lugano EM, Dauber JH, Elias JA, Bashey RI, Jimenez SA, Daniele RP. The regulation of lung fibroblast proliferation by alveolar macrophages in experimental silicosis. Am Rev Respir Dis 1984; 129:767–771.
114. Bateman ED, Emerson RJ, Cole PJ. A study of macrophage-mediated initiation of fibrosis by asbestos and silica using a diffusion chamber technique. Br J Exp Pathol 1982; 63:414–425.
115. Aalto M, Kulonen E, Pikkarainen J. Isolation of silica-dependent protein from rat lung with special reference to development of fibrosis. Br J Exp Pathol 1989; 70:167–182.
116. Dubois CM, Bissonnette E, Rola-Pleszczynski M. Asbestos fibers and silica particles stimulate rat alveolar macrophages to release tumor necrosis factor: Autoregulatory role of leukotriene B_4. Am Rev Respir Dis 1989; 139:1257–1264.
117. Mohr C, Gemsa D, Hemenway DR, Leslie KE, Absher M, Davis GS. Systemic immunostimulation in rats with silicosis: Remote effects of localized dust. Am Rev Respir Dis 1990; 141:417a.
118. Kawada H, Horiuchi T, Shannon JM, Kuroki Y, Voelker DR, Mason RJ. Alveolar type II cells, surfactant protein A (SP-A), and the phospholipid components of surfactant in acute silicosis in the rat. Am Rev Respir Dis 1989; 140:460–470.
119. Adams DO. The granulomatous inflammatory response: A review. Am J Pathol 1976; 84:164–191.
120. Kasahara K, Kobayashi K, Shikama Y, Yoneya I, Kaga S, Hashimoto M, Odagiri T, Soejima K, Ide H, Takahashi T, Yoshida T. The role of monokines in granuloma formation in mice: The ability of interleukin 1 and tumor necrosis factor-α to induce lung granulomas. Clin Immunol Immunopathol 1989; 51:419–425.
121. Kindler V, Sappino AP, Grau GE, Piguet PF, Vassalli P. The inducing role of tumor necrosis factor in the development of bactericidal granulomas during BCG infection. Cell 1989; 56:731–740.
122. Zambon P, Simonato L, Mastrangelo G, Winkelmann R, Saia B, Crepet M. Mortality of workers compensated for silicosis during the period 1959–1963 in the Veneto region of Italy. Scand J Work Environ Health 1987; 13:118–123.
123. Finkelstein M, Liss GM, Krammer F, Kusiak RA. Mortality among workers receiving compensation awards for silicosis in Ontario 1940–85. Br J Ind Med 1987; 44:588–594.
124. Infante-Rivard C, Armstrong B, Petitclerc M, Cloutier LG, Theriault G. Lung cancer mortality and silicosis in Quebec, 1938–85. Lancet 1989; 2:1504–1507.
125. Mastrangelo G, Zambon P, Simonato L, Rizzi P. A case-referent study investigating the relationship between exposure to silica dust and lung cancer. Int Arch Occup Environ Health 1988; 60:299–302.

5

Bronchiolitis Obliterans

Gary R. Epler

Bronchiolitis obliterans was first described in 1901.[1] Scattered reports of the disorder caused by fumes and other agents appeared until the 1980s, when a cascade of publications began to appear on idiopathic bronchiolitis obliterans organizing pneumonia (BOOP),[2-6] idiopathic bronchiolitis obliterans,[7] marrow and heart-lung transplant bronchiolitis obliterans,[8-14] diffuse panbronchiolitis,[15,16] and respiratory bronchiolitis.[17,18] This chapter will discuss the clinical and pathologic perspectives of diffuse panbronchiolitis, respiratory bronchiolitis, and the obliterative lesions—bronchiolitis obliterans (BrOb) and bronchiolitis obliterans organizing pneumonia (BOOP).

ANATOMY OF THE BRONCHIOLE AIRWAYS

A standard classification of bronchiolar anatomy has not yet been universally adopted, but there is some general agreement. **Bronchioles** are conducting airways that do not have cartilage or submuscosal glands. They begin at about the fourth generation of airway branching at 4 mm in diameter, proceed to the seventh generation at 2 mm, and the tenth at 1 mm in diameter.[19] Smooth muscle persists until the distal bronchioles are reached. The **terminal bronchioles** represent the final conducting bronchioles at the 16th generation and have a diameter of 0.6 mm. There are about 28,000 terminal bronchioles.[20] The **respiratory bronchioles** are distinctive because they contain alveolar sacs. There are 224,000 respiratory bronchioles, which are about 0.4 mm in diameter. The bronchioles conclude with **alveolar ducts** and **alveolar sacs**.

PATHOLOGIC CONSIDERATIONS

The pathologist can identify several distinct lesions. **Bronchiolitis** is defined as cellular inflammation of the bronchioles.[21] Diffuse **panbronchiolitis** is defined as a chronic

156

cellular infiltrate of the terminal and respiratory bronchioles in which walls are thickened by infiltrating lymphocytes, plasma cells, and histiocytes.[15,16] **Respiratory bronchiolitis–interstitial lung disease** is characterized by pigmented macrophages within respiratory bronchioles and neighboring alveolar ducts and alveoli. Alveolar septa show a mild chronic inflammatory cell infiltrate and hyperplasia of the alveolar lining cells.[17,18] **Bronchiolitis obliterans** consists of granulation tissue plugs within the lumens of small airways that may heal without a scar (an early lesion) or heal with a scar, sometimes with complete obstruction of small airways (a late, irreversible lesion).[7,22] **Bronchiolitis obliterans organizing pneumonia** (BOOP) is defined as granulation tissue plugs within lumens of small airways that sometimes completely obstruct the airways and extend into alveolar ducts and alveoli.[2]

CLINICAL CONSIDERATIONS

Clinicians and pathologists see patients from different perspectives. For example, the Japanese physician may see a patient who displays severe sinusitis, a cough, a radiograph with bilateral small nodular opacities, and a poor response to aminoglycoside antibodies and corticosteroid therapy, and the pathologist will see diffuse panbronchiolitis.[15,16] A smoker may develop crackles on examination, a low diffusing capacity, and a radiograph showing diffuse nodular opacities. The syndrome, referred to as respiratory bronchiolitis–interstitial lung disease, disappears after cessation of smoking.[17,18] A worker may develop cough, dyspnea, and airflow obstruction and have a normal chest radiograph 2 to 4 weeks after exposure to sulfur dioxide in a gas explosion. The illness, bronchiolitis obliterans, may not respond to corticosteroid therapy.[23,24] The same pathologic findings of bronchiolitis obliterans can also occur after bone marrow transplantation[9–11] or heart-lung transplantation[12–14] and in rheumatoid arthritis.[22,25] Finally, the clinician may see a patient with a cough and a flu-like illness that persists for 1 to 2 weeks and then progresses 1 to 2 weeks later to dyspnea and a chest roentgenogram showing bilateral patchy infiltrates. Crackles are heard on examination and physiological studies show a slight reduction in the vital capacity with a moderate to severe reduction in the diffusing capacity. This syndrome, idiopathic bronchiolitis obliterans organizing pneumonia, or BOOP, shows complete recovery in 65% of patients treated with corticosteroid therapy.[2–6] The syndrome may also occur in patients who are cocaine abusers.[26]

CLASSIFICATION

As just described, what to the pathologist is bronchiolitis obliterans or bronchiolitis obliterans organizing pneumonia may represent five distinctly different clinical situations. Consequently, the classification of bronchiolar diseases has been slow to develop. As more information becomes available, a uniform classification should emerge. In the meantime, the most appropriate classification is a combination of histologic findings as main categories and clinical settings as subcategories (Table 5-1).

TABLE 5-1. Diseases of the Bronchioles

Acute and chronic bronchiolitis
  Respiratory syncytial virus in infants
  Viral bronchiolitis in adults
Diffuse panbronchiolitis
Respiratory bronchiolitis
Bronchiolitis obliterans
  Idiopathic
  Fume exposure
  Postinfection
  Connective tissue disorder
  Drugs
  Focal nodule
  Bone marrow transplantation
  Heart-lung transplantation
  Activated charcoal
Bronchiolitis obliterans organizing pneumonia
  Idiopathic
  Fume exposure (early)
  Postinfection (early)
  Connective tissue disorders
  Focal nodule
  Cocaine

Three of the bronchiolar lesions do not have a major obliterative component: acute and chronic bronchiolitis, diffuse panbronchiolitis, and respiratory bronchiolitis–interstitial lung disease. Two of the lesions are obliterative: bronchiolitis obliterans (Fig. 5-1A) and bronchiolitis obliterans organizing pneumonia (Fig. 5-2A). Pure bronchiolitis obliterans is associated with the clinical findings of airflow obstruction whereas bronchiolitis obliterans organizing pneumonia is associated with the clinical findings of interstitial lung disease. Although there is some overlap, the pathologist can usually distinguish the two lesions. The clinician can distinguish the airway process by a syndrome of early inspiratory crackles, abnormal FEV_1/FVC ratio, and a normal chest radiograph (Fig. 5-1B) The clinician can also distinguish the interstitial lung disease process in patients with a flu-like illness, crackles, abnormal diffusing capacity, and patchy infiltrates on the chest film (Fig. 5-2B). In other situations, especially with the chronic airway obstruction process, the clinician may have more difficulty, because several months of monitoring are required before the process of pure bronchiolitis obliterans is established. The lesion of bronchiolitis obliterans organizing pneumonia tends to be an "early" process and often responds to corticosteroid therapy, whereas the late, irreversible scarring of the airways in bronchiolitis obliterans does not.

BRONCHIOLITIS

Bronchiolitis may be acute or chronic. Acute bronchiolitis is usually thought of as a disease of infants caused by the respiratory syncytial virus. Chronic bronchiolitis in the

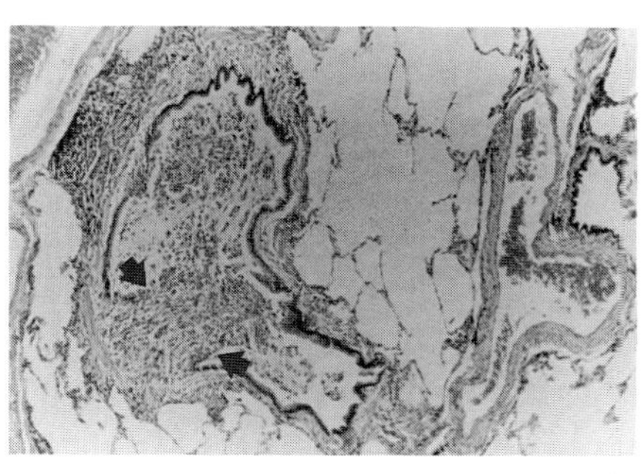

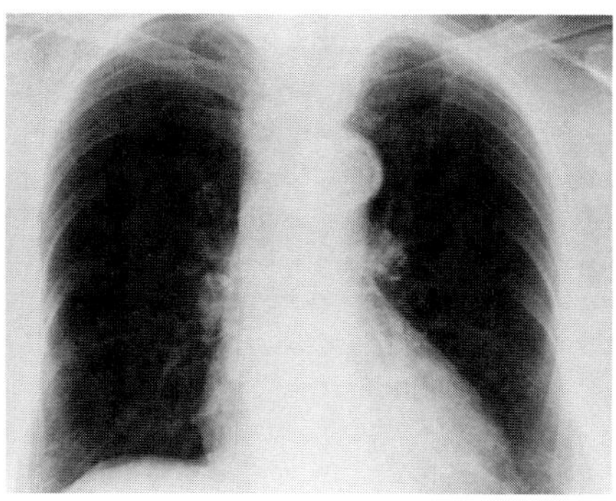

A   **B**

Figure 5-1. Bronchiolitis obliterans. (*A*) This photomicrograph shows a focal ulceration of the bronchiolar mucosa (*arrows*) in a proliferation of mixed inflammatory cells. Fibroblasts extend into the lumen. There is focal chronic inflammation in the wall of the bronchiole. Significantly, the surrounding alveolar parenchyma is unremarkable. (*B*) This radiograph is from a 55-year-old woman with severe dyspnea, early inspiratory crackles, and an FEV_1 of 0.88 liters. The radiographic appearance is normal. The illness did not respond to corticosteroid therapy.

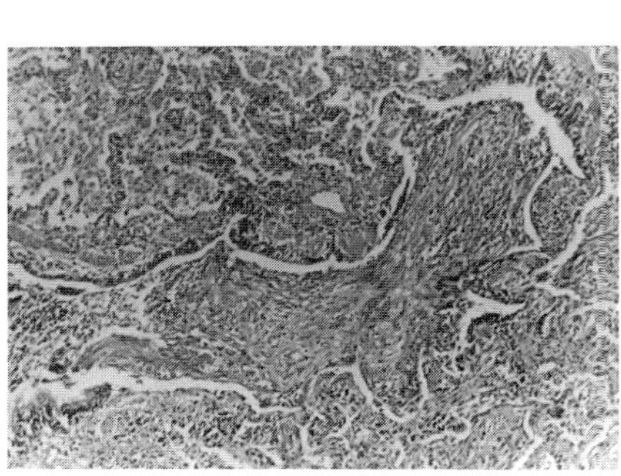

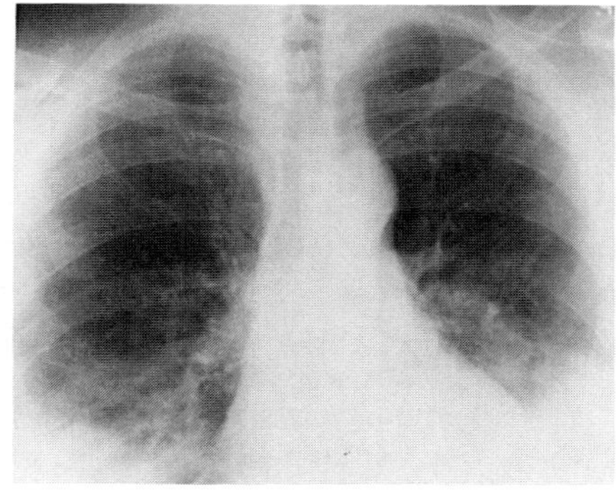

A   **B**

Figure 5-2. Bronchiolitis obliterans organizing pneumonia. (*A*) This photomicrograph shows a polyp of granulation tissue cut longitudinally in a bronchiolar lumen. The surrounding alveolar parenchyma shows prominent interstitial infiltrate and accumulations of cells within their lumens. (*B*) This radiograph is from a 61-year-old man who developed a flu-like illness, late inspiratory crackles, and an abnormal diffusing capacity. Bilateral patchy infiltrates are apparent on the lower lung fields. The patient recovered completely after 1 year of prednisone therapy.

adult may be seen in lung biopsy specimens as part of chronic bronchitis or as a non-specific finding associated with primary lung disorders such as infectious pneumonias, lung cancer, or chronic interstitial pneumonias. The incidence of viral bronchiolitis in the adult is not known for several reasons. Lung biopsies are rarely obtained except in the most advanced form. Adenovirus and rhinovirus infections may be common causes, but the degree of severity may be so mild that patients do not seek medical advice. Finally, there have been no systematic studies of viral bronchiolitis in the adult.

Clinically, it is difficult if not impossible to distinguish severe bronchiolitis from idiopathic bronchiolitis obliterans. The illness occurs equally in men and women of all ages. Most patients have a cough without sputum production. The chest roentgenogram is normal or shows hyperinflation. Pulmonary function shows airflow obstruction. In a group of 11 patients with biopsy-proven adult bronchiolitis, symptoms were chronic with an average duration of almost 5 years.[7] Dyspnea and cough without sputum production occurred in all patients, and many had an FEV_1 of less than 1 liter. The prognosis is variable; most patients have irreversible fixed airflow obstruction, but patients in whom bronchoalveolar lavage shows a high percentage of neutrophils may respond to prednisone therapy.[7]

DIFFUSE PANBRONCHIOLITIS

Panbronchiolitis occurs among Japanese, Chinese, and Koreans. The disorder is histologically characterized by thickening of the wall of the respiratory bronchiole with infiltration of lymphocytes and plasma cells.[15,16] The inflammatory changes often extend into the peribronchiolar tissue. The alveolar septa and lumens remain intact. In the advanced stage, narrowing and constriction of the respiratory bronchioles cause ectasia of proximal terminal bronchioles. Cor pulmonale develops in the terminal stages of the disease.

Most patients range from 30 to 70 years of age. The disease is more prevalent in younger males, but after ages 50 to 60 the sex distribution is equal. Dyspnea, chronic cough with sputum production, and wheezing are common symptoms. Importantly, more than 75% of those affected have paranasal sinusitis. There is no preponderance of smokers. Crackles and rhonchi are commonly heard on physical examination. Pseudomonas detected in the sputum often suggests that patients have progressed to the terminal stage. The chest roentgenogram may be normal or show hyperinflation in some patients, but the majority show bilateral small nodular opacities, at the lung bases in the early stages and then diffusely throughout the lungs. Ring shadows and cystic structures are seen at the lung bases at the terminal stage. Chest CT findings show that the ring-shaped opacities are connected to the proximal bronchovascular bundles and the large cystic opacities are accompanied by dilated proximal bronchi.[16] Pulmonary function studies show airflow obstruction with associated reduction in the vital capacity during the late stage. The diffusing capacity is usually decreased. Hypercapnia is seen at late stages. The prognosis is poor: survival at 10 years for patients with pseudomonas infection is only 30%.[15]

RESPIRATORY BRONCHIOLITIS–INTERSTITIAL LUNG DISEASE

Respiratory bronchiolitis is a distinct but uncommon entity in smokers that has the appearance of an interstitial lung disorder.[17,18] Patients are aged 30 to 60 years and all are heavy smokers. Cough is an early symptom. Dyspnea then develops that causes patients to seek a medical evaluation. End-inspiratory fine crackles are frequently heard on examination. The vital capacity may be normal or decreased, but the diffusing capacity is decreased in virtually all patients. There may be mild airflow obstruction. The chest roentgenogram shows bilateral small reticular nodular opacities. The lung biopsy is characterized by the accumulation of pigmented macrophages within respiratory bronchioles and neighboring alveolar ducts and alveoli. Alveolar septa may show nonspecific thickening due to fibrosis, a mild chronic inflammatory cell infiltrate, and hyperplasia of the alveolar lining cells. The peribronchiolar interstitium is focally involved by a mild infiltrate of lymphocytes and histiocytes. Ultrastructural examination may demonstrate needle-like electron-lucent particles, so-called smokers inclusions, within phagolysosomes.[17] The illness is reversible if the patient stops smoking. Some patients may require an initial course of corticosteroid therapy.

A study of 18 patients with respiratory bronchiolitis–interstitial lung disease indicated that all were smokers and that the mean age was 36 years.[18] Patients with desquamative interstitial pneumonia (DIP), by comparison, were older, had more severe dyspnea and more severely abnormal pulmonary function tests, and often had progressive respiratory disease.

BRONCHIOLITIS OBLITERANS

The Chronic Airflow Obstruction Disease

Idiopathic Bronchiolitis Obliterans.   This disorder occurs in individuals with no obvious inciting agent and no associated connective tissue disorder. There have been scattered reports of this disorder over the years. Although there is a distinct difference pathologically between bronchiolitis and obliterative bronchiolitis. clinically the two are indistinguishable except that an irreversible, fixed airflow obstruction probably represents the obliterative lesion. In such individuals, cough is the presenting symptom and is soon followed by dyspnea. Early inspiratory crackles are often heard and are probably related to scarring of airways. The lungs on chest roentgenogram are normal or hyperinflated and physiological studies show severe irreversible airflow obstruction with a marked reduction in FEV_1. Prognosis is poor despite corticosteroid therapy, although among five patients with biopsy-proven bronchiolitis obliterans, the presence of neutrophils in the bronchoalveolar lavage fluid may have indicated responsiveness to prednisone.[7] Three months of high-dose prednisone (1 mg/kg) is often needed to determine effectiveness with tapering doses for 3 more months and lower dosages for at least 1 year. Patients who survive the initial episode may stabilize for several years or progress to end-stage lung. It is difficult to determine whether progression is a continual process such as that seen in usual interstitial pneumonia (UIP) or is due to intermittent infections with disabling loss of function. Lung transplantation may be effective for patients who do not respond to corticosteroid therapy and develop irreversible chronic respiratory failure.[27]

Toxic Fume Exposure.   Exposure to nitrogen dioxide, sulfur dioxide, and other toxic fumes can cause a spectrum of symptoms from mild eye, nose, and throat irritation to immediate asphyxiation and death. Some patients develop acute respiratory failure after a 4- to 6-hour latency period. One to three weeks later, some of these patients develop irreversible airflow obstruction due to bronchiolitis obliterans. This is a late lesion, and lung biopsy reveals irreversible scarring of the bronchioles. The chest examination may reveal early inspiratory crackles but no wheezing. By chest radiography the lungs appear normal or show hyperinflation.

The degree of permanent functional impairment is related directly to the number of bronchioles that have been irreversibly scarred, which is also related to the type and amount of fume inhalation, being most severe after accidents involving exposure to sulfur dioxide.[23,24] A different perspective on silo-filler's disease is emerging: In the past it was thought that bronchiolitis obliterans was common and often inevitable, but with early recognition, the nitrogen dioxide–related acute alveolar injury and the bronchiolitis obliterans lesion are treatable with corticosteroid therapy.[28]

Post Infectious Bronchiolitis Obliterans.   This disorder may occur after a viral or mycoplasmal infection. Cough develops several days after the initial infection. Chest radiographs may show diffuse reticular nodular opacities early but are normal or show hyperinflation in the late phase of the illness. The diagnosis is often suspected clinically. Lung specimens may show granulation tissue that heals without a scar with complete clinical resolution or irreversible, extensive scarring that obliterates many of the bronchioles, which correlates with severe airflow obstruction clinically. Among the latter group of patients the illness may be fatal, although there has been success with a double lung transplant.[27]

Bronchiolitis Obliterans in the Connective Tissue Diseases.   Bronchiolitis obliterans has been seen in patients with rheumatoid arthritis, scleroderma, lupus erythematosus, eosinophilic fasciitis, and polymyalgia rheumatica.[22,25,29] Bronchiolitis obliterans associated with rheumatoid arthritis has a particularly poor prognosis; death within 3 years is common.[25,30] Dyspnea is severe in these patients, early inspiratory crackles are heard,[22] the chest film is normal or shows hyperinflation, and physiologically there is severe airflow obstruction. In general, bronchiolitis obliterans is a poor prognostic sign in the connective tissue disorders—whether it is the combination of two disorders or an accelerated, progressive form of bronchiolitis obliterans that is responsible is not known. The underlying disorder must be managed as well as possible, and a course of high-dose corticosteroid therapy (prednisone 1 mg/kg) can be used for severe pulmonary involvement or for exacerbations of the pulmonary lesion. Long-term corticosteroid therapy appears to have no beneficial effect on the natural course of the illness.

Drug-Related Bronchiolitis Obliterans.   This may occur in patients with the connective tissue disorders, especially rheumatoid arthritis. Penicillamine is associated with a pure bronchiolitis obliterans.[22,25,31] Cough with no sputum production is the first symptom, soon followed by dyspnea. Early inspiratory crackles are heard,[22] the chest roentgenogram is normal, and there is severe airflow obstruction, with FEV_1 values often less than 1 liter. The lesion also has a poor prognosis[25] although discontinuing the penicillamine and instituting prednisone therapy may result in stabilization.[31]

Gold therapy for patients with rheumatoid arthritis may cause bronchiolitis obliterans, but the relationship has not been firmly established. There has been a report of a woman with rheumatoid arthritis in whom severe airflow obstruction developed after 1.125 g of gold therapy; autopsy showed extensive obliterative bronchiolitis.[32] An additional report indicated that irreversible airway obstruction developed in a woman with severe rheumatoid arthritis while she was receiving oral gold therapy; a lung biopsy showed bronchiolitis with an obliterative component.[33]

The cause-and-effect relationship between penicillamine, gold therapy, and bronchiolitis obliterans is difficult to establish because bronchiolitis obliterans occurs in patients with rheumatoid arthritis who have not been treated,[25] and airflow obstruction as measured by pulmonary function testing is common. In addition, these agents, especially gold, cause interstitial pneumonitis usually associated with eosinophils and responsive to corticosteroid therapy. Most patients with drug-induced lung toxicity do not have an open lung biopsy; thus, the histologic lesion is not definitively characterized—that is, the lesion may represent an acute alveolitis with or without fibrosis, usual interstitial pneumonia, or perhaps bronchiolitis obliterans organizing pneumonia.[2,34] An HLA antigen study of 28 patients did not show an increase in a specific antigen for patients with suspected gold or penicillamine toxicity.[35] Regardless of whether these lesions are caused by these agents, by the rheumatoid arthritis, or by both, patients who develop unexplained cough or dyspnea must be evaluated immediately.

Bone Marrow Transplantation Bronchiolitis Obliterans.   This disorder was reported in 1982 in a 22-year-old patient who received an allogenic bone marrow graft for aplastic anemia.[9] Review of this complication[8,10] indicates that obliterative bronchiolitis may occur in 10% of patients who develop chronic graft-versus-host disease and in about 5% of patients receiving marrow transplantation. The lesion can occur at any age and in either sex. It is preceded by typical findings of graft-versus-host disease, including skin rash, mucositis, and angiitis, which usually occur within 3 months after transplantation. Six months later a cough will develop, soon followed by severe and progressive dyspnea. The chest radiograph is normal in 80% of patients.[10] Crackles are generally heard at this time. The FEV_1 is severely reduced and there is usually no improvement after bronchodilator inhalation. Response to therapy has been poor once severe airflow obstruction has been established. Mortality was 65% at 3 years after transplant although long-term survival was achieved in more than 25% of patients.[10] Pneumothorax may be a complication. In patients who have airway disease associated with chronic graft-versus-host disease, therapy is directed at controlling the graft-versus-host disease and at preventing infection with antibiotics and intravenous immunoglobulin. If primary treatment with prednisone fails to result in a complete response, the early addition of azathioprine or cyclosporine is recommended.[10]

Among the possible mechanisms of bronchiolitis obliterans in marrow recipients are repeated respiratory tract infections and immunologic mechanisms. Investigators have suggested that the lung may be a specific target organ for immunologically mediated damage—that is, lung damage may be a manifestation of graft rejection.[11] Experimental studies have shown that epithelium can express Ia antigens that may activate donor T cells among bronchi-associated lymphatic tissue (BALT), making the airways a target for immunologically mediated injury.[11]

Heart-Lung Transplant Bronchiolitis Obliterans was reported in 1984,[12] and airway disease soon emerged as the most important clinical complication among heart-lung transplant recipients. There are several clinical differences between this complication and that associated with marrow transplantation. The typical patients are men aged 20 to 40 years. They develop cough and dyspnea sometimes associated with fever. The chest roentgenogram shows patchy infiltrates or bilateral nodular opacities. In some, the respiratory illness occurred after evidence of cardiac rejection, but there were no skin lesions, mucositis or liver abnormalities consistent with typical signs of chronic graft-versus-host disease. The respiratory illness may begin from 3 to 28 months after transplantation. Lung specimens show extensive bronchiolitis obliterans with some interstitial fibrosis. All of the lung specimens show marked pleural fibrosis. The prognosis is variable. One study indicated that obliterative bronchiolitis developed in one-half of twenty long-term survivors: four died, three had functional limitation with disabling irreversible airflow obstruction, and two responded successfully to corticosteroid therapy.[13]

Mechanisms of heart-lung–related bronchiolitis obliterans include repeated viral or bacterial infections, which may result in chronic inflammation with squamous metaplasia and loss of surface cilia, leading to more infection, more inflammation, and obliterative bronchiolitis. Inflammation itself also impairs the secretion of IgA, an important agent for lung defense. The mucociliary clearance may also be altered because of ciliary dysfunction or abnormal mucus chemistry and viscosity. Ligation of the bronchial circulation may alter repair of the bronchioles. It has been proposed that bronchiolitis obliterans after lung transplantation is a form of allograft rejection related to augmented expression of class II major histocompatibility complex antigens on the airway epithelium and mediated by activated T cells.[14]

Aspiration of Activated Charcoal has been reported as a cause of bronchiolitis obliterans.[36] Profound dyspnea, severe airflow obstruction, hypercapnia, a chest radiograph showing upper lung pneumatocoeles, and death may occur. The pathogenesis is not known, but massive amounts of activated charcoal found in the bronchiolar scars suggest a pathogenetic role for the charcoal itself, although gastric contents adsorbed to its surface may be a contributing factor.

BRONCHIOLITIS OBLITERANS ORGANIZING PNEUMONIA

The Interstitial Lung Disease

Idiopathic bronchiolitis obliterans organizing pneumonia (BOOP) was described from a review of 94 patients in whom lung biopsy revealed bronchiolitis obliterans.[2] Among these patients there were 50 who had an organizing pneumonia component histo-

TABLE 5-2. Bronchiolitis Obliterans (BrOb) and Bronchiolitis Obliterans Organizing Pneumonia (BOOP)

PARAMETER	BrOb	BOOP
Dyspnea	Yes	Yes
Cough	Yes	Yes
Wheezing	+/−	No
Hemoptysis	No	No
Crackles	Early Inspiratory	Late Inspiratory
Wheezing on exam	+/−	No
Chest radiograph	Normal or hyperinflation	Bilateral patchy
Vital capacity	Nl or dec	Decreased
FEV$_1$/FVC	Decreased	Normal
Diffusing cap	Nl or dec	Decreased
Pathology	Airways	Airways and parenchyma
Prognosis	Poor to fair	Fair to good

pathologically and who had a distinct clinical entity. The illness occurs in men and woman aged 20 to 70 years and is not related to smoking. A flu-like illness occurs in one-third, cough in one-third, and cough or dyspnea in the remaining patients. Dyspnea is mild. Hemoptysis and wheezing do not occur. The duration of illness is less than 2 months in 75% of patients. On physical examination, finger clubbing is not seen, but fine end-inspiratory crackles are heard in two-thirds of patients. The chest radiograph shows bilateral patchy infiltrates. Bilateral linear or nodular opacities are seen in less than 20% of cases. Linear opacities may be associated with a poor prognosis.[5] Cavities and effusions occur in less than 5% of cases. Pulmonary function studies show an abnormally low vital capacity in one-half of patients, no airflow obstruction except in smokers, and an abnormal diffusing capacity in virtually all patients. Prednisone, 1 mg/kg, is the treatment of choice. This regimen should continue for a minimum of 3 months, followed by tapering doses for 1 year. Relapse is frequent with a short-duration treatment course, but patients will respond to an additional treatment course without any escalation in the amounts of prednisone. The management resembles that of sarcoidosis. In more than 65% of patients the disease resolves completely. Some of the remaining patients experience resolution without therapy, some require maintenance doses of prednisone every other day for several years, and others may stabilize with chronic symptoms and pulmonary dysfunction. Death occurs in 5% of patients.

BOOP is a distinctly different pathological and clinical syndrome from a usual interstitial pneumonia (UIP).[3] In the past, pathologists described an inflammatory process with scarring that was clinically represented by idiopathic pulmonary fibrosis, but systematic review of the histologic specimens has revealed that the scarring is not random but represents obliteration (ghosts) of branching or *en face* circular bronchioles. There are several distinct clinical differences between BOOP and UIP. In UIP a flu-like illness is not seen and dyspnea is more severe. Finger clubbing is common in UIP but rare with BOOP. The chest radiograph shows linear opacities and honeycombing in UIP but patchy infiltrates in BOOP. Prednisone therapy rarely leads to complete recovery in UIP.

Ultrastructural features of BOOP show extensive epithelial damage involving peribronchiolar alveolar septa, with necrosis and sloughing of alveolar lining cells.[4] These changes involving the interstitium resemble those occurring in the interstitial pneumonias, a suggestion that BOOP also represents an acute epithelial injury.

A study of 16 patients with BOOP suggested subcategories.[5] Patients with patchy infiltrates and elevated erythrocyte sedimentation rate recover completely with a sufficient amount and duration of corticosteroid therapy. Patients with diffuse small opacities had a more chronic illness and more severe dyspnea; even though some recovered with corticosteroid therapy, two patients died. Bronchoalveolar lavage (BAL) showed an increased number of cells, lymphocytes, and eosinophils in patients with patchy infiltrates but not in those with diffuse interstitial process. The high percentage of neutrophils seen in the BAL fluid of patients with bronchiolitis obliterans[7] were not seen in BOOP.

BOOP may occur in patients with **connective tissue diseases** such as lupus erythematosus, dermatomyositis, and Sjögren's syndrome.[2] Such patients develop a nonproductive hacking cough, and dyspnea soon follows. End-inspiratory crackles are heard on examination. The chest roentgenogram shows bilateral patchy infiltrates. Pulmonary function studies show a slight decrease in the vital capacity and a reduction in the diffusing capacity. The response to corticosteroid therapy and the prognosis are variable. Patients have a better prognosis than patients with rheumatoid arthritis plus bronchiolitis obliterans airway disorder but do not respond as well as those with idiopathic BOOP. A trial of prednisone at 1 mg/kg is advised.

BOOP is sometimes seen in a **localized lesion** in a resected pulmonary nodule.[5] Many cases are thought to be the end result of an inflammatory or infectious process. In these cases the lesion is localized to one area of the lungs and resection is curative.

SUMMARY

Bronchiolar diseases should not be combined together as bronchiolitis or bronchiolitis obliterans. There are several distinct entities with different pathologic and clinical findings. Respiratory bronchiolitis is seen in smokers whereas bronchiolitis obliterans and bronchiolitis obliterans organizing pneumonia may be idiopathic or result from fume exposure or infection. Bronchiolitis obliterans has a poor prognosis, especially in association with rheumatoid arthritis and after bone marrow transplantation. Bronchiolitis obliterans organizing pneumonia is usually idiopathic and is often responsive to corticosteroid therapy, although it has a slightly worse prognosis when associated with the connective tissue disorders.

ACKNOWLEDGEMENT

The author would like to thank Dr. Thomas V. Colby for the interpretation of Figures 5-1A and 5-2A.

REFERENCES

1. Lange W. Über eine eigenthumliche Erkrankung der kleinen Bronchien und Bronchilen. Dtsch Arch Klin Med 1901;70:342–364.
2. Epler GR, Colby TV, McLoud TC, Carrington CB, Gaensler EA. Bronchiolitis obliterans organizing pneumonia. N Engl J Med 1985; 312:152–158.
3. Guerry-Force ML, Muller NL, Wright JL, Wiggs B, Coppin C, Pare PD, Hogg JC. A comparison of bronchiolitis obliterans with organizing pneumonia, usual interstitial pneumonia, and small airways disease. Am Rev Respir Dis 1987; 135:705–712.
4. Myers JL, Katzenstein AA. Ultrastructural evidence of alveolar epithelial injury in idiopathic bronchiolitis obliterans-organizing pneumonia. Am J Pathol 1988; 132:(1):102–109.
5. Cordier JF, Loire R, Brune J. Idiopathic bronchiolitis obliterans organizing pneumonia. Chest 1989; 96:999–1004.
6. Bartter T, Irwin RS, Nash G, Balikian JP, Hollingworth HH. Idiopathic bronchiolitis obliterans organizing pneumonia with peripheral infiltrates on chest roentgenogram. Arch Intern Med 1989; 149:273–279.
7. Kindt GC, Weiland JE, Davis WB, Gadek JE, Dorinsky PM. Bronchiolitis in adults: A reversible cause of airway obstruction associated with airway neutrophils and neutrophil products. Am Rev Respir Dis 1989; 140:483–492.
8. Epler GR. Bronchiolitis obliterans and airways obstruction associated with graft-versus-host disease. Clin Chest Med 1988; 9:551–556.
9. Roca J, Granena A, Rodriguez-Roisin R, Alvarez P, Agusti-Vidal A, Rozman C. Fatal airway disease in an adult with chronic graft-versus-host disease. Thorax 1982; 37:77–78.
10. Clark JG, Crawford SW, Madtes DK, Sullivan KM. Obstructive lung disease after allogeneic marrow transplantation. Ann Intern Med 1989; 111:368–376.
11. Clark JG, Schwartz DA, Flournoy N, Sullivan KM, Crawford SW, Thomas ED. Risk factors for airflow obstruction in recipients of bone morrow transplants. Ann Intern Med 1987; 107:648–656.
12. Burke CM, Theodore J, Dawkins KD, Yousem SA, Blank N, Billingham ME, Van Kessel A, Jamieson SW, Oyer PE, Baldwin JC, Stinson EB, Shumway NE, Robin ED. Post-transplant obliterative bronchiolitis and other late lung sequelae in human heart-lung transplantation. Chest 1984; 86:824–829.
13. Burke, CM, Baldwin JC, Morris AJ, Shumway NE, Theodore J, Tazelaar HD, McGregor C, Robin ED, Jamieson SW. Twenty-eight cases of human heart-lung transplantation. Lancet 1986; i:517–519.
14. Burke CM, Glanville AR, Theodore J, Robin ED. Lung immonogenicity, rejection, and obliterative bronchiolitis. Chest 1987; 92:547–549.
15. Homma H, Yamanaka A, Tanimoto S, Tamura M, Chijimatsu Y, Kira S, Izumi T. Diffuse panbronchiolitis: A disease of the transitional zone of the lung. Chest 1983; 83:63–70.
16. Akira M, Kitatani F, Yong-Sik L, et al. Diffuse panbronchiolitis: Evaluation with high-resolution CT. Radiology 1988; 168:433–438.
17. Myers JL, Veal CF, Shin MS, Katzenstein AA. Respiratory bronchiolitis causing interstitial lung disease. Am Rev Respir Dis 1987; 135:880–884.
18. Yousem SA, Colby TV, Gaensler EA. Respiratory bronchiolitis-associated interstitial lung disease and its relationship to desquamative interstitial pneumonia. Mayo Clin Proc 1989; 64:1373–1380.
19. Weibel ER, Taylor CR. Design and structure of the human lung. In: Fishman AP, ed. Pulmonary diseases and disorders. New York: McGraw-Hill 1988; V:11–60.
20. Fraser RB, Pare JAP, Pare PD, Fraser RS, Genereux GP. Diagnosis of diseases of the chest. Philadelphia:WB Saunders 1988:4.
21. Wohl MEB, Chernick V. State of the art: Bronchiolitis. Am Rev Respir Dis 1978; 118:759–781.

22. Epler GR, Snider GL, Gaensler EA, Cathcart ES, FitzGerald MX, Carrington CB. Bronchiolitis and bronchitis in connective tissue disease. JAMA 1979; 242:528–532.

23. Charan NB, Myers CG, Lakshminarayan S, Spencer TM. Pulmonary injuries associated with acute sulfur dioxide inhalation. ARRD 1979; 119:555–560.

24. Rabinovitch S, Greyson ND, Weiser W, Hoffstein V. Clinical and laboratory features of acute sulfur dioxide inhalation poisoning: Two-year follow-up. Am Rev Respir Dis 1989; 139:556–558.

25. Geddes DM, Corrin B, Brewerton DA, Davies RJ, Turner-Warwick M. Progressive airway obliteration in adults and its association with rheumatoid disease. Q J Med 1977; 46:427–444.

26. Patel RC, Dutta D, Schonfeld SA. Free-base cocaine use associated with bronchiolitis obliterans organizing pneumonia. Ann Intern Med 1987; 107:186–187.

27. Cooper JD, Patterson GA, Grossman R, Maurer J. Double-lung transplant for advanced chronic obstructive lung disease. Am Rev Respir Dis 1989; 139:303–307.

28. Epler GR. Silo-filler's disease: A new perspective. Mayo Clin Proc 1989; 64:368–370.

29. Epler GR, Mark EJ. A 65-year old woman with bilateral pulmonary infiltrates. N Engl J Med 1986; 314:1627–1635.

30. Cooney TP. Interrelationship of chronic eosinophilic pneumonia, bronchiolitis obliterans, and rheumatoid disease: A hypothesis. J Clin Pathol 1981; 34:129–137.

31. Murphy KC, Atkins CJ, Offer RC, Hogg JC, Stein HB. Obliterative bronchiolitis in two rheumatoid arthritis patients treated with penicillamine. Arthritis Rheum 1981; 24:557–560.

32. Holness L, Tenenbaum J, Cooter NBE, Grossman RF. Fatal bronchiolitis obliterans associated with chrysotherapy. Ann Rheum Dis 1983; 42:593–596.

33. O'Duffy JD, Luthra HS, Unni KK, Hyatt RE. Bronchiolitis in a rheumatoid arthritis patient receiving auranofin. Arthritis Rheum 1986; 29:556–559.

34. Hakala M. Poor prognosis in patients with rheumatoid arthritis hospitalized for interstitial lung fibrosis. Chest 1988; 93:114–118.

35. Sweatman MC, Markwick JR, Charles PJ, Jones SE, Prior JM, Maini RN, Turner-Warwick MEH. Histocompatibilitiy antigens in adult obliterative bronchiolitis with or without rheumatoid arthritis. Dis Mark 1986; 4:19–26.

36. Elliott CG, Colby TV, Kelly TM, Hicks HG. Charcoal lung: Bronchiolitis obliterans after aspiration of activated charcoal. Chest 1989; 96:672–674.

6

Pulmonary Complications of Lung Transplantation

James H. Dauber
Adriana Zeevi

Although transplantation of the lung was first attempted early this century[1] and enjoyed a resurgence with the success of cardiac transplantation in the 1960s,[2] it was not until the availability of cyclosporine A in 1979 that it became a true therapeutic option for the treatment of end-stage cardiopulmonary disease.[3] Since that time activity has increased dramatically. As of 1988, over 300 pulmonary transplants had been performed worldwide and by the end of 1990 this number will have doubled.[4] Much has been learned in the last 10 years about the complications that beset these patients and limit the application of this approach. The focus of this chapter will be on those complications that are encountered after the perioperative period, since these are the conditions that internists and pulmonary physicians are most likely to be asked to diagnose and treat. These complications also have much to teach us about the mechanisms of lung defense and pulmonary inflammation. For this reason they are under intensive investigation at many of the centers where pulmonary transplantation is performed.

Although there are several approaches to pulmonary allografting that involve transplantation of either a single lung, two lungs, or a heart-lung bloc, the types (and probably the frequency) of complications involving the transplanted lung after the perioperative period tend to be similar. For this reason, no distinction between the surgical approaches will be made here. In reality, only two complications account for the vast majority of the postoperative morbidity and mortality: infection and chronic rejection of the lung allograft. In the experience at the University of Pittsburgh, infection has been the major cause for two-thirds of all deaths. Initially the magnitude of the problem caused by the appearance of bronchiolitis obliterans was underestimated. As experience has accumulated, this syndrome, which probably is a manifestation of chronic rejection,[5,6] seems to occur in up to half of the long-term survivors and clearly represents a major threat to their continued survival and quality of life. Surprisingly, these two complications often are intertwined. Certain infections, particularly those due to cytomegalovirus (CMV)[7] and *Pneumocystis carinii,* seem to predispose the recipient to rejection,[8] and once established, chronic rejection clearly predisposes to recurrent bacterial bronchopneumonia.[9]

Transplantation of the lung, although potentially more difficult and currently less successful in the short term[4] than transplantation of other major organs, such as the heart, enjoys one distinct advantage from the viewpoint of establishing diagnoses of infection and rejection. This is the relatively safe and easy access to cells and tissue from the allograft. Fiberoptic bronchoscopy is well tolerated even in critically ill recipients. This approach provides cells and alveolar fluid through the technique of bronchoalveolar lavage (BAL) and small, but nonetheless valuable, pieces of tissue for histologic evaluation through transbronchial lung biopsy.[10,11] More importantly, this procedure can be performed sequentially and the results used to establish a "profile" for each recipient. The outcome of various treatments can be assessed not only from a clinical standpoint (chest radiographs and lung function) but also from cytologic and histologic criteria. For investigators interested in the pathogenesis of infection and rejection of the allograft, sequential bronchoscopy has provided previously unheard-of of numbers of immune effector cells to study in vitro. The authors of this chapter have been fortunate to have access to cells and tissue obtained repetitively by bronchoscopy from most of the recipients who underwent pulmonary transplantation at the University of Pittsburgh. In this chapter we will attempt to highlight how this information has guided the therapy of these patients and improved our understanding of the pathogenesis of infection and rejection of the allograft.

INFECTIOUS COMPLICATIONS

General Considerations

Virtually any pathogen is capable of causing infection in these recipients, but with a few exceptions the causes and time courses of the respective infections are similar to those encountered in immunosuppressed recipients of other major organs.[4] In the early experience at both Stanford University[12] and the University of Pittsburgh,[13] the lung allograft was most often the target of infection. This pattern continues today, but prophylactic measures (described below) have had a beneficial effect on the frequency and severity of most life-threatening pulmonary infections. BAL has proved to be particularly useful in the early diagnosis of infection and has provided insight into the type of cellular response mounted by the lung to major pathogens.[8] Despite our improved ability to prevent, detect, and treat it, infection remains the leading cause of death in lung recipients.

This chapter will focus on the most common causes of pneumonia in the lung allograft, namely bacteria, cytomegalovirus, and *P. carinii*. Other viruses, such as adenovirus and respiratory syncytial virus, have been implicated particularly in children but are distinctly uncommon. The lung allograft is also susceptible to infection with fungi, but fungal pneumonia usually is a manifestation of disseminated infection and instability of the airway anastomosis. These issues, although important, will not be treated further here.

Bacterial Pneumonia

Prevalence

Bacterial pneumonia is the first life-threatening infection the recipient encounters in the early postoperative course, but it can strike at any time and has become distressingly frequent in the late postoperative period of patients with obliterative bronchiolitis. The overall prevalence at the University of Pittsburgh as of late 1989 was 66% (43 of 65 patients at risk). Recurrence is a feature: there have been a total of 66 episodes in the 43 patients. Prior to 1988, the prevalence in the first 2 postoperative weeks was 42% (21 episodes in 50 subjects). Following institution of broader spectrum prophylactic antibiotic therapy (ceftazidime and clindamycin vs. cephamandole) and specific treatment for organisms cultured from the donor trachea at the time of harvest even in the absence of clinical pneumonia,[14] the prevalence appears to have declined (2 episodes in 15 subjects). The apparent reduction may also have reflected better selection of donors, whose lungs may harbor subclinical pneumonitis that has the potential to blossom into a full-blown pneumonia following transplantation.[15]

Diagnosis

Gram-negative rods from the *Enterobacteriaceae* and *Pseudomonas* families are the most frequent cause of infection, particularly in the first two postoperative weeks. *Staphylococcus aureus* (coagulase positive), *Hemophilus pneumoniae*, *Legionella pneumophilia,* and polymicrobial mouth flora have also been isolated. Diagnostic efforts should begin with a careful examination and culture of the sputum and blood cultures. In many instances this approach yields the diagnosis. When these measures are unsuccessful, we resort to BAL. Since the organisms identified on Gram stain and by culture of the concentrated pellet from the BAL fluid usually seem to be the causative agents, we have not found it necessary to perform semiquantitative cultures.[9]

Treatment and Outcome

Broad-spectrum antibiotics are given parenterally until the etiology is established. Once the sensitivities of the organisms are determined, appropriate drugs are selected. Although antibiotics are clearly the mainstay of therapy, we routinely institute postural drainage with chest percussion to assist in the clearance of secretions in both the early and late postoperative periods. Some of the pneumonias occurring in the late postoperative course are associated with bronchospasm. In these instances beta agonist drugs are given by metered dose inhaler. The duration of therapy required for adequate control is often prolonged, particularly for episodes occurring in association with the syndrome of bronchiolitis obliterans. Recipients with bronchiolitis obliterans may mimic patients with cystic fibrosis and bronchiectasis, having chronic bacterial colonization of their airways and recurrent episodes of bronchopneumonia. Despite effective prophylaxis and treatment, bacterial pneumonia extracts a high toll, being the direct cause or leading factor in just over 42% of all deaths in our program. Clearly, more effective measures to prevent and treat this complication are needed.

Cytomegalovirus Pneumonia

Prevalence

The rate of infection with CMV depends on the preoperative serologic status of the recipients and the degree of selection of donor organs and blood products. Recipients who are seronegative at the time of transplantation contract a primary infection mainly from the donor organs or contaminated blood products. After a policy of giving only seronegative blood products to allograft recipients who had not been previously infected with CMV was instituted, the rate of primary infection at the University of Pittsburgh declined from 71% to 34%.[9] The recipients who contracted a primary infection after this precaution all received organs from seropositive donors. At present it is not feasible to avoid transplanting lungs from a seropositive donor into a seronegative recipient because the supply of suitable allografts is too limited.

Recipients who are seropositive for CMV at the time of transplantation have about a 75% chance of becoming infected a second time, either from reactivation of a latent infection or from a second infection with a different strain of virus.[16] Such secondary infections occurred even when the organs came from a seronegative donor. Thus, in the absence of some form of prophylaxis, the majority of seropositive recipients will contract a secondary infection.

The first isolation of CMV from any source most commonly occurs around the sixth postoperative week. The range at the University of Pittsburgh was 13 to 94 days with a median of 39 days. Infection may be recurrent or chronic, with virus being shed for many years in asymptomatic subjects.

Clinical Manifestations

In fully half of the recipients at Pittsburgh infected with CMV, pneumonia is the major clinical manifestation. The frequency of pneumonia remains high despite the reduction in the overall prevalence of infection achieved by the use of seronegative blood products in seronegative recipients. It continues to be greater than the rate encountered in comparably immunosuppressed recipients of a cardiac allograft.[13] About 25% of infected individuals are asymptomatic. The remainder have either a syndrome of viral illness characterized by fever, myalgias, fatigue, and leukopenia or clinically apparent disease of one or several organs.[9]

Symptoms in recipients with CMV pneumonia range from those of a very mild respiratory tract infection to acute respiratory failure. Findings on the chest radiograph usually correlate well with the severity of symptoms. The cough is usually nonproductive unless there is superimposed bacterial infection, a situation that has occurred in several of our recipients.

Diagnosis

Documenting that pneumonitis is due to CMV is absolutely essential for several reasons. First, and most important, is that early rejection produces the same clinical picture, but treatment of the two conditions is radically different. Second, as therapy with ganciclovir carries risks of renal and hematologic toxicity in patients whose kidney and bone marrow function may already be impaired by immunosuppressive agents,[17] the need for this agent must be firmly established. Finally, CMV infection seems to predispose to chronic rejection.[7] Documenting an episode of CMV pneumonia necessitates careful monitoring of the recipient for this complication after resolution of the infection.

A staged approach is used at the University of Pittsburgh to establish a diagnosis. All recipients have routine cultures performed of their urine and buffy coat after the second postoperative week. Positive results from these cultures indicate an active infection and raise the possibility that pneumonia will develop in the ensuing 6 weeks. If symptoms or findings of pneumonia arise, the recipient undergoes BAL and transbronchial lung biopsy if the coagulation status permits. In our hands cultures of BAL cells are very sensitive for detecting CMV pneumonia but lack specificity,[18] a finding reported by others.[19] The presence of nuclear inclusions in cytologic preparations of BAL cells is very specific (98%) but not very sensitive (21%). The detection of viral antigen in lung lavage cells by immunocytochemical techniques is nearly as sensitive as culture but equally nonspecific. The advantages offered by the latter technique are rapidity and a high negative predictive value.[18] Lately, transbronchial lung biopsy has assumed a more important role in the diagnosis. This approach, when feasible, allows for a more definitive demonstration of either viral inclusion bodies or acute rejection. In rare instances an open lung biopsy may be necessary.

Treatment and Outcome

Treating clinically apparent infection is challenging. A major reduction in the level of immunosuppression, an approach often used in recipients of other solid organs, is not felt to be an option here because it may lead to life-threatening rejection of the lung allograft. Ganciclovir should be used when the diagnosis is confirmed, but we have not found the drug to be particularly effective in patients with far advanced pneumonia.[9] Because the drug has considerable toxicity,[17] we have not used it to treat asymptomatic pneumonitis. In view of the strong relationship between CMV pneumonitis and chronic rejection, this stance is being reconsidered at the University of Pittsburgh. Prophylaxis with oral acyclovir seems to reduce mortality and morbidity from primary and probably secondary infection in renal allograft recipients.[20] We have recently instituted a similar regimen in our lung allograft recipients, but it is too early to assess the efficacy of this approach.

Prior to therapy with ganciclovir and prophylaxis with acyclovir, the toll exacted by CMV infection was high. Nearly one-quarter of the infections were fatal, and this disease accounted for 16% of all deaths in our recipients. The toll was highest in those recipients whose primary infection was complicated by pneumonia. Nearly 80% of these patients succumbed. Such statistics highlight the need for more effective prevention and treatment.

Pneumocystis Carinii

Time Course and Prevalence

P. carinii is most often recovered from the lung allograft from 3 to 6 months after surgery but has been found as early as the 60th postoperative day and as late as 3 years after transplantation. Prior to the rigorous application of prophylaxis with trimethoprim/sulfamethoxazole (TMP/SMZ) in 1986, nearly 75% of recipients at risk developed an infection at the University of Pittsburgh. Since then, the rate has fallen to less than 5%, and in all instances the recipients who contracted an infection had not been following the prescribed prophylactic regimen.[9]

Clinical Manifestations

Only one-third of our recipients infected with *P. carinii* had findings of a pneumonia, such as fever, cough, hypoxemia, and radiographic infiltrates.[8] Nearly half were truly asymptomatic and had a normal chest radiograph. The remainder experienced symptoms of an upper respiratory tract infection near the time of diagnosis but had no radiographic infiltrates or physical findings of pneumonia.

Diagnosis

Demonstrating the presence of *P. carinii* organisms in the lung by biopsy or in BAL fluid is the most sensitive approach.[21] We have relied almost solely on BAL at the University of Pittsburgh,[8] reserving biopsy for unusual cases. Although Grocott's methenamine silver stain enjoys considerable popularity for detecting the cysts, we have found that the modified toluidine-O technique is faster and as sensitive.[22] The profile of cells in BAL fluid is highly suggestive. There is usually a striking increase in the percentage of lymphocytes,[8] but as this finding may occur in the absence of infection or with a CMV infection (Dauber JH, Paradis IL, unpublished results), it is not conclusively diagnostic of infection with pneumocystis. The majority of lymphocytes express the cytotoxic-suppressor phenotype. Their level of spontaneous proliferation when cultured along with the alveolar macrophages is very high. A greater than expected proportion of these cells also appear to be activated, as judged by their proliferative response to interleukin-2 in vitro. Before and after the infection, the proportion of lymphocytes is lower and they appear to be less activated.[8] This sequential change in the bronchoalveolar lymphocyte populations was seen in both symptomatic and asymptomatic infections.

Treatment and Outcome

Oral therapy (TMP 160 mg and SMZ 800 mg twice daily) eradicates organisms from the lavage fluid and causes the BAL cell count and differential to return to baseline values in recipients whose infection is not clinically evident. This form has also remitted spontaneously, even though immunosuppression was not reduced.[8] Symptomatic infection requires more aggressive intervention with intravenous TMP/SMZ. Bacterial superinfection occurred in 40% of recipients with symptomatic disease and was prominent in two of our three fatal infections.

A variety of prophylactic regimens with TMP/SMZ appear to be effective in preventing infection. A double-strength tablet every other day or one tablet twice daily for 1 week of each month seems to be equally potent in our experience.

Predisposition of the Allograft to Infection

Bacterial Pneumonia

Factors unique to pulmonary transplantation appear to predispose the lung allograft to bacterial pneumonia in the early postoperative period. These factors involve both the mechanical clearance of organisms from the allograft and the immunologic response to them.

Bacteria are found in the trachea of the majority of donor lungs at the time of harvest. These organisms seem to be a harbinger of pneumonia that develops in the early postoperative period.[14] Ischemic injury to the airway mucosa impairs mucociliary function in the distal airways, and the airway anastomosis may act as a dam for secretions in the proximal airways.[23] Denervation eliminates the cough reflex, allowing secretions to accumulate in the dependent airways of the lung.

Lymphatic drainage to regional lymph nodes is abrogated for a time after transplantation. For a normal primary systemic humoral immune response to occur after deposition of antigen in the airspaces, the antigen must reach regional lymph nodes.[24] Failure of this to occur may explain why the primary humoral response to particulate antigen injected into the allograft is diminished in a canine model of pulmonary transplantation.[25] In addition some of the phagocytic cells that present antigen to responsive lymphocytes in regional lymph nodes may express an incompatible class II MHC phenotype, because macrophages derived from an intrapulmonary pool in the donor lung persist for months.[26] Finally, in preliminary studies we have found that alveolar macrophages from the lung allograft have lower than expected uptake of *Candida* organisms in vitro (Paradis IL, Dauber JH, unpublished results). A similar defect for the uptake of bacteria by these cells in vivo may be yet another factor predisposing to bacterial pneumonia.

Chronic rejection seems to be another, albeit later, risk factor for this type of infection. In this setting the small and large airways are chronically inflamed and obstructed with inflammatory cells, secretions, and granulation tissue. Airway colonization with potential pathogens is not uncommon, and these bacteria may eventually cause overt infection. Finally, the level of systemic immunosuppression is usually increased both acutely and chronically in an attempt to control this process. In recipients of a cardiac allograft, such a therapeutic maneuver is associated with a higher than expected rate of infection in the lung.[27] Presumably the risk of infection in lung allograft recipients also rises after the level of immunosuppression is increased.

CMV and Pneumocystis Pneumonia

Although humoral immune responses are important in the control of pneumonias due to CMV and pneumocystis, the cellular immune system is thought to play the leading role. Immunosuppressive regimens employed to prevent rejection are particularly effective at blunting a cellular immune response. But since the lung allograft seems to be more susceptible to infections with the above agents than are the lungs of comparably immunosuppressed recipients of other major organs, explanations in addition to systemic immunosuppression must be sought. Incompatibility between infiltrating lymphocytes and infected parenchymal cells may be one possibility, since this may lead to slowed recognition and an inadequate overall cellular response to the infecting agents.

By the time these infections strike the transplanted lung, most of the lymphocytes recovered by BAL express the MHC class I phenotype of the recipient,[26] but the parenchymal cells continue to express the phenotype of the donor (Yousem S, unpublished results). At the outset of infection, there may be a problem with the presentation of antigen to responsive lymphocytes. Viral and protozoal antigens presented on the surface of infected parenchymal cells may not stimulate the proliferation of recipient-derived cytotoxic T lymphocytes because of mismatch of the class I MHC determinants and may fail to stimulate the proliferation of T-helper cells because of mismatch of class II determinants.

Pneumonia due to both CMV and pneumocystis is eventually associated with expansion and activation of bronchoalveolar lymphocyte populations.[8] Some of these cells probably are capable of mediating cytotoxicity toward infected cells in the lung, because subclinical infections resolve spontaneously[8] and not all recipients with CMV pneumonia succumb to this infection. It is also possible that humoral mechanisms assume a more important role in the control of these infections because the response of the cellular immune system is frustrated by immunosuppression. Because the majority of airspace macrophages express the MHC phenotype of the recipient by the time these infections become prevalent, they may be able to present antigen properly to the recipient-derived lymphocytes, which still are capable of generating sufficient levels of specific antibodies. Until more is learned about how the host responds to these infections in general, this line of reasoning remains speculative. But, the view through the window afforded by this "experiment in nature" tends to confirm prevailing theories regarding mechanisms by which the lung defends itself against these types of infection.

ALLOGRAFT REJECTION

The lung is no different from any other transplanted organ in that rejection will set in within a few days if the recipient is not exactly matched to the donor or adequately immunosuppressed. Despite receiving what appears to be adequate amounts of immunosuppressive drugs, some recipients still develop signs of pulmonary allograft rejection as soon as the tenth postoperative day. This type of rejection is often referred to as early, "acute" rejection and causes a recognizable syndrome of diffuse lung disease that may be seen for up to 6 weeks after transplantation. After this time the syndrome of bronchiolitis obliterans may develop. Many investigators, including those at the University of Pittsburgh, associate this form of injury with allograft rejection. For this reason we and others use the terms "chronic rejection" and bronchiolitis interchangeably. The evidence supporting the notion that obliterative bronchiolitis is a manifestation of allograft rejection will be reviewed below, but our understanding of why the small airways of the allograft become the target for rejection is rudimentary at present. Whether the syndrome of bronchiolitis obliterans is due solely to rejection remains to be established, but for the purpose of this discussion it has been included in this section.

Acute Rejection

Time Course and Prevalence

As noted above, rejection may set in within a few days of the transplant in the absence of sufficient immunosuppression. But, for the most part, it does not become clinically evident until after the tenth postoperative day if the recipient is receiving the regimen of immunosuppression used in the early postoperative period at most centers, which includes cyclosporine A, antilymphocyte globulin, and azathioprine. At the University of Pittsburgh, approximately 50% of recipients who survive longer than 2 weeks will develop some degree of clinically evident acute rejection. A similar prevalence of rejection has been encountered at Papworth Hospital in the United Kingdom.[28]

Clinical Manifestations

In mild cases the recipient is usually asymptomatic and the condition is suspected because of widening of the alveolar–arterial oxygen gradient, the advent of an unexplained leukocytosis, or the appearance of reticular interstitial infiltrates on the chest radiograph. Persistent fever in the absence of findings suggestive of infection may be the first and only sign of acute rejection. In more advanced situations, the recipients complain of tightness in the chest, a nonproductive cough, and dyspnea on exertion. As the situation progresses the radiographic infiltrates coalesce and an alveolar filling pattern eventually develops. Respiratory symptoms intensify and, at this stage, the recipient is in danger of lapsing into respiratory failure. Interpretation of the plain chest film, both the standard posteroanterior and particularly the portable, may be confounded by the presence of large pleural effusions, which at times may be loculated. Because such effusions develop in the same time frame in the absence of clinically evident acute rejection, their occurrence does not always denote this complication. However, they may either mask significant interstitial infiltrates or intensify normal bronchovascular markings. Computed tomography (CT) is helpful in evaluating the lung parenchyma in this setting. Pulmonary function testing is of limited value at this stage in the postoperative course because most recipients have a relatively large restrictive impairment. Acute rejection usually is associated, however, with a decline in the forced vital capacity in patients whose function has been steadily improving during their convalescence.

Differential Diagnosis

Volume overload and infection produce a picture resembling acute rejection. Excluding volume overload is usually not difficult but at times requires measurement of the pulmonary capillary wedge pressure. The most important causes of the infections that masquerade as acute rejection are bacteria and virus, particularly CMV. Bacterial infection occurring in the setting of resolving diffuse lung injury as a consequence of poor allograft preservation is especially difficult to distinguish from very early acute rejection. CMV pneumonia may produce a clinical picture identical to acute rejection in the third to sixth postoperative weeks. BAL is helpful in identifying the cause of infection, but we have not found the total cell or differential count to be pathognomonic for acute rejection (Paradis IL, Dauber JH, unpublished results). Detecting organisms by Gram stain in the concentrated cell pellet of the fluid correlates strongly with clinically significant bacterial pneumonia.[9] Failure to demonstrate the presence of CMV early antigen in bronchoalveolar cells by immunohistochemistry essentially excludes this type of pneumonia in our experience.[18]

Confirmation of the diagnosis requires tissue. In most instances transbronchial lung biopsy is well tolerated and the specimens are sufficient.[11] In particularly complex cases or clinically unstable patients an open biopsy may be unavoidable.[5] The histopathologic findings in acute rejection depend on the severity of the process at the time of biopsy. Perivascular mononuclear cell infiltrates are the earliest and most frequent finding (Fig. 6-1). Initially only the subpleural and intraseptal venules are affected, but

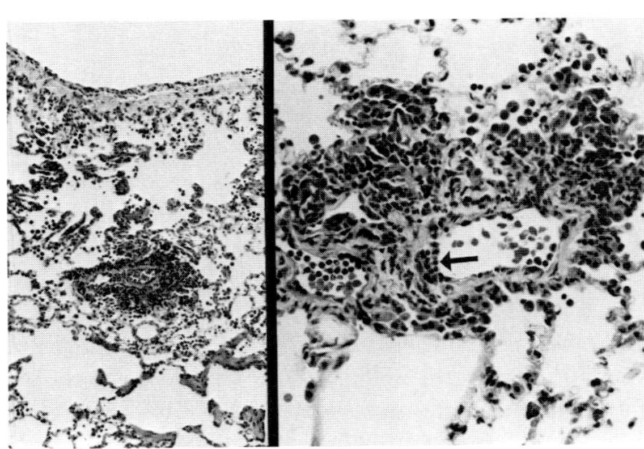

Figure 6-1. The histopathology of acute human lung allograft rejection. The insert on the left is a low-power view showing a mononuclear cell infiltrate around a subpleural venule. There is light infiltration of the alveolar walls that is most notable adjacent to the involved venule. The insert on the right is a high-power view of an infiltrated venule. There is typical permeation of lymphocytes into the sub-endothelial space (*arrow*). (Photomicrograph courtesy of Dr. Samuel A. Yousem)

as the process accelerates, larger veins and arteries and even the pulmonary capillaries become involved and polymorphonuclear leukocytes become more prominent. If the reaction advances further, pulmonary edema ensues. In more advanced situations, the airways are also the focus of inflammation, but within the first 6 postoperative weeks we have encountered fully established bronchiolitis obliterans in only one of 48 recipients. The latter finding is usually not seen until at least the sixth postoperative month.

Treatment and Outcome

Once the diagnosis of acute rejection is certain, treatment with enhanced immunosuppression may be undertaken safely. Most centers have found pulsed methylprednisolone therapy (1 g IV daily for 1 to 3 days) highly effective. Radiographic infiltrates and symptoms may recede within hours of the first dose. The vast majority of cases will respond to the full 3 days of treatment. Rarely, symptoms and findings of acute rejection will persist in the face of this therapy. In these instances a second course of anti-lymphocyte globulin is effective. If recognized and treated promptly, acute rejection poses little risk. There have been no fatalities due to this complication at the University of Pittsburgh. The major threat to the recipient comes from mistaking the diagnosis. Increasing the level of immunosuppression in the face of infection has potentially disastrous consequences, especially for CMV pneumonia.

Bronchiolitis Obliterans

Time Course and Prevalence

In all but a few instances the predominant histologic finding of bronchiolar inflammation with or without compromise of lung function and respiratory symptoms does not begin to appear until the fourth to sixth postoperative month. Although this syndrome, which has been called bronchiolitis obliterans, has several features to suggest that its pathogenesis involves immunologically mediated injury to cells expressing antigens of the donor, there is still some controversy about whether or not it represents a classic rejection reaction. In the opinion of the authors, there is sufficient evidence (to be discussed later) to implicate rejection as the underlying mechanism. For this reason and the late appearance of this complication, we usually refer to it as chronic rejection.[5] Bronchiolitis obliterans affects up to 50% of long-term survivors of heart-lung transplantation.[1] The prevalence in single- and double-lung transplants has been reported to be lower than that in heart-lung transplants.[29,30] In these series, however, biopsies were not performed unless there was clinical evidence of disease. For this reason asymptomatic cases would have been overlooked and the true prevalence of this complication underestimated.

Clinical Manifestations

There is a wide spectrum of findings in bronchiolitis obliterans. As noted above, some affected recipients may be asymptomatic and have normal pulmonary function test results. This was the case in about one-third of the recipients with bronchiolitis obliterans at the University of Pittsburgh. Most of the asymptomatic recipients were detected after August of 1987, when we adopted sequential transbronchial biopsy to monitor the status of the allograft. Prior to this time, we routinely performed sequential BAL on all recipients but reserved biopsy for symptomatic individuals. The most common symptoms are cough, which is usually productive, and dyspnea on exertion. Systemic symptoms are rare unless infection supervenes. Physical examination may be normal or reveal bibasilar rhonchi and rales. Wheezing is uncommon but can be provoked by infection or instrumentation of the airway. At the outset the chest radiograph is often unchanged from studies done before the disease was detected. Careful examination of sequential films may reveal a subtle loss of lung volume, however. In more advanced cases, interstitial markings are accentuated and rarely there are nodular infiltrates. Pleural effusion is rare and suggests some other complication, such as heart failure or empyema. When bacterial infection supervenes, most often bilateral infiltrates consistent with diffuse bronchopneumonia are seen.

Lung function testing reveals a combined obstructive and restrictive impairment in symptomatic individuals. About one-third of these recipients respond to inhaled bronchodilator. Changes in the single-breath diffusion capacity for carbon monoxide are more variable, but this value usually declines in concert with flow rates and lung volumes.[10] Initially the degree of impairment in lung function is mild, but if the condition fails to respond to therapy and progresses, severe airflow obstruction and resting hypoxemia ensue with affected recipients becoming respiratory cripples for a second and usually last time. Death due directly to the obliterative bronchiolitis is rare; these recipients usually succumb to infection.

Most affected individuals will produce sputum. Initially it is mucoid in appearance, but it generally becomes purulent if the disorder persists. At the outset of the productive cough, isolation of respiratory pathogens even when the sputum is purulent is uncommon. If the condition progresses, the airways usually become colonized with *Staphylococcus aureus* or *Pseudomonas* species. Recurrent bronchopneumonia eventually ensues, and at this stage the recipient's condition begins to resemble bronchiectasis. Because anesthesia of the airway appears to be complete and permanent, these individuals can accumulate large amounts of secretions in dependent airways. An abnormal quantity of thick tenacious secretions found at bronchoscopy is an excellent indicator of bronchiolitis obliterans.

Diagnosis

In the absence of the findings described above, the diagnosis is made solely on the presence of typical histopathology. Transbronchial biopsy usually provides adequate tissue and is the only practical approach to diagnosis in asymptomatic recipients. For this reason it is difficult to define precisely the sensitivity and specificity of transbronchial biopsy results, but there is general agreement that this approach is very useful.[10,11]

The earliest lesion appears to be peribronchiolar inflammation. Mononuclear cells accumulate around affected terminal and respiratory bronchioles, infiltrating the entire thickness of the wall. Epithelial cell injury is prominent. Cellular debris, fibrin, inflammatory cells—and neutrophils in particular—are present in the lumen. As the process progresses, buds of young granulation tissue emanate from the submucosa into the lumen of the denuded airway (Fig. 6-2). When this plug matures into dense collagen, the bronchiole may become completely obliterated, being identifiable with certainty only by the demonstration of elastic tissue remnants with special stains. Healing of less severely involved airways leads to eccentric or concentric collections of dense collagen in the submucosa that narrow the lumen (Fig. 6-3). The epithelial lining cells in such airways often lack cilia. Perivascular mononuclear cell infiltrates may be seen but appear in a minority of cases. Larger bronchi are also affected (Fig. 6-4), demonstrating changes of bronchiectasis.[31] Biopsy samples obtained during an episode of bronchopneumonia may show a similar pattern of acute bronchiolitis. For this reason, the presence of bacteria should always be sought with appropriate special stains. Not to be overlooked are vascular changes.[32] Although found in the absence of bronchiolitis obliterans, patchy atherosclerotic plaques are more frequent and severe in recipients with this complication (Figs. 6-4, 6-5). These plaques are often infiltrated with lymphocytes, histiocytes, and plasma cells, producing a picture of endovasculitis (Fig. 6-5). Small venules may be affected by the same process, but the degree of intimal sclerosis tends to be greater and the frequency of endovasculitis is smaller than in affected ar-

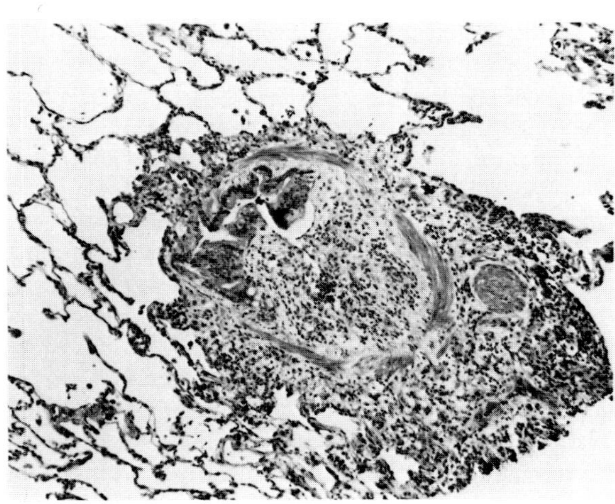

Figure 6-2. Early and severe bronchiolitis obliterans. Mononuclear cells have invaded the wall of this affected airway, and young granulation tissue, heavily infiltrated by inflammatory cells, nearly occludes the lumen. Only a remnant of columnar epithelial cells remain. It is likely that this airway will become totally obliterated in the near future and be recognizable only with special stains for elastin and smooth muscle. (Photomicrograph courtesy of Dr. Samuel A. Yousem)

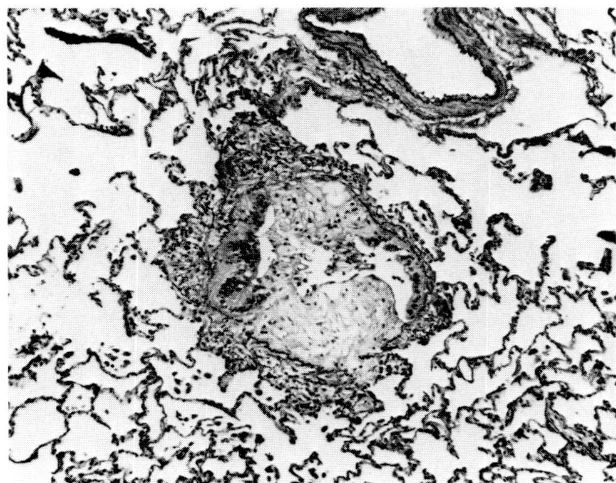

Figure 6-3. Bronchiolitis obliterans that is more mature but less severe than that in Figure 6-2. The mucosa and lumen are better preserved and the intraluminal granulation tissue is less cellular. Nonetheless, a large portion of the epithelial lining is denuded and the lumen is severely narrowed. It is likely that this airway will remain patent but that eccentric scar tissue will compromise airflow and the clearance of secretions. (Photomicrograph courtesy of Dr. Samuel A. Yousem)

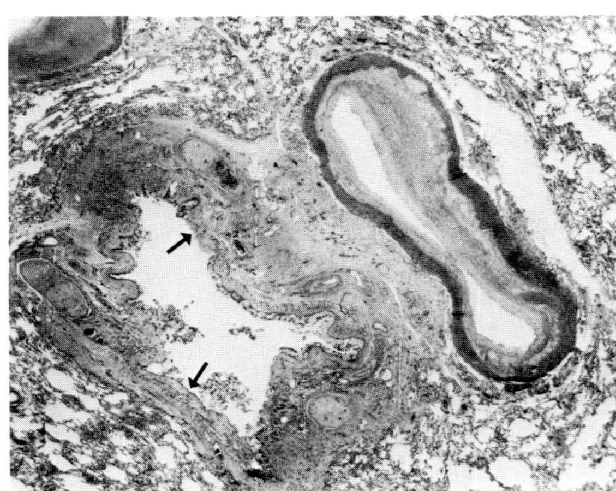

Figure 6-4. Bronchiolitis obliterans. A low-power view of a small bronchus and associated artery demonstrates two additional histologic findings of obliterative bronchiolitis, bronchiectasis, and arteriosclerosis. A portion of the mucosa of this airway is missing (*arrows*) and the wall is inflamed. Eccentric fibrointimal thickening of the artery narrows its lumen. (Photomicrograph courtesy of Dr. Samuel A. Yousem)

teries. Interstitial fibrosis is not uncommon but is usually not extensive. Some airspaces and small airways may be filled with foamy macrophages, suggesting obstruction of proximal airways.

Treatment and Outcome

Supervening infection should always be diagnosed and treated first since it may be the major cause for symptoms and the decline in lung function. Once this issue has been resolved, attention may be turned to the persistent bronchiolitis obliterans. Because most centers believe that immunologic mechanisms play an important role in this disorder, the prevailing approach to therapy is to increase immunosuppression. We have

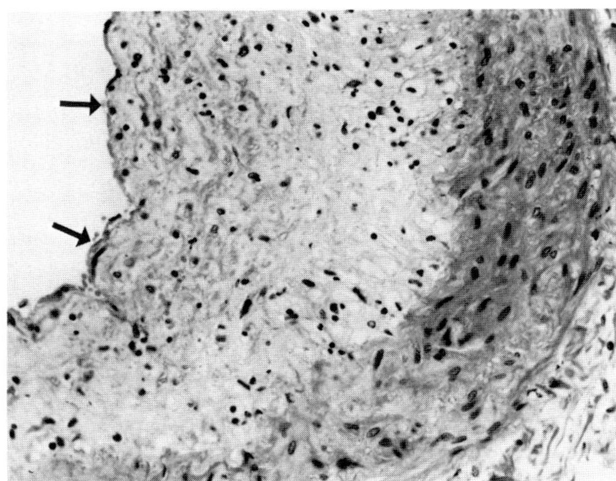

Figure 6-5. Endovasculitis. A high-power view of an involved artery detailing the fibrointimal thickening and scattered round cell infiltration typical of the endovasculitis of obliterative bronchiolitis. Arrows point to the endothelial surface of this vessel. Proliferation of myofibroblasts is thought to lead to widening of the intima. (Photomicrograph courtesy of Dr. Samuel A. Yousem)

found a short course of polyclonal antilymphocyte globulin to produce the largest and most sustained improvement in histologic findings, symptoms, and pulmonary function.[5] Temporarily increasing the dose of steroids[10] and pushing azathioprine to tolerance[6] have also been reported to be effective.

Because the approach to diagnosis and treatment has evolved considerably in the last 7 years at the University of Pittsburgh, it is difficult to say with certainty that the outcome of these patients is improving, but the trend is encouraging. In the early years of the program, there was a much longer delay than there is now in establishing a histologic diagnosis because the patients did not routinely undergo sequential transbronchial biopsy, and open lung biopsy was reserved only for evaluating the most advanced cases. By the time obliterative bronchiolitis was confirmed by biopsy in that era, the recipient had become overtly symptomatic and had lost a considerable amount of lung function. For the most part these early cases were treated with pulsed doses of corticosteroids and received polyclonal antilymphocyte globulin only after they failed to respond to the steroid treatment.

At present we favor treating the first occurrence of active bronchiolitis with polyclonal antiserum even when the recipient is asymptomatic. Relapses are usually treated with another course of antilymphocyte globulin from the same source (rabbit antihuman thymocyte) or with antiserum from a different source (horse antihuman lymphocyte) if the peripheral blood lymphocyte count failed to decline sufficiently after the former antiserum was given. Following the acute increase in the level of immunosuppression, the cyclosporine level in whole blood is maintained above 700 μg/ml (by radioimmunoassay) whenever possible, azathioprine is increased until the peripheral blood neutrophil count falls below 1500, and the dose of prednisone is kept above 0.2 mg/kg unless side effects preclude this level.

Of 48 recipients at risk, a total of 26 had developed this complication in our program as of late 1989. There were 5 affected recipients encountered early in the program who either died before adequate treatment could be started (3 subjects) or were lost to follow-up (2 subjects). If this group of inadequately treated recipients is excluded, the following generalizations regarding outcome in the 21 subjects who were treated appropriately can be made. About two-thirds will have a clearcut clinical response with improvement in symptoms and lung function. In two-thirds of this responding subgroup, the response has been sustained and there have been no relapses. In the remainder, there were relapses that responded to additional therapy. The level of function in this group of responders is generally good but most did not regain the highest level of function achieved before this complication set in.

The other, less fortunate one-third of affected recipients have failed to respond to this approach. About half of this subgroup have already developed severe impairment of lung function that dramatically limits their activity. One subsequently died from sepsis. The other half continue to experience a gradual decline in function despite multiple courses of antilymphocyte globulin and pulsed doses of corticosteroids. Without some other approach, they will likely become respiratory cripples as well. Alternative forms of treatment, such as inhaled cyclosporine, vincristine, or total nodal lymph node irradiation, are being considered in this group, but none has been implemented to date. Although such an outcome is discouraging to both the recipient and concerned physicians, the life expectancy and the quality of existence of affected recipients are still far in excess of what they would have been without a transplant.

Pathogenesis of Rejection

Acute Rejection

The histologic changes in the human lung allograft undergoing acute or early rejection are quite similar to those of unmodified rejection in the canine[33] and rat[34] models of unilateral lung transplantation, but the exact sequence of events is not as well established as those in the model systems for obvious reasons. The earliest response in the animal models appears to be a mononuclear cell inflammatory reaction centered around venules but eventually involving all vessels. The bronchus-associated lymphoid tissue (BALT) is also the focus of intense mononuclear cell infiltration. As the process continues, the airways become markedly inflamed and the alveolar walls become infiltrated and thickened. Eventually the alveoli fill with inflammatory cells, fibrin, and red cells. By this stage the allograft is no longer functional.[34] During the development of acute rejection in these models, cytotoxic antibodies and lymphocytes that recognize donor antigens can be detected in BAL fluid and blood. Prop and his colleagues have accumulated convincing evidence that both local and systemic cellular immune reactions play a role in unmodified rejection of the rat lung allograft.[35] In their experience removal of "passenger leukocytes," including dendritic cells that are found primarily in BALT, slowed the rate of unmodified rejection.[34] They postulated that the large amount of donor-derived lymphoid tissue present in the permissive environment of BALT was the reason that a local rejection response could develop and that this local response was the explanation for why the lung allograft rejects more rapidly than a heart allograft in the same model system. In addition, BALT served as a source of donor-derived cells that circulate from the allograft to distant lymphoid tissue, where they stimulate the systemic rejection response.

A similar cellular reaction appears to occur in the human lung allograft during early rejection, but the amount of histologic material for evaluation is limited since open lung biopsy is rarely required for the diagnosis. In addition, the response is clearly modified by intense systemic immunosuppression mediated by a combination of agents with differing mechanisms of action. Whether there is a strong local rejection response is not known. But as BALT is not well developed in the human lung, it is unlikely that exactly the same type of local response as that seen in the rat occurs in the human.

On the other hand, we have demonstrated that allograft lymphocytes obtained during acute rejection almost always showed a brisk proliferative response after 3 days in culture with irradiated donor cells—a response we call a positive primed lymphocyte test, or PLT.[36] In contrast, peripheral blood cells showed a positive PLT half as often. The allograft lymphocytes also proliferated well when cultured with IL2. After resolution of acute rejection, the response to IL2 declined and the PLT became negative in most instances for both allograft and blood lymphocytes. These findings strongly support the notion that activated, alloreactive lymphocytes accumulate preferentially in the allograft during acute rejection. Most of these cells probably came from systemic lymphoid tissue, but some may have been derived from local proliferation. We have shown that donor-derived lymphocytes and macrophages may still be recovered from the allograft during this time.[26] These cells could drive a local immune reaction to the allograft by stimulating a mixed leukocyte reaction as postulated in the rat model,[37] and they may circulate to distant lymphoid tissue to stimulate a systemic rejection response. In addition, cells from the rejecting human allograft demonstrate cellular cytotoxicity that is restricted by class II MHC antigens. The exact targets of these cells have not been determined, but they seem to be able to inflict injury on the allograft. Thus, acute rejection of the human lung allograft modified by continuous immunosuppression resembles that seen in more systematically studied animal models.

Why some recipients reject their allograft acutely despite intense immunosuppression remains unclear. Presumably this tendency could be reduced by closer matching of the MHC phenotypes as noted for the rat, but at present this is not clinically feasible. Another consideration is the inherent response of the recipient to any type of immunologic stimulus. Weakly responding rats retain their allografts for a longer period than do strongly responding recipients.[37] It is possible that a similar situation pertains in humans. Some recipients may also be less sensitive to the effects of immunosuppression. A final consideration is endogenous or exogenous stimulants of inflammation and the immune response. In non-immunosuppressed rats, removal of bowel bacteria and maintenance of recipients in a clean environment prolonged graft survival. In contrast, deposition of nonspecific irritants and of specific antigens in the airways of previously sensitized recipients shortened graft survival.[38] Similar factors may affect the incidence of acute rejection in humans, but we have been unable to identify risk factors for this complication in our program. There are still too few recipients to be certain that compatibility at the MHC loci prolongs graft survival in humans, but given the growth of the field in the last few years, this issue should be clarified soon.

Bronchiolitis Obliterans

Evidence presented above lends support to the notion that immunologically mediated inflammation underlies bronchiolitis obliterans. Recent experimental results to be presented below add convincing weight to this argument. On the other hand, if this syndrome is a manifestation of rejection, one must explain why the small airways are the primary focus of inflammation and injury whereas in the early form of rejection perivascular infiltrates are universal and interstitial inflammation is more global.

In our experience the syndrome is almost always associated with the reappearance of a positive PLT due to the presence of alloreactive lymphocytes in both the blood and, more frequently, the lung.[36] When the response to augmented immunosuppression is favorable, alloreactive lymphocytes disappear, but when the recipient fails to respond, these cells persist (Zeevi A, unpublished results). In addition, when transbronchial lung biopsy samples are maintained in culture in the presence of IL2, alloreactive cells are found in the expanded lymphocyte populations derived from patients with bronchiolitis obliterans but not in those from clinically quiescent recipients. The presence of a positive PLT for tissue-derived lymphocytes correlates exceedingly well with a positive test for cells in lavage fluid obtained at the time of biopsy (Rabinowich H, unpublished results). Cells in the tissue-derived population also mediate cellular cytotoxicity that is restricted by essentially the same loci that govern the proliferative response for the PLT. In recipients in whom the PLT or the CML, or both, were positive but no evidence of bronchiolitis was found, follow-up studies done on average 3 months later revealed acute bronchiolitis. These findings suggest not only that these studies have clinical utility but also that bronchiolitis obliterans is a manifestation of rejection.

Additional but more circumstantial evidence supporting a role for immunologically mediated injury comes from the observation that infection with CMV or *P. carinii*—agents that stimulate a strong cell-mediated immune response but do not injure bronchioles—often precedes the appearance of bronchiolitis. All of our recipients to date who have contracted CMV or *P. carinii* following transplantation have eventually developed bronchiolitis obliterans.[7] About two-thirds of recipients who contracted an infection with *P. carinii* did the same. Fortunately prophylaxis with TMP/SMZ has nearly eliminated this risk factor. The association between CMV and bronchiolitis warrants more aggressive prophylactic measures, which we recently have adopted. In some instances the PLT for allograft lymphocytes becomes positive during these infections, suggesting that the host's response to the infection leads to the nonspecific expansion of alloreactive lymphocytes. The infection may also up-regulate the expression of donor antigens in the allograft and promote their release to distant lymphoid tissue, reactivating the immunologic response toward them.

There are many potential explanations for why small airways bear the brunt of this process, but all are highly speculative. Because of the prolonged delay in the appearance of this complication and the fact that it occurs even in recipients who have not experienced acute rejection or infection with CMV or *P. carinii,* there is growing sentiment that anatomical changes in the airways that occur as a manifestation of transplantation, such as the loss of the bronchial circulation and anesthesia of the airway mucosa, may contribute. The inhalation of irritants and specific antigens is known to aggravate acute rejection in the rat model.[38] Perhaps the same is true for chronic rejection in humans, particularly if the clearance of such agents is impaired from absence of the cough reflex and inadequate mucociliary action. Their prolonged retention may lead to chronic inflammation in the small airways and up-regulation of class II MHC antigen expression on epithelial cells (Yousem SA, unpublished results) or endothelial cells in the vicinity of affected bronchioles. These cells may then be able to stimulate a local mixed leukocyte reaction (MLR) and become a target of this response. Lymphokines and cytokines generated during an MLR may further up-regulate the expression of class I and II MHC antigens and locally activate macrophages. Interstitial macrophages derived from the donor may localize to these sites of inflammation, become activated, and stimulate the proliferation of alloreactive lymphocytes. Once significant inflammation sets in around the bronchioles, it may disrupt blood flow to more proximal airways that is derived from the pulmonary-bronchial artery anastomoses. The resulting ischemia may contribute to development of bronchiectasis and recurrent bronchopneumonia.

Because of the complexity of the potential cellular interactions in the lung allograft, many other mechanisms leading to inflammation and injury of the small airways may be possible. Until some of the more obvious explanations have been evaluated, however, further speculation seems unwarranted.

SUMMARY

Although pulmonary transplantation is becoming widely accepted as a form of treatment for end-stage lung disease and its 5-year survival nearly equals that of cardiac transplantations,[4] sobering complications continue to plague the field and limit the success rate of this technique. Better preventive measures, earlier diagnosis, and more effective treatment should push the rate of infection even lower. Nonetheless the rate of pulmonary infection is likely to always remain higher than expected because of impairment of clearance mechanisms and incompatibility of immune effector and parenchymal cells in the allograft. Acute rejection of the human lung allograft has features typical of a classic transplantation response and resolves rapidly after transient increases in the level of immunosuppression. The syndrome of bronchiolitis obliterans occurs frequently in the late postoperative period and if untreated or poorly responsive leads to slow but progressive loss of allograft function. Evidence is accumulating that suggests an underlying role for rejection in this process, but the mechanisms leading to the relatively selective injury of small airways in the early stages are poorly understood. Certain infections clearly predispose to bronchiolitis obliterans, but it is likely that other factors peculiar to pulmonary transplantation account for the full expression of this syndrome. A better understanding of these mechanisms must be achieved because raising the level of immunosuppression is not consistently effective and may further aggravate the risk for bacterial pneumonia, which is all too common following this complication. Although these challenges seem formidable, they will eventually yield to our efforts and allow lung transplantation to occupy a legitimate niche in the treatment of end-stage cardiopulmonary disease.

REFERENCES

1. Tuna I, Jamieson S: Human heart and lung transplantation. Adv Surg 1989;22:251.
2. Hardy JD, Webb WR, Dalton ML Jr, Walker GR Jr. Lung homotransplantation in man. JAMA 1963;186:1065.

3. Reitz BA, Wallwork J, Hunt SA, et al. Heart-lung transplantation: A successful therapy for patients with pulmonary vascular disease. N Engl J Med 1982;306:557.

4. Griffith BP. Pulmonary transplantation status in 1989. In: Thompson ME, ed. Cardiovascular clinics, vol 22. Philadelphia: FA Davis, 1989:249.

5. Griffith BP, Paradis IL, Zeevi A, et al. Immunologically mediated disease of the airways after pulmonary transplantation. Ann Surg 1988;208:371.

6. Glanville AR, Baldwin JC, Burke CM, et al. Obliterative bronchiolitis after heart-lung transplantation: Apparent arrest by augmented immunosuppression. Ann Int Med 1987;107:300.

7. Keenan R, Zeevi A, Rabinowich H, et al. CMV status and donor specific alloreactivity of BAL cells correlates with risk of developing chronic rejection after pulmonary transplantation. J Heart Transplantation 1990;(in press).

8. Gryzan S, Paradis IL, Zeevi A, et al. Unexpectedly high incidence of *Pneumocystis carinii* infection after lung-heart transplantation. Am Rev Resp Dis 1988;137:1268.

9. Dauber JH, Paradis IL, Dummer SJ. Infectious complications in pulmonary allograft recipients. In: Grossman R, Mauer J, eds. Clinics in chest medicine. Philadelphia: WB Saunders, 1990; (in press).

10. Higenbottam T, Stewart S, Penketh A, Wallwork J. Transbronchial lung biopsy for the diagnosis of rejection in heart-lung transplant patients. Transplantation 1989;46:532.

11. Yousem SA, Paradis IL, Dauber JH, Griffith BP. Efficacy of transbronchial lung biopsy in the diagnosis of bronchiolitis obliterans in heart-lung transplant recipients. Transplantation 1989;47:893.

12. Brooks RG, Hofflin JM, Jamieson SW, Stinson EB, Remington JS. Infectious complications in heart-lung recipients. Am J Med 1985;79:412.

13. Dummer SJ, Montero CG, Griffith BP, et al. Infections in heart lung recipients. Transplantation 1986;41:725.

14. Zenati M, Dowling RB, Armitage JM, et al. Organ procurement for pulmonary transplantation. Ann Thorac Surg 1989;48:882.

15. Zenati M, Dowling R, Dummer S, et al. Influence of the donor lung on the development of early infections in lung transplant recipients. J Heart Transplant 1990;(in press).

16. Grundy JE, Lui SF, Super M, et al. Symptomatic cytomegalovirus infection in seropositive kidney recipients: Reinfection with donor virus rather than reactivation of recipient virus. Lancet 1988; ii:132.

17. Keay S, Bisset J, Merigan T. Ganciclovir treatment of cytomegalovirus infections in iatrogenically immunocompromised patients. J Infect Dis 1987;156:1016.

18. Paradis IL, Grgurich WF, Dekker A, et al. Rapid detection of cytomegalovirus pneumonia by evaluation of bronchoalveolar cells. Am Rev Resp Dis 1988;38:697.

19. Crawford SW, Bowden RA, Hackman RC, et al. Rapid detection of cytomegalovirus pulmonary infection by bronchoalveolar lavage and centrifugation culture. Ann Int Med 1988;108:180.

20. Balfour HH Jr, Chace BA, Stapleton JT, et al. Randomized, placebo controlled trial of oral acyclovir for the prevention of cytomegalovirus disease in recipients of renal allografts. N Engl J Med 1989;320:1381.

21. Hughes WT. *Pneumocystis carinii* pneumonitis, vol 2. Boca Raton:CRC Press, 1988:49.

22. Paradis IL, Ross C, Dekker A, Dauber JH. A comparison of methenamine silver and modified toluidine blue stains for the detection of *Pneumocystis carinii* in bronchoalveolar lavage. Acta Cytol 1990;34:511.

23. Mancini MC, Tauxe WN. Assessment of pulmonary clearance in heart-lung transplant recipients using technicium-99 minimicronized albumin colloid. Am Rev Respir Dis 1986;133:A11.

24. Bice DE, Harris DL, Hill JO, Muggenberg BA. Regional immunologic responses following localized deposition of antigen in the lung. Exp Lung Res 1980;1:33.

25. Muggenberg BA, Bice DE, Haley PJ, et al. Immune response in the transplanted canine lung. Am Rev Respir Dis 1986;133:A103.
26. Paradis IL, Marrari M, Zeevi A, et al. HLA phenotype of lung lavage cells following heart lung transplantation. J Heart Transplant 1985;4:442.
27. Mason JW, Stinson EB, Hunt SA, et al. Infections after cardiac transplantation: Relation to rejection therapy. Ann Int Med 1976; 85:69.
28. Hutter JA, Despins P, Higenbottam T, Stewart S, Wallwork J. Heart-lung transplantation: Better use of resources. Am J Med 1988; 85:4.
29. Pearson FG. Lung transplantation. Arch Surg 1989;124:535.
30. McGregor CGA, Dark JH, Hilton CJ, et al. Early results of single lung transplantation in patients with end-stage fibrosis. J Thorac Cardiovasc Surg 1989;98:350.
31. Yousem SA, Burke CM, Billingham ME. Pathologic pulmonary alterations in long-term human heart-lung transplantation. Hum Pathol 1985;16:911.
32. Yousem SA, Paradis IL, Dauber JH, et al. Pulmonary arteriosclerosis in long-term human heart-lung transplant recipients. Transplantation 1989;47:564.
33. Kirby JA, Pepper JR, Reader JA, Corbishley CM, Hudson L. Precursor frequency of donor-specific lymphocytes recovered from canine lung transplants. Clin Exp Immunol 1986;63:334.
34. Prop J, Nieuwenhuis P, Wildevuur CRH. Lung allograft rejection in the rat. I. Accelerated rejection caused by graft lymphocytes. Transplantation 1985;40:25.
35. Prop J, Wildevuur CRH, Nieuwenhuis P. Lung allograft rejection in the rat. II. Specific immunological properties of lung grafts. Transplantation 1985;40:126.
36. Rabinowich H, Zeevi A, Paradis IL, et al. Proliferative responses of bronchoalveolar lavage lymphocytes from heart-lung transplant recipients. Transplantation 1990;49:115.
37. Prop J, Wildevuur CRH, Nieuwenhuis P. Lung allograft rejection in the rat. III. Corresponding morphological rejection phases in various rat strain combinations. Transplantation 1985;40:132.
38. Prop J, Jansen HM, Wildevuur CRH, Nieuwenhuis P. Lung allograft rejection in the rat. V. Inhaled stimuli aggravate the rejection response. Am Rev Respir Dis 1985;132:68.

7
Sarcoidosis

Joseph P. Lynch III
Robert M. Strieter

Sarcoidosis is a granulomatous disease of uncertain etiology in which pulmonary manifestations typically predominate, but which exhibits protean extrapulmonary and systemic manifestations.[1-7] Despite exhaustive investigations and a variety of hypotheses regarding causative agents, the etiology of sarcoidosis remains unknown.[1,8,9] Within the past decade, tremendous insights into the pathogenic mechanisms and factors modulating this disorder have been gained by the application of bronchoalveolar lavage (BAL) and a variety of cellular and molecular biological techniques that have allowed better characterization of the relevant immune effector cells composing the sarcoid granuloma.[8-10]

IMMUNOPATHOGENESIS

The histologic hallmark of sarcoidosis is the noncaseating (non-necrotizing) granuloma (NCG), which is composed of a central core of histiocytes, epithelioid cells, and multinucleated giant cells surrounded by lymphocytes, scattered plasma cells, and varying quantities of fibroblasts and collagen deposition in the periphery (Figs. 7-1, 7-2).[8-10] Progressive granulomatous inflammation and accumulation of collagen may injure and disrupt the architecture of involved organs. The precise signals dictating the course of the granulomatous process have not been clarified, but complex interactions between activated T cells, mononuclear phagocytes, fibroblasts, and possibly other immune effector cells are responsible for the induction, evolution, and immunoregulation of the granulomatous inflammation.[8,9] The evolution of the sarcoid granuloma represents a tightly orchestrated event regulated by activated T lymphocytes and mononuclear phagocytes. There is a marked preponderance of T-helper cells, with few suppressor cells, in association with aggregates of mononuclear phagocytes (epithelioid cells) in the center of the sarcoid granuloma, whereas suppressor T cells predominate in the

"

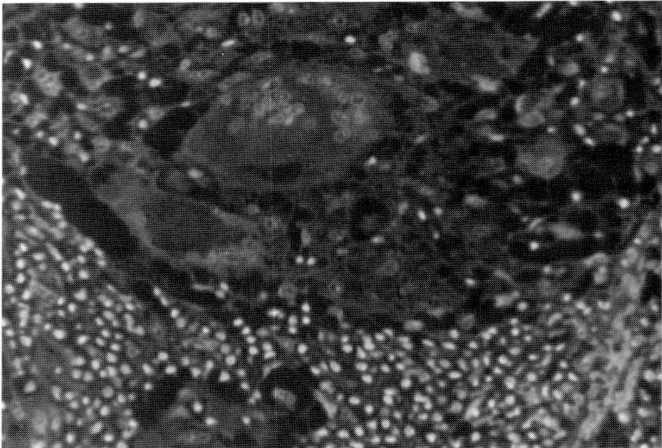

Figure 7-1. Multinucleated giant cell. This high-power photomicrograph of a lung biopsy sample demonstrates a large multinucleated giant cell in the center of a granuloma, with numerous lymphocytes and mononuclear cells in the periphery.

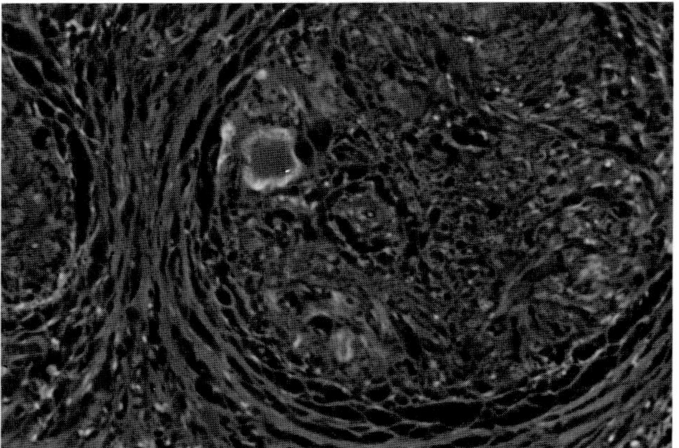

Figure 7-2. "Burned out" granuloma. This high-power photomicrograph of a lung biopsy sample demonstrates a "burned out" granuloma containing multinucleated giant cells and epithelioid cells in the center. In the periphery, no significant inflammatory cells are present but concentric rings of collagen encircle the granuloma.

lymphocytic mantle in the periphery.[8,11] This immune response in sarcoidosis is compartmentalized, however, as immune cells derived from different sites exhibit striking differences in phenotype or function.[8–10,12–14] In the peripheral blood, lymphopenia, impaired T-cell responsiveness to mitogens, increased numbers of T-suppressor cells, decreases in T-helper cells, and a reduced T-helper to T-suppressor ratio, consistent with impaired cellular immunity, have been demonstrated.[8–10,12,13]

The pulmonary lesion in sarcoidosis begins as an alveolitis with activated T lymphocytes and alveolar macrophages infiltrating the alveolar septae and airspaces.[8–10,12] Significant insights into the pathogenesis of the pulmonary lesion in sarcoidosis have been gained over the past 15 years by bronchoalveolar lavage (BAL), a technique that permits retrieval of immune effector cells from the alveolar spaces.[8–10] Increased numbers of activated T lymphocytes, T helper/inducer (Leu 3+ or CD4+) cells, immunoglobulin (Ig) secreting cells, and activated mononuclear phagocytes, with reduced numbers of suppressor/cytotoxic (Leu 2+ or CD8+) cells, have been demonstrated in BAL fluid and lung tissue in patients with active pulmonary sarcoidosis.[8-14] Lung T cells from patients with active pulmonary sarcoidosis display enhanced expression of class Ia antigen and express the helper/inducer phenotype[15]; spontaneously release several lymphokines, including monocyte chemotactic factor and macrophage inhibitory factor (MIF; which may recruit and activate mononuclear phagocytes); and induce blood mononuclear cells to differentiate and produce IgM.[8-10] In this context, increased levels of lung lymphocytes bearing the CD4+ TQ1− phenotype (the major helper subset for B-cell Ig synthesis) have been demonstrated in active pulmonary sarcoidosis.[16] Rossi and co-workers,[13] using a monoclonal antibody 5/9, demonstrated that the 5/9 (+) subset of T cells was preferentially expanded in active sarcoidosis and was primarily responsible for the release of specific lymphokines (such as monocyte chemotactic factor and B-cell differentiation factor) in this disorder.

Lung, but not blood, T cells from patients with active sarcoidosis spontaneously secrete IL2[17,18] and contain mRNA transcripts for IL2,[14] a lymphokine that may activate T cells and induce T-cell proliferation. This increased release of IL2 by sarcoid T cells may be a mechanism by which the T-cell population within the lung is expanded and perpetuated. In this context, it is of interest that corticosteroids, the cornerstone of therapy in sarcoidosis, dramatically suppress spontaneous release of IL2 and proliferation of T cells in sarcoidosis.[19] Lung T cells from patients with active pulmonary sarcoidosis spontaneously incorporate tritiated thymidine,[8,17] exhibit an altered distribution of RNA and DNA,[20] and display increased expression of a cell-cycle–related nuclear antigen, Ki67,[21] supporting the concept that replicating T cells exist in the lung in sarcoidosis. The lack of detectable IL2 on circulating sarcoid blood lymphocytes suggests that sarcoid T cells are not activated in the blood, but are probably activated at local sites of disease. Augmented expression of the receptor for IL2 (IL2R) has also been demonstrated in serum, BAL fluid, and lung immune cells (T lymphocytes and alveolar macrophages) from patients with active pulmonary sarcoidosis.[22-25] Recent studies using a cDNA probe for the 55 kDa chain of IL2R demonstrated that sarcoid blood T cells (CD4+) expressed functional surface IL2R and contained IL2R mRNA transcripts, whereas normal blood T cells did not.[22] This suggests that sarcoid blood cells expressing IL2R may have a proliferative advantage over normal T cells, particularly if these cells circulate to local sites rich in IL2. The inciting signal responsible for initial activation of T cells is not known. However, T-cell activation via local mononuclear phagocytes or accessory cells following as yet to be identified inhaled or circulating antigens is plausible. Circulating serum immune complexes (possibly reflecting antibody complexes to one or more specific antigens) have been demonstrated early in the course of sarcoidosis, when acute inflammatory manifestations are present, but were absent in more chronic phases of the disease.[26]

The importance of antigenic stimulation in other cell-mediated immune processes (such as berylliosis, tuberculosis, histoplasmosis) is well recognized. Exposure to inhaled beryllium salts may result in a granulomatous pneumonitis clinically and histologically indistinguishable from sarcoidosis.[10,27] The pathogenesis of berylliosis closely mimics sarcoidosis: increased numbers of activated T cells, T-helper cells, and an increased CD4+/CD8+ (T4/8) ratio have also been demonstrated on BAL in patients with berylliosis.[10,27] A delayed hypersensitivity cutaneous reaction to beryllium compounds may be elicited in patients with chronic berylliosis, and blood lymphocytes from patients with chronic berylliosis undergo blast transformation on exposure to beryllium salts in vitro, whereas normal lymphocytes do not.[10,27] The importance of local immune cell activation is underscored by the finding that lung lymphocytes from patients with berylliosis display a greater blastogenic response than do autologous blood monocytes.[10] This compartmentalization of the immune response in berylliosis, by which immune cells are locally activated, lends credence to the hypothesis that sarcoidosis may be a manifestation of a granulomatous response to an inhaled antigen. Sarcoid lung T-helper lymphocytes express the "very late activation antigen" (VLA-1), a protein complex typically expressed on T cells 2 to 3 weeks after activation.[28] This complex is not expressed on sarcoid lung suppressor cells or blood lymphocytes, suggesting that the VLA-1 + T-helper subset may reflect a population of cells that may have been previously stimulated, possibly by an inhaled antigen. Molecular biological techniques using specific DNA probes directed against various gene segments of the T-cell receptor have demonstrated that a subset of patients with active pulmonary sarcoidosis have increased proportions of lung T cells expressing surface determinants for the β variable (V) region of the T-cell antigen receptor (Ti3A+ lymphocytes). These cells express mRNA transcripts of the Vβ8 family and are compartmentalized with CD4+ lymphocytes.[29] Although many possible explanations exist for the expansion of Ti3A+ T cells in sarcoidosis, it is possible that specific sarcoid antigens may select for Vβ8-encoded T cell receptors. The fact that Vβ8-expressing T cells were found on only a subgroup of patients with sarcoidosis suggests that sarcoid is not due to a single antigen, but may result from a multiplicity of antigens, all capable of eliciting sarcoid granulomas. If specific antigens are responsible for sarcoidosis, it may be possible to identify specific clones of antigen-stimulated T cells by characterizing distinct clonal or oligoclonal patterns of rearranged genes encoding for specific antigen receptors.

The interaction of activated CD4+ lymphocytes with mononuclear phagocytes and other cell types results in a complex and carefully orchestrated series of molecular signals that drive the granulomatous response.[8-10] Although the T cell has little intrinsic ability to injure the lung parenchyma directly, T-cell–derived lymphokines influence the migration, differentiation, and activation of mononuclear phagocytes.[8-10] Sarcoid lung T cells release monocyte chemotactic factor (which recruits blood monocytes to sites of activity), MIF (which may activate macrophages), and other lymphokines that activate mononuclear phagocytes and induce the release of specific mononuclear phagocyte products.[8,9] T-helper cells and alveolar macrophages from patients with active pulmonary sarcoidosis display increased expression of a cell-cycle–related nuclear antigen (Ki67) on immunohistochemical stains, a feature of proliferating cells, whereas epithelioid cells and giant cells do not.[21] This suggests that both replicating T lymphocytes and mononuclear phagocytes (probably recently derived from circulating blood monocytes) participate in the induction and evolution of the granulomatous process, but that the epithelioid cells and giant cells are the end-stage products of effete macrophages.[21]

The macrophage is a key cell in granuloma development by virtue of its potency as a secretory cell and its ability to interact with T lymphocytes.[8,9] T-cell–dependent mononuclear phagocyte activation may then result in the release of a variety of endogenous mediators that may contribute to the inflammatory process and promote fibrogenesis. Alveolar macrophages from patients with active pulmonary sarcoidosis are activated,[8,9] contain increased amounts of lysozyme and angiotensin converting enzyme (ACE),[8] release increased amounts of oxygen radicals in response to stimulation,[8] display increased expression of transferrin (which may reflect activation) and HLA-DQ (involved in antigenic recognition by helper T cells),[30] and exhibit increased surface expression of several surface antigens of monocyte/macrophage lineage (63D3, MoP-9, MoS-1, MoS-39) compared to alveolar macrophages from controls or from patients with inactive sarcoidosis.[31] These antigens are progressively lost in culture, and are not re-expressed following addition of lymphokine-rich media or interferon-gamma.[31] These findings suggest that the sarcoid alveolar macrophages expressing these surface antigens represent newly recruited cells (i.e., derived from blood monocytes) rather than cells activated locally within the T-cell lymphokine milieu.

Sarcoid alveolar macrophages display several features that may promote T-cell replication and perpetuate the T-cell alveolitis of sarcoidosis. Sarcoid alveolar macrophages exhibit enhanced antigen-presenting capacity,[8,32] release increased amounts of interferon-gamma,[33] express IL2 receptors in the absence of in vitro stimulation,[24,25] and may spontaneously secrete IL1,[34] although this latter point remains controversial.[35,36] Epithelioid cells, multinucleated giant cells, and infiltrating T-helper cells within sarcoid granulomas express IL2, IL2R, and interferon-gamma on their cell surface, whereas macrophages from normal lymph nodes do not.[24] However, normal alveolar macrophages can be induced to express IL2R following stimulation with interferon-gamma, IL2, or lymphokine-conditioned media.[25] Thus, IL2R expression by sarcoid mononuclear phagocytes in vivo in sarcoidosis may be a consequence of high levels of interferon-gamma or other cytokines and may be involved in the pathogenesis of the granulomatous lesion. Sarcoid alveolar macrophages release increased amounts of fibronectin,[8] interferon-gamma,[37] and alveolar macrophage–derived growth factor (AMDGF),[8,38] factors that promote fibroblast recruitment and replication and may be involved in the fibrotic component of the sarcoid lesion.

The release of monokines by activated sarcoid alveolar macrophages may exert pleomorphic effects on a variety of cell types in addition to lymphocytes and fibroblasts. For example, sarcoid alveolar macrophages exhibit increased procoagulant activity,[39] may induce angiogenesis,[40] and release increased levels of tumor necrosis factor alpha (TNF_α),[41,42] a polypeptide that has potent effects on diverse arms of the immune system, including lymphocyte/mononuclear phagocyte–driven processes.[43] Thus, the macrophage has the capacity to secrete an array of cytokines that may have phlogistic effects and may drive the granulomatous process.

The role of the macrophage, however, may be more complex than simply initiation of the inflammatory response in sarcoidosis. Macrophages may exert bidirectional effects on inflammatory processes. In addition to their immune-potentiating properties, macrophages have the capacity to release endogenous mediators, such as E series prostaglandins (PGs), that may suppress several important lymphocyte and mononuclear phagocyte functions and inhibit the release of lymphokines and monokines, including IL1 and TNF_α.[43] Sarcoid alveolar macrophages exhibit a generalized down-regulation of arachidonate metabolism and a blunted ability to release PGE compared to normal controls.[44] Changes in the profile of endogenous mediators released by mononuclear phagocytes at sites of disease may be important in modifying the course of inflammatory processes. For example, reduced release of PGE_2 may intensify or perpetuate the heightened cellular immunity evident in sarcoid, whereas endogenous release of PGEs by mononuclear phagocytes may serve to autoregulate the inflammatory processes and modulate the extent of injury. Thus, macrophages may play a pivotal role not only in initiating and perpetuating the inflammatory process in sarcoidosis, but in modulating or turning off this granulomatous process.

EPIDEMIOLOGY

Although the incidence of sarcoidosis varies among geographical regions, prevalence rates of between 10 to 20 cases per 100,000 population have been reported in North America, Europe, and Japan.[1-6,45,46] For reasons that are not clear, over 80% of cases occur in individuals between ages 20 and 45 years.[1-6,45,46] A genetic predisposition likely exists, as the disease is eight times more common in blacks, and slightly more common in females.[1-6] Occasional clustering of cases within families has been described.[1,2,8] Genetic factors may determine the expression of the disease, as patients with HLA-B8 major histocompatibility loci have been associated with the acute inflammatory manifestations of sarcoidosis, such as erythema nodosum, arthritis, and bilateral hilar lymphadenopathy (Löfgren's syndrome), whereas patients with HLA-B13 more commonly exhibit a progressive and protracted course.[47] An increased frequency of HLA-DR5J antigen in Japanese patients with sarcoidosis and a lower rate of spontaneous resolution among DR5J-positive patients has been noted.[48] Conflicting data exist, however, among various ethnic and geographic groups, and the importance of tissue histocompatibility antigens and HLA-DR antigens in the evolution and expression of sarcoidosis remains to be clarified.

CLINICAL FEATURES

The clinical expression and natural history of sarcoidosis are extraordinarily variable. Spontaneous remissions occur in nearly two-thirds of patients, and a waxing and waning course is common.[1-6,46] Pulmonary manifestations typically dominate, but virtually any organ system can be involved.[1-8] Abnormalities on chest radiograph can be demonstrated in 90% to 95% of cases of sarcoidosis, but 40% to 60% of patients are asymptomatic.[1-6,8,49] Fever, polyarthritis, erythema nodosum, and bilateral hilar lymphadenopathy (Löfgren's syndrome) are common early features of the disease, and have been associated with an excellent prognosis.[8,50,51] However, chronic, progressive sarcoidosis involving one or more organs may lead to irreversible injury, and even death.[1-8] The overall mortality rate for sarcoidosis as assessed by most investigators at referral institutions has been 2% to 6%[1-6,45] but lower mortality rates have been reported in nonreferral settings.[49] The organ systems most commonly involved, apart from the lung, include lymph nodes (both intrathoracic and extrathoracic), skin, and eye, but symptomatic neurologic, myocardial, renal, hepatic, or splenic involvement occurs in 2% to 5% of cases.[1-8] Asymptomatic involvement of specific organ systems may be quite common, however, as noncaseating granulomas have been detected by liver biopsy or necropsy in 20% to 80% of cases even in the absence of specific symptoms.[2,5-8] The extrapulmonary manifestations of sarcoidosis have been well reviewed in previous publications[1-8] and will not be extensively addressed in this chapter.

DIAGNOSTIC TECHNIQUES

The presence of symmetric bilateral hilar lymphadenopathy in an asymptomatic individual strongly suggests the diagnosis of sarcoidosis. Winterbauer and co-workers[52] reviewed 100 patients with bilateral hilar lymphadenopathy on chest radiograph and noted that all 43 patients who were asymptomatic or had only erythema nodosum or uveitis had sarcoidosis. All 11 with neoplasm as a cause of bilateral hilar lymphadenopathy were symptomatic, and 9 had easily identifiable extrathoracic tumor on physical examination. Only 2 of 52 with bilateral hilar lymphadenopathy and a normal physical examination had neoplasm. Thus, in patients with asymptomatic bilateral hilar lymphadenopathy (or with only symptoms of uveitis or erythema nodosum), biopsy may not be necessary to corroborate the presumptive diagnosis of sarcoidosis, as long as physical examination is normal, there is no prior history of malignancy, and significant laboratory aberrations (such as anemia) are absent. This practice has been followed widely in Europe, and misdiagnoses in this context have been exceedingly rare.[45,46] Nonetheless, bilateral hilar lymphadenopathy may be a presenting feature of infectious granulomatous disorders such as histoplasmosis or tuberculosis, and these entities must be excluded, particularly if patients are febrile or have constitutional symptoms. Serum complement fixation studies for fungi and tuberculin skin testing are appropriate in this context. We have required biopsy confirmation of the diagnosis in any patient in whom systemic corticosteroid therapy is required, as well as in any patient with atypical features. Although open lung biopsy or mediastinoscopy have diagnostic yields of 80% to 100%[1,4-6] their morbidity and requirement for general anaesthesia make them undesirable as initial diagnostic procedures of choice. Scalene node or liver biopsies are diagnostic in 70% to 80% of cases, but have potential morbidity.[1,4-6] Conjunctival biopsy has been advocated by some, with diagnostic yields as high as 15% to 20% but experience with this procedure is limited and we have found it to be less helpful. Fiberoptic bronchoscopy with transbronchial lung biopsy is the initial preferred invasive procedure of choice, with diagnostic yields of 60% to 70% among patients with stage 1 disease and yields of 80% to 90% with stage 2 or 3 disease.[8,53] Endobronchial biopsies are also frequently diagnostic, owing to the frequent submucosal location of granulomas (Fig 7-3). When significant endobronchial granulomatous inflammation is evident, a diffuse cobblestone appearance on gross endoscopic examination may be observed.

LABORATORY FEATURES

Laboratory features of sarcoidosis are nonspecific. Historically, the Kveim test was originally utilized to corroborate the diagnosis of sarcoidosis.[54,55] However, the long delay required (4 to 6 weeks) for interpretation and the lack of a commercially available

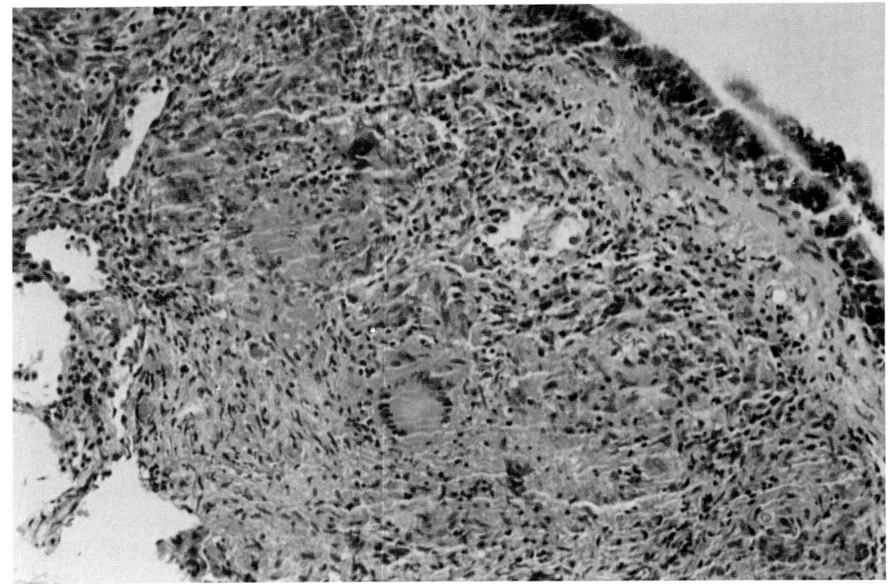

A

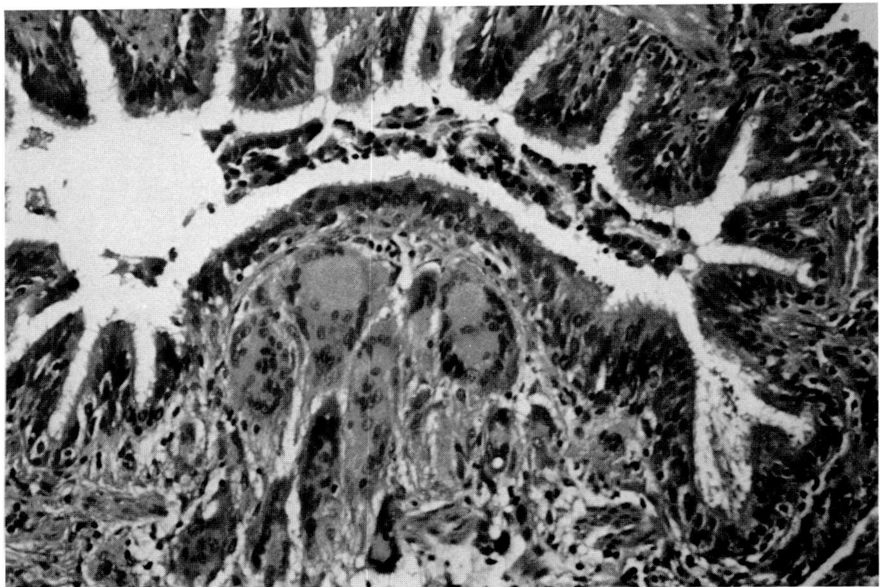

B

Figure 7-3. Endobronchial biopsy sample. (*A*) This low-power photomicrograph of an endobronchial biopsy sample demonstrates multinucleated giant cells, scattered mononuclear inflammatory cells, and collagen within the submucosa of a bronchiole. (*B*) This high-power photomicrograph of an endobronchial biopsy sample demonstrates prominent multinucleated giant cells within the submucosa underlying the bronchiole.

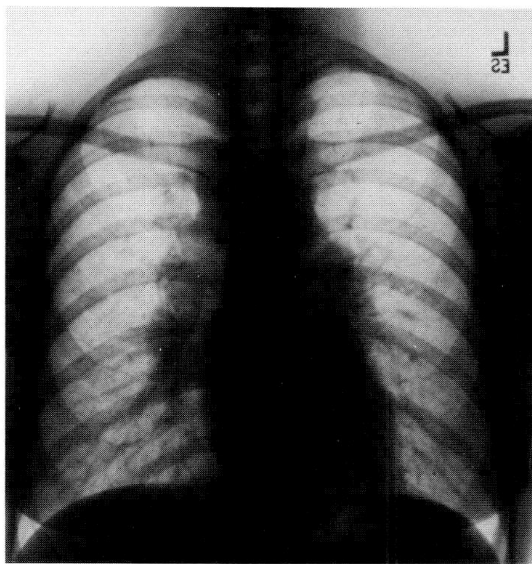

Figure 7-4. Stage 1 sarcoidosis. This chest radiograph demonstrates extensive bilateral hilar and right paratracheal lymphadenopathy.

antigen with satisfactory specificity have rendered this test obsolete.[56,57] Although no laboratory feature is pathognomonic for sarcoidosis, several laboratory aberrations may be observed in this disorder. Hypergammaglobulinemia, a reflection of generalized B-cell activation, has been reported in 30% to 80% of cases.[2,5,8,9] The erythrocyte sedimentation rate may be elevated in some patients, but is not consistently reliable in assessing disease activity. More recently, measurements of serum angiotensin converting enzyme (SACE) have been used as better indicators of disease activity,[58–68] a subject which will be addressed later in the chapter. Hypercalcemia has been reported in 10% to 20% of cases in retrospective studies,[2–5] but more recent prospective studies suggest that only 2% to 6% of patients exhibit chronic hypercalcemia.[46,69] Hypercalcuria is more common, occurring in 20% to 50% of cases.[1–8,69] The abnormalities of calcium metabolism in sarcoidosis reflect an enhanced sensitivity to vitamin D.[8,70] Elevated serum levels of 1,2-dihydrocholecalciferol have been demonstrated in sarcoid patients exhibiting hypercalcemia. These may reverse with corticosteroid therapy.[70] Mild elevation in transaminases or alkaline phosphatase occurs in 5% to 10% of sarcoid patients, reflecting hepatic involvement, but serious hepatic dysfunction is rare.[1–6] Leukopenia occurs in 5% to 10% of patients, but significant anemia is uncommon.[1–6,52]

CHEST RADIOGRAPHIC FEATURES

Bilateral hilar lymphadenopathy, the classic radiographic feature of sarcoidosis, is present in nearly three-quarters of patients, with or without concomitant parenchymal infiltrates (Fig. 7-4, 7-5).[1,8,46] Right paratracheal lymphadenopathy is a common associated feature, seen in up to 50% of cases. Enlargement of left paratracheal, paraaortic, and subcarinal lymph node groups may be present concomitantly but is rarely a dominant finding on plain chest radiograph. Intrathoracic lymphadenopathy, which may be inapparent or subtle on conventional chest radiographs, may be easily demonstrated

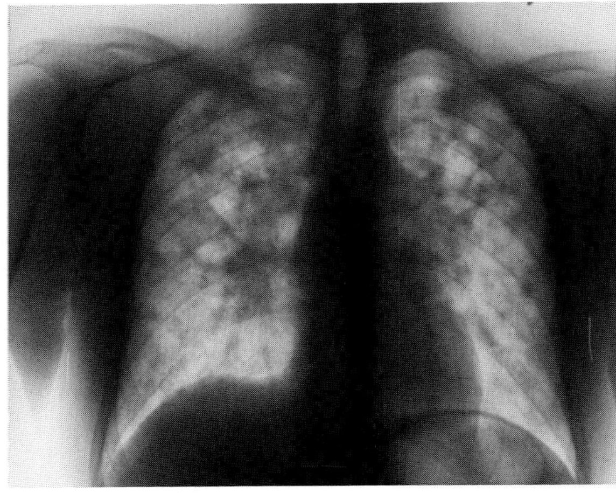

Figure 7-5. Stage 2 sarcoidosis. This chest radiograph demonstrates extensive patchy infiltrates, some of which have a nodular appearance. Bilateral hilar adenopathy is also present.

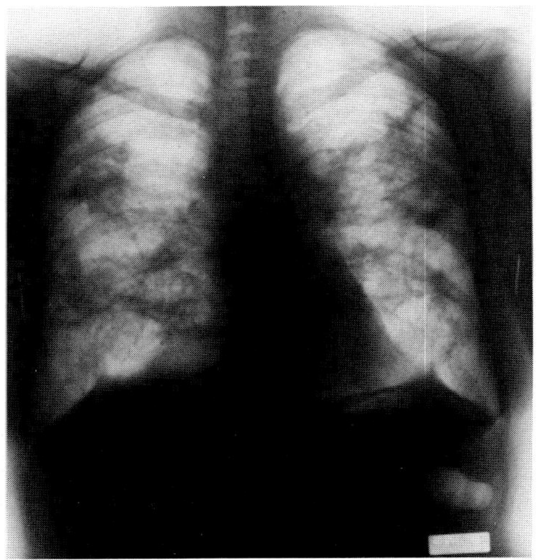

Figure 7-6. Stage 3 sarcoidosis. This chest radiograph demonstrates patchy parenchymal infiltrates, with a slight mid and upper lung zone predominance, associated with cystic changes, honeycombing, and linear fibrotic bands.

on computed tomographic (CT) scanning, although we see little reason for routine CT scanning in the staging or evaluation of sarcoidosis. Calcification of hilar or mediastinal lymph nodes may sometimes be a feature in patients with long-standing sarcoidosis. Parenchymal infiltrates are present in 20% to 50% of cases and may assume a variety of patterns.[1–8,46,71] Infiltrates may be patchy or diffuse, with a predilection for the mid and upper lung zones (Fig. 7-6). The spectrum of radiographic manifestations is extraordinarily broad. Diffuse reticulonodular infiltrates ranging from 1 mm to 4 mm in diameter may reflect interstitial granuloma or inflammation. A diffuse miliary pattern suggests early alveolitis (Fig. 7-7),[8] and dense focal airspace disease with air bronchograms may reflect more intense alveolitis.[8,9,72] However, chest radiographs distinguish

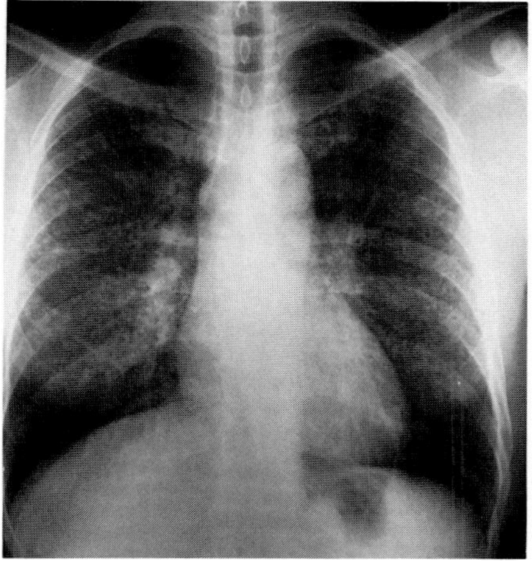

A

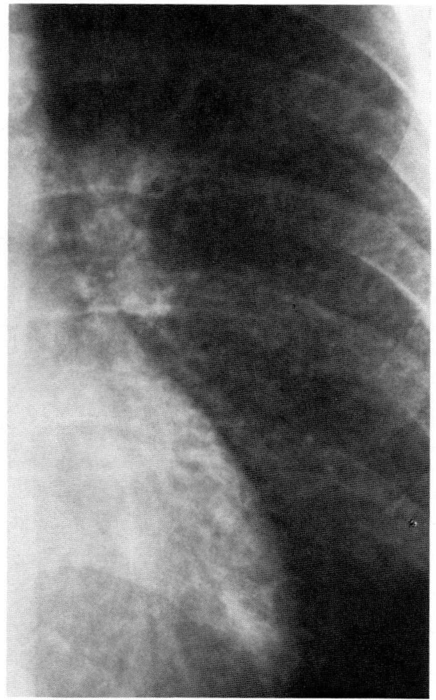

B

Figure 7-7. Stage 3 sarcoidosis. (*A*) This chest radiograph demonstrates a fine miliary pattern throughout all lung fields in a 28-year-old male who 8 months earlier had presented with bilateral hilar lymphadenopathy alone. (*B*) An enlargement of a chest radiograph from the same patient demonstrates the fine miliary pattern.

poorly between fibrosis and alveolitis.[8,9] In patients with significant volume restriction, "shrinking" lungs on chest radiographs may be a dominant feature. Although this manifestation typically occurs in patients with chronic disease, often progressing over several years, the course may be quite rapid, progressing to severe volume restriction and end-stage pulmonary insufficiency within a matter of several months in a small percentage of cases. When fibrosis occurs, retraction of hilae, volume loss, and coarse linear fibrous bands may be observed on chest radiograph. Atypical features such as unilateral hilar adenopathy, large nodular infiltrates (simulating metastases), marked upper mediastinal lymphadenopathy (simulating malignant lymphoma), and pleural effusions have been described in 1% to 2% of cases.[2,5,46,71] In the presence of such atypical findings, alternative etiologic diagnoses should be rigorously excluded before the diagnosis of sarcoidosis is accepted. Lobar atelectasis (due to severe endobronchial involvement leading to bronchostenosis)[73] and extensive bullous emphysematous changes from severe destructive parenchymal sarcoidosis with airways obliteration occur in 1% to 3% of cases (Fig. 7-8).[2–7,46] Patients with upper lobe bullous or cavitary disease from long-standing destructive pulmonary sarcoidosis may also develop aspergillomas or fungal mycetomas.[74] Enlargement of the cardiac silhouette or pulmonary vasculature may be observed in patients with far-advanced pulmonary hypertension and cor pulmonale (approximately 1% to 4% of cases).[1–7,47,71]

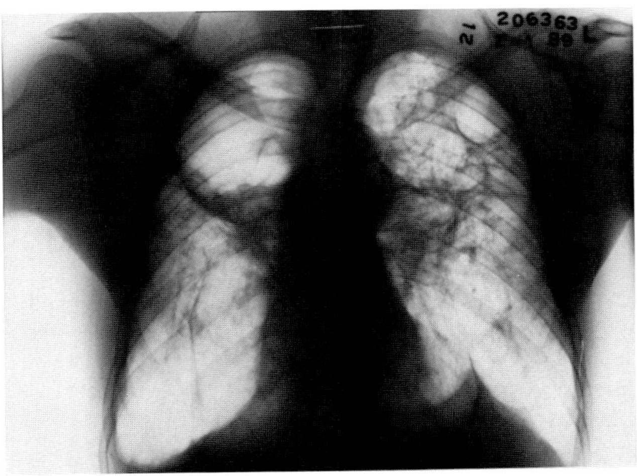

Figure 7-8. Progressive pulmonary sarcoidosis. This chest radiograph demonstrates extensive emphysematous and bullous changes and patchy parenchymal infiltrates, reflecting a severe case of progressive pulmonary sarcoidosis.

The chest radiographic staging system as espoused by Siltzbach may be useful as a prognostic guide (stage 0 = normal; stage 1 = bilateral hilar lymphadenopathy [BHL]; stage 2 = BHL plus parenchymal infiltrates; stage 3 = pulmonary infiltrates without BHL).[6] The radiographic criteria applied in the literature have not always been uniform, however. Some investigators have accepted stage 1 through 3 but have added a stage 4 to reflect pulmonary infiltrates associated with significant fibrosis, honeycombing, or cystic changes consistent with end-stage disease.[45] Chretien and associates[75] have adopted a modified staging system is which stage 1 refers to bilateral hilar lymphadenopathy, but two subgroups A and B are recognized within stage 2 to designate, respectively, bilateral hilar lymphadenopathy with pulmonary infiltrates and pulmonary infiltrates without bilateral hilar lymphadenopathy (what others have termed stage 3). In their classification schema, stage 3 refers to radiographic evidence for fibrosis. As much of the literature has referred to stages 1 through 3 of the Siltzbach classification, we believe this schema has greatest applicability.

Although exceptions occur, stage 1 identifies a subset of patients with the best overall prognosis, whereas stage 3 patients are least likely to remit. In several large series, spontaneous resolution has occurred in 50% to 80% of cases of stage 1 sarcoid, compared to remission rates of less than 60% for stage 2 and less than 30% for stage 3 disease.[3–6,45] In one recent study of 210 cases of sarcoidosis followed for 1 to 10 years in a Danish urban area, the radiographic staging classification had major prognostic significance.[46] Among 116 patients with stage 1 disease, radiographic abnormalities resolved completely in 57% and only 10% progressed to stage 2; none developed stage 3 disease. By contrast, normalization of chest radiograph occurred in only 1 of 10 patients with stage 3 disease, and 80% remained in stage 3. The prognosis for stage 2 was intermediate, as complete resolution of disease occurred in 48% and an additional 38% exhibited improvement or stability. Some interesting observations regarding rate of resolution are worthy of note. With few exceptions, the course of the disease was dictated within the first 12 to 24 months of diagnosis. Most remissions occurred within the first year of observation and 85% of all remissions had occurred within 2 years. Among patients who remained in stage 2 after 2 years of observation, eventual normalization of the chest radiograph was achieved in only 12%, and the disease progressed in 30%. Late relapses were also rare, however, in patients exhibiting stable disease for the first 2 years. Among 63 patients in initial radiographic stage 1 followed for longer than 2 years, only one demonstrated disease progression after the second year. Notwithstanding these clinical trends, the rate of resolution (or progression) may be quite variable, as evidenced by a Swedish study in which 505 patients with sarcoidosis (both treated and untreated) were followed over a 15-year period.[45] Radiographic normalization was achieved within 15 months in 50% of 308 patients with initial stage 1 disease, but 25 patients remained in stage 1 for more than 6 years. Progression to stage 2 occurred in 29 of 308 (9%) of stage 1 patients, and only five patients (1.6%) progressed to stage 3. By contrast, among 128 patients with initial radiographic stage 2 disease, chest radiographs had normalized in only 22% of cases and 21% progressed to stage 3 by 1 year. After 5 years, however, radiographs had normalized in 68% of patients (both treated and untreated). Radiographic normalization occurred in 37% of 49 patients with initial stage 3 disease over the course of the observation period. The impact of corticosteroid therapy on eventual outcome was not clear.

Although imperfect, the Siltzbach classification scheme is clinically useful, as it identifies subsets of patients most likely to improve spontaneously (i.e., stage 1) as compared to stage 2 or 3 disease, where spontaneous remission is less likely. Nevertheless, several limitations of the system are apparent. Abnormalities on chest radiograph do not distinguish alveolitis from fibrosis and fail to correlate with either pulmonary function or symptoms.[8,76] Occasional patients with stage 1 disease develop progressive disease and require therapy, whereas others with stage 3 disease remit spontaneously. Thus, additional parameters and clinical data are required upon which to base therapeutic decisions. The presence of acute inflammatory manifestations, such as erythema nodosum, acute polyarthritis, and fever, characteristically predicts an excellent long-term outcome.[2,46,50] Clinical factors associated with a poorer prognosis include the presence of chronic extrathoracic disease,[3,5,46,77] hypercalcemia,[3,46] cor pulmonale,[3] age at onset greater than 40 years,[46] and black race.[5,77]

PULMONARY FUNCTION TESTS (PFTs)

Reductions in lung volumes (vital capacity [VC] and total lung capacity [TLC]) or diffusing capacity for carbon monoxide (D$_L$CO) occur in 40% to 70% of cases, and even more commonly in stage 2 or 3 disease.[2,8–9,74,76] Although changes in the D$_L$CO may be a more sensitive indicator of activity of disease in some cases, the D$_L$CO appears to be less sensitive than lung volumes (VC and TLC) as an indicator of the underlying parenchymal pathology in sarcoidosis.[78] Measurements of resting and exercise gas exchange (D$_L$CO and alveolar–arterial O_2 gradient) are relatively well preserved in sarcoidosis compared to idiopathic pulmonary fibrosis (IPF) at comparable degrees of reduction in lung volumes (VC and TLC).[78] Significant hypoxemia is uncommon in sarcoidosis except in far advanced disease. Nevertheless, in chronic sarcoidosis associated with severe parenchymal fibrosis, the physiological aberrations may mirror IPF, with striking hypoxemia and reductions in DlCO. The predilection of sarcoidosis to involve the airways and bronchial submucosa may also lead to reduction in the FEV_1 (1-second forced expiratory volume) and expiratory flow rates and to clinically significant airways obstruction in 20% to 30% of patients.[8,76,79,80] Most patients exhibiting airways obstruction due to sarcoidosis also have a concomitant restrictive defect, although an isolated obstructive defect mimicking asthma may occur. This obstructive component represents a striking contrast to IPF, where expiratory flow rates are normal or often supranormal. When sensitive tests of airways obstruction have been performed (such as frequency dependence of compliance, airways resistance, closing volumes, and so on), some element of airways obstruction has been documented in virtually all sarcoid patients exhibiting the characteristic physiological changes of restrictive lung disease.[80] In addition to compromise of the bronchial lumen by granulomatous inflammation or fibrosis within the bronchi and bronchioles, abnormal bronchial hyperreactivity in response to methacholine has been documented in subsets of patients with sarcoidosis.[79] Clinically, this may result in chronic, hacking cough as a dominant manifestation of endobronchial disease. In some cases, administration of bronchodilators may ameliorate the symptoms, but corticosteroids are often required.

Unfortunately, pulmonary function studies fail to correlate with either histologic severity of disease or the extent of alveolitis.[8,9.76] Baseline pulmonary function tests are most useful to assess the extent of physiological aberration but do not predict long-term prognosis and may not reflect activity of disease.[8,9,76] However, sequential studies are important to follow the course of the disease longitudinally. Changes in vital capacity appear to be most sensitive indicators of disease progression (or resolution).[8,74,76,78] Corticosteroid therapy may be warranted in patients exhibiting sustained decreases or deterioration in pulmonary function, irrespective of whether symptoms or changes on chest radiograph are present.

NEWER STAGING TECHNIQUES (BAL AND GALLIUM-67 SCANNING)

Bronchoalveolar Lavage

Since its introduction in the mid-1970s, enthusiasm for bronchoalveolar lavage (BAL) as a clinical tool has waned. Although BAL has permitted great insights into the pathogenesis of a variety of interstitial lung diseases, its clinical value in the staging and management of sarcoidosis is unproven. Initial reports from the National Institutes of Health demonstrated increases in the number and percentage of lymphocytes (typically 25% to 60%) in patients with pulmonary sarcoidosis, with higher levels in patients with clinically active or radiographic stage 2 or 3 disease.[9] Subsequent studies from several centers corroborated marked increases in activated T lymphocytes or T-helper cells on BAL from patients with pulmonary sarcoidosis, but wide variation and considerable overlap between patients with active and inactive disease have been found.[81–95] French investigators[81] performed serial lavages in 23 patients and noted that BAL lymphocytosis was characteristic of active disease and usually normalized as the patients entered clinical remission (either spontaneously or in response to therapy). However, a few patients with clinically active disease exhibited normal BAL values.[81] In addition, a subgroup of patients with advanced radiographic stage 3 disease exhibited elevations in both BAL lymphocyte and neutrophil counts, suggesting that BAL neutrophilia may reflect irreversible scarring.[81] Several prospective studies analyzing the prognostic role of BAL in sarcoidosis have been done, with conflicting results. Keogh and associates[88] stratified patients on the basis of initial BAL and gallium scan findings into either low-intensity alveolitis (LIA; arbitrarily defined as having fewer than 28% T lymphocytes on BAL or a negative gallium-67 scan) or high-intensity alveolitis (HIA; defined as greater than 28% T lymphocytes on BAL and a positive gallium scan) and prospectively performed BAL, gallium scans, and pulmonary function tests every 6 months in 19 patients with untreated pulmonary sarcoidosis. The rate of pulmonary functional deterioration was lower among 14 patients with LIA than in the 5 with HIA even though the two groups had the same clinical features at the outset.[88] Although the authors suggested that stratifying patients into LIA or HIA may be prognostically useful, changes in pulmonary function were small, and spontaneous reversion to LIA or HIA occurred in several cases. Hollinger and colleagues[60] studied 21 patients before and after therapy with corticosteroids and noted that pretreatment BAL lymphocyte counts correlated better with corticosteroid responsiveness than other pretreatment parameters such as clinical score, forced vital capacity (FVC), quantitative gallium score, and SACE. FVC improved in 10 of 11 patients with pretreatment BAL lymphocyte counts greater than 35%, whereas among 10 patients with initial BAL lymphocyte counts of less than 35%, FVC improved in five and deteriorated in five.[60] However, several investigators have found that initial BAL lymphocyte counts are of no clinical value in predicting prognosis or corticosteroid responsiveness. Lawrence and co-workers[89] found that serial BAL lymphocyte counts (CD4+/CD8+ subtyping was not done) performed before and 6 weeks after corticosteroid therapy failed to correlate with clinical course in 12 patients with clinically active pulmonary sarcoidosis. The level of BAL IgG-secreting cells served as a better marker of disease activity, but was less accurate than SACE or gallium scans.[89] Buchalter and associates[84] noted that initial BAL percentage lymphocyte counts failed to correlate with changes in any parameter of pulmonary function among 29 patients with clinically active pulmonary sarcoidosis (15 of whom subsequently received therapy with corticosteroids), and predicted neither the evolution of the disease nor response to treatment. Turner-Warwick and associates[91] performed serial BAL, gallium scans, and SACE in 32 patients with pulmonary sarcoidosis before and after initiation of corticosteroid therapy and concluded that none of these parameters were useful in predicting change in chest radiographs or pulmonary function. In 7 patients, substantial radiographic improvement occurred even though the initial BAL lymphocyte counts were normal. BAL lymphocytes, SACE, and gallium uptake tended to decline in patients whose chest radiographs cleared, but these parameters frequently remained elevated even in patients whose radiographs and pulmonary function test scores normalized for extended periods.[91] Israel-Biet and co-workers[87] prospectively followed 73 patients with recently diagnosed stage 1 or 2 sarcoidosis for 2 years without treatment, 84% of whom had BAL lymphocytosis at the outset. The degree of lymphocytosis at the initial lavage failed to predict subsequent outcome at 2 years. However, persistence of BAL lymphocytosis at 12 months was prognostically helpful; resolution of disease had occurred at 24 months in only 3 of 21 (13%) patients exhibiting

BAL lymphocytosis at 12 months, whereas the recovery rate at 24 months was 81% among 23 patients exhibiting a normal BAL lymphocyte count at 12 months.[87] Bjermer and associates[83] performed serial BAL cell counts at time 0, 6, and 12 months in 45 patients with newly diagnosed sarcoidosis, 35 of whom (77%) exhibited initial BAL lymphocytosis (>30%). Initial BAL lymphocyte count bore no relationship to subsequent prognosis as assessed at 2 years. Increases in BAL mast cells, a cell type not extensively investigated in sarcoidosis, were associated with a greater rate of deterioration in pulmonary function. BAL mastocytosis (>0.5% of all cells) was found in 4 of 14 patients who had complete spontaneous remission, so was not specific for deterioration. The combination of two serial lavages demonstrating mastocytosis and lymphocytosis (>30%) or mastocytosis and neutrophilia (>15%) was seen in 9 of 16 patients with persistently active disease, but in none of 14 patients who made a complete recovery and in none of nine with inactive disease with sequelae. The association of BAL mastocytosis and subsequent functional deterioration is of interest, but further studies are required to assess whether measurements of yet another cell type will have any predictive value.

Several investigators have found that BAL T4/T8 ratio is a better reflection of disease activity than lymphocyte or T-lymphocyte count alone. Ceuppens and associates[85] determined T-cell subsets in 35 patients with sarcoidosis, 12 of whom had sequential lavages (3 treated, 9 untreated). Whereas the percentage of BAL lymphocytes fell in only 6 of 10 patients who exhibited clinical improvement, changes in the T-helper to T-suppressor cell (T4/T8) ratio mirrored disease activity in every case.[85] Bauer and associates[82] performed serial BALs on eight patients with sarcoidosis (four HIA and four LIA) and noted that the number of BAL T-helper and activated T-helper cells decreased in all four patients with HIA who remitted (three in response to corticosteroids) whereas cell counts remained stable in four untreated patients with LIA. Baughman and colleagues[58] noted that the BAL T-helper cell count, but not the absolute number of T lymphocytes, correlated well with the response of the vital capacity to therapy in 16 patients with clinically active pulmonary sarcoidosis treated with corticosteroids. Costabel and associates demonstrated that initial BAL T4/T8 ratios predicted subsequent functional deterioration much better than pulmonary function tests, SACE, gallium scans, or BAL lymphocyte counts without subtyping.[86] Only 2 of 15 patients with normal T4/T8 ratios on initial BAL deteriorated, whereas 10 of 16 patients with initial high T4/T8 levels deteriorated and required corticosteroid therapy.[86] Although quantitation of T-cell subsets may better reflect disease activity than other parameters at a given point in time, the spontaneous variability of sarcoidosis, with its tendency to wax and wane, makes the clinical applicability of BAL cell counts of limited value. High levels of activated T cells and an increased T4/T8 ratio may indicate high-intensity alveolitis, but this has no significant prognostic value unless persistence of HIA can be demonstrated. Gerli and co-workers[16] demonstrated that sarcoid patients exhibiting the highest levels of CD4+ TQ1− cells and IgM on BAL (consistent with the most active alveolitis) also had a shorter duration of symptoms (typically <1 year), whereas lower levels of BAL CD4+ TQ1− cells and IgM (often within the normal range) were noted in patients with more prolonged symptoms.[16] This study did not correlate BAL data with pulmonary function tests or specifically analyze the prognostic value of BAL, but it suggests that HIA may simply reflect an earlier phase of disease and may have no significant predictive value, because normalization of the alveolitis may occur spontaneously over time. The type of clinical presentation dictates to a great extent the degree of alveolitis as assessed by BAL.

In a recent study, patients exhibiting an acute onset of sarcoidosis with erythema nodosum or acute uveitis had a higher percentage of T-helper cells and higher T4/T8 ratios than patients presenting with pulmonary symptoms or studied after resolution of erythema nodosum.[94] The T-lymphocyte percentage and T4/T8 ratio also appeared to diminish with time following onset of erythema nodosum. Valeyre and co-workers[51] previously had shown that BAL performed within 3 months of onset of erythema nodosum and acute sarcoidosis revealed striking lymphocytosis (consistent with HIA) in 13 of 14 patients, even though the disease remitted spontaneously in all but one patient over the next 12 months. As it is well recognized that patients with an acute onset with erythema nodosum or uveitis have a markedly improved prognosis, including such patients in studies of the predictive value of BAL on outcome will fail to demonstrate any useful correlations. Inclusion of patients with differing clinical presentations may explain in part some of the widely discrepant results reported by different centers regarding the predictive value of BAL for outcome. Regional heterogeneity may also occur, particularly in patients with focal disease.[8,72] In cases where asymmetric radiographic findings are evident, normal cell counts may be found in some regions, whereas HIA may be documented in areas characterized by greater radiographic involvement.[72] Given the inherent variability of the clinical course of sarcoidosis, no single parameter can be expected to correlate with long-term prognosis.

High levels of T lymphocytes or other markers of HIA in BAL fluid may be a reflection of active alveolitis, but do not imply that deterioration will inevitably occur. Further, some patients with LIA on BAL deteriorate in the absence of therapy or respond to corticosteroids,[81,89,91] suggesting that current functional and phenotypic markers are not accurate enough to serve as the basis for clinical decisions. If BAL is to have any clinical role, it will be in the subset of patients with chronic but stable symptoms or radiographic infiltrates in whom clinical parameters of disease activity are uncertain. In such cases, marked increases in T-helper cells consistent with HIA would suggest that the patients would be more likely to respond to corticosteroids than patients exhibiting LIA. Nevertheless, owing to the invasive nature of bronchoscopy, its expense, and the need for serial studies to more objectively assess disease activity over time, we do not believe that BAL has an established clinical role in the management of sarcoidosis.

GALLIUM-67 CITRATE SCANNING

Gallium-67 scanning has been used to assess the degree of alveolitis in a variety of inflammatory and immunologic pulmonary disorders, including sarcoidosis, because ^{67}Ga is taken up avidly by activated inflammatory cells within the lung.[8–10] In initial studies at the National Institutes of Health, increased intrapulmonary uptake of ^{67}Ga was observed in 25 of 41 (61%) of patients with sarcoidosis and correlated with the proportion of lymphocytes and T cells on BAL.[95] Other investigators have reported increased intrapulmonary uptake of ^{67}Ga in 60% to 94% of cases,[58–61,91] but the value of ^{67}Ga scanning in predicting prognosis is controversial. Disparate results have been reported by different investigators. In some studies, the degree of intrapulmonary uptake of ^{67}Ga correlated better with activity of disease and responsiveness to corticosteroid therapy than BAL lymphocyte count,[58,59,89] SACE,[59,90] or clinical parameters,[9,59,61] whereas in others, ^{67}Ga scans did not predict recovery among patients with stage 2 or 3 sarcoidosis[77,91] and did not predict responsiveness to corticosteroids.[60,86,91] Enthusiasm for the use of ^{67}Ga in the staging of sarcoidosis has waned because there is no convincing evidence that data derived from this study greatly enhance predictive value over more conventional techniques. In addition, several factors, including expense, exposure to a radioisotope that makes repeated measurements potentially dangerous, inconvenience (scanning follows the injection by 48 hours), differences in techniques, interobserver variability, and the lack of a reproducible "gold standard" make ^{67}Ga scanning unsuitable for routine use.

SERUM ANGIOTENSIN CONVERTING ENZYME

Elevated levels of serum angiotensin converting enzyme (SACE) in sarcoidosis were first reported by Lieberman in 1975.[64] In that landmark study, SACE levels were elevated in 15 of 17 patients with active untreated sarcoidosis but were normal in all 11 patients with inactive disease or receiving corticosteroid therapy.[64] Although endothelial cells may produce ACE, increased levels or production of ACE have been found in sarcoid lymph nodes, granulomas, and alveolar macrophages, suggesting that cells of the mononuclear phagocyte system are the primary source of the increased SACE in sarcoidosis.[8-10] Since Lieberman's original report, several investigators have confirmed elevated SACE levels in 30% to 80% of cases, with false-positive rates ranging from 1% to 5% in non-sarcoid controls.[62,63,65-68,91] Higher levels have been found in patients with clinically active disease, and the level may fall in response to corticosteroid therapy.[61,63,65,67,91] In one British study,[67] SACE was elevated in only 1 of 19 patients with stable sarcoid, but in 8 of 13 (62%) with progressive disease. Klech and associates[61] reported elevated SACE levels in 77% of 35 patients with clinically active sarcoid, but in only 12% of those with inactive sarcoid. Although SACE levels usually agree with clinical assessment of activity,[65] changes in SACE appear to be more sensitive in predicting clinical relapse (or remission) than conventional parameters such as pulmonary function tests or chest radiographs.[61,63,65,68] However, patients with a normal SACE level may still have active disease that may be responsive to corticosteroids; in such cases, falls in SACE may parallel radiographic clearing.[62,65,68] The predictive value of SACE in sarcoidosis is controversial, however; some investigators have found that SACE is not a sensitive indicator of alveolitis. Rossman and associates[66] noted increases in SACE in only 7 of 17 patients with recently diagnosed sarcoidosis exhibiting lymphocytosis on BAL. Others have observed that SACE fails to correlate with the degree of BAL T lymphocytosis,[58,90-93] intrapulmonary uptake on ^{67}Ga scan,[58,90] or responsiveness to corticosteroid therapy.[58,60,91] The inability of SACE to mirror activity of a single organ (such as the lung) is perhaps not surprising when one considers that serum levels likely reflect the total body burden of granulomas rather than the inflammatory component at a single site. In addition, SACE, ^{67}Ga scans, and BAL may reflect different stages or components of the disease process.[59] Alveolar macrophages are responsible for the increased intrapulmonary uptake of ^{67}Ga observed in cases of active alveolitis,[8–10] and SACE correlates better with ^{67}Ga uptake than does BAL lymphocytosis,[59] suggesting that SACE and ^{67}Ga scans reflect the macrophage component. This hypothesis is supported by the observation that SACE is frequently normal within the first 4 weeks of Löfgren's syndrome, when lymphocytic alveolitis is present, but SACE levels then increase over the next 2 to 3 months, even when the BAL lymphocytosis is resolving.[51] Although SACE appears to be less sensitive as an indicator of alveolitis than ^{67}Ga or BAL, the clinical significance of this remains unclear because patients exhibiting asymptomatic alveolitis most likely do not require therapy. Given the propensity of sarcoidosis to wax and wane spontaneously, no single parameter can be expected to reliably predict long-term prognosis. Therapeutic decisions should not be based solely on SACE levels, but SACE may provide ancillary information—particularly in patients whose disease is of uncertain activity clinically. Asymptomatic elevations in SACE level do not warrant therapy per se, but may identify patients who have active disease or are more likely to develop disease progression.

EFFICACY OF CORTICOSTEROIDS IN SARCOIDOSIS

Corticosteroids are the cornerstone of therapy in patients with severe or progressive sarcoidosis and often produce dramatic resolution of disease. The long-term impact of corticosteroids is less clear, as relapses may occur when therapy is tapered or discontinued.[1–6,96,97] Because of the high rate of spontaneous remission in this disorder, most patients do not require treatment, and indications for corticosteroid therapy are controversial. Several retrospective studies have assessed the efficacy of corticosteroids in sarcoidosis.[2–5,74] Unfortunately, most of these studies reflect the bias and individual management approaches of individual investigators, and utilize differing indications for treatment, parameters of disease activity, dosage and duration of treatment, and so on. The lack of reliable indicators of disease activity, the lack of standardized or objective criteria for response, and the high rate of spontaneous resolution characteristic of sarcoidosis have made interpretation of the efficacy of steroid therapy difficult. Nevertheless, by a variety of criteria, including changes in chest radiographs and pulmonary function tests, systemic corticosteroids have achieved favorable response rates in 70% to 90% of patients with symptomatic pulmonary sarcoidosis, although relapses have occurred in 30% to 50% of patients following discontinuation of the drug.[4–6,8,74] Owing to the lack of controls in these studies, the precise impact of corticosteroid therapy on long-term prognosis cannot be assessed. Several prospective studies have suggested that corticosteroids may result in temporary improvement but may not influence the ultimate outcome. In one early prospective study, which randomized patients to receive 20 mg prednisolone daily or 400 mg oxyphenbutazone or placebo daily for 6 months, both treatment groups exhibited greater radiographic improvement than placebo-treated controls.[98] However, long-term outcome or pulmonary function tests were not evaluated. Israel and associates[97] randomized 90 patients with pulmonary sarcoidosis to no therapy or 15 mg prednisone daily for 3 months. At 3 months, there was greater improvement in pulmonary function tests in corticosteroid-treated patients with stage 2 or 3 but not stage 1 disease, suggesting a beneficial effect of corticosteroids in treated patients. However, there was no difference between groups at 5 years. Although this have been interpreted as showing that steroids fail to modify long-term prognosis, it is plausible that the failure to demonstrate differences at 5 years reflected premature discontinuation of corticosteroids. Harkleroad and co-workers[99] prospectively randomized 25 patients with pulmonary sarcoidosis and abnormal pulmonary function on an alternate-case basis to receive either corticosteroids (for a minimum of 6 months) or no therapy. Although individual patients improved in both groups, follow-up pulmonary function tests at 6 months, 1 to 2 years, and 10 to 15 years did not differ between treated and untreated patients. However, the degree of pulmonary dysfunction was mild at the outset in both groups, and 4 of 13 treated patients were asymptomatic at the outset. Several prospective studies in the United States,[97,99,100] Europe,[96,101] and Japan[102] have failed to demonstrate any beneficial long-term effects of corticosteroids on the course of pulmonary sarcoidosis. A recent prospective, double-blind trial of 183 patients with sarcoidosis randomized to receive prednisone or placebo for at least 2 years failed to demonstrate any benefit in corticosteroid-treated patients as assessed by chest radiographs or pulmonary functions tests.[100] The dose of prednisone (40 mg daily for 3 months, followed by a maintenance dose of 20 mg daily for at least 2 years) should have been adequate to demonstrate any salutory effect. Eule and associates[96] randomized patients with asymptomatic pulmonary sarcoidosis and normal pulmonary function to placebo or therapy with steroids for 6 or 12 months. At the end of follow-up (mean duration of 9 years), approximately 80% of cases in both treatment groups had normal pulmonary functions tests and chest radiographs, with no significant differences between groups. It should be emphasized, however, that among patients who demonstrated progression of their disease, introduction of corticosteroids was effective in inducing remissions. Together, these studies suggest a conservative approach to the treatment of sarcoidosis, as early initiation of corticosteroid therapy may not avert pulmonary fibrosis or permanent impairment of pulmonary function. Aggressively treating every patient with sarcoidosis who exhibits pulmonary dysfunction or chest radiographic findings irrespective of the presence or absence of symptoms is inappropriate. However, these studies do not assess the impact of therapy in patients with severe pulmonary symptoms, chronic persistent pulmonary dysfunction, disabling extrapulmonary symptoms, or a deteriorating course. There is little doubt that steroids can temporarily suppress or reverse disease in at least some such cases. Although indications for therapy should be circumscribed and focused, we believe that a trial of corticosteroid therapy is indicated for patients exhibiting severe or progressive pulmonary or extrapulmonary symptoms or organ dysfunction. Aggressive corticosteroid therapy is mandatory for patients exhibiting cardiac, central nervous system, or ocular involvement or chronic hypercalcemia. While the optimal dose and duration of therapy have not been well defined, we usually initiate prednisone in a dosage of 60 mg/day for the first 1 to 2 weeks for patients with active, symptomatic sarcoidosis requiring therapy. The dose can then be tapered by 10 mg decrements every 1 to 2 weeks according to the clinical response and severity of disease. Objective criteria (such as pulmonary function tests, chest radiographs, SACE, and so on) must be defined and followed to ensure adequacy of therapy. In most cases, the dose can be converted to 60 mg every other day within 4 to 8 weeks, at which time a more gradual tapering program is appropriate. Once patients are on an alternate-day regimen, we taper by 10 mg decrements monthly for the first 3 months, but often maintain patients for extended periods at dosages of 20 or 30 mg prednisone every other day. Although corticosteroids can sometimes be successfully discontinued within 6 to 9 months in selected patients exhibiting an initial acute inflammatory component that promptly resolves with therapy, a more protracted course (often extending beyond 12 months) is generally recommended for patients with chronic disease requiring treatment. In some instances, repeated relapses occur on discontinuation of corticosteroid therapy. In such cases, prolonged (and sometimes indefinite) maintenance therapy with 15 to 20 mg prednisone every other day may be necessary to suppress the disease. The dose of corticosteroid must be modified, however, according to the severity and site of the disease process. In some patients with mild but symptomatic disease, a lower initial starting dose—in the range of 40 mg prednisone every other day for 3 months, with a gradual taper by 5 to 10 mg decrements every 2 to 3 months thereafter—may be effective.

ALTERNATIVE AGENTS

Although information on agents other than prednisone is limited, anecdotal successes have been claimed with a variety of antiinflammatory and immunosuppressive regimens. Chloroquine has been reported to be efficacious in cutaneous sarcoidosis in uncontrolled studies, but its efficacy in pulmonary or systemic sarcoidosis appears to be limited.[103,104] Phenylbutazone was associated with a higher remission rate than placebo in one study,[98] but its efficacy is unproven. A variety of immunosuppressive agents, including chlorambucil,[97,105] azathioprine,[106] methotrexate,[107] cyclophosphamide,[108] and cyclosporin A,[109–112] have been used in patients with progressive disease refractory to corticosteroids or with steroid side effects with anecdotal claims for success, but no controlled studies have been done. Owing to the lack of controlled studies and the limited number of patients treated with these immunosuppressive regimens, no single agent has been proven to be superior. Favorable responses have been achieved with chlorambucil in 8 of 10[105] and 4 of 8 patients[97] who previously failed to respond to corticosteroids, in two separate studies. Cyclophosphamide has been effective in cases refractory to corticosteroids,[108] but its potential toxicity limits its usefulness. Methotrexate has been utilized largely for the treatment of severe cutaneous sarcoidosis refractory to corticosteroid therapy, but a recent report[107] suggests that oral methotrexate may induce remissions in patients with pulmonary or severe systemic sarcoidosis as well. Cyclosporin A, a fungal cyclic peptide whose immunosuppressive effects derive largely from its ability to specifically inhibit T-lymphocyte activation, represents a logical agent that should be ideally suited for the treatment of sarcoidosis, a disorder in which T-cell activation plays a central role in the pathogenesis. Although there are anecdotal reports of remissions achieved with the use of cyclosporin A for the treatment of sarcoidosis,[110–112] data confirming its efficacy in large numbers of patients are lacking. In one study, the addition of cyclosporin to short-term cultures of sarcoid lung lymphocytes in vitro suppressed their spontaneous release of lymphokines (IL2 and monocyte chemotactic factor), and inhibited T-cell replication.[109] Despite its in vitro efficacy, however, oral cyclosporin A administered in conventional doses (10 mg/kg/day) to eight patients with active pulmonary sarcoidosis failed to suppress the T-cell alveolitis or lymphokine release or to improve pulmonary function over the 6-month study period.[109] It has been suggested that the failure of cyclosporin to suppress alveolitis in vivo may reflect reduced tissue levels of cyclosporin in the lung, but other mechanisms, including the inability of cyclosporin to override local stimuli for T-cell activation, may be operative.[109]

HEART-LUNG TRANSPLANTATION

Owing to the excellent prognosis in most patients with sarcoidosis, and the usual excellent response to corticosteroids in symptomatic patients with progressive pulmonary sarcoidosis, heart-lung or lung transplantation is rarely warranted. Nevertheless, successful lung transplants have been performed in patients with end-stage sarcoidosis with severe, life-threatening respiratory insufficiency. Although recrudescence of disease in the transplanted lung remains a concern, lung transplantation may be a viable option in patients with disabling pulmonary insufficiency and cor pulmonale refractory to medical therapy in whom life expectancy is greatly curtailed. However, indications for heart-lung or lung transplantation in this setting are evolving, and appropriate criteria for patient selection need to be defined.

REFERENCES

1. Mitchell DN, Scadding JG. Sarcoidosis: State of the art. Am Rev Respir Dis 1974:110;774–802.
2. Mayock RL, Bertrand P, Morrison CE, et al. Manifestations of sarcoidosis: Analysis of 145 patients with a review of nine series selected from the literature. Am J Med 1963:35;67–89.
3. Neville E, Walker AN, James DG. Prognostic factors predicting the outcome of sarcoidosis: An analysis of 818 patients. Q J Med 1983:205;525–538.
4. Scadding JG. Prognosis of intrathoracic sarcoidosis in England: A review of 136 cases after five years observation. Br Med J 1961:1165–1172.
5. Siltzbach LE, James DG, Neville E, Turiaf J, et al. Course and prognosis of sarcoidosis around the world. Am J Med 1974:57;847–852.
6. Siltzbach LE. Sarcoidosis: Clinical features and management. Med Clin North Am 1967:51; 483–502.
7. Longcope WT, Freiman DG. A study of sarcoidosis based on a combined investigation of 160 cases including 30 autopsies from the Johns Hopkins Hospital and Massachusetts General Hospital. Medicine 1952:31;1–128.
8. Thomas PD, Hunninghake GW. Current concepts of the pathogenesis of sarcoidosis. Am Rev Respir Dis 1987:135;747–760.
9. Crystal RG, Roberts WC, Hunninghake GW, Gadek JE, Fulmer JD, Line BR. Pulmonary sarcoidosis: A disease characterized and perpetuated by activated lung T lymphocytes. Ann Intern Med 1981:94;73–94.
10. Daniele RP, Elias JA, Epstein PE, Rossman MD. Bronchoalveolar lavage: Role in the pathogenesis, diagnosis, and management of interstitial lung disease. Ann Intern Med 1985:102; 93–108.

11. Modlin RL, Hofman FM, Meyer PR, Sharma OP, Taylor RR, Rea TH. In situ demonstration of T lymphocyte subsets in granulomatous inflammation: Leprosy, rhinoscleroma and sarcoidosis. Clin Exp Immunol 1983:51;430–438.
12. Hunninghake GW, Crystal RG. Pulmonary sarcoidosis: A disorder mediated by excess helper T-lymphocyte activity at sites of disease activity. N Engl J Med 1981:305;429–434.
13. Rossi GA, Sacco O, Cosulich E, Risso A, Balbi B, Ravazzoni C. Helper T-lymphocytes in pulmonary sarcoidosis: Functional analysis of a lung T-cell subpopulation in patients with active disease. Am Rev Respir Dis 1986:133;1086–1090.
14. Muller-Quernheim J, Saltini C, Sondermeyer P, Crystal RG. Compartmentalized activation of the interleukin-2 gene by lung T-lymphocytes in active pulmonary sarcoidosis. J Immunol 1986:137;3475–3483.
15. Costabel U, Bross KJ, Ruhle KH, Lohr GW, Matthys H. Ia-like antigens on T-cells and their subpopulations in pulmonary sarcoidosis and in hypersensitivity pneumonitis. Am Rev Respir Dis 1985:131;337–342.
16. Gerli R, Darwish S, Broccucci L, Spinozzi F, Rambotti P. Helper inducer T cells in the lungs of sarcoidosis patients: Analysis of their pathogenic and clinical significance. Chest 1989:95;811–816.
17. Hunninghake GW, Bedell GN, Zavala DC, Monick M, Brady M. Role of interleukin-2 release by lung T cells in active pulmonary sarcoidosis. Am Rev Respir Dis 1983:128;634–638.
18. Saltini C, Spurzem JR, Lee JJ, Pinkston P, Cyrstal RG. Spontaneous release of interleukin 2 by lung T lymphocytes in active pulmonary sarcoidosis is primarily from the Leu3+DR+ T cell subset. J Clin Invest 1986:77;1962–1970.
19. Pinkston P, Saltini C, Muller-Quernheim J, Crystal RG. Corticosteroid therapy suppresses interleukin 2 release and spontaneous proliferation of lung T lymphocytes of patients with active pulmonary sarcoidosis. J Immunol 1987:139;755–760.
20. Pacheco Y, Cordier G, Perrin-Favolle M, Rossman MD. Flow cytometry analysis of T lymphocytes in sarcoidosis. Am J Med 1982:73;82–88.
21. Chilosi M, Menestrina F, Capelli P, Montagna L, et al. Immunochemical analysis of sarcoid granulomas: Evaluation of Ki67+ and interleukin+ cells. Am J Pathol 1988:131;191–198.
22. Konishi K, Moller DR, Saltini C, Kirby M, Crystal RG. Spontaneous expression of the interleukin-2 receptor gene and presence of functional interleukin-2 receptors on T-lymphocytes in the blood of individuals with active pulmonary sarcoidosis. J Clin Invest 1988:82;775–781.
23. Lawrence EC, Brousseau KP, Berger MB, Kurman CC, Marcon L, Nelson DL. Elevated concentrations of soluble interleukin-2 receptors in serum samples and bronchoalveolar lavage fluids in active sarcoidosis. Am Rev Respir Dis 1988:137;759–764.
24. Hancock WW, Kobzik L, Colby AM, O'Hara CJ, Cooper AG, Godlescki JJ. Detection of lymphokines and lymphokine receptors in pulmonary sarcoidosis. Am J Pathol 1986:123;1–8.
25. Hancock WW, Muller WA, Cotran RS. Interleukin-2 receptors are expressed by alveolar macrophages during pulmonary sarcoidosis and are inducible by lymphokine treatment of normal human lung macrophages, blood monocytes, and monocyte cell lines. J Immunol 1987:138;185–191.
26. Daniele RP, McMillan LJ, Dauber JH, Rossman MD. Immune complexes in sarcoidosis. A correlation with activity and duration of disease. Chest 1978:74;261–264.
27. Saltini C, Winestock K, Kirby M, Pinkston P, Crystal RG. Maintenance of alveolitis in patients with chronic beryllium disease by beryllium-specific helper T cells. N Engl J Med 1989:320;1103–1109.
28. Saltini C, Hemler M, Crystal RG. Expression of the "very late activation antigen" (VLA-1) complex on lung T-cells characterizes a population of activated nonproliferating T-cells compartmentalized in the normal lung. Clin Immunol Immunopathol 1988:46;221–233.

29. Moller D, Konishi K, Kirby M, Balbi B, Crystal RG. Bias towards use of a specific T cell receptor β-chain variable region in a subgroup of individuals with sarcoidosis. J Clin Invest 1988:82;1183–1191.

30. Agostini C, Trentin L, Zambello R, Luca M, Masciarelli M, Cipriani A, Marcer G, Semenzato G. Pulmonary alveolar macrophages in patients with sarcoidosis and hypersensitivity pneumonitis: Characterization by monoclonal antibodies. J Clin Immunol 1987:7:64–70.

31. Hance AJ, Douches S, Winchester RJ, Ferrans J, Crystal RG. Characterization of mononuclear phagocyte subpopulations in the human lung by using monoclonal antibodies: Changes in alveolar macrophage phenotype associated with pulmonary sarcoidosis. J Immunol 1985:134;284–292.

32. Venet A, Hance AJ, Saltini C, Robinson BWS, Crystal RG. Enhanced alveolar macrophage–mediated antigen-induced T lymphocyte proliferation in sarcoidosis. J Clin Invest 1985:75; 293–301.

33. Robinson BWS, McLemore TL, Crystal RG. Gamma interferon is spontaneously released by alveolar macrophages and lung T lymphocytes in patients with pulmonary sarcoidosis. J Clin Invest 1985:75;1488–1495.

34. Hunninghake GW. Release of interleukin-1 by alveolar macrophages of patients with active pulmonary sarcoidosis. Ann Rev Respir Dis 1984:129;569–572.

35. Kern JA, Lamb RJ, Reed JC, Elias JA, Daniele RP. Interleukin-1-β gene expression in human monocytes and alveolar macrophages from normal subjects and patients with sarcoidosis. Am Rev Respir Dis 1988:137:1180–1184.

36. Wewers MA, Saltini C, Sellers S, Tocci MJ, Bayne EK, Schmidt JA, Crystal RG. Evaluation of alveolar macrophages in normals and individuals with active pulmonary sarcoidosis for the spontaneous expression of the interleukin-1-β gene. Cell Immunol 1987:107;479–488.

37. Moseley PL, Hemken C, Monick M, Nugent K, Hunninghake GW. Interferon and growth factor activity for human lung fibroblasts. Chest 1986:89;657–662.

38. Bitterman PB, Slatzman LE, Adelberg S, Ferrans VJ, Crystal RG. Alveolar macrophage replication: One mechanism for the expansion of the mononuclear phagocyte population in the chronically inflamed lung. J Clin Invest 1984:74;460–469.

39. Hasday JD, Bachwich PR, Lynch JP, Sitrin RS. Tissue thromboplastin and urokinase activities in bronchoalveolar lavage fluid of patients with pulmonary sarcoidosis. Exp Lung Res 1988:14;261–278.

40. Meyer KC, Kamininski MJ, Calhoun WJ, Auerbach R. Studies of bronchoalveolar lavage cells and fluids in pulmonary sarcoidosis: Enhanced capacity of bronchoalveolar lavage cells from patients with pulmonary sarcoidosis to induce angiogenesis in vivo. Am Rev Respir Dis 1989:140;1446–1449.

41. Bachwich PR, Lynch JP, Larrick J, Spengler M, Kunkel SL. Tumor necrosis factor production by human sarcoid alveolar macrophages. Am J Pathol 1986:125;421–425.

42. Spatafora M, Merendino A, Chiappara G, Gjomarkaj M, et al. Lung compartmentalization of increased TNF releasing ability by mononuclear phagocytes in pulmonary sarcoidosis. Chest 1989:96;542–549.

43. Le J, Vilcek J. Tumor necrosis factor and interleukin 1: Cytokines with multiple overlapping biological activities. Lab Invest 1987:56;234–248.

44. Bachwich PR, Lynch JP, Kunkel SL. Arachidonic acid metabolism is altered in sarcoid alveolar macrophages. Clin Immunol Immunopathol 1987:42;27–37.

45. Hillerdal G, Nou E, Osterman K, Schmekel B. Sarcoidosis: Epidemiology and prognosis. A 15 year European study. Am Rev Respir Dis 1984:130;29–32.

46. Romer FK. Presentation of sarcoidosis and outcome of pulmonary changes: A review of 243 patients followed for up to 10 years. Dan Med Bull 1982:29;27–32.

47. Rochat T, Hunninghake GW. Sarcoidosis. In: King T, Schwarz M, eds. Interstitial lung disease. Philadelphia: BC Decker, 1988:229–238.

48. Abe S, Yamaguchi E, Makimura S, et al. Association of HLA-DR5J antigen with sarcoidosis: Correlation with clinical course. Chest 1987:92;488–490.

49. Reich JM, Johnson RE. Course and prognosis of sarcoidosis in a nonreferral setting: Analysis of 86 patients observed for 10 years. Am J Med 1985:89;61–66.

50. Löfgren S. Primary pulmonary sarcoidosis: Early signs and symptoms. Acta Med Scand 1953:145;424–431.

51. Veleyre D, Saumon G, Georges R, et al. The relationship between disease duration and noninvasive pulmonary explorations in sarcoidosis with erythema nodosum. Am Rev Respir Dis 1984:129;938–943.

52. Winterbauer RH, Belic N, Moores KD. A clinical interpretation of bilateral hilar adenopathy. Ann Intern Med 1973:78;65–71.

53. Gilman MJ, Wang KP. Transbronchial lung biopsy in sarcoidosis. An approach to determine the optimal number of biopsies. Am Rev Respir Dis 1980:122;721–724.

54. Siltzbach LE. The Kveim test in sarcoidosis: A study of 750 patients. JAMA 1961:178;476–482.

55. Williams WC, Seal RE, Davies KJ, Chapman JS. International Kveim histology trail. Ann NY Acad Sci 1976;687–699.

56. Douglas AC, Wallace A, Clark J, Stephens JH, Smith IE, Allan NC. The Edinburgh spleen: Source of a validated Kveim-Siltzbach test material. Ann NY Acad Sci 1976;670–680.

57. Israel HL, Goldstein RA. Relation of Kveim-antigen reaction to lymphadenopathy: Study of sarcoidosis and other diseases. N Engl J Med 1971:284;345–349.

58. Baughman RP, Fernandez M, Bosken CH, Manitl J, Hurtubise P. Comparison of gallium-67 scanning, bronchoalveolar lavage, and serum angiotensin-converting enzyme levels in pulmonary sarcoidosis: Predicting response to therapy. Am Rev Respir Dis 1984:129; 676–681.

59. Beaumont D, Herry JY, Sapene M, Bourguet P, Larzul JJ, DeLabarthe B. Gallium-67 in the evaluation of sarcoidosis: Correlations with serum angiotensin-converting enzyme and bronchoalveolar lavage. Thorax 1982:37;11–18.

60. Hollinger WM, Staton GW, Fajman WA, Gilman MJ, Pine JR, Check IJ. Prediction of therapeutic response in steroid-treated pulmonary sarcoidosis: Evaluation of clinical parameters, bronchoalveolar lavage, gallium-67 scanning, and serum angiotensin-converting enzyme levels. Am Rev Resp Dis 1985:132;65–69.

61. Klech H, Kohn H, Kummer F, Mostbeck A. Assessment of activity in sarcoidosis: Sensitivity and specificity of 67 Gallium scintigraphy, serum ACE levels, chest roentgenography, and blood lymphocyte subpopulations. Chest 1982:82;732–738.

62. DeRemee RA, Rohrbach MS. Normal serum angiotensin converting enzyme activity in patients with newly diagnosed sarcoidosis. Chest 1984:85;45–48.

63. DeRemee RA, Rohrbach MS. Serum angiotensin-converting enzyme activity in evaluating the clinical course of sarcoidosis. Ann Intern Med 1980:92;361–365.

64. Lieberman J. Elevation of serum angiotensin-converting enzyme (ACE) level in sarcoidosis. Am J Med 1975:59;365–372.

65. Rohatgi PK, Ryan JW, Lindeman P. Value of serum measurement of serum angiotensin converting enzyme in the management of sarcoidosis. Am J Med 1981:70;44–50.

66. Rossman MD, Dauber JM, Cardillo ME, Daniele RP. Pulmonary sarcoidosis: Correlation of serum angiotensin-converting enzyme with blood and bronchoalveolar lymphocytes. Am Rev Respir Dis 1982:125,366–369.

67. Turton CW, Grundy E, Firth G, Mitchell D, Rigden BG, Turner-Warwick M. Value of measuring serum angiotensin 1 converting enzyme and serum lysozyme in the management of sarcoidosis. Thorax 1979:34;57–62.

68. Ueda E, Kawabe T, Tachibana T, Kokubu T. Serum angiotensin-converting enzyme activity as an indicator of prognosis in sarcoidosis. Am Rev Respir Dis 1980:121;667–671.

69. Goldstein RA, Israel HL, Becker KL, Moore CF. The infrequency of hypercalcemia in sarcoidosis. Am J Med 1971:51;21–30.
70. Meyrier A, Valeyre D, Bouillon R, Paillard F, Battesti JP, Georges R. Resorptive versus absorptive hypercalciuria in sarcoidosis: Correlations with 25-dihydroxy vitamin D_3 and 1,25-dihydroxy vitamin D_3 and parameters of disease activity. Q J Med 1985:215;269–281.
71. Romer FK. Sarcoidosis with large nodular lesions simulating pulmonary metastases: An analysis of 126 cases of intrathoracic sarcoidosis. Scand J Respir Dis 1977:58;11–16.
72. Cantin A, Begin R, Rola-Pleszczynski M, Boileau R. Heterogeneity of bronchoalveolar lavage cellularity in stage 3 pulmonary sarcoidosis. Chest 1983:83;485–486.
73. Olsson T, Bjornstad-Petterson H, Stjernberg NL. Bronchostenosis due to sarcoidosis. Chest 1979:75;663–666.
74. Johns CJ, Zachary JB, Macgregor I, Ball WC. Extended experience in the long-term corticosteroid treatment of pulmonary sarcoidosis. Ann NY Acad Sci 1976:278;722–731.
75. Chretien J, Stanislas-Lequern G, Saltiel JC, Huchon G, Marsac J. Course and treatment of sarcoidosis in 350 patients. In: Japan Medical Research Foundation, ed. Sarcoidosis. Tokyo: University of Tokyo Press, 1981.
76. Winterbauer RH, Hutchinson JF. Use of pulmonary function tests in sarcoidosis. Chest 1980:78;640–647.
77. Israel HI, Karlin P, Menduke H. Factors affecting outcome of sarcoidosis: Influence of race, extrathoracic involvement, and initial radiologic lung lesions. Ann NY Acad Sci 1986:465; 609–618.
78. Dunn TL, Watters LC, Hendrix C, Cherniack RM, Schwarz MI, King TE Jr. Gas exchange at a given degree of volume restriction is different in sarcoidosis and idiopathic pulmonary fibrosis. Am J Med 1988:85;221–224.
79. Bechtel JJ, Starr T, Dantzker DR, Bower JS. Airway hyperreactivity in patients with sarcoidosis. Am Rev Respir Dis 1981:124;759–761.
80. Levinson RS, Metzger LF, Stanley NN, et al. Airway function in sarcoidosis. Am J Med 1977:62;51–59.
81. Arnoux A, Marsac J, Stanislas-Leguern G, Huchon G, Chretien J. Bronchoalveolar lavage in sarcoidosis: Correlation between alveolar lymphocytosis and clinical data. Pathol Res Pract 1982:175;62–79.
82. Bauer W, Gorny MK, Baumann HR, Morell A. T-lymphocyte subsets and immunoglobulin concentrations in bronchoalveolar lavage of patients with sarcoidosis and high and low intensity alveolitis. Am Rev Respir Dis 1985:132;1060–1065.
83. Bjermer L, Rosenhall L, Angstrom T, Hallgren R. Predictive value of bronchoalveolar lavage cell analysis in sarcoidosis. Thorax 1988:43;284–288.
84. Buchalter S, App W, Jackson L, Chandler D, Jackson R, Fulmer J. Bronchoalveolar lavage cell analysis in sarcoidosis: A comparison of lymphocyte counts and clinical course. Ann NY Acad Sci 1986:465;679–684.
85. Ceuppens JL, Ludovicus M, Lacquet GM, Maurits D, Andre VDE, Stevens E. Alveolar T-cell subsets in pulmonary sarcoidosis: Correlation with disease activity and effect of steroid treatment. Am Rev Respir Dis 1984:129;563–569.
86. Costabel U, Bross KJ, Guzman J, Nilles A, Ruhle KH, Matthys H. Predictive value of bronchoalveolar T cell subsets for the course of pulmonary sarcoidosis. Ann NY Acad Sci 1986:465; 418–426.
87. Israel-Biet D, Venet A, Chretien J. Persistent high alveolar lymphocytosis as predictive criterion of chronic pulmonary sarcoidosis. Ann NY Acad Sci 1986:465;395–406.
88. Keogh BA, Hunninghake GW, Line BR, Crystal RG. The alveolitis of pulmonary sarcoidosis: Evaluation of natural history and alveolitis-dependent changes in lung function. Am Rev Respir Dis 1983:128;256–265.

89. Lawrence EC, Teague RB, Gottlieb MS, Jhingran SG, Lieberman J. Serial changes in markers of disease activity with corticosteroid treatment in sarcoidosis. Am J Med 1983:74;747–756.

90. Schoenberger CI, Line BR, Keogh BA, et al. Lung inflammation in sarcoidosis: Comparison of serum angiotensin-converting enzyme levels with bronchoalveolar lavage and gallium-67 scanning assessment of the T lymphocyte alveolitis. Thorax 1982:37;19–25.

91. Turner-Warwick M, McAllister W, Lawrence R, et al. Corticosteroid treatment in sarcoidosis: Do serial lavage lymphocyte counts, serum angiotensin converting enzyme measurements and gallium-67 scans help management? Thorax 1986:41;903–913.

92. Valeyre D, Aumon G, Bladier D, J Amouroux, et al. The relationship between noninvasive exploration in pulmonary sarcoidosis of recent origin as shown by bronchoalveolar lavages, serum angiotensin converting enzyme, and pulmonary function tests. Am Rev Respir Dis 1982:126;41–45.

93. Wallaert B, Ramon P, Fournier E, Tonnel AB, Voisin C. Bronchoalveolar lavage, serum angiotensin converting enzyme, and ^{67}Ga scanning in extrathoracic sarcoidosis. Chest 1982:82;553–555.

94. Ward K, O'Connor C, Odlum C, Fitzgerald MX. Prognostic value of bronchoalveolar lavage in sarcoidosis: The critical influence of disease presentation. Thorax 1989:44;6–12.

95. Line BR, Hunninghake GW, Keogh BA, Jones AE, Johnston GS, Crystal RG. Gallium-67 scanning to stage the alveolitis of sarcoidosis: Correlation with clinical studies, pulmonary function studies, and bronchoalveolar lavage. Am Rev Respir Dis 1981:123;440–446.

96. Eule H, Weinecke A, Roth I. The possible influence of corticosteroid therapy on the natural course of pulmonary sarcoidosis. Ann NY Acad Sci 1986:465;695–701.

97. Israel HL, Fouts DW, Beggs RA. A controlled trial of prednisone treatment of sarcoidosis. Am Rev Respir Dis 1973:107;609–614.

98. James DG, Carstairs LS, Trowell J, Sharma OP. Treatment of sarcoidosis: Report of a controlled therapeutic trial. Lancet:1967:2;526–528.

99. Harkleroad LE, Young RL, Savage PJ, Jenkins DW, Lordon RE. Pulmonary sarcoidosis: Long-term follow-up of the effects of steroid therapy. Chest 1982:82;84–87.

100. Zaki MH, Lyons HA, Leilop L, Huang CT. Corticosteroid therapy in sarcoidosis: A five-year, controlled follow-up study. NY State J Med 1987:87;496–499.

101. Selroos O, Sellergren TL. Corticosteroid therapy of pulmonary sarcoidosis: A prospective evaluation of alternate day and daily dosage in stage II disease. Scand J Respir Dis 1979:60;215–221.

102. Yamamoto M, Saito N, Tachibana T, et al. Effects of an 18 month corticosteroid therapy to stage I and stage II sarcoidosis patients (a control trial). In: Chretien J, Marsac J, Saltiel JC, eds. Sarcoidosis and other granulomatous disorders. Paris: Pergamon Press, 1980:470–474.

103. Siltzbach LE, Teirstein AS. Chloroquine therapy in 43 patients with intrathoracic and cutaneous sarcoidosis. Acta Med Scand (suppl) 1964:425;302–308.

104. British Tuberculosis Association: Chloroquine in the treatment of sarcoidosis. Tubercle 1967:48;257–272.

105. Kataria YP. Chlorambucil in sarcoidosis. Chest 1980:78;36–43.

106. Sharma O, Hughes DTD, Geraint-James D, Naish P. Immunosuppressive therapy with azathioprine in sarcoidosis. In: Levinsky L, Macholda F, eds. Fifth International Conference on Sarcoidosis. Prague: Universita Karlova; 1971;635–637.

107. Lower EE, Baughman RP. The use of low dose methotrexate in refractory sarcoidosis. Am J Med Sci 1990:299;153–157.

108. Demeter SL. Myocardial sarcoidosis unresponsive to steroids. Treatment with cyclophosphamide. Chest 1988:94;202–203.

109. Martinet Y, Pinkston P, Saltini C, Spurzem J, Muller-Quernheim J, Crystal RG. Evaluation of the in vitro and in vivo effects of cyclosporine on the lung T-lymphocyte alveolitis of active pulmonary sarcoidosis. Am Rev Respir Dis 1988:138;1242–1248.

110. Rebuck AS, Stiller CR, Braude AC, Laupacis A, Cohen RD, Chapman KR. Cyclosporin (CyA) in the treatment of pulmonary sarcoidosis. In: Schindler R, ed. Cyclosporin in autoimmune diseases. Berlin: Springer-Verlag, 1985:193–196.
111. York EL, Mann SFP, Sproule BJ. Cyclosporin-A in a case of refractory systemic and cutaneous sarcoidosis. Chest 1986:89 (suppl):519.
112. Bielory L, Holland C, Gascon P, Frohman L. Uveitis, cutaneous and neurosarcoid: Treatment with low-dose cyclosporin A. Transplant Proc 1988:20 (suppl 4(3));144–148.

8

Chronic Beryllium Disease

Milton D. Rossman

Chronic beryllium disease (CBD) is a pulmonary granulomatous disorder caused by a cell-mediated immune reaction to beryllium. Although involvement of other organ systems, such as skin and liver, has been reported, the lungs are the principal organ affected. Chronic beryllium disease is the preferred name for this disorder to distinguish it from acute beryllium disease, an acute toxic pneumonitis.[1] The terms "berylliosis" and "chronic beryllium poisoning" are inappropriate because a dose-response relationship has never been demonstrated.

EPIDEMIOLOGY

The clinical syndrome of CBD was first reported by Hardy and Tabershaw in 1946.[2] Seventeen beryllium workers in the fluorescent lamp industry developed a syndrome that was characterized by a long delay between initial exposure and the onset of symptoms. Sources of cases of occupational CBD reported to the beryllium case registry through 1980[3] have been observed in a variety of industrial settings. Workers using beryllium phosphors in lamp manufacture (319 cases or 57%) represent the largest single occupational exposure. Since beryllium has not been used in lamp manufacture since 1950, this source of exposure is largely of historical interest.

Other industrial sources of cases of CBD identified by the beryllium case registry include beryllium extraction (101 cases), research laboratories (29 cases), beryllium copper foundries (22 cases), beryllium metal machining (47 cases), beryllium ceramics (11 cases), and other (17 cases).[3] Since 1980, cases of CBD have continued to be identified in beryllium extraction,[4] beryllium copper and precious metal foundries,[5,7] beryllium machining in nuclear plants,[6] and in the aircraft industry.[8] In addition, the first case of CBD in a dental technician that was probably secondary to heat treatment of a

TABLE 8-1. Occupations with Significant Beryllium Risk Potential

Production and maintenance work in:
    Beryllium extraction plants
    Basic beryllium plants producing:
        1. metallic beryllium
        2. beryllium alloys
        3. beryllium oxide powders
Work in foundries melting beryllium alloys
Work in beryllium machine shops
Work in plants in which beryllium oxide powders are processed
Operations involving:
    Grinding, lapping, or otherwise abrading beryllium-containing materials
    Welding, brazing, or melting beryllium-containing materials
    Beryllium oxide furnace cleaning, or rebuilding
    Laser cutting, scribing, or trimming
    Dental laboratory operations utilizing beryllium alloys
    Beryllium oxide pressing or extrusion
    Heat treating beryllium alloys
    Chemical milling of beryllium

beryllium alloy will shortly be reported (Rossman M, unpublished). Table 8-1 lists occupations that have a significant beryllium hazard if proper precautions are not observed.

Nonoccupational cases of CBD have also been reported to the beryllium case registry. These cases have been attributed to air pollution (42 cases) and to household exposure of dust brought home on work clothes (23 cases). However, no cases have occurred among individuals exposed after 1950. Thus, like the occupational cases in lamp manufacture, nonoccupational cases of CBD appear to be largely of historical interest.[3]

PREVALENCE

The prevalence of CBD among a number of occupational exposures was reviewed in 1983[3] and ranged from 0% to 4.9% of exposed workers. These numbers are suspect, however, because the number of exposed workers was only estimated and the true number of cases of CBD may have been underestimated because of the difficulty of making a diagnosis of CBD. The exposure to beryllium in all these cases occurred before 1950. Since occupational exposures to beryllium are much lower today, the prevalence of CBD among all beryllium workers is much less. However, in two recent series of occupational exposures to probable excessive levels of beryllium (i.e., above the OSHA standards), a prevalence of CBD of 3.6%[5] and 8%[6] was observed. Thus, among workers exposed to airborne beryllium above the OSHA standards, the prevalence of CBD is still about 5%.

In addition to the relatively low prevalence of CBD among exposed workers, another factor that has made the identification of cases of CBD difficult is the long time interval between initial exposure to beryllium and the onset of symptoms. In the original series of 17 cases of CBD, 12 of those affected had onset of symptoms between 6 months and 3 years after they had stopped working.[2] In the 1983 review of the beryllium case registry,[3] the duration from initial exposure until first symptoms or diagnosis ranged from 1 to 41 years, with a mean of 11 years.

The low prevalence and long latency of CBD not only make the identification of cases difficult but also make it difficult to determine the relationship between airborne concentration of beryllium and disease. Because of the long latency, even in current outbreaks of CBD, the airborne concentrations of beryllium that existed during working conditions must be estimated retrospectively.[5] As secondary users of beryllium proliferate, adequate environmental controls may not be installed in small operations and air samples may not be determined. The long interval from the first identification that adequate environmental controls were not being used in dental laboratories[9] to the first identified case of CBD in a dental technician in 1989 (Rossman M, personal communication) illustrates this problem.

The current OSHA standards[10] for acceptable beryllium exposures are:

1. The daily weighted average exposure during an 8-hour working day may not exceed 2 $\mu g/m^3$.
2. Short-term exposures above 5 $\mu g/m^3$ but not greater than 25 $\mu g/m^3$ are permissible for a total of not more than 30 minutes per 8-hour working day.

Although these standards were originally proposed for the control of acute beryllium disease, they are probably reasonable recommendations for the control of chronic beryllium disease. The rarity of CBD today in major beryllium processing plants (reference 3 and Preuss O, personal communication) and the probable association between current cases and excessive beryllium exposure[4–6] are strong evidence that if the OSHA standards are maintained, CBD should not occur.

IMMUNOPATHOGENESIS

When CBD was first described, the initial hypothesis concerning the pathogenesis of CBD was that it was a delayed chemical pneumonitis.[2] Although an acute tracheobronchial pneumonia had already been described,[1] certain findings in CBD were inconsistent with this theory. First, beryllium levels in tissue did not correlate with the presence of CBD.[11] Second, the incidence of CBD did not correlate with exposure histories.[3] Thus, the theory that CBD was a delayed chemical pneumonitis or due to beryllium poisoning was suspect.

Immunological Studies in Chronic Beryllium Disease

Sterner and Eisenbud[12] in 1951 were among the first to propose that CBD was immunologically mediated. Their reasons for suggesting an immunologic cause were based on the epidemiologic evidence that (1) severe cases have occurred with low exposures; (2) tissue levels of beryllium have not correlated with the extent of disease; (3)

at low atmospheric concentrations of beryllium, there was a correlation with disease, but at high concentrations there was not; (4) the onset of symptoms may occur many years after the termination of beryllium exposure; and (5) the pulmonary lesions have not been easily reproduced in animals. In addition, animal studies have demonstrated that various species can become sensitized to beryllium.[13–18]

Curtis in 1951 was the first to demonstrate that beryllium could be sensitizing to humans.[19] Application of 2% beryllium sulfate or fluoride salts to the skin (patch or skin test) produced, within 48 hours, a local allergic eczematous reaction that was positive in all 13 beryllium extraction workers with a history of dermatitis. This test also sensitized 8 of 16 controls with no previous history of dermatitis. In a later study,[20] the test was positive in 32 patients with pulmonary beryllium disease and negative in 14 controls including some with sarcoidosis. Though some cases may give negative results, skin testing has been positive in the majority of patients with CBD.[21,22]

Despite these positive findings, skin testing of patients with CBD has not been widely used because of two major drawbacks. As mentioned above, the test may cause sensitization of those who have been previously unsensitized. In addition, the possibility exists that severe anaphylactoid reactions may result from the test.[23] Thus, skin testing is not considered suitable to screen an otherwise healthy, potentially exposed working population, and it may be dangerous to test patients with symptoms.

With the development of in vitro tests for delayed hypersensitivity in the late 1960s, Hanifin[24] was the first to apply an in vitro test for delayed hypersensitivity to beryllium in the investigation of CBD. He studied seven individuals with a delayed hypersensitivity response to patch testing. A blastogenic transformation of their peripheral blood lymphocytes was observed when these cells were cultured in vitro in the presence of beryllium oxide or beryllium sulfate. In addition, an important role of macrophages in mediating this response was demonstrated by incubating macrophages with beryllium, washing them, and then observing that autologous lymphocytes would proliferate when added to the washed beryllium-pulsed macrophages. In 1973, in the first larger series of patients with CBD, Deodhar[25] observed that the lymphocytes from 21 of 35 patients (60%) receiving corticosteroid therapy would undergo blast transformation in the presence of beryllium salts. Similar responses were noted with beryllium sulfate and beryllium fluoride but no response was observed with magnesium or sodium sulfate. Later results from some of the same workers[26] showed a positive response in 57% of 47 patients. Using the uptake of tritiated thymidine for detecting lymphocyte transformation or proliferation, 21 of 26 patients (80%) had positive results (Jones-Williams and Williams, unpublished). Similar positive rates, 10 of 12 (83%), were reported from Denver.[27] However, in Philadelphia only 6 of 14 (42%) patients were positive,[4] and at the National Institutes of Health in Bethesda, Maryland, only 1 of 8 patients was positive.[28] Part of the discrepancy between these findings can be attributed to the use of different cutoff points to determine a positive test. Nevertheless, in all studies, a population of patients was identified that did not have evidence of cell-mediated immunity to beryllium.

Peripheral blood lymphocyte testing has also been done on healthy beryllium workers with weak positive reactions being observed in 6% of 571 workers in the United States,[26] and in less than 2% of 117 workers in the United Kingdom.[29] To date, none of these workers has developed CBD. One of 45 healthy beryllium workers near

Denver was also observed to have a false-positive result on blood lymphocyte testing[6] since repeat testing failed to confirm an initially positive result.

Macrophage migration inhibitory factor (MIF) is a secretory product of lymphocytes that is produced after immune stimulation. This reaction has been established as an in vitro test of cellular immunity.[30] Henderson[31] in 1972 showed that the lymphocytes from three patients with experimentally induced positive patch tests to beryllium would produce MIF after they were cultured with beryllium oxide. Marx[32] in 1973 observed that the peripheral blood from six of seven patients with CBD produced MIF, whereas MIF production was not observed from the blood of controls.

Thus, one in vivo (patch test) and two in vitro tests (blast transformation and MIF producton) demonstrated that a specific immunologic response to beryllium can occur in humans and in patients with CBD. The significance and importance of these immune responses remained uncertain because of the variation in the incidence of positive responses.[26,29,33] Was the immune response to beryllium of etiologic significance or just an epiphenomenon?

With the development of bronchoalveolar lavage, a new approach was available for analyzing the significance of the immune response in CBD. For the first time, cells from areas of active inflammation could be harvested and studied. The initial study[34] demonstrated that the inflammatory response in CBD was characterized by an increased recovery of T lymphocytes. In addition, the proliferative or blastogenic response of the lung cells to beryllium salts was greater than that of peripheral blood. This initial report was confirmed in Germany,[35] Japan,[36] and in two other centers in the United States.[27,28]

The positive response of the lung cells to beryllium salts may be a universal response to the lung cells from patients with chronic beryllium disease (Table 8-2). Fourteen patients with an unequivocal exposure to beryllium and evidence of granulomatous pulmonary disease had positive lung proliferation responses whereas six normal controls and 16 patients with sarcoidosis had negative lung proliferation responses.[4]

TABLE 8-2. Comparative Finding in Chronic Beryllium Disease (CBD), Sarcoidosis, and Hypersensitivity Pneumonitis

	CBD	SARCOIDOSIS	HYPERSENSITIVITY PNEUMONITIS
Lavage			
Lymphocytes	↑ ↑	↑	↑ ↑
T cells	↑ ↑	↑	↑ ↑
Helper cells (CD4+)	↑ ↑	↑	↓
Suppressor cells (CD8+)	↓	↓	↑
Be prolif.	↑ ↑	—	—
Pathology			
Granulomas	↑ ↑	↑ ↑	↑
Alveolitis	↑ ↑	↑	↑ ↑

In addition, test results were negative in four beryllium workers with biopsy evidence of non-beryllium disease. Finally, the problem of false-negative studies that plagued peripheral blood studies has not been observed. Lavage studies have demonstrated that CBD patients have evidence of an immune response to beryllium despite negative blood studies in some.[4,27,28]

Further evidence that also supported an immune basis for CBD was the observation that the bronchoalveolar lymphocytosis (see Table 8-2) was due to an accumulation of helper T cells (CD4+).[4] To further understand the immune processes in the lung in CBD, Saltini and associates[28] analyzed the properties of subpopulations of T cells from the lungs of patients with CBD. In eight patients with CBD, 57% of the lavage cells were lymphocytes. Of these lymphocytes, 87% were T lymphocytes and 66% were helper T (CD4+) lymphocytes. Only 18% of the lymphocytes were suppressor/cytotoxic (CD8+) T lymphocytes. When the CD4+ cells were separated from the CD8+ T cells, the CD4+ T cells were able to proliferate in response to beryllium salts, whereas the CD8+ T cells did not. In addition, when T-cell lines were generated from lung cells cultured with beryllium, all the T-cell lines generated were of the CD4+ T-cell phenotype. Thus, beryllium appeared to specifically stimulate CD4+ T lymphocytes.

Major histocompatibility complex (MHC) surface antigens are thought to play an important role in the presentation of antigen by macrophages to lymphocytes. Class I MHC antigens are thought to have the major role in presenting antigens to CD8+ cells while class II MHC antigens are thought to have the major role in presenting antigens to CD4+ cells. Monoclonal antibodies against class II MHC but not class I MHC could block the proliferative response of lung cells to beryllium.[28] In addition, blocking the interleukin-2 pathway with anti-IL2 also suppressed the proliferative response. These observations suggest that beryllium stimulates CD4+ T lymphocytes through normal immunologic signals and corroborates the assumption that beryllium functions as a hapten.

Although there is evidence for nonspecific increases in immunoglobulin production in CBD,[25] specific antibody production against beryllium has not been observed. Thus, CBD may have a unique importance as an immunologic disease in which only cell-mediated immunity is active.

Proposed Immunopathogenesis

From the above discussion, there seems to be little doubt that certain individuals can develop a cell-mediated immune response to beryllium and that this response has been associated with the development of a pulmonary granulomatous reaction. The pathogenesis of CBD might best be explained as follows (Table 8-3). Beryllium is first deposited in the lungs. Acting as a hapten, beryllium binds to some unknown proteins in the lung. CD4+ cells become sensitized and proliferate after beryllium is presented to them in association with class II antigens on the surface of macrophages. CD4+ cells then produce a variety of lymphokines that activate macrophages and accelerate their differentiation into epithelioid cells. These activated, differentiated macrophages are responsible for the production of angiotensin converting enzyme activity that can be measured in the blood of patients with CBD and also for the positive gallium scans. Because beryllium is poorly excreted and not metabolized, the immune response per-

TABLE 8-3. Immunopathogenesis of Chronic Beryllium Disease

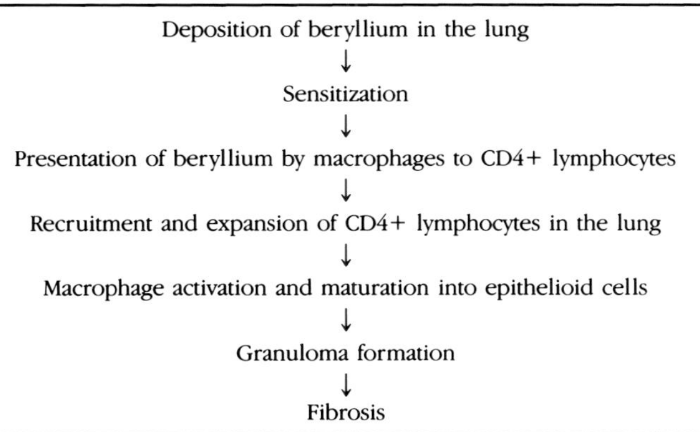

sists and granulomas develop. Epithelioid cells and lymphocytes within the granulomas produce fibrogenic factors, fibroblasts proliferate, and net collagen production is increased. Eventually, scarring and retraction may lead to a destroyed lung and respiratory failure.

However, this proposed pathogenesis does not explain the low incidence of CBD. There are two theories that could explain this. One is that only a small proportion of the population can become sensitized by beryllium. If enough beryllium is deposited in their lungs, these individuals will become sensitized to the metal and develop CBD. Support for this theory comes from animal studies that suggest a genetic predisposition for the ability to develop beryllium sensitization.[14]

A second hypothesis that could explain the low incidence of CBD is that the process of sensitization in the lung may be difficult. Normal lung cells demonstrate a poor antigen proliferation response compared with peripheral blood cells.[37,38] Sensitization in the lung may require a concurrent inflammatory event analogous to the effect of Freund's adjuvant in sensitizing animals. This second theory could explain several observations about CBD. First, the long latency period could be due to the difficulty of becoming sensitized by beryllium. Second, the occasional sudden onset of symptoms of CBD after a long latency period could reflect the onset of sensitization. Third, the difficulty of pulmonary sensitization could explain why a relatively high proportion of normals can develop skin sensitivity[19,31] but less than 5% of exposed beryllium workers develop CBD.[3] Finally, this second theory could explain the different incidences of CBD noted in several studies.[3,5,6] Lastly, it is important to realize that these two theories are not necessarily mutually exclusive.

Another important variable to consider in the immunopathogenesis of CBD is the route of sensitization. The above discussion focused on sensitization in the lung. Sensitization can also occur in the skin. These individuals would have evidence of blood proliferative responses to beryllium without any lung disease or granuloma. The reports in the literature[19,31] of experimentally produced positive patch tests indicate that this is possible. It is not known whether these individuals may be more or less likely to develop CBD. Their sensitization to beryllium could lead to accelerated removal of inhaled beryllium and decrease the likelihood of beryllium deposition in the lung. However, if these individuals were exposed to a quantity of beryllium sufficient to overload their ability to clear inhaled beryllium, an acute hypersensitivity reaction to beryllium could develop. This reaction could subsequently develop into CBD or clear if the immune response prevented the retention of beryllium in the lung.

Supporting the above hypothesis are recent observations in a patient who developed an insidious form of acute beryllium disease after exposure to soluble beryllium salts (Peuss O, personal communication). This patient developed an acute pulmonary reaction with a positive lung proliferative response to beryllium. After the patient was removed from further exposure to beryllium, the pulmonary infiltrates spontaneously cleared radiologically and, on repeat testing, the lung proliferative response to beryllium also reverted to normal. Thus, it is possible that this individual developed an acute hypersensitivity reaction to beryllium after exposure to soluble beryllium fumes (i.e., beryllium fluoride).

It is important to realize that the demonstration of an immune response to beryllium is not synonymous with chronic beryllium disease. Two beryllium workers have been described who had evidence of a positive lung proliferative response to beryllium, yet had no evidence of a pulmonary granulomatous disease.[27] For an immunopathologic reaction to occur, not only must there be the ability to respond to beryllium but beryllium must be present. Thus, the extent of the granulomatous inflammatory reaction will depend not only on the amount of beryllium deposited in the lungs but also on the vigor of the cell-mediated immune response to beryllium.

CLINICAL FEATURES

Symptoms usually develop insidiously in chronic beryllium disease. The first symptoms may not occur until months or years (up to 40 years) after the initial exposure to beryllium. Sudden exacerbations of pulmonary symptoms have been described and may follow surgery, pregnancy, respiratory infection, or re-exposure to beryllium. Dyspnea is the most common and often the only symptom. The next most frequent symptom is a nonproductive cough. This symptom can be most irritating and, on occasion, associated with the production of mucoid or purulent sputum; hemoptysis is rare. Fever, night sweats, malaise, anorexia, and weight loss usually develop in the setting of more advanced disease. Skin rashes and renal colic can also occur.

Individuals with mild CBD may appear completely normal on physical examination. However, fever, tachycardia, tachypnea, and dry crackles on chest auscultation can often be appreciated. In severe disease, central cyanosis, finger clubbing, and cor pulmonale may be present. Skin granulomas, which are indistinguishable from those found in sarcoidosis, can also be observed. Lupus pernio and erythema nodosum have not been seen.

A variety of roentgenographic abnormalities have been described.[39] The most common is disseminated small round or reticular opacities (Fig. 8-1). These opacities are usually symmetric but can be localized. Mild to moderate hilar adenopathy can be observed in one-third of cases but the large potato nodes that on occasion can be seen

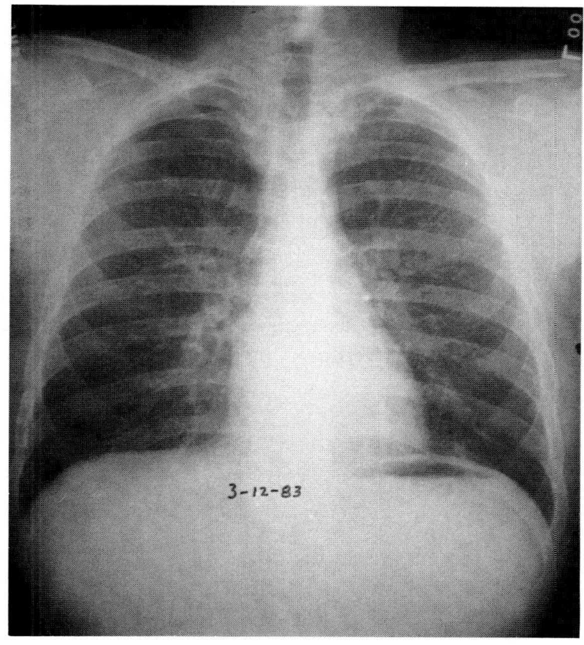

Figure 8-1. Chest radiograph of a 23-year-old beryllium oxide machinist. His first exposure to beryllium was 5 years previously. Pulmonary function revealed a vital capacity of 70% of predicted and a diffusing capacity of 60% of predicted. A gallium scan revealed diffuse uptake in the lung. The angiotensin converting enzyme level was normal. Biopsies of skin nodules and lung revealed noncaseating granulomas. Large amounts of beryllium were identified in lung biopsy samples. Beryllium caused a blood proliferative response; a year later beryllium induced a proliferative response in bronchoalveolar cells despite negative results on a blood study at that time. Diffuse small nodules are present on the chest radiograph. These nodules and the pulmonary function abnormalities cleared completely while the patient remained on corticosteroid therapy but returned whenever the therapy was discontinued.

in lymphoma or sarcoidosis have not been described in CBD (Fig. 8-2). On occasion, conglomerate nodules, linear scars, and pleural disease can occur.

The most common abnormalities observed by pulmonary function testing are a restrictive pattern and a diminished diffusing capacity.[4,39] At least one of these abnormalities is usually present in early disease. Late in the disease, when there is probable extensive destruction of the lung parenchyma, an obstructive pattern can be present.[40] Resting hypoxemia is often associated with a reduced diffusing capacity.

CBD has laboratory findings that resemble those of sarcoidosis. The angiotensin converting enzyme level is frequently elevated. Gallium scans of the lung will show increased uptake. Hypercalcemia and hypercalciuria have been reported. An elevated urinary level of beryllium is helpful for confirming a history of exposure to beryllium but is usually not useful in making the diagnosis of CBD, since most patients will have a normal urinary beryllium level.

HISTOPATHOLOGY

Chronic beryllium disease is characterized by noncaseating granulomas and a diffuse cellular infiltration of the interstitium. The cellular infiltrate consists of lymphocytes, plasma cells, and varying numbers of histiocytes. The histiocytes occur in groups

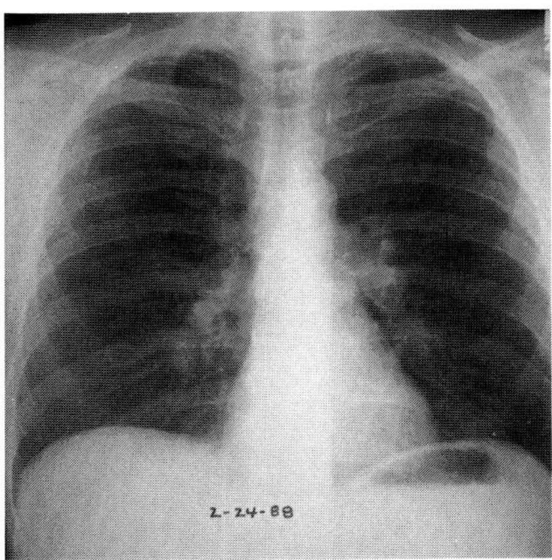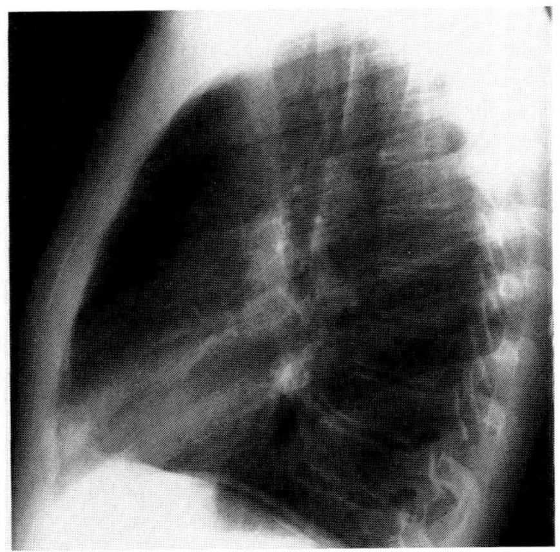

A   **B**

Figure 8-2. Posteroanterior (*A*) and lateral (*B*) chest radiographs of a 38–year-old former beryllium foundry worker. His exposure to beryllium began 17 years previously but symptoms of cough and shortness of breath only developed in the last 6 months. He was a cigarette smoker and had pulmonary function studies that demonstrated a vital capacity of 79% of predicted, residual volume of 161% of predicted, and an FEV_1/FVC of 68%. A diffusing capacity test could not be performed and he had a resting pO_2 of 63 torr. His angiotensin-converting enzyme level was elevated at 76.7 (nl < 52). Bronchoalveolar lavage revealed 23% lymphocytes. Beryllium did not induce a blood proliferative response but did induce a proliferative response in bronchoalveolar cells, a stimulation index of 19.8 (normal < 5.0). Transbronchial biopsy was inadequate. Bilateral hilar adenopathy is apparent on the radiograph. No parenchymal nodules were detected.

ranging from a few cells to large cell-demarcated granulomas. In their review of 124 cases of chronic beryllium disease, Freiman and Hardy[11] classified their cases into two main groups (Table 8-4). Group 1 consisted of 99 cases (80%) that had widespread cellular infiltration. In 55 of these cases granulomas were poorly formed or absent, and 44 had well-formed granulomas. Group 2 consisted of 25 cases that had predominantly well-formed granulomas with little cellular infiltration. The significance of this classification is that the patients with group 1 histology (absent or poorly formed granuloma) did poorly. Of the 53 patients for whom follow-up data were available, 45 died. In these patients, the mean life span from the time of diagnosis was 8.3 years.

The granulomas are scattered throughout the lung and can be found in subpleural, septal, peribronchial, and perivascular areas (Fig. 8-3). In addition, since beryllium is distributed throughout the body, granulomas can also be found in the spleen, liver, skin, and kidney. These granulomas are indistinguishable from the granulomas observed in sarcoidosis. However, recent studies using laser ion mass analysis (LIMA) identified beryllium within the granulomas in 13 of 14 patients with CBD.[41] Beryllium was not identified in specimens from seven cases of sarcoidosis, one case of tuberculosis, or two normal controls. However, beryllium was identified within the granuloma from two cases of coal workers' pneumoconiosis. The ultrastructural localization of

Figure 8-3. Transbronchial biopsy sample from a 53-year-old man who had worked in a beryllium plant for 30 years. His employment included chemical extraction, beryllium metal rolling, hot and cold beryllium copper rolling, health and safety inspection, and preventive maintenance inspection. His symptoms of cough and shortness of breath had only developed in the last 5 months. Results of pulmonary function studies, including diffusing capacity, were normal. The angiotensin converting enzyme level was also normal. Chest radiograph showed only slight upper lobe nodulation. Bronchoalveolar lavage revealed 20% lymphocytes with 67% T cells. Beryllium did not induce a blood proliferative response but did induce a proliferative response in bronchoalveolar cells, with a stimulation index of 19.1 (normal < 5.0). A well-formed granuloma with multinucleated giant cells and an area of alveolar exudate are evident.

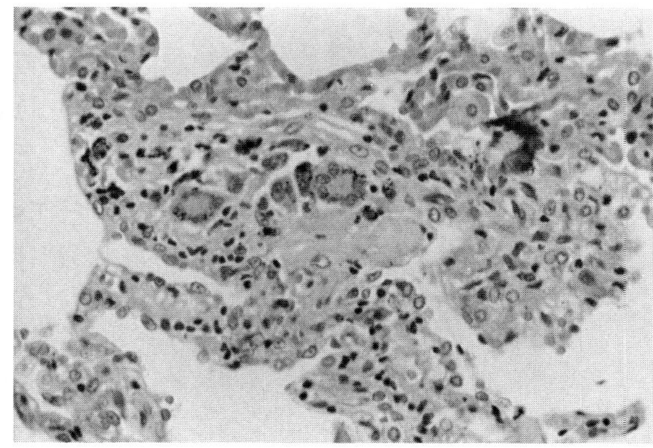

beryllium can be identified by energy-loss spectrometry.[42] This method was used to show that rat Kupffer cells accumulated beryllium phosphate particles within secondary lysosomes. The ultrastructural localization of beryllium within human tissues is unknown. These approaches, however, promise to increase our understanding of the pathogenesis of CBD.

A striking feature of the granuloma associated with beryllium disease is the calcific inclusions (Fig. 8-4). These calcifications have been termed conchoidal bodies, calcospherites, or Schaumann bodies. Characteristically, they appear as single or multiple, concentrically laminated bodies with a shell-like contour. Although these calcific inclusions usually occur within giant cells, they can also be found in extracellular locations.

Hyalinized nodules are also observed in about 33% of cases. These may be seen only occasionally or may be quite numerous. The etiology of these nodules is unknown. They consist of a narrow ring of fibrosis with a central core of hyaline. Ghosts

TABLE 8-4. Histologic Classification of Chronic Beryllium Disease

	1A	1B	2
Histology			
Interstitial infiltrates	Moderate to marked		Slight or absent
Granulomas	Few or absent	Well formed	Numerous and well formed
Calcific inclusions	Frequently present and numerous		Few or absent
Prognosis			
Percent survival	16	40	95

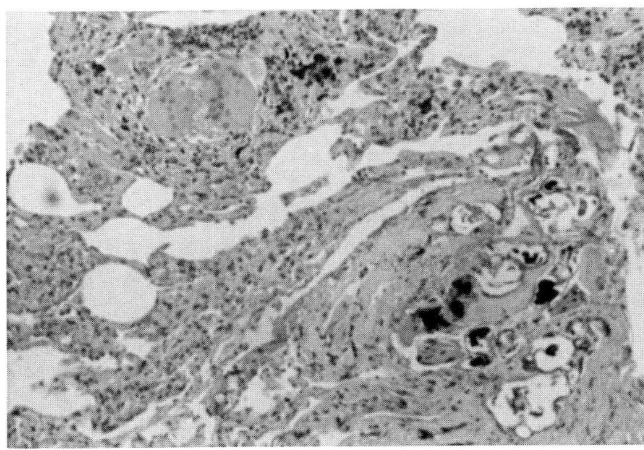

Figure 8-4. Another transbronchial biopsy sample from the same patient as in Figure 8-3. Well-formed granulomas, calcific densities within granulomas, and interstitial infiltrates are apparent.

of cells may be seen within the hyaline. These nodules are thought to represent a form of inflammatory exudate since granulomas can frequently be seen in the peripheral zones of the nodules. These nodules are not usually seen in sarcoidosis, and their presence suggests further evaluation for the possibility of CBD.[11]

DIAGNOSIS

Because the immune basis for CBD has only recently been demonstrated (see above), the diagnosis of CBD has traditionally been made using a variety of epidemiologic, clinical, and pathologic criteria. The criteria developed by the beryllium case registry have been most useful for identifying workers with CBD.[43] The case registry required a history or documentation of excessive exposure to beryllium and evidence of chronic lower respiratory tract disease (Table 8-5). Although none of the six criteria used by the beryllium case registry was specific for CBD, when used in combination the registry guidelines were helpful in differentiating most other lung disorders from CBD.

Documentation of exposure history can now be accomplished by three means. First, surveillance records can prove that a worker has been in an environment where

TABLE 8-5. Beryllium Case Registry Criteria for Inclusion of Cases

1. Evidence of significant beryllium exposure.
2. Clinical syndrome compatible with chronic lower respiratory tract disease.
3. Abnormal chest radiograph.
4. Abnormal pulmonary function tests with either obstructive or restrictive changes.
5. Histology consistent with chronic beryllium disease.
6. Evidence of elevated tissue levels of beryllium.

To be included in the beryllium case registry, a possible case must meet four of the six criteria, including at least no. 1 or no. 6.

the airborne beryllium concentration has been above the OSHA standards. Documentation requires the availability of recorded data indicating that within a specified period, the worker's environment did or was likely to contain excessive concentrations of beryllium. Unfortunately, it is frequently not possible to obtain this kind of technical information even if the worker has experienced such exposure.

A second means to document exposure to beryllium is by tissue analysis. In lieu of surveillance records, a positive beryllium analysis of a patient's tissue can provide evidence of exposure. However, the results of tissue analysis have been disappointing for several reasons. First, beryllium can be a normal contaminant of air and coal smoke, so the concentrations of beryllium detected in the lung, lymph nodes, or urine must be compared to normal values.[44] Second, an inexact relationship exists between beryllium levels in tissue or urine and the exposure history because beryllium is slowly excreted. Thus, certain patients with presumed CBD have had normal tissue beryllium levels. These normal levels do not prove the absence of exposure. Laser ion mass analysis (LIMA) appears to be a promising new technique for the detection of beryllium in small samples[41] and may help to resolve the problem of cases of CBD without abnormal amounts of beryllium in the lung. Nevertheless, elevated tissue levels of beryllium have been accepted as evidence of exposure. It must be emphasized, since a dose-response relationship has not been clearly demonstrated for CBD, that elevated beryllium levels in tissues or in urine alone cannot be considered as an indicator of disease, but only of exposure. Proof of this is that elevated beryllium levels were found in the urine of healthy beryllium workers and in the lung tissues of beryllium-exposed individuals who died of other causes but had normal lungs.

A third means to document exposure to beryllium is the demonstration of a hypersensitivity reaction to beryllium. A positive proliferative response of peripheral blood cells or lung cells to beryllium has been observed only in individuals exposed to beryllium.[4,6] Although it is possible to develop a positive skin test to beryllium after trivial skin exposures,[19] experience with proliferation testing suggests that a high stimulation index for blood or lung cells should be accepted as evidence of exposure to beryllium.

The second major criterion used by the beryllium case registry for the diagnosis of CBD was documentation of a clinical illness compatible with CBD (see Table 8-5). Presumptive evidence of pulmonary granulomatous disease was based on clinical, radiologic, and physiological criteria or compatible histology. At the time the case registry criteria were first developed, open lung biopsy was the only means available to obtain histologic samples. Thus, histologic evidence was not an absolute requirement to document the clinical disease. The safety of transbronchial biopsy and its high yield in sarcoidosis and CBD[4,27] now make this the procedure of choice for obtaining tissue in CBD. Because every patient with CBD should have a trial of corticosteroid therapy, it is always necessary to obtain tissue to rule out other (i.e., infectious) causes of pulmonary granulomas.

Thus, a probable diagnosis of CBD (Table 8-6) can be made using a modification of the classic criteria established by the beryllium case registry. This is based on the demonstration of pulmonary granulomas and a history or documentation of beryllium exposure. When the presumptive criteria for CBD are utilized, a beryllium worker with sarcoidosis may be mislabeled as having CBD. This mislabeling may have medical as

TABLE 8-6. Diagnosis of Chronic Beryllium Disease

A definite diagnosis of CBD requires:
1. Positive proliferative response of bronchoalveolar cells to beryllium
2. Histologic evidence of pulmonary granulomas
A probable diagnosis of CBD can be made if there is:
1. Histologic evidence of pulmonary granulomas
2. History of excessive exposure or documentation of exposure by:
   a. Positive blood proliferative response to beryllium
   b. Elevated urine beryllium levels
   or
   c. Elevated beryllium in lung or mediastinum

well as social and economic implications. Granulomatous involvement of certain organs (e.g., uveitis or carditis) may not be appreciated or investigated if a patient is labeled as having CBD rather than sarcoidosis. Therefore, any patient with a presumptive diagnosis of CBD should still have a complete evaluation for systemic involvement with sarcoidosis. Nevertheless, since the medical treatment of sarcoidosis and CBD (i.e., corticosteroid therapy) are so similar, there may be little difference in the medical management of these patients.

For the definite diagnosis of CBD (Table 8-6), a positive proliferative response of bronchoalveolar cells to beryllium may be sufficient.[4] However, two cases with a positive bronchoalveolar cell proliferative response to beryllium have been observed that had no evidence of granulomatous lung disease.[27] Whether these beryllium-sensitized individuals will develop CBD is uncertain. In addition, because the numbers of patients who have had proliferation testing is still relatively small (less than 50), a demonstration of granulomas should still be required for diagnosis. Thus, a definitive diagnosis of CBD requires the presence of pulmonary granulomas and evidence of a proliferative response of bronchoalveolar cells to beryllium.

THERAPY

As with any allergic or hypersensitivity disorder, the first therapeutic intervention should be the prompt removal of the worker from any environment where he or she can be further exposed to beryllium. This should be initiated as early as possible in the diagnostic work-up. Thus, any beryllium worker who is suspected of having CBD should be removed from the work environment until the diagnosis of CBD is either confirmed or ruled out. If the diagnosis of CBD is confirmed, the worker should not be allowed to enter any area where he or she might be exposed to beryllium. The OSHA standards were designed for the prevention of disease, but it is not known if these standards are sufficient to prevent exacerbations or progression of disease once an individual has become sensitized. However, workers have been successfully managed by placing them in locations in a beryllium plant where they will not have any significant exposure to respirable beryllium (Preuss O, personal communication).

Corticosteroids are the drugs of choice for the treatment of symptomatic CBD. Subclinical cases of CBD have been described. Because the natural history of subclinical CBD is not known, corticosteroids are not recommended for subclinical disease. However, for all other forms of the disease, corticosteroids are the only drugs that can alter the natural course of the disease. As in sarcoidosis, controlled trials documenting the beneficial effects of corticosteroids have not been performed. In contrast to corticosteroid therapy for sarcoidosis, one should assume that a lifetime of therapy will usually be required in patients with CBD because withdrawal of corticosteroids is associated with exacerbations of symptoms, progression of radiographic infiltrates, and progression of pulmonary function abnormalities. However, doses should be titrated to the lowest possible dose that will control the progression of the disease. On occasion, patients have been successfully withdrawn from corticosteroid therapy without progressive disease. The effectiveness of corticosteroid therapy in relieving symptoms probably relates to the proportion of active inflammation versus fibrosis that is contributing to the symptoms.

Supportive suplemental therapy should also be used, as in any chronic interstitial lung disorder. Immunizations should be offered for the prevention of influenza and pneumococcal infections. Oxygen therapy will improve arterial oxygen saturation and should be offered when the arterial oxygen saturation falls below 90%. In severe cases, right-sided heart failure may develop and should be treated in a conventional manner. While heart-lung transplantation has not been performed in any patient with CBD, if a patient with CBD had symptoms severe enough to warrant a transplantation, theoretically the procedure should be curative.

PROGNOSIS

Because so few cases of CBD are seen today, it is not known if the natural history of the disease has changed since the original description of the disease. At that time, environmental controls were nonexistent and cases may have represented a combination of acute and chronic beryllium disease. In addition, because the disorder was just being described, identified cases were more likely to represent advanced disease. In the best description of these cases,[11] patients with extensive interstitial infiltrates with poor granuloma formation had the worst prognosis (see Table 8-4). Patients with well-formed granulomas and little interstitial infiltrate had the best prognosis. Although this latter group contained less than 20% of the cases originally described, most cases described in the last decade appear to fall in this category. This is most encouraging, because 95% of these patients were still alive after a mean duration of illness of 11 years.

REFERENCES

1. VanOrdstrand HS, Hughes R, Carmody MG. Chemical pneumonia in workers extracting beryllium oxide: Report of three cases. Cleveland Clin 1943;10:10–18.
2. Hardy HL, Tabershaw IR. Delayed chemical pneumonitis occurring in workers exposed to beryllium compounds. J Indust Hygiene Toxicol 1946;28:197–211.

3. Eisenbud M, Lisson J. Epidemiological aspects of beryllium-induced nonmalignant lung disease: A 30 year update. J Occup Med 1983;25:196–202.

4. Rossman MD, Kern JA, Elias JA, Cullen MR, Epstein PE, Preuss OP, Markham TN, Daniele RP. Proliferative response of bronchoalveolar lymphocytes to beryllium. Ann Intern Med 1988;108:687–693.

5. Cullen MR, Kominsky JR, Rossman MD, Cherniack MG, Rankin JA, Balmes JR, Kern JA, Daniele RP, Palmer L, Naegel GP, McManus K, Cruz R. Chronic beryllium disease in a precious metal refinery: Clinical, epidemiologic and immunologic evidence for continuing risk from exposure to low-level beryllium fume. Am Rev Respir Dis 1987;135:201–209.

6. Kreiss K, Newman LS, Mroz MM, Campbell PA. Screening blood test identifies subclinical beryllium disease. J Occup Med 1989;31:603–608.

7. U.S. Department of Health Hazards and Safety. Public Health Service. Health hazard evaluation report. Atlanta: Centers for Disease Control, National Institute for Occupational Health and Safety, 1982. DHHS (NIOSH) Publication No. 82-024.

8. Beryllium disease among workers in a spacecraft manufacturing plant—California. MMWR 1983;32:419–425.

9. Rom WN, Lockey JE, Lee JS, Kimball AC, Bang KM, Leaman H, Johns RE, Perrota D, Gibbons HL. Pneumoconiosis and exposures of dental laboratory technicians. Am J Public Health 1984;74:1252–1257.

10. NIOSH recommendations for occupational safety and health standards. MMWR 1985;34:9s.

11. Freiman DG, Hardy HL. Beryllium disease. Hum Pathol 1970;1:25–44.

12. Sterner JH, Eisenbud M. Epidemiology of beryllium intoxication. Arch Indust Hygiene Occup Med 1951;4:123–157.

13. Barna BP, Deodhar SD, Chiang T, Gautam S, Edinger M. Experimental beryllium-induced lung disease I: Differences in immunologic responses to beryllium compounds in strains 2 and 13 guinea pigs. Int Arch Allergy Appl Immunol 1984;73:42–48.

14. Barna BP, Deodhar SD, Gautam S, Edinger M, Chiang T, McMahon JT. Experimental beryllium-induced lung disease II: Analysis of bronchial lavage cells in strains 2 and 13 guinea pigs. Int Arch Allergy Appl Immunol 1984;73:49–55.

15. Alekseeva OG. [Ability of beryllium compounds to produce delayed allergy]. Gidg Trud Prof Zabol 1965;11:20–25.

16. Alekseeva OG, Volkova AO, Ssvinkina NV. [Mechanism of action of beryllium on the organism]. Farmakol Toksikol 1966;3:353–355.

17. Cirla AM, Barbiano di Belgiojoso G, Chiappino G. [Hypersensitivity to compounds of beryllium: Passive transfer in guinea pigs with lymphoid cells]. Boll Ist Sieroter Milan 1968; 47:663–668.

18. Chiappino G, Cirla AM, Vigliani EC. Delayed-type hypersensitivity reactions to beryllium compounds. Arch Pathol 1969;87:131–140.

19. Curtis GH. Cutaneous hypersensitivity due to beryllium: A study of 13 cases. AMA Arch Dermatol Syph 1951;64:470–482.

20. Curtis GH. The diagnosis of beryllium disease with special reference to the patch test. Arch Indust Health 1959;19:150–153.

21. Stoeckle JD, Hardey HL, Weaver AL. Chronic beryllium disease. Am J Med 1969;46:545–561.

22. Jones Williams W, Nosworthy SE, Williams WR. UK beryllium case registry. In: Jones Williams W, Davies BH, eds. Eighth international conference on sarcoidosis and other granulomatous diseases. Cardiff, Wales: Alpha Omega Publishing Limited, 1980:771.

23. Sneddon IB. Berylliosis: A case report. Br Med J 1955;1:1488–1489.

24. Hanifin JM, Epstein WL, Cline MJ. In vitro studies of granulomatous hypersensitivity to beryllium. J Invest Dermatol 1970;55:284–288.

25. Deodhar SD, Barna B, VanOrdstrand HS. A study of the immunologic aspects of chronic berylliosis. Chest 1973;63:309–313.

26. Preuss OP, Deodhar SD, VanOrdstrand HS. Lymphoblast transformation in beryllium workers. In: Jones Williams W, Davies BH, eds. Eighth international conference on sarcoidosis and other granulomatous diseases. Cardiff, Wales: Alpha Omega Publishing Limited, 1980:711–714.

27. Newman LS, Kreiss K, King TE Jr, Seay S, Cambell PA. Pathologic and immunologic alteration in early stages of beryllium disease. Am Rev Respir Dis 1989;139:1479–1486.

28. Saltini C, Winestock K, Kirby M, Pinkston P, Crystal RG. Maintenance of alveolitis in patients with chronic beryllium disease by beryllium-specific helper T cells. N Engl J Med 1989;320:1103–1109.

29. Jones Williams W, Williams WR. Value of beryllium lymphocyte transformation tests in chronic beryllium disease and in potentially exposed workers. Thorax 1983;38:41–44.

30. Bloom BR, Bennett B. Mechanism of a reaction "in vitro" associated with delayed type hypersensitivity. Science 1966;153:80–82.

31. Henderson WR, Fukuyama K, Epstein WL, Spitler LE. In vitro demonstration of delayed hypersensitivity in patients with berylliosis. J Invest Dermatol 1972;58:5–8.

32. Marx JJ Jr, Burrell R. Delayed hypersensitivity to beryllium compounds. J Immunol 1973;111:590–598.

33. Price CD, Jones Williams W, Pugh A, Joynson DH. Role of in vitro and in vivo tests of hypersensitivity in beryllium workers. J Clin Pathol 1977;30:24–28.

34. Epstein PE, Dauber JH, Rossman MD, Daniele RP. Bronchoalveolar lavage in a patient with chronic berylliosis: Evidence for hypersensitivity pneumonitis. Ann Intern Med 1982;97:213–216.

35. Chihara J, Najai S, Fujmura N, Hirata R, Izumi T. Bronchoalveolar lavage lymphocyte findings in chronic beryllium disease. Am Rev Respir Dis 1983;127(suppl):64.

36. Buhl R, Rust M, Bargon J, Kronenberger H, Bergmann L, Meier-Sydow J. Cytologic and immunologic findings in bronchoalveolar lavage and peripheral blood of a patient with chronic beryllium disease. Presented at Chronic Beryllium Disease: A Diagnostic Workshop, May 8, 1986, Cleveland, OH.

37. Lipscomb MF. The alveolar macrophage: Role in antigen presentation and accessory cell function. In: Daniele RP, ed. Immunology and immunologic diseases of the lung. Cambridge, MA: Blackwell Scientific, 1988:79–96.

38. Ferro TJ, Kern JA, Elias JA, Kamoun M, Daniele RP, Rossman MD. Alveolar macrophages, blood monocytes and density-fractionated alveolar macrophages differ in their ability to promote lymphocyte proliferation to mitogen and antigen. Am Rev Respir Dis 1987;135:682–687.

39. Aronchick JM, Rossman MD, Miller WT. Chronic beryllium disease: Diagnosis, radiographic findings, and correlation with pulmonary function tests. Radiology 1987;163:677–682.

40. Andrews JL, Kazemi H, Hardy HL. Pattern of lung dysfunction in chronic beryllium disease. Am Rev Respir Dis 1969;100:791–800.

41. Jones Williams W, Kelland D. New aid for diagnosing chronic beryllium disease (CBD): Laser ion mass analysis (LIMA). J Clin Pathol 1986;39:900–901.

42. Dinsdale D, Bourdillon AJ. The ultrastructural localization of beryllium in biological samples by electron energy-loss spectrometry. Exp Molec Pathol 1982;36:396–402.

43. Sprince NL, Kazemi H. Beryllium disease. In: Rom W, ed. Environmental and occupational medicine. Boston: Little Brown, 1983;481–490.

44. Colby TV. Berylliosis. In: Churg A, Green FHY, eds. Pathology of occupational lung disease. New York: Igaku Shoin, 1988;73–87.

9

Vasculitides of the Polyarteritis Nodosa Group

Craig A. Wolfe
Gary W. Hunninghake

The polyarteritis nodosa group of systemic vasculitides includes classic polyarteritis nodosa, allergic angiitis and granulomatosis (Churg-Strauss syndrome), and the "overlap syndrome."[1-5] Each disorder can affect virtually any organ system. As a result, a myriad different clinical presentations can occur. For this reason, the predominant findings and symptoms in a given patient depend on the type and extent of vascular involvement in specific tissues. Localized inflammation and ischemia distal to vasculitic lesions are the two major processes by which involvement of specific organ systems is expressed. In this review, we will focus on classic polyarteritis nodosa and the overlap syndrome, since Churg-Strauss syndrome is covered in another chapter.

Polyarteritis nodosa (PAN) was first reported in 1852 when von Rokitansky[6] described a case with characteristic findings. The term "periarteritis nodosa" was originated by Kussmaul and Maier in 1866, when they described a 27-year-old man with symptoms of a systemic vasculitis, including fever, abdominal pain, renal disease, and peripheral neuropathy.[7] Palpable nodules noted at branching points of medium-sized muscular arteries resulted in the addition of "nodosa." Ferrari noted, in 1903, that these nodules were the result of aneurysmal, transmural vascular inflammation and coined the currently used term, "polyarteritis nodosa."[8] Zeek, in 1948, further classified PAN into two subgroups, classic or macroscopic polyarteritis nodosa and hypersensitivity or microscopic polyarteritis nodosa. The latter syndrome is also referred to as the overlap syndrome.[9,10]

Classic polyarteritis nodosa was described as a segmental necrotizing process affecting medium-sized muscular arteries and showing a predilection for bifurcations of vessels. Small vessels are not involved in the disease process. Lesions at various stages of development may be present. Hypertension, renal artery aneurysms, and infarcts are frequent complications of classic polyarteritis nodosa,[11] whereas glomerulonephritis is rarely seen. Classic polyarteritis, as originally described, is much less common than the overlap syndrome.

234

The overlap syndrome is, in many ways, similar to both hypersensitivity vasculitis, which affects smaller arteries, arterioles, and veins, and classic PAN, which affects larger vessels only. Renal lesions in the overlap syndrome may be characterized by a focal necrotizing glomerulonephritis, as well as hypertension, renal artery aneurysms, and infarcts. The diagnosis may be complicated by the fact that many diseases, such as Henoch-Schönlein purpura, Goodpasture's disease, cryoglobulinemia, and poststrepto-coccal glomerulonephritis, may present with renal and other organ lesions that clinically resemble those of PAN.

Polyarteritis nodosa is an uncommon disease, with an annual incidence of about 0.7 per 100,000.[12] It is less common than other disorders that may be associated with vasculitis, such as systemic lupus erythematosus, scleroderma, or polymyositis. The mean age of onset is in the fifth decade of life, although persons of any age may be affected. There is a 2.5:1 male predominance.[1] Five-year survival in untreated PAN may be as low as 13%.[1,13,14]

Due to the wide variety of organ systems that may be affected, the presenting signs and symptoms of PAN are many and varied. Nonspecific signs and symptoms, such as weight loss, fatigue, fever, and malaise are seen in more than half of the patients.[1] PAN frequently presents as a confusing picture of fever associated with evidence of multi-system disease. The manifestations may be mild, chronic, or rapidly fatal. The most frequently affected organ systems are the kidneys, the heart, and the nervous and gas-trointestinal systems. The most negative prognostic indicators are involvement of the gastrointestinal and renal sytstems. Peripheral neuropathy and hypertension do not pre-dict survival.[15]

MANIFESTATIONS OF PAN IN VARIOUS ORGAN SYSTEMS

Pulmonary Manifestations

Classic PAN does not involve the lung. However, more than half of patients with the overlap syndrome demonstrate pulmonary involvement.[4,16,17] Pulmonary vasculitis is documented in 54% of patients[4] and in this group chest radiographic abnormalities are common (Fig. 9-1).[4,18] Chest radiographic abnormalities include diffuse interstitial in-filtrates, nodules with or without cavitation, transient diffuse patchy infiltrates, and dif-fuse alveolar infiltrates, which are usually due to alveolar hemorrhage (Fig. 9-2).[4,19,20]

Renal Manifestations

The renal system is most frequently affected by PAN, and renal failure is the most important cause of morbidity and mortality.[1,21,22] Renal involvement may be limited to medium-sized muscular arteries or may be predominantly manifested as a necrotizing glomerulonephritis. It is not uncommon, as noted above, for both types of disease to be present in the same patient.

Acute lesions, in larger vessels, are characterized by polymorphonuclear cell in-filtrates that are segmental and occur more frequently at branching points. These le-sions may be limited to the intima and media, with associated intimal denudation and

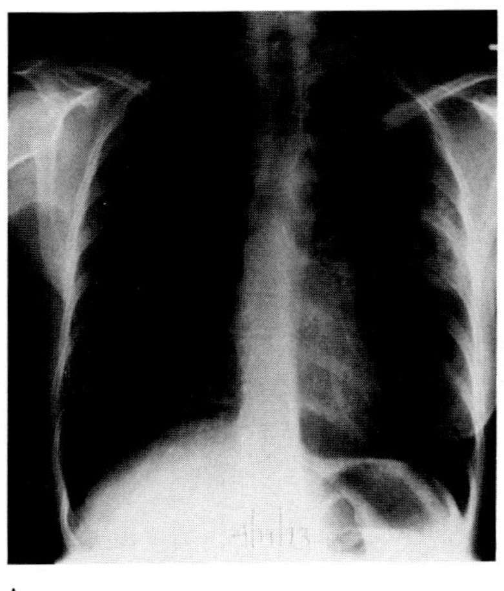

A

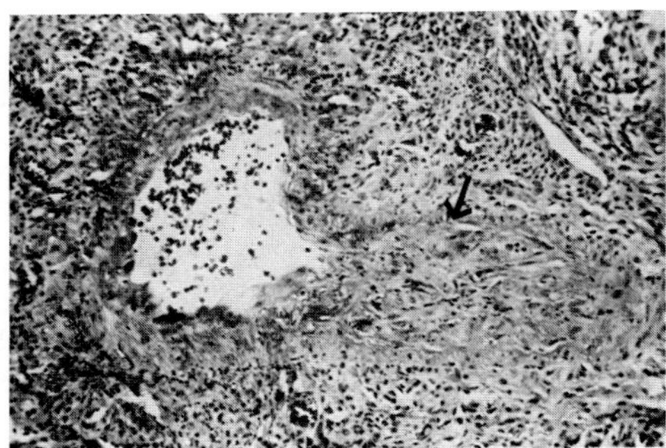

B

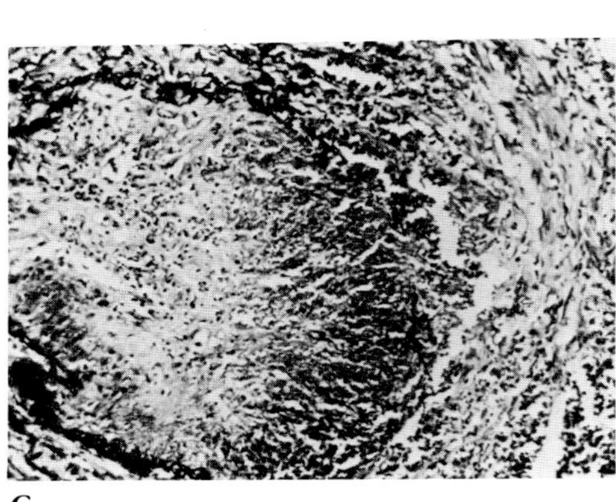

C

Figure 9-1. Polyarteritis nodosa. (*A*) Chest radiograph of a patient with PAN reveals a patchy alveolar left upper lung infiltrate. (*B*) Low-power micrograph of pulmonary tissue from the same patient reveals perivascular inflammation with aneurysm formation (*arrow*). (*C*) High-power micrograph of pulmonary tissue reveals perivascular inflammation and partial destruction of the elastic lamina.

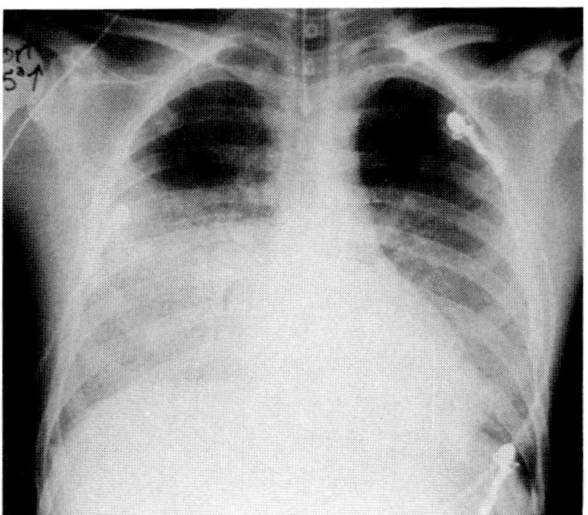

A

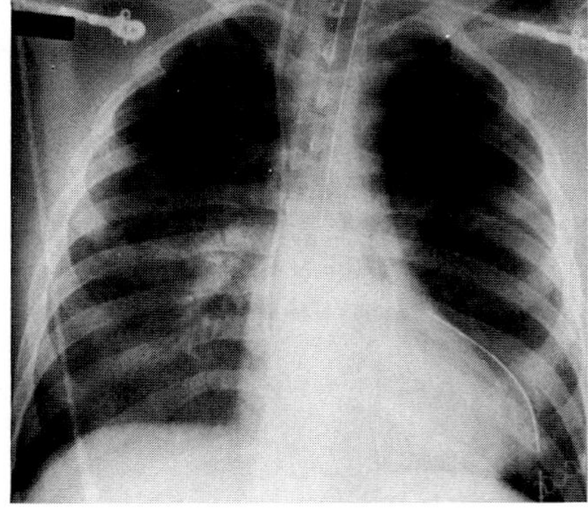

B

Figure 9-2. Polyarteritis nodosa. Chest radiograph of a patient with PAN reveals a diffuse alveolar infiltrate (*A*), which partially resolves after 2 days (*B*).

fibrinoid necrosis, or they may exhibit transmural involvement. Immunoglobulin is infrequently detected in the walls of involved renal vessels, either by immunofluorescence or by electron microscopy.[23] As the lesions mature, mononuclear cells become more prominent and intimal proliferation with fibrinoid necrosis may lead to vascular thrombosis, resulting in distal ischemia. The end result of this process may be infarction, aneurysm formation, or vascular obliteration. When only smaller vessels are involved, all lesions tend to be of similar age.[23] They tend to be circumferential rather than segmental. Glomerulonephritis is a common complication in this setting. When there is diffuse involvement of smaller vessels, in addition to larger vessels, the prognosis is usually poor—worse than that of the classic disease.

The clinical effects of renal involvement are mediated through several pathologic processes. These include the local effects of the vasculitis (i.e., glomerulonephritis), ischemia distal to obstructing vasculitic lesions, hemorrhage secondary to the rupture of aneurysms or in infarcted tissue, systemic hypertension due to renal hypoperfusion, and uremia due to end-stage disease.

Abnormal urine sediment or renal function is found in 70% of patients with PAN. Hypertension is the most frequent sign of renal involvement and is seen in 60% of cases, followed by proteinuria in 60% of cases, oliguria in 50% of cases, and hematuria in 40% of cases.[1,24] Hypertension may be due to renal vascular obliteration, which results in increases in circulating levels of renin and aldosterone.[1] Consequently, the hypertension may persist despite resolution of the vasculitis and cause further nonvasculitic renal damage. Renal function, however, tends to stabilize or improve in patients who survive the acute illness. In one series, only 3 of 26 patients with PAN and renal involvement required chronic dialysis.[21] Aneurysm rupture or renal infarction may result in pain, gross hematuria, retroperitoneal hemorrhage, or signs of acute blood loss.

Cardiac Manifestations

Cardiac involvement in PAN was first reported in 1866 by Kussmaul and Maier in their description of a young man with coronary arteritis and symptoms of a systemic vasculitis.[7] Cardiac involvement may be present in more than half of the patients with PAN,[9,22,25] but symptomatic cardiac disease occurs less frequently.[22]

Morphologic abnormalities in the heart usually consist of arteritis of intramural and extramural coronary arteries, myocardial infarction, pericarditis, and hypertensive cardiomyopathy.[22] Vasculitic lesions of PAN typically involve small subpericardial vessels just as they enter the myocardium. Lesions may represent active or healed disease. Active cardiac disease is associated with increased mortality. Some of this increased mortality is due to the associated increase in systemic disease activity, however, since not all of the deaths in these patients are cardiac in origin.[22] Histologically, inflammation of the vascular media and adventitia are characteristic.[22] Advanced lesions may show transmural vascular necrosis, with occlusion and aneurysm formation.[22,26]

Clinically, cardiac involvement in PAN may result in myocardial infarction, cardiac arrhythmias, pericarditis, or congestive heart failure. Pericarditis may result from direct involvement of the pericardium or from damage to adjacent myocardial tissue, or it may be a sequela of renal failure with uremia. Cardiac arrhythmias have several etiologies. The disease may damage the conducting system or cause "irritable foci" in the myocardium. Nutrient arteries that supply the sinoatrial and atrioventricular nodes are often affected by PAN, explaining the supraventricular origin of most arrhythmias seen in this disease.[25,27]

Congestive heart failure may also be due to direct myocardial damage or to fluid overload following renal failure.[9,25,27] The electrocardiogram is abnormal in up to 85% of patients with PAN. The most frequent abnormalities are nonspecific ST–T wave changes and sinus tachycardia out of proportion to body temperature.[9]

Nervous System Manifestations

80% of patients with PAN exhibit evidence of either central or peripheral nervous system involvement.[28,29] Peripheral involvement is more frequent than central involvement and usually occurs earlier in the course of the disease.[28,29,30] In the majority of cases, vascular lesions cause axonal degeneration of the wallerian type—that is, degeneration of both the axon and the myelin sheath distal to the lesion.[31] Four patterns of neuropathy may occur: mononeuritis multiplex; extensive mononeuritis; cutaneous neuropathy; and polyneuropathy.[29]

Mononeuritis multiplex, the most common pattern,[1,28,29,31] consists of motor or sensory deficits in the distribution of one or more peripheral nerves. Extensive mononeuritis with flaccid motor weakness and multimodality sensory loss in the extremities is the next most common type of presentation. One or more extremities may be involved, with the lower extremities usually being affected more severely. Cutaneous neuropathy consists of areas of hypesthesia or paresthesia in the distribution of small cutaneous nerves.

Central nervous system involvement occurs in approximately 40% of patients with PAN. It is usually a late complication, often occurring 2 to 3 years after the initial diagnosis of the disease.[29] Two general patterns of presentation of central nervous system disease occur: diffuse disease and focal or multifocal disease.[28,29] Diffuse disease in the form of encephalopathy is common and may be associated with focal or generalized seizures.[1,28,29,32,33] Electroencephalography usually reveals diffuse slowing.[28,29] Computed tomograms of the head, brain scans, and analysis of the cerebrospinal fluid usually yield normal results. However, cerebrospinal fluid analysis may reveal increased protein levels or white blood cell counts. Red blood cells may be seen in the cerebrospinal fluid when subarachnoid hemorrhage is present.[28,29,33] Other manifestations of central nervous system disease include meningoencephalitis, vascular parkinsonism, and psychiatric disturbances.[33–36] Although the spinal arteries may be affected, the spinal cord is rarely involved.[37]

Focal disease is frequently acute in onset, and the result of ischemic or hemorrhagic stroke.[29] These manifestations are usually cerebral in location but may affect the cerebellum or brainstem.[28] With therapy, most nervous system deficits resolve in a period of days to weeks.[29] Residual deficits are more frequent in the lower extremities and are usually sensory rather than motor.[28]

Ocular Manifestations

A long list of ocular manifestations of PAN has been compiled. The reported frequency of ocular involvement ranges from 1% to 20%.[38,39] The plexiform structure and extensive network of collaterals in the vascular supply to the eye may serve to minimize the frequency of ocular manifestations. Injury may result from the effects of systemic hypertension or from vasculitic lesions.[39] Ocular complications are usually late sequelae of PAN,[38] but they may be presenting complaints.[39]

The most frequently affected structures of the eye are the choroidal and posterior ciliary arteries.[39,40] Involvement may result in choroidal insufficiency, infarcts, or retinal detachment.[38,39,41] Choroidal insufficiency may, in turn, lead to transient ischemic attacks.[39] Peripheral nervous system disease may result in multiple forms of ocular dysfunction, including extraocular muscle palsies,[28,39] homonymous hemianopsia, amaurosis, nystagmus, and Horner's syndrome.[28] Involvement of the optic nerve may result in papilledema, papillitis, and decreased visual acuity.[28,39] Both anterior and posterior ischemic optic neuropathy have been reported.[38,39] Orbital disease may produce exophthalmos or pseudotumor, which may be a presenting complaint.[39] Corneoscleral changes include keratitis, necrotizing scleritis and episcleritis, and corneal and scleral ulcerations. Iritis and anterior uveitis are uncommon.[28,39] Other ocular complications of PAN include central retinal artery and vein occlusion,[40,42] retinal hemorrhages, exudates and cotton wool spots,[40] and retinal artery irregularities and aneurysms.[40]

Testicular Manifestations

The testes and epididymis are frequently involved in patients with PAN, but clinical symptoms are rare.[2,3,43] Autopsy studies with careful analysis of the testes reveal involvement in up to 86% of patients.[1,3,44] Clinical presentations include orchitis and epididymitis, which are seen in 2% to 18% of patients with PAN.[13,44] In light of the frequency of involvement of the testes at autopsy, testicular biopsy has been proposed as a diagnostic procedure. However, due to the limited amount of tissue available by this route, a firm diagnosis is established in only 20% of patients. For this reason, testicular biopsy should be reserved for patients with clinical symptoms.[1,43]

Musculoskeletal Manifestations

The musculoskeletal system is involved in approximately 75% of patients with PAN.[45] Myalgias and weakness are common presenting symptoms, and muscle biopsy is a useful means of establishing the diagnosis. Histologic changes of PAN in muscle consist of perivascular inflammatory infiltrates with minimal coincident inflammation of muscle fibers. This differs from polymyositis, in which both vessels and muscle fibers reveal marked inflammation.[46] Likewise, the homogeneity of the muscle damage seen in PAN separates it from the patchy involvement that is characteristic of polymyositis.[46] The vascular lesions that are seen in muscle in PAN resemble those seen with rheumatoid arthritis.[46]

The causative mechanism for the muscle damage seen in PAN is unclear, but it may be due to ischemic damage distal to occluded vessels or to denervation of the muscle tissue.[46] Electromyographic changes are minimal and frequently not helpful in making a diagnosis.[47]

Among the common clinical sequelae of these processes are arthralgia, weakness, and arthritis. Arthritis is rarely destructive and occurs less frequently than arthralgia.[45] Lower extremity claudication due to proximal vascular compromise, periosteal bone formation, and soft tissue swelling have also been reported in patients with PAN.[47,48] Although most musculoskeletal symptoms resolve with therapy, pain due to periostitis frequently persists.[47]

Gastrointestinal Manifestations

Up to 85% of patients with PAN exhibit some evidence of gastrointestinal tract involvement. This may range from mild chronic abdominal pain to acute onset of a surgical abdomen. Gastrointestinal disease usually appears in concert with other evidence of systemic vasculitis.[49]

Histologic changes in the gastrointestinal tract consist of a characteristic infiltration of polymorphonuclear cells into the vascular wall. This infiltration is rarely documented on endoscopic biopsy, which usually detects only nonspecific inflammation.[49] Intramucosal hemorrhage, suggestive of a vasculitic process, may be seen, however. The lack of utility of endoscopic biopsy may simply reflect the fact that small and medium-sized arteries, those most affected by PAN, are located more deeply in the intestinal mucosa and are, therefore, not accessible. Direct visualization by endoscopy is currently the best method of evaluating the extent of disease.[49]

Clinically, PAN of the gastrointestinal tract may manifest itself as abdominal pain due to serosal inflammation or perforation of an abdominal viscus, diarrhea due to inflammation or ischemia, or liver disease.[49–51] Ischemic disease most often affects the small intestine or colon.[52,53] Ischemic colitis may be associated with abdominal pain, nonbloody diarrhea, perforation, or pseudomembrane formation.[53] Mortality approaches 100% in patients who suffer intestinal infarction.[52,54] Other complications include intraperitoneal hemorrhage, hemorrhage into the lumen of an abdominal viscus,[55] pancreatic abscess formation,[56] spontaneous splenic rupture,[57,58] intraparenchymal rupture of hepatic artery aneurysms,[55] mural ulceration or perforation in ischemic areas, and massive intraperitoneal hemorrhage secondary to rupture of visceral artery aneurysms.[18,59] Hemorrhage into the peritoneal cavity carries a high mortality rate and is an indication for emergency surgical exploration. If the patient is sufficiently stable, a preoperative angiogram may help to confirm the diagnosis and identify the source of bleeding.[50] PAN may present as an acute abdomen and mimic acute appendicitis, cholecystitis, salpingitis, pancreatitis, or small bowel obstruction.[18,59–61] It may also affect the liver directly, leading to parenchymal artery aneurysms, abnormal results on liver function studies, and nodular regenerative hyperplasia in the absence of cirrhosis.[50,51,62] PAN of the gastrointestinal tract may be indistinguishable from primary ulcerative colitis, ischemic colitis, or Crohn's disease.[49,63] These diseases share many pathologic and clinical characteristics, which accounts for the similarity of their clinical presentations.

Skin Manifestations

The frequency of skin involvement in PAN is unclear, as reports have cited frequencies ranging from 5% to 56%.[1,64–69] The most common skin manifestations in this disease are nonspecific purpura or a maculopapular rash.[1,64] Other manifestations include nodules, ecchymosis, edema, livedo reticularis, and ulcerations. Nodules are the most characteristic lesion for PAN but occur in only 15% to 25% of cases.[1,64,65] Nodules tend to occur in waves, lasting from days to months before resolution. They may be palpated along the course of an artery.[1,65] Nodules may be single or multiple, are tender to palpation, and may pulsate. They are more frequent on the lower extremity, where the overlying skin may be shiny and atrophic.[1,64,65] The skin over these nodules may ulcerate. Ecchymoses may result from subcutaneous hemorrhage or, more rarely, rupture of subcutaneous aneurysms.[64,65]

Edema occurs at some time during the course of the disease in 50% of patients with PAN. It may be a result of renal or cardiac dysfunction.[64] Livedo reticularis is a network of red-blue mottling that is usually seen on the lower extremities but which may involve the entire body surface.[1,65,67] It may occur in normal individuals as a result of exposure to cold.[64] In PAN, the pattern is probably due to compromise of blood flow.[64] The production of livedo reticularis is a chronic process and indicates the disease has entered a chronic phase.[64]

Ulceration may occur in areas of acute ischemia in skin or over subcutaneous nodules.[64,65] Ulcerations may have a characteristic "punched-out" circumference with necrotic-appearing tissue in the center. They are usually small and occur most frequently on the lower extremities.[65]

PATHOGENESIS

The pathogenesis of PAN remains unclear. It is generally accepted that immune complex deposition in vessel walls triggers the disease process.[1,4,69–74] However, direct evidence of damage to vessel walls from the deposition of immune complexes is lacking.

That immune complexes might cause PAN is suggested by the following observations: circulating immune complexes have been identified in the sera of patients with PAN.[71,75–81] The presence of circulating immune complexes roughly correlates with disease activity.[71,80] It is not always possible, however, to demonstrate immune complexes in tissue.[78,82] There are several factors that may influence whether immune complexes are found in patients with PAN. First, different assays measure different types of immune complexes. Polyethylene glycol precipitation detects total immune complexes, whereas other assays, such as conglutinin-anticonglutinin precipitation, measure only complexes that bind complement.[78] A variety of studies suggest that there are different types of immune complexes in patients with PAN.[71,73,78] The timing of sampling for immune complexes also has a marked effect on the results of these studies. For example, animal studies have shown that immune complexes are only transiently found in the blood following exposure to relevant antigen.[83] In humans, immune complexes are also quickly removed from the bloodstream by reticuloendothelial cells or granulocytes.[72,73,83]

Other studies also suggest that immune complexes trigger the vasculitis in PAN. These include a number of animal studies, using serum sickness as a model,[83,85–87] which show that immune complexes can cause vasculitis. In addition to circulating immune complexes, immune complexes are detected in reticuloendothelial cells of patients with PAN. These contain immunoglobulin, complement, and antigen in about the same proportions as circulating immune complexes.[88] Hypocomplementemia usually occurs when immune complexes are present in the circulation,[71,78,88,89] and the presence of complement in vessel walls suggests that immune complexes triggered the deposition of these proteins.[71,78,88] Consistent with the animal models of vasculitis, some studies have shown that immune complexes are present in vessel walls during acute disease and that they are decreased as the disease becomes more chronic.[73] Finally, an association has been suggested between PAN and diseases such as hepatitis B antigenemia,[75–78,80,81,88,90–93] hairy cell leukemia,[94–98] serous otitis media,[99,100] and methamphetamine abuse.[93,101] Immune complexes in these diseases may contain relevant antigen, such as hepatitis B viral antigens.[75] However, the presence of immune complexes in tissue does not always cause detectable disease since, at autopsy, studies have shown that immune complexes may be deposited in glomeruli of patients with hepatitis B without evidence of vasculitis.[84]

Positive hepatitis B serologies have been reported in up to 68% of patients with PAN.[30,75,88] HB_sAg immune complexes have also been identified in the sera of patients with PAN.[30,75,77] Circulating immune complexes composed of HB_sAg and HB_sAb, as well as deposits of similar composition in the reticuloendothelial cells of more than 70% of patients with hepatitis B, have been reported.[88] Deposits of similar composition to the HB_sAg/Ab complexes were found on autopsy in the spleen and lymph nodes of five of seven patients with clinically diagnosed PAN.[88] Large deposits of material with similar composition to HB_sAg/Ab immune complexes have also been identified in vessel walls of patients with PAN. Not all investigations, however, have noted such a high incidence of hepatitis B infection. Nevertheless, the presence of these deposits in acute lesions, their gradual diminution with time, and their absence in healed lesions also suggest a role for HB_sAg/Ab immune complexes in some patients with this disease.[88]

Hairy cell leukemia is a disease of B cells that has also been linked to PAN. Asplenia and pancytopenia are often present and may affect the patient's ability to clear circulating immune complexes.[98] Evidence for a role of immune complexes in this disorder is also indirect. An alternative mechanism of vasculitis in this disease may involve direct toxicity to vessel walls by leukemic cells. The leukemic cells may directly invade vessel walls.[98] A monoclonal antibody has identified a common antigen on the surface of the leukemia cells, endothelial cells, and epidermal basal cells.[102] Thus, hairy leukemia cells may also initiate an immune response that crossreacts with vessel walls, leading to vasculitis.[98]

Many of the findings of PAN could be attributed to vasculitic lesions mediated by immune complexes. The proposed mechanism would involve deposition of circulating immune complexes in the walls of blood vessels in susceptible areas. This would be enhanced by an increase in vascular wall permeability, which would allow localization of the immune complexes within the vessel wall. The increased permeability might result from the release of vasoactive substances from platelets or activated basophils. In conjunction with complement, immune complexes would cause the generation of chemotactic factors that would result in the infiltration of vessel walls by polymorphonuclear leukocytes. Localized vascular damage and inflammation would result, leading to further recruitment of other inflammatory cells, such as mononuclear cells.

Many of the mechanisms by which immune complexes could cause damage were elucidated using animal models of the Arthus reaction.[83] In the classic Arthus reaction, an experimental animal is exposed to a foreign antigen, resulting in production of antibody to that antigen. After 10 to 14 days, the animal is re-exposed to the antigen, causing formation of immune complexes. This results in the development of a syndrome consisting of arthritis, glomerulonephritis, and vasculitis.[103]

Certain characteristics of immune complexes affect their pattern of deposition and their ability to cause vascular damage. These include the size of the complex and the ratio of antigen to antibody. The ability of immune complexes to fix complement, and thus to cause inflammation, is inversely related to the proportion of antigen present in the complex.[86] The most damaging complexes are those formed in a slight antigen excess.[104] As the relative amount of antigen rises, the ability to fix complement decreases. When the antigen concentration reaches three to six times equivalence, the ability of the immune complexes to cause inflammation by activating the complement cascade is markedly reduced.[86] The larger, more insoluble complexes, however, may trigger a granulomatous process in the vessels. Deposition appears to be independent of the charge on the complex or of complement activation.[1] Thus, it is clear that immune complexes can cause a variety of types of vasculitis, including both granulomatous and nongranulomatous vasculitis.

Inflammatory cells are activated by exposure to immune complexes or complement proteins activated by immune complexes.[83,85] This results in the production of toxic compounds by the cells. In the polymorphonuclear leukocyte there are two major types of toxins. The first is a family of oxygen free radicals, including superoxide ion, O_2^-; hydrogen peroxide, H_2O_2; singlet oxygen; and hypochlorous ion, HOCL.[105] In addition to the oxygen free radicals, proteolytic enzymes are released from intracellular granules into the extracellular space. These enzymes and oxygen free radicals are toxic to cells, increase membrane permeability, and destroy the connective tissues of the vessel wall. The end result of these changes is aneurysm formation or obliteration of the vascular lumen or both.[106,107]

DIAGNOSIS

There are no laboratory tests that are diagnostic for PAN. An increased erythrocyte sedimentation rate, anemia, thrombocytosis, proteinuria, and red blood cells casts in the urine are suggestive of PAN but may be seen in any systemic vasculitis as well as in many malignancies or infections. Confirmation of the diagnosis depends on appropriate demonstration of typical lesions (Fig. 9-3) in various tissues.[70] This tissue may be obtained from easily accessible areas of involvement, including the skin, muscle, testicles, or sural nerve. Biopsy of muscle near symptomatic subcutaneous nodules less than 6 months old has a sensitivity of 50% and a specificity of 100%.[108] The kidney and liver are alternative biopsy sites, but biopsy of these sites may result in an increased rate of complications.

When visceral involvement is suspected, angiography may be used. Findings of areas of vascular narrowing and multiple intraparenchymal aneurysms are virtually pathognomic for PAN. Aneurysms of the renal, hepatic, splenic, mesenteric, and cerebral arteries have also been reported.[109] Other modalities, such as computed tomography and ultrasonography may aid in the diagnosis of parenchymal infarcts, hypoperfusion, and hemorrhage. Malignant or infectious processes, however, may yield a similar picture.[110]

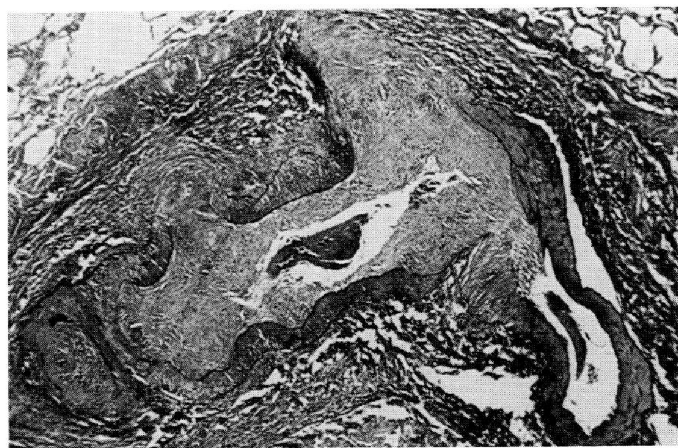

Figure 9-3. Polyarteritis nodosa. Photomicrograph of pulmonary blood vessel displays thrombosis and a complicated aneurysm.

TREATMENT

A reasonable treatment approach is to initiate prednisone therapy at a dosage of 1 mg/kg/day. Corticosteroids, alone, however, have improved 5-year survival to only 50%, while the combination of corticosteroids and cyclophosphamide have improved survival to 90% at 5 years.[111] Cyclophosphamide, therefore, should also be initiated in a single dose of 1.5 to 2 mg/kg/day. Rapidly progressive or severe disease may be treated with intravenous cyclophosphamide at a dosage of 4 mg/kg/day for the first 3 days, followed by an oral dose of 1.5 to 2 mg/kg/day. Since cyclophosphamide does not exert significant effects for 2 to 3 weeks, the dosage of corticosteroids is usually not decreased for the first 6 weeks. If the disease stabilizes, the dosage of prednisone is decreased to an alternate-day regimen (usually 15 mg to 20 mg, every other day). The doses of cyclophosphamide are monitored by measuring total white blood cell and granulocyte counts, which should be maintained above 3,000 cells/mm^3 and 1,500 cells/mm^3, respectively. Doses of cyclophosphamide adjusted in this manner are not associated with an increased incidence of opportunistic infections.[1] Adverse effects of cyclophosphamide, in addition to marrow suppression, include hemorrhagic cystitis, alopecia, gonadel and ovarian dysfunction, and predisposition to malignant disease.[1,111] The duration of therapy depends on the clinical course in each patient. Cyclophosphamide is continued for at least 1 year following complete disease remission.[112] Patients who relapse following discontinuation of therapy may be successfully retreated with the same regimen. When therapy is discontinued because of side effects, azathioprine or chlorambucil may be used.[111]

REFERENCES

1. Cupps TR, Fauci AS. In: Lloyd H, Smith MD Jr, eds. The vasculitides. Philadelphia: WB Saunders, 1981:211.
2. Kitridou RC. Polyarteritis and related disorders. In: Katz W, ed. Rheumatic diseases: Diagnosis and management. Philadelphia: JB Lippincott, 1977:1057.
3. Alarcon-Segovia D. Clinics in rheumatic diseases. In: Alarcon-Segovia D, ed. The necrotizing vasculitides. Philadelphia: WB Saunders, 1980:241.

4. Leavitt RY, Fauci AS. Pulmonary vasculitis. Am Rev Resp Dis 1986;134:149.
5. Fulmer JD, Kaltreider HB. The pulmonary vasculitides. Chest 1982;82:615.
6. Von Rokitansky C. Über einige der wichtigsten krankheitin der arterien. Denkscher d k Akad d Wissensch 1852;4:49.
7. Kussmaul A, Maier K. Über eine bischer nicht beschreibens eigenthümliche arterienerkrankung (periarteritis nodosa), die mit morbus brightii und rapid fortschreitender allgemeiner muskellähmung einhergeht. Deutsches Arch Klin Med 1866;1:484.
8. Ferrari E. Über polyarteritis acuta nodosa (sogenannte periarteriitis nodosa) und ihre beziehungen zur polymyositis und polyneuritis acuta. Beitr Pathol Anat 1903;34:350.
9. Holsinger DR, Osmundson PJ, Edwards JE. The heart in periarteritis nodosa. Circulation 1962;25:610.
10. Hunninghake GW, Fauci AS. Pulmonary involvement in the collagen vascular diseases. Am Rev Resp Dis 1979;119:471.
11. Zeek PM. Periarteritis nodosa and other forms of necrotizing angiitis. N Engl J Med 1953;248:764.
12. Kurland LT, Hauser WA, Ferguson RH, Holley KE. Epidemiologic features of diffuse connective tissue disorders in Rochester, MN, 1951–1967, with special reference to systemic lupus erythematosus. Mayo Clin Proc 1969;44:649.
13. Frohnert PP, Sheps SG. Long-term follow-up study of periarteritis nodosa. Am J Med 1967;43:8.
14. Coward RA, Hamdy NAT, Shortland JS, Brown CB. Renal micropolyarteritis: A treatable condition. Nephrol Dial Transplant 1986;1:31.
15. Cohen RD, Conn DL, Ilstrup DM. Clinical features, prognosis, and response to treatment in polyarteritis. Mayo Clin Proc 1980;55:146.
16. Zeek PM, Smith CC, Weeter JC. Studies on periarteritis nodosa. III: The difference between the vascular lesions of periarteritis nodosa and hypersensitivity. Am J Pathol 1948;24:889.
17. Fauci AS, Haynes BF, Katz P. The spectrum of vasculitis: Clinical pathologic, immunologic, and therapeutic considerations. Ann Intern Med 1978;89:660.
18. McCauley RL, Johnston MR, Fauci AS. Surgical aspects of systemic necrotizing vasculitis. Surgery 1985;97(1):104.
19. Leatherman JW, Davies SF, Hoidal JR. Alveolar hemorrhage syndromes: Diffuse microvascular lung hemorrhage in immune and idiopathic disorders. Medicine (Baltimore) 1984:63,343–361.
20. Mark EJ, Ramirez JF. Pulmonary capillaritis and hemorrhage in patients with systemic vasculitis. Arch Pathol Lab Med 1985:109;413–418.
21. Adu D, Howie AJ, Scott DGI, Bacon PA, McGonigle RJS, Michael J. Polyarteritis and the kidney. Q J Med 1987;62(239):221.
22. Schrader ML, Hochman JS, Bulkley BH. The heart in polyarteritis nodosa: A clinicopathologic study. Am Heart J 1985;109:1353.
23. D'Agati V, Chander P, Nash M, Mancilla-Jimenez R. Idiopathic microscopic polyarteritis nodosa: Ultrastructural observations on the renal vascular and glomerular lesions. Am J Kidney Dis 1986;7:95.
25. James TN, Birk RE. Pathology of the cardiac conducting system in polyarteritis nodosa. Arch Intern Med 1966;117:561.
26. Cassling RS, Lortz JB, Olson DR, Hubbard TF, McManus BM. Fatal vasculitis (periarteritis nodosa) of the coronary arteries: Angiographic ambiguities and absence of aneurysms at autopsy. J Am Coll Cardiol 1985;6:707.
27. Thiene G, Valente M, Rossi L. Involvement of the cardiac conducting system in panarteritis nodosa. Am Heart J 1978;95:716.
28. Moore PM, Cupps TR. Neurological complications of vasculitis. Ann Neurol 1983;14:155.
29. Moore PM, Fauci AS. Neurologic manifestations of systemic vasculitis. Am J Med 1981;71:517.
30. Goeke DJ, Hsu K, Morgan C, Bombardieri S, Lockshin M, Christian CL. Association between polyarteritis and australia antigen. Lancet 1970;ii:1149.

31. Vital A, Vital C. Polyarteritis nodosa and peripheral neuropathy. Acta Neuropathol (Berlin) 1985;67:136.
32. Prescott JE, Johnson JE, Dice WH. Polyarteritis nodosa presenting as seizures. Ann Emerg Med 1983;12:642.
33. Smith C, Rae SA, Berry H. Polyarteritis nodosa presenting as meningoencephalitis. R Soc Med 1987;80:704.
34. Mayo J, Arias M, Leno C, Berciano J. Vascular parkinsonism and periarteritis nodosa. Neurology 1986;36:874.
35. Weddington WW Jr, Cook EH, Denson MW. Periarteritis nodosa mimicking an affective disorder. Psychosomatics 1986;27:449.
36. Rogers C, Paranassus W, Noguchi TT. Suicide in a patient with undiagnosed periarteritis nodosa. Am J Forensic Med Pathol 1987;8:51.
37. Ojeda VJ. Polyarteritis nodosa affecting the spinal cord arteries. Aust NZ J Med 1983;13:287.
38. Hutchinson CH. Polyarteritis nodosa presenting as posterior ischemic optic neuropathy. J R Soc Med 1984;77:1043.
39. Morgan CM, Foster CS, D'Amico DJ, Gragoudas ES. Retinal vasculitis in polyarteritis nodosa. Retina 1986;6:205.
40. Leung ACT, McLay A, Boulton-Jones JM. Polyarteritis presenting with thrombocytosis and central retinal vein thrombosis. Scott Med J 1987;32:024.
41. Saraux H, Laroche L, Foels A, Martin-Gousset D. Ischemic algue posterieure du nerf optique. J François d'Ophthalmol 1982;5:167.
42. Ford RG, Siekert RG. Central nervous system manifestations of periarteritis nodosa. Neurology 1965;15:114.
43. Wright LF, Bicknell SL. Systemic necrotizing vasculitis presenting as epididymitis. J Urol 1986;136:1094.
44. Dahl EV, Baggenstoss AH, Deweerd JH. Testicular lesions of periarteritis nodosa with special reference to diagnosis. Am J Med 1960;28:222.
45. Ferreiro JE, Saldana MJ, Azevedo SJ. Polyarteritis manifesting as calf myositis and fever. Am J Med 1986;80:312.
46 Matsubara S, Mair WGP. Ultrastructural changes of skeletal muscles in polyarteritis nodosa and in arteritis associated with rheumatoid arthritis. Acta Neuropathol (Berlin) 1980;50:169.
47. Golding DN, Letcher RGM. Polyarteritis involving the lower limbs associated with periosteal new bone formation. Br J Hosp Med 1986;36:59.
48. Meredith GS, Mitnick HJ, Burstin HE, Zimmerman SS. Polyarteritis nodosa presenting with migratory soft tissue swelling. NY State J Med 1987;87:402.
49. Camilleri M, Pusey CD, Chadwick VS, Rees AJ. Gastrointestinal manifestations of systemic vasculitis. Q J Med 1983;206:141.
50. Sellke FW, Williams GB, Donovan DL, Clarke RE. Management of intra-abdominal aneurysms associated with periarteritis nodosa. J Vasc Surg 1986;4:294.
51. Ahmed HA, Arulambalam KJ, Nickols CD. Polyarteritis nodosa of the liver: A case report and review of the literature. Mater Med Pol 1986;18:231.
52. Buffo GC, Deitch JS. Pneumatosis intestinalis in a patient with polyarteritis nodosa. Gastrointest Radiol 1986;11:286.
53. Lee EL, Smith HJ, Miller GL, Burns DK, Weiner H. Ischemic pseudomembranous colitis with perforation due to polyarteritis nodosa. Am J Gastrol 1984;79:35.
54. Karp DR, Kantor OS, Halverson JD, Atkinson JP. Successful management of catastrophic gastrointestinal involvement in polyarteritis nodosa. Arthritis Rheum 1988;31:683.
55. Alleman MJA, Janssens AR, Spoelstra P, Kroon HMJA. Spontaneous intrahepatic hemorrhages in polyarteritis nodosa. Ann Int Med 1986;105:712.
56. Hadary A, Haskel Y, Nissan S. Pancreatic abscess complicating periarteritis nodosa. Am J Gastroenterol 1986;81:501.

57. Fallinborg J, Laustsen J, Jakobsen J, Winther P, Svanholm H. Atraumatic rupture of the spleen in periarteritis nodosa. Acta Chir Scand 1985;151:85.
58. Ford GA, Bradley JR, Appleton DS, Thiru S, Calne RY. Spontaneous splenic rupture in polyarteritis nodosa. Postgrad Med J 1986;62:965.
59. Harvey MH, Neoptolemos JP, Fossard DP. Abdominal polyarteritis nodosa: A possible surgical pitfall? Br J Clin Pract 1984;38:282.
60. Lombard CM, Moore MH, Seifer DB. Diagnosis of systemic polyarteritis nodosa following total abdominal hysterectomy and bilateral salpingo-oophorectomy: A case report. Int J Gyn Pathol 1986;5:63.
61. Piette JC, Bourgault I, Legrain S, et al. Systemic polyarteritis nodosa diagnosed at hysterectomy. Am J Med 1987;82:836.
62. Nakanuma Y, Ohta G, Sasaki K. Nodular regenerative hyperplasia of the liver associated with polyarteritis nodosa. Arch Pathol Lab Med 1984;108:133.
63. Silvermann MH. Polyarteritis nodosa associated with ulcerative colitis. J Rheumatol 1984;11:377.
64. Lyell A, Church R. The cutaneous manifestations of polyarteritis nodosa. Br J Dermatol 1954;66:335.
65. Belisario JC. Cutaneous manifestations in polyarteritis (periarteritis) nodosa. Arch Dermatol 1960;82:526.
66. Gilliam JN, Smiley JD. Cutaneous necrotizing vasculitis and related disorders. Ann Allergy 1976;37:328.
67. Reeves A, Bresnihan B. Clinical features, treatment and outcome of polyarteritis nodosa. Ir J Med Sci 1987;156:90.
68. Leung ACT, McLay A, Mosley H, Boulton Jones JM. Polyarteritis group of systemic vasculitis: New diagnostic criteria. Scott Med J 1985;30:225.
69. Alarcon-Segovia D, Brown AL. Classification and etiologic aspects of necrotizing angiitides. Mayo Clin Proc 1964;39:205.
70. Conn DL. Update on systemic necrotizing vasculitis. Mayo Clin Proc 1989;64:535.
71. Leib ES, Hibrawi H, Chia D, Blaker RG, Barnett EV. Correlation of disease activity in systemic necrotizing vasculitis with immune complexes. J Rheumatol 1981;8:258.
72. Dreisin RB. Lung diseases associated with immune complexes. Am Rev Respir Dis 1981;124:738.
73. Conn DL, McDuffie FC, Holley KE, Schroeter AL. Immunologic mechanisms in systemic vasculitis. Mayo Clin Proc 1976;51:511.
74. Henson PM, Daniele RP. Immune complex injury of the lung. Am Rev Resp Dis 1981;124:739.
75. Trepo CG, Zuckerman AJ, Bird RC, Prince AM. The role of circulating hepatitis B antigen/antibody immune complexes in the pathogenesis of vascular and hepatic manifestations in polyarteritis nodosa. J Clin Pathol 1974;27:863.
76. Gooke DJ, Hsu K, Morgan C, Bombardieri S, Lockshin M, Christian CL. Vasculitis in association with Australia antigen. J Exp Med 1971;134:330S.
77. Prince AM, Trepo C. Role of immune complexes involving SH antigen in pathogenesis of chronic hepatitis and polyarteritis nodosa. Lancet 1971;i:1309.
78. Gupta RC, Kohler PF. Identification of HB$_s$Ag determinants in immune complexes from hepatitis B virus–associated vasculitis. J Immunol 1984;132:1223.
79. Van de Pette JEW, Jarvis JM, Wilton JMA, MacDonald DM. Cutaneous periarteritis nodosa. Arch Dermatol 1984;120:109.
80. Fye KH, Becker MJ, Theofilopoulos AN, Moutsopoulos H, Feldman J, Talal N. Immune complexes in hepatitis B antigen–associated periarteritis nodosa. Am J Med 1977;62:783.
81. Gupta RC. Characterization of antigen moiety of Hb$_s$Ag in the complement fixing immune complexes of hepatitis B virus positive chronic active hepatitis. Clin Exp Immunol 1982;49:543.

82. Ronco P, Verroust P, Mignon F, et al. Immunopathological studies of polyarteritis nodosa and Wegener's granulomatosis: A report of 43 patients with 51 renal biopsies. Q J Med 1983;206:212.

83. Cochrane CG, Weigle WO, Dixon FJ. The role of polymorphonuclear leukocytes in the initiation and cessation of the Arthus vasculitis. J Exp Med 1959;110:481.

84. Sutherland JC, Markham RV Jr, Mardiney MR Jr. Subclinical immune complexes in the glomeruli of kidneys postmortem. Am J Med 1974;57:536.

85. Kniker WT, Cochrane CG. Pathogenic factors in vascular lesions of experimental serum sickness. J Exp Med 1965;122:83.

86. Scherzer H, Ward PA. Lung injury produced by immune complexes of varying composition. J Immunol 1978;121:947.

87. Kniker WT, Cochrane CG. The localization of circulating immune complexes in experimental serum sickness. J Exp Med 1968;127:119.

88. Michalak T. Immune complexes of hepatitis B surface antigen in the pathogenesis of periarteritis nodosa. Am J Pathol 1978;90:619.

89. Lewis EJ, Schur PH, Busch GJ, Galvanek E, Merrill JP. Immunopathologic features of a patient with glomerulonephritis and pulmonary hemorrhage. Am J Med 1973;54:507.

90. Duffy J, Lidsky MD, Sharp JT, et al. Polyarthritis, polyarteritis and hepatitis B. Medicine (Baltimore) 1976;55:19.

91. Sergent JS, Lockshin MD, Christian CL, Goeke DJ. Vasculitis with hepatitis B antigenemia. Medicine (Baltimore) 1976;55:1.

92. Trepo CG, Magnius LO, Schaefer RA, Prince AM. Detection of e antigen and antibody: Correlations with hepatitis B surface and hepatitis B core antigens, liver disease, and outcome in hepatitis B infections. Gastroenterology 1976;71:804.

93. Koff RS, Widrich WC, Robbins AH. Necrotizing angiitis in a methamphetamine user with hepatitis B: Angiographic diagnosis, five month follow-up results and localization of bleeding site. N Engl J Med 1973;288:946.

94. Lie JT. Isolated polyarteritis of testis in hairy-cell leukemia. Arch Pathol Lab Med 1988;112:646.

95. Krol T, Robinson J, Bekeris L, Messmore H. Hairy cell leukemia and a fatal periarteritis nodosa-like syndrome. Arch Pathol Lab Med 1983;107:583.

96. Elkon KB, Hughes GRV, Catovsky D, et al. Hairy cell leukemia with polyarteritis nodosa. Lancet 1979;ii:280.

97. Lowe J, Russell NH. Cerebral vasculitis associated with hairy cell leukemia. Cancer 1987;60:3025.

98. Gabriel SE, Conn DL, Phyliky RL, Pittelkow MR, Scott RE. Vasculitis in hairy cell leukemia: Review of literature and consideration of possible pathogenic mechanisms. J Rheumatol 1986;13:1167.

99. Sergent JS, Christian CL. Necrotizing vasculitis after acute serous otitis media. Ann Intern Med 1974;81:195.

100. Thomson JG, Karsh J. Polyarteritis nodosa presenting as serous otitis media in a patient receiving hyposensitization therapy. J Rheumatol 1986;13:958.

102. Posnett DN, Marboe CC, Knowles DM, Jaffe EA, Kunkel HG. A membrane antigen (HCl) selectively present on hairy cell leukemia cells, endothelial cells, and epidermal basal cells. J Immunol 1984;132:2700.

103. Dixon FJ, Vazquez JJ, Weigle WO, Cochrane CG. Pathogenesis of serum sickness. Arch Pathol 1958;65:18.

104. Ishizaka K, Ishizaka T, Campbell DH. Biological activity of soluble antigen-antibody complexes. J Immunol 1959;83:105.

105. Weiss SJ. Tissue destruction by neutrophils. N Engl J Med 1989;320:365.

106. Hay EA. Collagen and embryonic development. In: Hay E, ed. Cell biology of extracellular matrix. New York: Plenum Press, 1981:379–409.

107. Vracko R. Basal lamina scaffold: Anatomy and significance for maintenance of orderly tissue structure. Am J Pathol 1974;77:314.
108. Dahlberg PJ, Lockhart JM. Diagnostic studies for systemic necrotizing vasculitis. Arch Intern Med 1989;149:161.
109. Herschman A, Blum R, Lee YC. Angiographic findings in polyarteritis nodosa. Radiology 1970;94:147.
110. Hekali P, Kivisaari L, Standeitskjold-Nordenstam CG, Pajari R, Turto H. Renal complications of polyarteritis nodosa: CT findings. J Comp Assist Tomog 1985;9:333.
111. Leavitt RY, Fauci AS. Therapeutic approach to the vasculitic syndromes. Mt Sinai J Med 1986;53:440.
112. Fauci AS, Katz P, Haynes BF, Wolff SM. Cyclophosphamide therapy of severe systemic necrotizing vasculitis. N Engl J Med 1979;301:235.

10
Wegener's Granulomatosis

Richard A. DeRemee

Vasculitis is a fascinating subject. As the term implies, the simplest definition is inflammation of blood vessels. However, leaving the definition at such a primitive level is not helpful to the clinician who must deal with these often difficult problems. Thus, we must attempt to refine what we mean by vasculitis. Were there a unifying etiologic agent or pathogenic mechanism, our nosologic task would be greatly simplified. Wolfe and Hunninghake, elsewhere in this volume, discuss a number of hypotheses that have been raised concerning etiology and pathogenesis, but there are few concrete data in this regard. For the time being, we must rely on the construction of clinicopathologic syndromes in attempting to create order out of chaos.

A good beginning point is to determine whether or not the vasculitis in question is a local phenomenon or generalized and systemic in character. In the case of localized lesions, these may be encountered at sites of local trauma or immunologic challenge, such as a tuberculin skin test, a cut and abrasion complicated by secondary infection, an insect bite, or the lesion of erythema nodosum, as well as other examples. The consequences of such localized lesions are minor and ephemeral.

In contrast, generalized or systemic vasculitis holds the patient in peril of vital organ dysfunction or death. Among those patients having systemic vasculitis, there are a number of features that allow subgroupings to be made. These features include the kind and size of vessels involved, the nature of the inflammatory reaction, major organ systems affected, accompanying or pre-existing clinical syndromes (particularly the so-called collagen vascular diseases), and the presence of positive results for certain serologic blood tests. The purposes of classification are to (1) aid in recognition of a disease characterized by vasculitis; (2) allow an approximate prognostication regarding clinical course and outcome; and (3) direct proper treatment.

It is hoped that patients sharing a number of common features that allow them to be classified into specific diagnostic groups, as for instance Wegener's granulomatosis, Churg-Strauss syndrome, Behçet's syndrome, or other specific designations, share common etiologies or pathogenesis. When the specific etiology and pathogenesis have been discovered, treatment can be specifically directed or measures can be taken to prevent the disease in the first place.

I have taken this length in introducing the subject so as to dispel any illusions that terms such as Wegener's granulomatosis, Churg-Strauss syndrome, polyarteritis nodosa, and others have any immutable meaning. It could well be that the clinicopathologic syndrome of Wegener's granulomatosis, for instance, may be further subdivided or eliminated altogether when final data are available concerning etiology and pathogenesis. Thus, when one encounters patients with vasculitis, the features of which do not clearly conform to one of the well-established but admittedly arbitrary categories, it should not confound the observer, for it is clear we are groping for understanding. But then again, our syndromic constructions may be cogent, having ultimate etiologic meaning. Time will tell.

HISTORICAL PERSPECTIVES

We must return to the mid-19th century to find the progenitors of Wegener's granulomatosis. The famous German pathologist von Rokitansky[1] published, in 1852, perhaps the earliest description of what Kussmaul and Maier[2] subsequently called periarteritis nodosa in their classic paper of 1866. Today, the term polyarteritis nodosa seems to be preferred over the earlier one. Kussmaul and Maier described a 27-year-old man with fever and nephritis, in addition to intense muscular pain and weakness, who followed a rapidly deteriorating course to death within a few weeks. Subcutaneously in the anterior chest and abdomen were palpable pea-sized nodules, which on microscopic examination represented nodular aneurysmal inflammation of the arteries—hence the term "periarteritis nodosa." Similar widespread involvement was found in the arteries subserving the intestines, stomach, kidneys, heart, and voluntary muscle. Nodular lesions similar to those discovered subcutaneously were also seen in the substance of the voluntary muscle.

For approximately 70 years, periarteritis nodosa was the model of and the chief diagnosis given to cases of systemic vasculitis. Occasionally, isolated reports would appear delineating cases of vasculitis having features atypical for periarteritis nodosa. In 1931, Klinger[3] reported two cases with vasculitis involving the lung and spleen, unusual sites for periarteritis nodosa. The first case also had a granulomatous reaction in the upper airway. Klinger referred to these cases as *Grenzformen* (borderline forms) of periarteritis nodosa. Analysis of the first case, in retrospect, strongly suggests Wegener's granulomatosis.

Friedrich Wegener (Fig. 10-1) must be given credit for recognizing key differences in the detailed analyses of three patients he reported first in 1936[4] and again in greater detail in 1939.[5] These patients had in common necrotizing granulomas chiefly affecting the upper airways but also found in the lungs and major bronchi, together with focal necrotizing glomerulitis and systemic vasculitis resembling periarteritis nodosa. He was of the opinion that the anatomic locations in the upper and lower respiratory tracts and the prominent necrotizing granulomatous response were critical differences from the traditional conception of periarteritis nodosa. Wegener used the term "rhinogenic

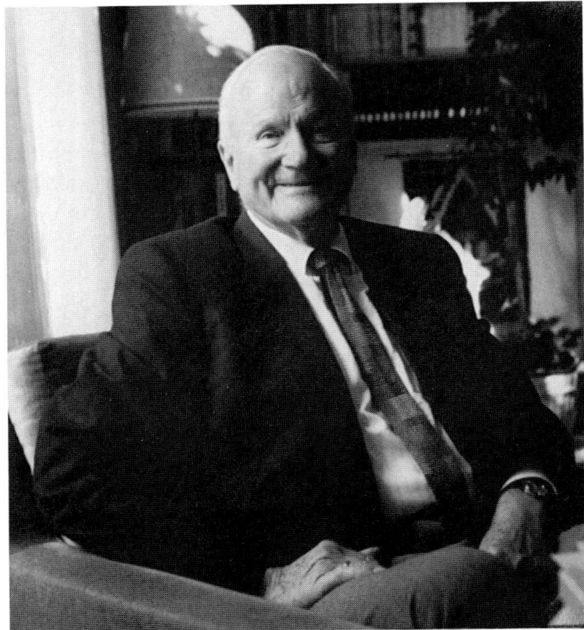

Figure 10-1. Dr. Friedrich Wegener, age 82, in his home in Lübeck, Federal Republic of Germany, October 1988. (used with permission of Dr. Wegener)

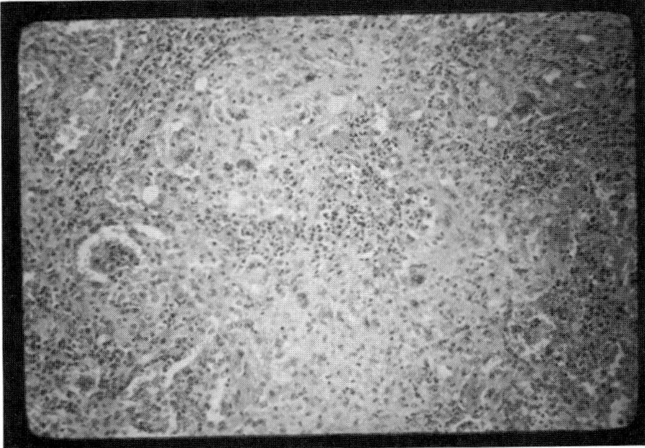

Figure 10-2. Necrotizing granuloma on biopsy of nasal mucosa.

granulomatosis" to designate these patients. Godman and Churg[6] in 1954 published their analysis of seven more cases, setting down criteria for the diagnosis of what they called "necrotizing respiratory granulomatosis and angiitis," giving Wegener due credit for the initial observations. The criteria they set down were three: (1) necrotizing granulomas of the upper or lower respiratory tract or both (Fig. 10-2); (2) generalized focal necrotizing vasculitis involving both arteries and veins, and almost always in the lungs and disseminated to other sites in various degrees; (3) focal necrotizing glomerulitis (Fig. 10-3). These three criteria have come to be called Wegener's triad. It was common

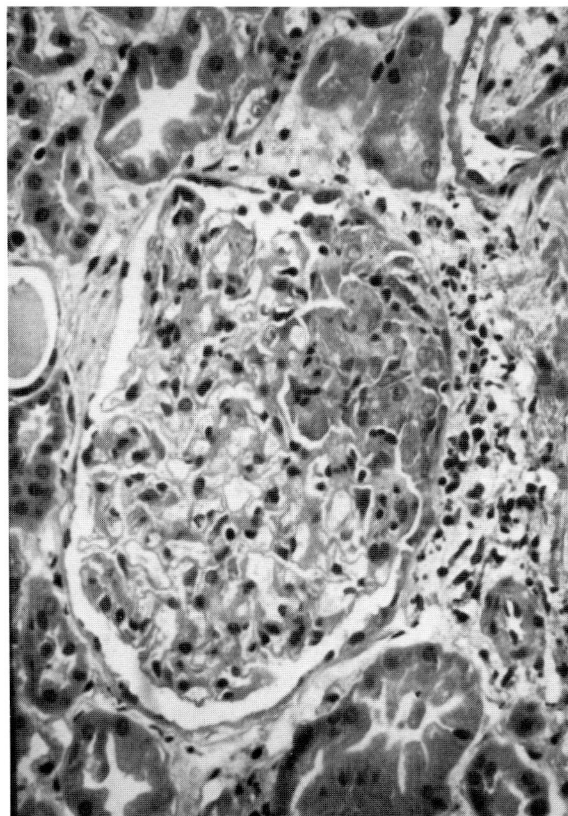

Figure 10-3. Focal necrotizing glomerulitis.

to insist that all features of the triad be present in order to make the diagnosis of Wegener's granulomatosis. However, Carrington and Liebow[7] in 1966 reported on 16 cases having typical pathology primarily in the lungs but no nephritis. They created the term "limited Wegener's granulomatosis," suggesting these patients had a better prognosis, probably due to the lack of serious kidney insult.

Early in my career, I encountered patients similar to those described by Carrington and Liebow, but in whom the typical necrotizing granulomas of the Wegener's type were confined to the upper respiratory tract (including the nose, paranasal sinuses, and subglottic area). At times, these patients had concomitant evidence of nephritis or subsequently developed it under observation, while not developing lung disease. These patients responded to the same treatment, namely cyclophosphamide and prednisone, as did those with the classic Wegener's triad. From this experience, I reasoned there must be a continuum of involvement of the three major sites, namely the upper respiratory tract or E (originally standing for ENT), lung or L, and kidney or K (Fig. 10-4). This was formalized into the ELK system,[8] which has proved extremely helpful, first in understanding the aforementioned ambiguous cases, and second in guiding the application of treatment at the earliest point in the course of the disease. Other than pathology and observation of clinical course, there was no other test to prove the

WEGENER'S GRANULOMATOSIS
Anatomic Sites

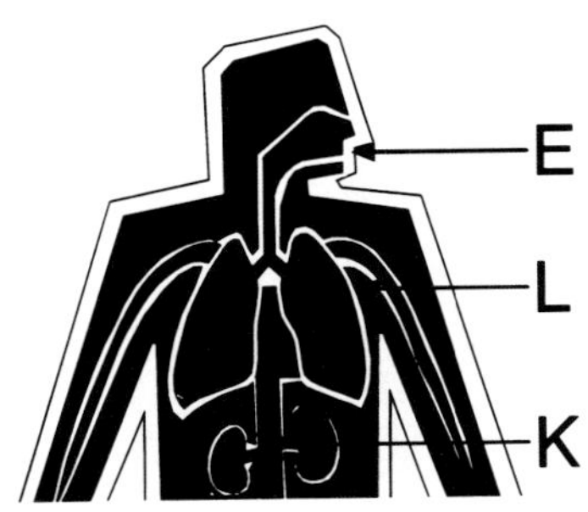

Figure 10-4. Wegener's granulomatosis, anatomic sites of the ELK classification.

validity of the ELK system until the advent of the anticytoplasmic autoantibody (ACPA), which is frequently present in the incomplete forms. More will be said of the ACPA test later. Thus, by the ELK system, Wegener's granulomatosis can manifest with any combination of ELK or singular occurrence in one of the major sites except that, by current criteria, involvement of the kidney alone is not accepted. There must be substantiating pathology elsewhere, particularly from E or L, to confirm the significance of the renal lesion of focal necrotizing glomerulitis, which is not specific for Wegener's granulomatosis. Tempering this view, however, is a recent report of nephritis antedating the fully declared picture of Wegener's granulomatosis[9] and isolated nephritis occurring with positive results for the ACPA test.[10]

Fienberg[11] has described long-standing lesions of the skin and mucous membranes consistent with Wegener's granulomatosis evolving over as long as 18 years. Thus, there has been a slow evolution of our concepts of Wegener's granulomatosis that continues to the present. The disease may be explosive in time and extent of lesions manifesting in all three major sites or ELK, or it may be indolent, involving one or two sites (particularly E) over long periods. Ostensibly, these extremes represent diseases of similar etiology and pathogenesis. The evidence of pathology, clinical course, response to treatment, and the ACPA test suggest this hypothesis is valid.

THE RELATIONSHIP OF LETHAL MIDLINE GRANULOMA TO WEGENER'S GRANULOMATOSIS

An essential perspective on Wegener's granulomatosis is provided by a consideration of lethal midline granuloma. In 1897, McBride[12] reported "photographs of a case of rapid destruction of the nose and face." This paper appears to have opened the discussion and ultimate controversy on lethal midline granuloma. From a contemporary vantage point, it is clear that the term was originally entirely clinical in character, without other

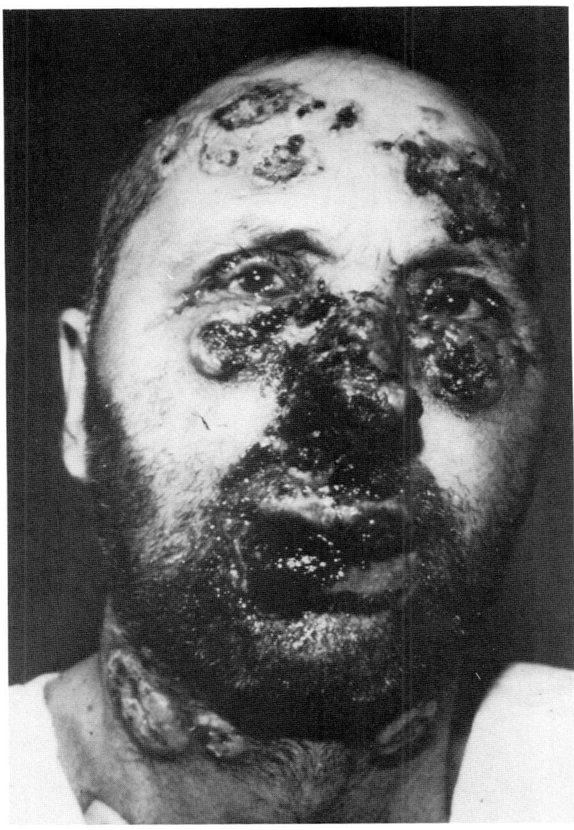

Figure 10-5. A 54-year-old man with fulminant Wegener's granulomatosis with prominent necrotizing skin lesions.

qualifying features, referring only to necrotizing lesions affecting the central face and its deeper appendages. Buried within this designation were at least three entities, namely Wegener's granulomatosis, polymorphic reticulosis/lymphomatoid granulomatosis, and conventional lymphoma. Similar lesions can also be caused by various bacterial and fungal infections, as well as by leishmaniasis.

A body of knowledge has gathered implicating polymorphic reticulosis/lymphomatoid granulomatosis as a lymphoproliferative disease, if not a frank lymphoma of the T-cell variety.[13,14] It is likely that this process was included under the older titles of malignant midline granulomatosis or nonhealing midline granuloma of the Stewart type.[15]

There are still some who contend there is an entity of midline granuloma apart from the specific lesions mentioned above. The term "idiopathic midline destructive disease" has been used to designate this group of patients.[16] Whether or not such a unique group does exist cannot at present be proved. What is most important is to understand that the term "lethal midline granuloma" has no specificity in modern parlance and should, therefore, be discarded except in historical context. It is clear that

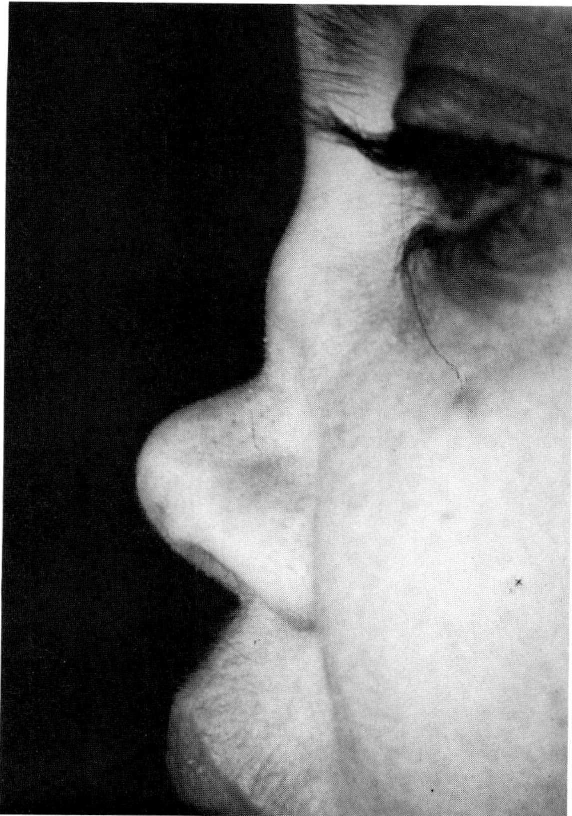

Figure 10-6. Saddle nose deformity in a 23-year-old woman with Wegener's granulomatosis.

Wegener's granulomatosis may begin and remain a locoregional disease confined to the upper respiratory tract, thus simulating "lethal midline granuloma." The proposition that Wegener's granulomatosis is always a systemic disease appears no longer tenable. Future discussions of lethal midline granuloma would be more aptly entitled "midfacial necrotizing lesions," as suggested by Batsakis and Luna.[17]

CLINICAL FEATURES

Wegener's granulomatosis is a disease of protean manifestations and clinical course. An extreme is the patient who becomes desperately ill over a one- to two-day period, arriving in the hospital in both respiratory and renal insufficiency covered by a profusion of necrotic skin lesions (Fig. 10-5). Or there may be a long history mounting over a number of years with the slow collapse of the nasal septum causing the so-called saddle nose deformity (Fig. 10-6).

TABLE 10-1. ELK Classification of Wegener's
Granulomatosis in 151 Patients

CLASS	NUMBER	% OF TOTAL
E	46	(30)
L	10	(7)
EL	33	(22)
EK	24	(16)
LK	14	(9)
ELK	25	(17)
	151	

E, upper respiratory tract; L, lung; K, kidney

Clinical presentation is strongly influenced by the anatomic location and extent of involvement. As was previously stated, there are three major sites to be considered, the upper respiratory tract or E, the lungs or L, and the kidney, K. Other less commonly affected sites or organ systems will be elaborated on later.

In an analysis of 151 patients seen at the Mayo Clinic from 1975 through 1985, we found that 128 (85%) had involvement of E; 81 (54%) had involvement of the lung; and 62 (41%) had involvement of the kidneys.[18] Table 10-1 shows the distribution of cases by the ELK classification scheme. The group included 69 men and 82 women, the median age being 49.8 years, with a range of 16 to 78 years. The difference in frequency between men and women is not statistically significant in this series, but the literature has tended to report a higher frequency in men. The following is a more detailed analysis of the kinds of involvement seen at various sites.

Upper Respiratory Tract (E)

Chronic nasal congestion, often with a serosanguineous discharge, is the classic representation of involvement at E. At times, both patient and physician may mistake the symptoms for mere chronic sinusitis or nasal allergy. However, when these symptoms persist for weeks or months, a more serious diagnosis should be entertained, particularly if the sedimentation rate is very high. An experienced otorhinolaryngologist can be of inestimable value in evaluation of these patients.[19] He or she will note on examination crusting that, on removal, reveals a friable underlying mucosa. There may be actual perforation of the nasal septum. A particularly reliable sign is ulceration of the vomer, as seen on nasopharyngoscopy. Paranasal sinus involvement can be demonstrated by sinus roentgenograms. Patients with paranasal sinus involvement will frequently complain of deep-seated central facial pain. Collapse of the nasal septum with saddling raises not only the diagnosis of Wegener's granulomatosis, but also that of relapsing polychondritis. The presence of ulcerated mucosa favors the diagnosis of Wegener's granulomatosis.

The ear and its appendages are involved in a number of ways. As in relapsing polychondritis, the pinna may be reddened and painful, but this is a decidedly uncommon

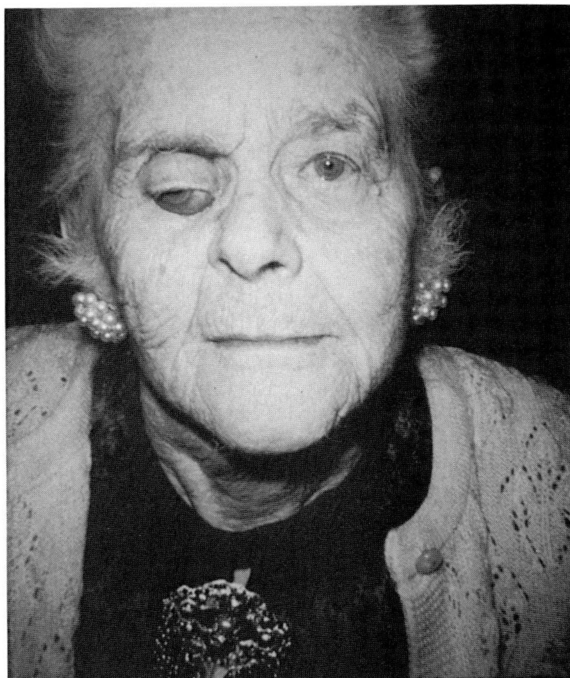

Figure 10-7. An 80-year-old woman with unilateral proptosis due to Wegener's granulomatosis.

finding. Chronic otitis media is perhaps the most frequent manifestation of ear pathology. This is, in part, fostered by dysfunction of the eustachian tube due to lesions of the nasopharyngeal mucosa. Mastoiditis and cholesteatoma may also be encountered. The cochlea can be involved with vasculitis so that not only a conductive hearing loss, but also a sensori neural hearing loss may be uncovered. Virtually any combination of the above mentioned pathologic manifestations can occur. As might be anticipated, nasal saddling and perforation are usually associated with long clinical courses. Subglottic stricture may be an isolated finding but is usually seen in concert with pathology of the nose. Such subglottic stricture may be mistaken by the clinician for asthma. Ulcerations of the gingiva and nasopharynx are uncommon.

The orbit and eye are affected almost invariably in association with nasal involvement.[20] Infiltration of the orbit with inflammatory tissue may cause proptosis, usually unilateral, but occasionally bilateral, simulating Grave's ophthalmopathy (Fig. 10-7). One patient referred to me with such bilateral involvement had undergone bilateral surgical orbital decompression for presumptive Grave's ophthalmopathy. The pathologist noted changes of necrotizing granuloma that led to a thorough examination by an otorhinolaryngologist that in turn yielded biopsy samples consistent with Wegener's granulomatosis.

One of the most dreaded ocular complications is necrotizing scleritis with "melt down," which may lead to perforation of the globe resulting in loss of sight. Such pathology may occur and recur while evidence of disease in other sites is under control. In other words, the inflammation at times is compartmentalized to the eye. A "red eye" indicative of conjunctivitis or episcleritis may occasionally be the first sign of an impending case of Wegener's granulomatosis. Other forms of ocular involvement include central artery occlusion, uveitis, and retinal and optic nerve vasculitis. Stenosis of the nasolacrimal ducts may result from inflammation and scarring of the nasal mucosa. Such patients are at risk for recurrent dacryocystitis. Major salivary glands, including the parotid and submaxillary, are rarely enlarged. On biopsy, they reveal typical necrotizing granulomas.

Lung (L)

The most characteristic finding in the lungs is the appearance of multiple nodules of variable size (1–5 cm) with or without cavitation and with variable definition (Fig. 10-8). Rarely, the patient may present with a diffuse alveolar filling pattern consistent with a diffuse alveolar hemorrhage (Fig. 10-9). Although mentioned in some articles, the presence of a pure interstitial pattern on chest roentgenogram has not been observed in my patients. An interstitial pattern may be seen, but it coexists and is dominated by the multiple nodular pattern. The chief differential diagnoses raised by the chest roentgenogram include metastatic malignancies, granulomas of specific microbial etiology, and the various alveolar hemorrhage syndromes. Strictures similar to those encountered in the subglottic area may occur in the major bronchi, leading to recurrent obstructive pneumonias.

The patient may be entirely unaware of lung pathology, having no symptoms, or may have rapidly progressive signs and symptoms of respiratory failure. Between these extremes there are variable degrees of cough and shortness of breath. Hemoptysis is, of course, suggestive of diffuse alveolar hemorrhage and of ulcerating lesions of the bronchi or upper airways.

Kidney (K)

Forty-one percent of 151 patients seen at the Mayo Clinic manifested kidney involvement.[18] Fauci and associates reported an 85% incidence.[21] The frequency of kidney involvement will vary according to the criteria used for diagnosis. If one insists on a complete Wegener's triad, then by definition there will be 100% incidence of kidney involvement. However, if one adheres to the criteria implicit in the ELK scheme, the frequency will be necessarily lower.

The classic kidney lesion found in Wegener's granulomatosis is focal necrotizing glomerulitis.[22] This is not specific for Wegener's, but may also be seen as a freestanding lesion or in the context of polyarteritis nodosa. When the urinalysis shows proteinuria and red blood cell casts, the diagnosis of kidney involvement can be accepted. Some would claim that a kidney biopsy is necessary to confirm the presence or absence of kidney disease. I consider that the urinalysis findings are adequate. The serum creatinine and creatinine clearance will be affected by the severity of the disease. Patients may present with advanced renal insufficiency or frank failure that occurs over a relatively short period, or there may be a history of slowly progressive kidney dysfunction.

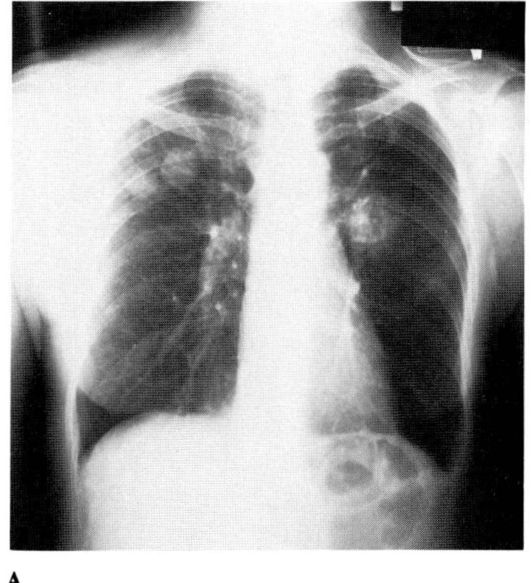

A

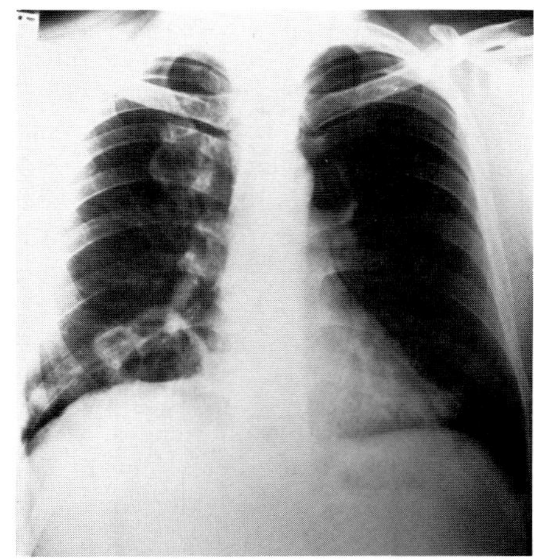

B

C

Figure 10-8. Typical chest roentgenograms of three patients with Wegener's granulomatosis.

Skin

After the big three sites, ELK, the skin is most frequently involved, involvement occurring in 15% to 50% of cases.[23] A broad range of lesions can be seen, including symmetric papulonecrotic lesions of the extremities, generalized urticaria, vesicles, and pyoderma gangrenosum. The histologic features have been divided into three distinct groups: necrotizing vasculitis, necrotizing palisading granuloma of the Churg-Strauss type, and granulomatous vasculitis. Activity of the skin lesions generally parallels disease activity in other sites.

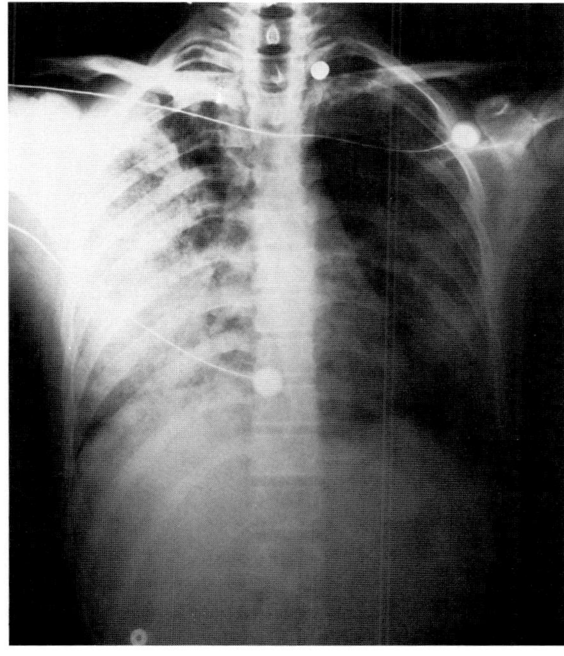

Figure 10-9. A chest roentgenogram of a 17-year-old boy demonstrating diffuse alveolar hemorrhage due to Wegener's granulomatosis.

Nervous System

Mononeuritis multiplex is the chief manifestation of neurologic involvement. It is probably due to nerve ischemia caused by vasculitis of the vasanervorum. Other neurologic lesions include multiple cranial nerve palsies, symmetric peripheral neuropathy, amaurosis fugax, cerebral infarction, seizures, and transverse myelitis.

Hansen and associates, reviewing a Mayo Clinic series of 106 patients, reported a 29% incidence of neurologic involvement.[24] Fauci reported a 27% rate from a study of 85 patients.[21] Of particular clinical interest from the Mayo series was the observation that no patient developed mononeuritis multiplex after effective treatment was started with glucocorticoids and/or cyclophosphamide. In addition, all patients with mononeuritis multiplex or generalized peripheral neuropathy had concomitant kidney involvement. Neurologic lesions usually do not regress following treatment that is effective in ameliorating lesions in other systems.

The Joints

Symmetric polyarthritis may be a feature of Wegener's granulomatosis, serving as a sensitive indicator of disease activity. Such arthritis may be observed in the wrists, shoulders, or knees, and in the small joints of the hands and feet. It is difficult to ascribe a firm incidence rate, but it is probably of the order of 20%. Although infrequently, a thorough joint history and inspection can produce very helpful lesions with which to monitor the clinical course. In contrast to rheumatoid arthritis, the arthritis seen in Wegener's granulomatosis is not deforming. Single inflamed joints may occasionally be observed.

Miscellaneous

As vasculitis may be systemic, virtually any organ can be subject to its consequences. We have seen perforations of the bowel, elevation of liver enzymes, and necrotizing granulomas involving the prostate.[25]

LABORATORY TESTING

Only a few tests are helpful in the evaluation and management of patients with Wegener's granulomatosis.

Anemia is common, but usually mild. Occasionally, levels of hemoglobin of the order of 8 to 9 g/dL can be observed. Blood morphology may disclose schistocytes and burr cells indicative of a traumatic hemolytic process. I have also observed microcytic hypochromic pictures consistent with iron deficiency, perhaps due to the loss of hemosiderin in the urine or lung.

A leukocytosis is seen in about one half of patients but is rarely greater than 18,000 per mm^3. Peripheral eosinophilia is not a feature of Wegener's granulomatosis but is a salient feature of the Churg-Strauss syndrome, a major differential diagnosis. Occasionally, an eosinophil count to 10% of the total may be seen. Most of the time the eosinophil percentage will be less than 5%.

Positive rheumatoid factors have been observed in approximately 40% of our patients. The titers may be high. The erythrocyte sedimentation rate is most valuable when it is in the very high range, which I would define as equal to or greater than 80mm/hr Westergren. A lower or normal sedimentation rate in no way excludes inflammatory activity. Measured in serial fashion, the sedimentation profile may be of value in monitoring the effect of treatment. There is an increasing likelihood of very high sedimentation rates in patients of higher ELK class.

Any of the immunoglobulin fractions, including IgE, may be elevated above the normal range. I know of no current significance to such aberrations and cannot recommend these tests as routine.

It cannot be overemphasized that a urinalysis with careful microscopic examination is one of the most important tests. In addition, measurements of renal function, such as serum creatinine and urea, should be done in every patient. I find that renal clearance studies give more sensitive data in the estimation of the degree of kidney impairment.

Measurement of pulmonary function does not usually play a decisive role in the evaluation of patients unless there are strictures involving the subglottic or major airways distally. The graphic display of a flow volume loop can indicate the degree and approximate location (e.g., extrathoracic versus intrathoracic) of the stricture. Tomography of the involved sites is useful in delineating the anatomic extent of the lesion.

APPROPRIATE CONSULTATIONS

As Wegener's granulomatosis is often a multisystem disease, it is inevitable that consultation from one or more medical specialists will be sought. This is particularly important in any suspected eye involvement, where an ophthalmologist should play an important role. A baseline fundus examination of the eye is a reasonable part of the evaluation of every patient with Wegener's granulomatosis. A dermatologist can be of great assistance, both in taking tissue for diagnosis and in advising on the local treatment of skin lesions. When there is manifest neurologic involvement, the neurologist can be very helpful both in assessing the extent of involvement and in the serial monitoring of the course of the disease. The neurologist may occasionally order an electromyogram when the extent and nature of the findings are in question.

ANTICYTOPLASMIC AUTOANTIBODY (ACPA)

Diseases of unknown etiology rarely have specific tests for their diagnosis. Such was the case for Wegener's granulomatosis until the mid 1980s, when the first reports appeared of autoantibodies directed against constituents in the cytoplasm of monocytes and neutrophils. Davies and colleagues,[26] and Hall and colleagues[27] first reported the phenomenon in patients with focal necrotizing glomerulonephritis, apparently not recognizing the possibility of Wegener's granulomatosis. Van der Woude and colleagues[28] linked the phenomenon with Wegener's granulomatosis and a closely related entity, microscopic polyarteritis nodosa.[29] Today the validity of the finding of anticytoplasmic autoantibodies (ACPA) in patients with Wegener's granulomatosis has been repeatedly confirmed. Not only does the test for these antibodies have high specificity for the diagnosis, but it can also be enlightening in assessing the clinical course.

The term antineutrophil cytoplasmic antibody or ANCA is equivalent to ACPA. The term ACPA is less restrictive, since the antibody may be found not only in neutrophils but in monocytes as well. For details concerning methodology for detecting ACPA, readers are referred to a number of authoritative publications.[28,30,31]

Three main patterns of cytoplasmic fluorescence are currently recognized: granular with central accentuation, perinuclear, and homogeneous. Proper recognition of the various patterns is of critical importance, as it is the granular pattern that has specificity for Wegener's granulomatosis. The perinuclear pattern has been identified with other vasculitides and connective tissue disorders. Thus, a reader of considerable experience is needed for proper interpretation. An enzyme linked immunosorbent assay (ELISA) is being developed that may ultimately replace the immunofluorescent technique, thereby avoiding the human observer element.

In a cooperative study with scientists at the University of Kiel, West Germany, we studied 222 biopsy-substantiated cases of Wegener's granulomatosis, comparing them with 1657 control patients.[31] Patients were divided into groups depending on ELK class and activity. Group 1 was designated locoregional and included ELK classes E, L, and EL. Group 2, or generalized disease, embraced patients in ELK classes LK and ELK. There were no patients in EK class, but if there were they would have been included in group 2, as the differentiating factor was the presence of kidney involvement taken as evidence of generalized disease. Activity was determined by clinical and laboratory assessment.

Patients in group 1 (locoregional) deemed to be active showed a 67% sensitivity, which dropped to 32% when the disease was in remission. Patients in group 2 (generalized) had a 96% sensitivity rate, declining to 41% upon remission.

What is perhaps of greater importance is that overall the test for ACPA had 99% specificity for Wegener's granulomatosis. ACPA was positive in a few cases of microscopic polyarteritis nodosa, a disease having a number of features in common with Wegener's granulomatosis and perhaps of similar pathogenesis. Control patients encompassed a number of diseases, including those with granulomatous features, such as sarcoidosis, other kidney diseases, and other forms of vasculitis.

I suggested at the outset of this discussion that since the mid 1980s we have had a specific test for Wegener's granulomatosis; certainly, 99% specificity is impressive. Yet, understanding that rarely do biologic systems yield such tight data, I would advise physicians for the time being to continue to base the diagnosis based on histologic evidence, using the ACPA test for confirmation. As previously intimated, the application of ACPA testing to various isolated expressions of Wegener's granulomatosis, such as nephritis, pulmonary hemorrhage, subglottic stricture, obscure skin lesions, and so on, has enlarged and probably will continue to enlarge the scope of the diagnosis.

In addition to their diagnostic importance, our data suggest that ACPA titers parallel clinical activity. The utility of this phenomenon is obvious. It helps in the determination of the adequacy of the treatment regimen. Also, complicating infections can often be differentiated from relapses of Wegener's granulomatosis based on ACPA titers.

Beyond its diagnostic and clinical implications, the ACPA has stimulated interest in its cause, in the antigen against which it is directed, and in what role, if any, it plays in pathogenesis. The antigen against which the antibody is directed has not, at this writing, been conclusively determined. Previous data indicated myeloperoxidase as the antigen for the perinuclear autoantibody.[32] Some investigators[33] have suggested alkaline phosphatase as the antigen, while others have presented data contradicting this claim.[34] When the origin is finally settled, a whole new era of investigation will probably be opened. Abbott and co-workers[35] have recently presented data showing that cytoplasmic autoantibodies can bind to cultured normal epithelial and endothelial cells from human kidneys. This would, of course, help to explain the renal lesion, but what of the pathology at other sites? What pathologic or teleologic function do the autoantibodies play in the monocytes and neutrophils? Are they merely epiphenomena? Such are the tantalizing questions raised by the advent of ACPA. The whole classification of vasculitis may be radically changed by subsequent investigations into the ACPA phenomenon.

MAKING THE DIAGNOSIS

Table 10-2 lists findings and symptoms that should alert the physician to the possibility of Wegener's granulomatosis. As with other rare conditions, a high index of suspicion is helpful in leading to the correct diagnosis, particularly in atypical or incompletely expressed cases. If at all possible, the diagnosis should be confirmed by tissue biopsy.

The nose often offers the best site for biopsy due to the overall frequency of involvement and its accessibility. Physicians should be aware that even after generous

TABLE 10-2. Findings or Symptoms Prompting Consideration
of Wegener's Granulomatosis

Upper Respiratory Tract—E (Including Orbit and Eye)
Nasal obstruction and epistaxis
Nasal septal perforation
Chronic sinusitis
Chronic otitis media
Saddle nose deformity
Mastoiditis, cholesteatoma
Subglottic stenosis (stridor)
Proptosis (particularly if unilateral)
Red eye (conjunctivitis, scleritis)
Uveitis
Retinal and optic nerve vasculitis
Nasolacrimal duct stenosis and epiphora
Enlarged salivary glands
Lower Respiratory Tract—L
Multiple nodules (with or without cavitation)
Diffuse alveolar filling pattern
Hemoptysis
Kidney—K
Glomerulonephritis
Kidney insufficiency or failure
Miscellaneous
Necrotizing skin lesions
Mononeuritis multiplex
Polyarthritis
Necrotizing vasculitis of arteries and veins in any organ

biopsies from seemingly promising areas, the pathologist may see only nonspecific inflammation. Then it becomes a matter of either performing more extensive biopsies in the nose or searching for sites elsewhere, particularly in the lung—or, if the clinical picture is typical, of simply making the diagnosis clinically. The latter course I would tend to discourage. An exception might be the patient having a positive ACPA test in whom no other sites for biopsy can be found.

Fienberg[36] has made a very persuasive case for the primacy of the necrotizing granuloma as the pathologic hallmark not requiring the presence of vasculitis. He has argued that vasculitis simply represents extension of the disease to another organ system. Although bacteriologic study of the tissue should be made, particularly for fungi and acid-fast bacilli, I have seen no case of classic Wegener's granulomatosis in which either of these kinds of organisms were cultured and held responsible for the clinicopathologic picture. Yet, caution must be exercised in localized and incomplete forms of the disease to exclude a specific microbial cause for the granuloma.

Occasionally, patients presenting with features suggestive of Wegener's granulomatosis have had surgery on the nose, sinuses, or mastoid sometime in the past. It is highly recommended that these tissues be reviewed with a specific eye toward the possibility of changes consistent with Wegener's granulomatosis. When there is proptosis of the orbit or abnormal infiltration of the orbit, orbital biopsies are recommended.

When the nose and other parts of the upper respiratory tract are not affected, the lung is usually the next biopsy source. Bronchoscopy with biopsy would appear to be a less invasive, safer technique than the open lung biopsies. Since the pieces of tissue obtainable by way of the bronchoscope are small, I have found this technique to be singularly disappointing. Thus, I have preferred open lung biopsy to ensure adequate tissue sampling, not only for histopathology, but for bacteriologic studies as well. Due to the often serious nature of the disease and the risks of therapy with glucocorticoids and alkylating agents, a firm diagnosis is mandatory, justifying the possible added risks of an open lung biopsy. In cases of diffuse alveolar hemorrhage due to Wegener's granulomatosis, pathologic section may reveal only so-called capillaritis and not the classic necrotizing granulomatous changes.

As alluded to earlier, an accurate urinalysis showing red blood cell casts and proteinuria is sufficient in my mind to implicate kidney involvement. This finding is strengthened by an increase in serum creatinine and a decrease in renal clearance. If the ACPA test allows us to recognize Wegener's granulomatosis localized to kidney, it may be reasonable to accurately diagnose the pathology by a biopsy. It may also be that a kidney biopsy will have already been done and the finding of focal necrotizing glomerulitis will trigger investigations for ACPA.

After the sites just mentioned, the skin is perhaps the next most frequently biopsied organ. A granulomatous vasculitis may be seen, but usually there is a nonspecific, leukocytoclastic vasculitis. Furthermore, I have never seen a case of Wegener's granulomatosis entirely confined to changes in the skin. It is doubtful that biopsies of joint synovia or of peripheral nerves will be helpful in making the specific diagnosis of Wegener's granulomatosis. One should be aware that any biopsy site revealing vasculitis, particularly involving arteries and veins or having granulomatous features, should cause a reflex consideration of Wegener's granulomatosis, thereby initiating appropriate investigations.

What I have just said about the use of bronchoscopic biopsy, the overall need for tissue confirmation, and Wegener's granulomatosis confined to the skin may all be shortly changed when and if the specificity of the ACPA test becomes unequivocally confirmed by further studies. The ACPA need not be positive to make the diagnosis but is extremely helpful in corroborating the diagnosis and, as mentioned earlier, in following the clinical course by way of serial titers.

TREATMENT

Historical Evolution

The first effective treatment for Wegener's granulomatosis was cortisone, reported by Moore and colleagues in 1951.[37] In 1950, Williams[38] reported a favorable response of a patient with mid-facial granuloma following treatment with cortisone. Although the clinical features were consistent, the description of the pathology is too vague to be certain if that patient did in fact have disease we would now consider Wegener's granulomatosis limited to E. Before the advent of cortisone, patients died mostly from kidney failure or sepsis, often within a few months of onset. The first patient treated with cortisone was started on 200 mg daily for 4 days and then switched to a maintenance of 100 mg per day for a total of 3 weeks. Shortly after cortisone was stopped, signs and symptoms recurred and the drug was restarted, resulting once again in control of the disease. Subsequently, other reports appeared of the use of glucocorticoids, ACTH, and various cytotoxic drugs, including nitrogen mustard, chlorambucil, azathioprine, methotrexate, and cyclophosphamide. Since the early 1970s, cyclophosphamide and prednisone have been the agents of choice. Drugs of second choice include azathioprine and chlorambucil. As will be discussed, trimethoprim/sulfamethoxazole (T/S) can now be considered an important addition to the armamentarium.

Clinical Course and Prognosis

At the time of Wegener's first description of the disease, death resulted in a few months as a rule. Shortly after the introduction of glucocorticoids, Walton[39] reported an 80% death rate at the first year following diagnosis and 93% at the second year. This certainly represented some, but not very impressive progress. In 1983, Fauci[21] and co-workers reported 93% complete remissions in 85 patients treated with a regimen of cyclophosphamide 2 mg/kg body weight per day, plus prednisone 1 mg/kg body weight per day. Our group[18] reported on 151 patients in 1987, showing an overall mortality of 28% (Fig. 10-10). Survivorship was 90% at 1 year, 87% at 2 years, and 76% at 5 years. The chief regimens included cyclophosphamide at 2 mg/kg body weight per day with variable doses of prednisone. It was conventional to consider kidney disease as the chief cause of death, with sepsis the second leading cause. From our series, we surprisingly found that involvement of the lung and the consequences thereof was the most important factor in overall survivorship. Kidney involvement was important, but only in the first year. Thus, if a patient survived insult to the kidneys over the first year, it was the course of the lung involvement that tended to decide the outcome.

Analysis of deaths showed 11 patients dead of kidney failure, seven within the first year. Twelve patients died of opportunistic infections, five of malignant neoplasms, two of cytotoxic lung, and one of bone marrow failure. The role of immunosuppression in these cases merits more than passing suspicion. It would appear that lung involvement provides an ideal portal of entry for infections that may thrive in the immunosuppressed patient. In addition, the development of malignant neoplasms may have been facilitated by depression of immune surveillance. It is of the greatest importance that the therapist exercise care in the application of cytotoxic drugs in the treatment of Wegener's granulomatosis.

Since the advent of trimethoprim/sulfamethoxazole (T/S), the possibilities of effective yet safe treatment have been expanded. In 1975, I made my first observations on the effectiveness of T/S in the treatment of Wegener's granulomatosis.[40] This experience, on last analysis,[41] has encompassed 46 patients, of whom 40 were judged to have responded positively to T/S either as monotherapy or as an additive to failing conventional regimens. A number of reports have appeared in the literature confirming these observations.[42–44] Experience has suggested that T/S is most effective when the

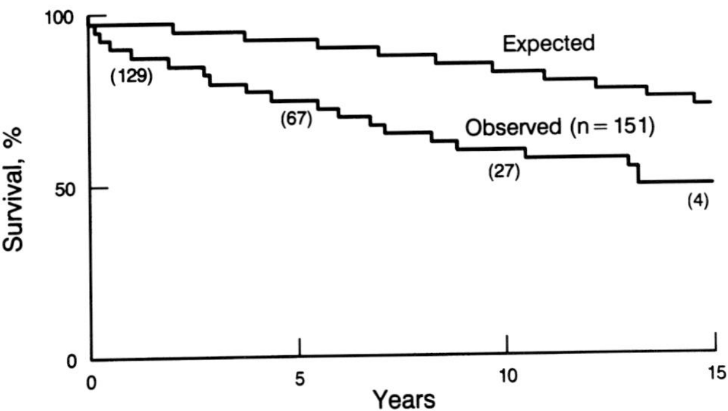

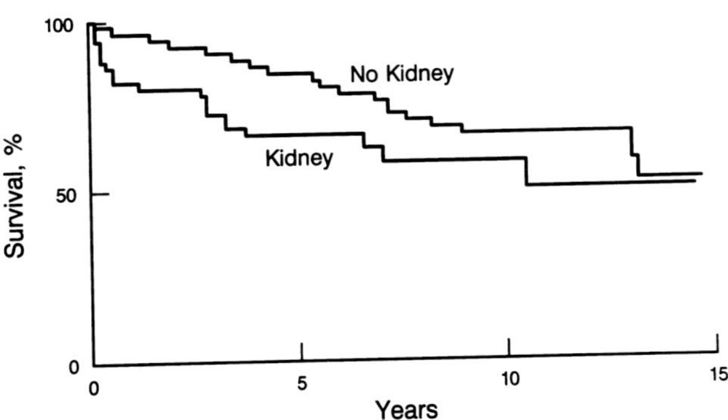

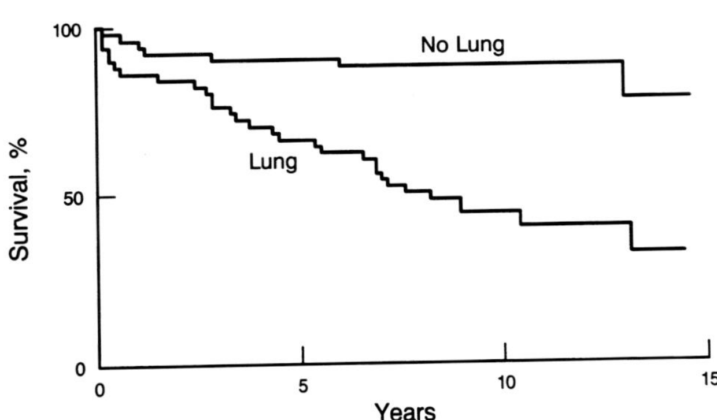

Figure 10-10. Wegener's granulomatosis, survival statistics. (*A*) Overall survival to death by Kaplan Meier method. (*B*) Overall survival with and without kidney involvement. (*C*) Overall survival with and without lung involvement.

disease is localized to the upper or lower respiratory tracts and in the absence of signs of disseminated vasculitis and, in particular, nephritis. It should be noted, however, that in my early series two patients with nephritis went into remission on T/S as monotherapy. Although T/S has shown promise, its use needs to be verified by rigorous control studies.

Graduated Treatment Regimens

I have come to the following graduated regimens based on the anatomic extent and clinical tempo. For patients having indolent clinical courses with disease confined to E, L, or EL, I would start T/S one double-strength tablet twice a day. I would maintain this dose, provided the patient is tolerating the medication and is not worsening, for 8 weeks before changing management. If the patient is improved, I would continue the drug indefinitely. At present, one of my patients has taken T/S for 14 years without discernible side effects. If there is no improvement after 8 weeks of observation, I would add prednisone 40 or 60 mg on alternate days. It is likely this regimen will be effective. If no response is observed, one might legitimately question the diagnosis. If the diagnosis is firm, then the addition of cyclophosphamide at 2 mg/kg body weight per day is a reasonable next step.

For patients presenting with more extensive disease, such as EK, LK, or ELK, it is likely that cyclophosphamide will be necessary to effect a cure. The decision to combine with alternate-day prednisone will depend on clinical tempo. Rapidly progressive disease requires combined treatment. Patients with indolent disease could be started on cyclophosphamide as the sole agent.

The patient with fulminant disease, usually with rapidly progressing nephritis and extensive vasculitis, demands more intensive treatment, which should include daily glucocorticoid in the form of prednisone 60 mg to 80 mg a day or equivalent thereof. Bolus administration of methylprednisolone 1 g daily for 2 to 3 days has been advocated, particularly for patients with diffuse alveolar hemorrhage.[45] I have found that the concomitant administration of high-dose glucocorticoid and cyclophosphamide leaves the patient unusually vulnerable to opportunistic infection. It is further my experience that high-dose glucocorticoid administration will bring the disease under control, at least temporarily. Therefore, it has been my custom to stabilize the acutely ill patient with glucocorticoid alone, adding cyclophosphamide in 10 to 14 days when widespread lesions have begun to heal. When cyclophosphamide has been established, it is recommended that prednisone be continued for 4 to 6 weeks and then converted to an alternate-day regimen by gradually reducing the alternate day dose by 5 mg to 10 mg decrements at 1- to 2-week intervals. Given a stable or improving course, the prednisone is gradually withdrawn while maintaining the cyclophosphamide at 2 mg/kg body weight per day orally. Like Fauci and co-workers,[21] we maintain cyclophosphamide for 1 year past last evidence of disease activity. When the decision to stop cyclophosphamide is made, the drug is withdrawn abruptly without taper. The leukocyte count is maintained above 3000/mm^3. If it goes below this level, cyclophosphamide is stopped and the white blood cell count is monitored at weekly intervals. When the count rises above 3000/mm^3, cyclophosphamide is reinstituted at one-half the previous dose. Monitoring of the white blood cell count and alteration of dose is continued based on a similar format.

Cyclophosphamide is taken as a single morning dose with instructions to drink about one quart of water above normal intake. This is done to promote excretion of the metabolic byproduct acrolein, which is implicated in the genesis of hemorrhagic cystitis and ultimately bladder carcinoma. Gross[42] has advocated intraveous bolus cyclophosphamide (15 mg/kg body weight) monthly for 6 months for patients failing the standard low oral dose regimens or experiencing complications such as leukopenia. I have not had occasion to use such a regimen and cannot, therefore, comment on its usefulness. When cyclophosphamide cannot be tolerated, chlorambucil may be substituted in doses of 4 mg to 12 mg per day. Leukocyte counts, platelet counts, and hemoglobin should be measured at weekly intervals at the beginning of treatment, subsequently prolonging the intervals to 2 to 3 weeks depending on the patient's tolerance. If chlorambucil is not a satisfactory substitution, one may employ azathioprine at 2 mg/kg body weight per day. The chief toxic effects of azathioprine are depression of leukocyte and platelet counts and injury to the liver. Appropriate monitoring for these untoward effects must be done.

Studies are planned to prospectively test the effect of T/S alone and in various combinations with prednisone and cytotoxic agents, particularly cyclophosphamide.

Surgical Treatment

Occasionally, surgery is employed, mainly in attempts to remedy otherwise irreversible fibrotic sequelae of a now arrested inflammation.

Subglottic stenosis has been, in my experience, the most frequently encountered irreversible fibrotic lesion for which surgical intervention may be employed. Frequently, tracheostomy is needed to ensure an adequate airway; often this tracheostomy may be for the life of the patient. If the stenotic lesion is short surgical resection may be entertained. It must be certain that the underlying disease is entirely arrested before considering such an option. We have attempted to open subglottic strictures with lasers but have found that the result was only temporary. I cannot, at this time, recommend it as anything but a temporizing procedure. In one patient, a pneumonectomy was performed because of severe strictures of the bronchial tree that led to repeated pulmonary suppuration.

Saddle nose deformity can be repaired surgically for cosmetic purposes. Nasolacrimal duct obstruction can at times be surgically corrected. A suppurative dacryocystitis may occasionally require surgical drainage. If there are problems with recurrent middle ear infections due to dysfunction of the eustachian tube, ventilating tubes may be placed through the tympanic membrane to alleviate this problem. The otorhinolaryngologist may additionally be involved in creating drainage of chronically infected paranasal sinuses.

Infrequently, an ophthalmologic surgeon may be involved in enucleation of a destroyed eye. Recently, one of my patients was submitted to multiple surgical procedures to cover thinned areas of sclera due to episcleritis. There was risk of perforation with consequent loss of vision. Patients who have sustained total kidney failure may be candidates for transplantation. Of interest is the fact that for two patients under my care who have undergone kidney transplantation, Wegener's granulomatosis ceased to be a problem, probably as a result of antirejection treatment. However, in another patient the disease reactivated while she was taking azathioprine, cyclosporine, and prednisone following renal transplantation.

NOTE

Friedrich Wegener died on July 9, 1990 six weeks following a stroke. He was a man of great joy, wisdom, and character, a legend in his own time.

REFERENCES

1. von Rokitansky C: Über einige der wichtigsten erkrankungen der arterien. Denkscher d k Akad d Wissensch 1852;4:49.
2. Kussmaul A, Maier R: Über eine bisher nicht beschriebene eigenthümliche arterienerkrankung (periarteritis nodosa), die mit morbus brightii und rapid fortschreitender allgemeiner muskellähmung einhergeht. Deutsches Arch f Klin Med 1866;1:484.
3. Klinger H: Grenzformen der periarteritis nodosa. Frankfurter Z Pathol 1931;42:455.
4. Wegener F: Über generalisierte, septische gefässerkrankungen. Verhandl Deutsch Pathol Gesellsch 1936;29:202.
5. Wegener F: Über eine eigenartige rhinogene granulomatose mit besonderer beteiligung des arteriensystems und der nieren. Beiträge zur Pathol Anat 1939;102:36.
6. Godman G, Churg J: Wegener's granulomatosis. Arch Pathol 1954;58:533.
7. Carrington CB, Liebow AA: Limited forms of angiitis and granulomatosis of Wegener's type. Am J Med 1966;41:497.
8. DeRemee RA, McDonald TJ, Harrison EG Jr, Coles DT: Wegener's granulomatosis: Anatomic correlates, a proposed classification. Mayo Clin Proc 1976;51:777.
9. Woodworth TG, Abuelo JG, Austin HA, Esparza A: Severe glomerulonephritis with late emergence of classic Wegener's granulomatosis. Medicine (Baltimore) 1987;66:181.
10. Hoare TJ, Rhys Evans PH: Antineutrophil cytoplasmic antibody assay in diagnosis of recurrent subglottic stenosis. Lancet 1988;2:1360.
11. Fienberg R: The protracted superficial phenomenon in pathergic (Wegener's) granulomatosis. Hum Pathol 1981;12:458.
12. McBride P: Photographs of a case of rapid destruction of the nose and face. J Laryngol Otol 1897;12:64.
13. DeRemee RA, Weiland LH, McDonald TJ: Polymorphic reticulosis, lymphomatoid granulomatosis, two diseases or one? Mayo Clin Proc 1978;53:634.
14. Jaffe ES, Lipford EJ Jr, Margolic JB, Longo DL, Fauci AS: Lymphomatoid granulomatosis and angiocentric lymphoma: A spectrum of post-thymic T-cell proliferations. Semin Resp Med 1989;10:167.
15. Stewart JP: Progressive lethal granulomatous ulceration of the nose. J Laryngol Otol 1933;48:657.
16. Tsokos M, Fauci AS, Costa J: Idiopathic midline destructive disease (IMDD). Am J Clin Pathol 1982;77:162.
17. Batsakis JG, Luna MA: Midfacial necrotizing lesions. Semin Diagn Pathol 1987;4:90.
18. DeRemee RA, McDonald TJ, Weiland LH: Aspekte zur therapie und verlaufsbeobachtungen der Wegenerschen granulomatose. Med Welt 1987;38:470.

19. McDonald TJ, DeRemee RA, Kern EB, Harrison EG Jr.: Nasal manifestations of Wegener's granulomatosis. Laryngoscope 1974;84:2101.

20. Bullen CL, Liesegang TJ, McDonald TJ, DeRemee RA: Ocular complications of Wegener's granulomatosis. Ophthalmology 1983;90:279.

21. Fauci AS, Haynes BF, Katz P, Wolff SM: Wegener's granulomatosis: Prospective clinical and therapeutic experience with 85 patients for 21 years. Ann Int Med 1983;98:76.

22. Weiss MA, Crissman JD: Renal pathologic features of Wegener's granulomatosis: A review. Semin Resp Med 1989;10:141.

23. DeRemee RA: Extrapulomonary manifestations of Wegener's granulomatosis and other respiratory vasculitides. Semin Resp Med 1988;9:403.

24. Hansen RB, Swanson JW, DeRemee RA, McDonald TJ, Weiland LH: Neurologic involvement in Wegener's granulomatosis. (Abstract) Neurology (Cleveland) 1983;33 (suppl 2):240.

25. Stillwell TJ, DeRemee RA, McDonald TJ, Weiland LH, Engen DE: Prostatic involvement in Wegener's granulomatosis. J Urol 1987;138:1251.

26. Davies DJ, Moran JE, Niall JF, Ryan GB: Segmental necrotizing glomerulonephritis with antineutrophil antibody: Possible arbovirus aetiology? Br Med J 1982;285:606.

27. Hall JB, Wadham BM, Wood CJ, Ashton V, Adam WR: Vasculitis and glomerulonephritis: A subgroup with an antineutrophil cytoplasmic antibody. Aust NZ J Med 1984;14:277.

28. van der Woude FJ, Rasmussen N, Labatto S, et al: Autoantibodies against neutrophils and monocytes: Tool for diagnosis and marker of disease activity in Wegener's granulomatosis. Lancet 1985;i:425.

29. Savage COS, Winearls CG, Evans DJ, Rees AJ, Lockwood CM: Microscopic polyarteritis: Presentation, pathology, and prognosis. Q J Med 1985;56:467.

30. Lüdemann G, Gross WL: Autoantibodies against cytoplasmic structures of neutrophil granulocytes in Wegener's granulomatosis. Exp Immunol 1987;69:350.

31. Nölle B, Specks U, Lüdemann J, Rohrbach MS, DeRemee RA, Gross WL: Anticytoplasmic autoantibodies: Their immunodiagnostic value in Wegener granulomatosis. Ann Intern Med 1989;111:28.

32. Falk RJ, Jennette JC: Anti-neutrophil cytoplasmic autoantibodies with specificity for myeloperoxidase in patients with systemic vasculitis and idiopathic necrotizing and crescentic glomerulonephritis. N Engl J Med 1988;318:1651.

33. Lockwood C, Bakes D, Jones S, Whitaker K, et al: Association of alkaline phosphatase with an autoantigen recognized by circulating anti-neutrophil antibodies in systemic vasculitis. Lancet 1987;i:716.

34. Rasmussen N, Borregard N, Wiik A: Anti-neutrophil-cytoplasm antibodies in Wegener's granulomatosis are not directed against alkaline phosphatase (letter). Lancet 1987;i:1488.

35. Abbott F, Jones S, Lockwood CM, Rees AJ: Autoantibodies to glomerular antigens in patients with Wegener's granulomatosis. Nephrol Dial Transplant 1989;4:1.

36. Feinberg R: A morphologic and immunohistologic study of the evolution of the necrotizing palisading granuloma of pathergic (Wegener's) granulomatosis. Semin Resp Med 1989;10:126.

37. Moore PM, Beard EE, Thoburn TW, Williams HL: Idiopathic (lethal) granuloma of the midline facial tissues treated with cortisone: Report of a case. Laryngoscope 1951;61:320.

38. Williams HL, Hochfilzer JJ: Effect of cortisone on idiopathic granuloma of the midline tissues of the face. Ann Otol Rhinol 1950;59:518.

39. Walton EW: Giant-cell granuloma of the respiratory tract (Wegener's granulomatosis). Br Med J 1958;2:265.

40. DeRemee RA, McDonald TJ, Weiland LH: Wegener's granulomatosis: Observations on treatment with antimicrobial agents. Mayo Clin Proc 1985;60:27.

41. DeRemee RA: The treatment of Wegener's granulomatosis with trimethoprim/sulfamethoxazole: Illusion or vision? Arthritis Rheum 1988;31:1068.

42. West BC, Todd JR, King JW: Wegener's granulomatosis and trimethoprim-sulfamethoxazole: Complete remission after a twenty-year course. Ann Intern Med 1987;106:840.
43. Israel HL: Sulfamethoxazole-trimethoprim therapy for Wegener's granulomatosis. Arch Intern Med 1988;148:2293.
44. Fukuda K, Yuasa K, Uchizono A, Matsuyama H, Shimada K, Ohyama M: Three cases of Wegener's granulomatosis treated with an antimicrobial agent. Arch Otolaryngol Head Neck Surg 1989;115:515.
45. Gross WL: Wegener's granulomatosis, new aspects of the disease course, immunodiagnostic procedures, and stage-adapted treatment. Sarcoidosis 1989;6:15.

11

Lymphomatoid Granulomatosis and Lymphoproliferative Disorders of the Lung

Elaine S. Jaffe
William D. Travis

The diagnosis and classification of pulmonary lymphoid infiltrates have undergone significant reassessment and revision in recent years. Among B-cell lymphoproliferative disorders many examples of lymphocytic interstitial pneumonitis have been recognized as small lymphocytic or well-differentiated lymphocytic lymphomas.[1] Similarly, most pulmonary nodules composed of small lymphocytes and residual germinal centers once would have been interpreted as pseudolymphomas. However, the recognition that the small lymphocytic component in these lesions was often monoclonal led to the reclassification of many of these lesions as low-grade lymphomas.[2] Similarly, there has been a reappraisal of certain T-cell infiltrates within the lung. Lymphomatoid granulomatosis, as described by Liebow and colleagues, was interpreted as an atypical reactive lymphoid infiltrate in the lung frequently associated with extensive necrosis, to be distinguished from Wegener's granulomatosis.[3] Although it was recognized that many of these patients were at risk to develop malignant lymphoma, the initial lesions were interpreted as reactive and benign. Subsequent studies led to the speculation that these lesions might represent lymphoma at onset and that the spectrum of histologic features represented progression from a low-grade to a high-grade lymphoid malignancy.[4]

This chapter will review the clinical and pathologic manifestations of lymphoproliferative disorders involving the lung. Because these disorders can best be understood in terms of their relationship to the normal immune system, they will be discussed in relation to the T- and B-cell lineages.

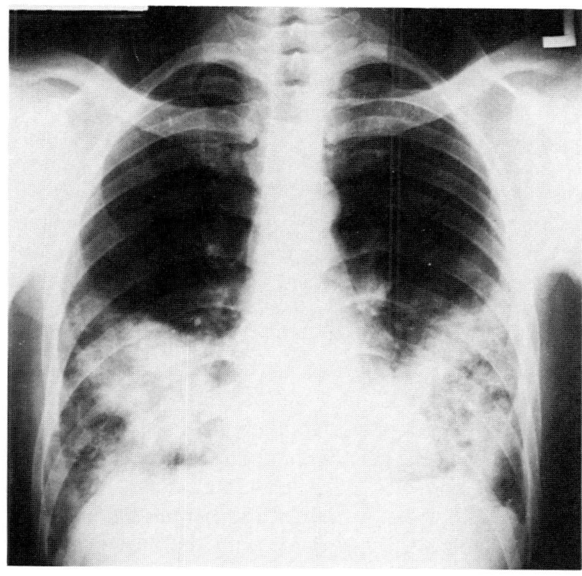

Figure 11-1. Chest radiograph from a patient with lymphomatoid granulomatosis (angiocentric immunoproliferative lesion, grade II). The lower lung fields contain multiple nodular densities.

PROLIFERATIVE DISORDERS OF T CELLS

Lymphomatoid Granulomatosis (LYG)— The Angiocentric Immunoproliferative Lesions (AIL)

Lymphomatoid granulomatosis (LYG) was first described by Liebow and colleagues as a process clinically resembling Wegener's granulomatosis, but pathologically mimicking lymphoma.[3] Although LYG is a systemic disease that can involve many organ systems, the lung is the most common site of presentation. Most patients present with bilateral multifocal nodular pulmonary densities (Fig. 11-1). Larger lesions may show central cavitation. Other common sites of involvement are the upper respiratory tract, skin, central and peripheral nervous systems, kidneys, and gastrointestinal tract. Lymph node involvement is conspicuous by its absence, and indeed, the absence of lymph node involvement prompted Liebow to conclude that the disorder probably was not malignant lymphoma. The diagnosis is usually established by open lung biopsy or biopsy of another involved site. Although fine-needle aspirate may show a lymphoid lesion, the unique architectural features of this process cannot be diagnosed cytologically.

As defined by Liebow and co-workers, LYG was characterized by a necrotizing angiocentric and angiodestructive pulmonary vasculitis.[3] In contrast to Wegener's granulomatosis, which had a conspicuous granulomatous component with palisading epithelioid cells and giant cells, LYG lacked true granulomas. Vessels showed a dense lymphoid infiltrate with an inflammatory background of plasma cells, polymorphonuclear leukocytes, and other inflammatory elements. Large bizarre and cytologically atypical cells were also noted. As a consequence of the angiodestructive character of the infiltrate, necrosis was conspicuous.

Although it is now recognized that LYG (AIL) commonly involves the upper respiratory tract, none of the original cases described by Liebow and co-workers manifested this finding. In 1966 Eichel and colleagues described polymorphic reticulosis as a variant of a malignant lymphoproliferative process presenting with the lethal midline granuloma syndrome.[5] Infiltration of blood vessels was noted as common and was associated with ischemic necrosis. The angioinvasive character of the infiltrate simulated a vasculitis. The process tended to remain localized to the upper respiratory tract and the majority of patients responded to local radiotherapy without peripheral dissemination.

Subsequently, DeRemee and colleagues, in reviewing the Mayo Clinic experience with polymorphic reticulosis, noted common histologic and clinical features between LYG and polymorphic reticulosis.[6] In their review pulmonary involvement was common and such cases were indistinguishable from LYG presenting exclusively with pulmonary disease. They proposed that both disorders were part of a single nosologic entity.

Katzenstein and colleagues expanded on the clinical and pathologic manifestations of LYG in a study of 152 cases.[7] They noted progression to overt malignant lymphoma involving lymph nodes in only 12% of patients. However, more importantly, nearly two-thirds of the patients died, with a median survival of only 14 months. Most of the patients developed disseminated disease, despite sparing of the lymphoreticular system, and central nervous system involvement was associated with shortened survival. In retrospect, we can recognize LYG as a unique form of disseminated and probably malignant lymphoproliferative process. Whereas Colby and Carrington had suggested that the architectural features of LYG might not be unique and that they could be encountered in many pulmonary lymphomas,[8] subsequent studies have supported the concept that LYG–AIL is a unique, usually systemic, disease entity.[9]

Jaffe proposed the term angiocentric immunoproliferative lesion (AIL) to encompass the clinical and pathologic spectrum of LYG and polymorphic reticulosis.[4] She proposed that AIL represented a unique T-cell lymphoproliferative process and perhaps a form of T-cell lymphoma. A T-cell phenotype has been demonstrated in LYG–AIL and in cases of nasal angiocentric lymphoma, which is part of the AIL spectrum.[9–11] It was noted that the inflammatory background often found in LYG is a feature of many peripheral T-cell lymphomas and thus does not necessarily connote a benign process.[4] AIL was proposed as a unifying concept for the diagnosis of LYG, polymorphic reticulosis, and a similar lesion affecting many organ systems, in that it conveys both the proliferative and probably neoplastic character of the process, as well as its cytologic composition and architectural distribution. "Lymphomatoid granulomatosis" is in reality a misnomer, since true granulomas are absent. Moreover, "lymphomatoid" suggests that the lymphoid proliferation is non-neoplastic.

Subsequently, a grading scheme for AIL was proposed to encompass the histologic spectrum of these lesions.[12] An earlier study by Katzenstein had suggested that histologic features might be of prognostic significance.[7] As proposed by Jaffe and associates, grade I lesions have a polymorphous cellular composition without cytologic atypia (Fig. 11-2). As with all AIL, they demonstrate an angiocentric and angiodestructive pattern of growth. Grade II AIL maintains a polymorphous cellular background, but some atypia is evident in the small lymphoid cells, and necrosis secondary to profound vascular involvement is more readily observed. Grade III lesions represent frank angiocentric lymphoma manifesting cytologic atypia diagnostic of a malignant lymphoma.

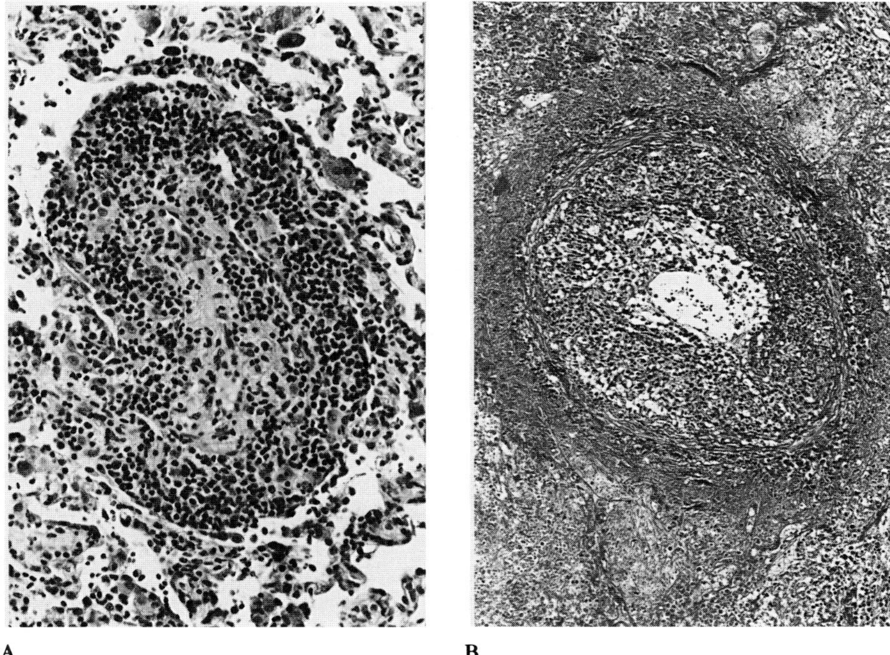

A   B

Figure 11-2. Lymphomatoid granulomatosis or angiocentric immunoproliferative lesion. (*A*) In this grade I example the infiltrate is composed primarily of small lymphocytes without cytologic atypia (H&E, × 400). (*B*) This grade III histology is characterized by an angioinvasive process composed of large atypical lymphoid cells. The surrounding lung parenchyma is extensively necrotic (H&E, × 250).

Grade III lesions can be further subclassified in the Working Formulation as malignant lymphoma, diffuse mixed cell type, or large cell, immunoblastic.

The histologic grading scheme proposed was shown to have prognostic value.[9] Only one-third of the patients with grade I AIL progressed to overt malignant lymphoma following conservative therapy with cyclophosphamide and prednisone. In contrast, two-thirds of the patients with grade II AIL progressed, with a median time to progression of 12 months, as compared to 23 months in grade I. Notably, when histologic progression did occur in patients with either grade I or grade II disease, most failed to respond to aggressive combination chemotherapy. Paradoxically, patients with grade III disease who were treated with aggressive combination chemotherapy, with or without radiation therapy, were able to sustain a complete remission without recurrence. The one patient who failed to achieve a complete remission died of his disease.

The clinical behavior of AIL, including angiocentric lymphoma, appears analogous in many respects to the follicular center cell lymphomas of the B-cell system.[13] Follicular cell lymphomas of low histologic grade present with an indolent clinical course, and patients may survive for many years either with or without aggressive therapy. However, if histologic progression occurs to a diffuse lymphoma of mixed or large cell type, the disease is associated with more aggressive clinical course.[14] Similarly, the high-grade follicular center cell lymphomas appear to be more responsive to aggressive combination chemotherapy. Patients who achieve an initial complete remission and sustain that remission for more than 2 years are frequently cured of their disease.

Immunophenotypic studies support the concept that AIL represents a single clinicopathologic entity. The proliferating cells have mature T-cell characteristics in all cases studied.[9-11] A predominance of CD4+ T cells is usually observed. However, the immunophenotypic studies have not been helpful in ascertaining if AIL is neoplastic at onset. Phenotypic abnormalities such as antigen-loss were absent in all grade I and grade II lesions studied,[9] but have been seen in angiocentric lymphomas or grade III AIL.[9,11]

More recently, molecular genetic analyses have not provided strong evidence for a clonal T-cell proliferation in AIL. One grade III lesion initially reported did show a clonal rearrangement of the gene for the beta chain of the T-cell receptor.[9] However, in a subsequent analysis with additional enzymes that finding could not be confirmed. Moreover, in an expanded series of six additional cases, clonal rearrangements of the T-cell receptor genes were seen in only one case, regardless of histologic grade.[15] Ferry and colleagues reported similar results.[16] Notably, in a study of peripheral T-cell lymphomas lacking beta or gamma gene rearrangement, 5 of 7 cases had features of angiocentric lymphomas.[17] Thus, utilizing current technology most cases of LYG–AIL are not demonstrably monoclonal, a fact that argues against a neoplastic character for this process. Although clonality does not necessarily imply malignancy, to date virtually all neoplasms have been monoclonal.

Clinical studies suggest that LYG–AIL may be associated with an immunologic deficit. Katzenstein and associates noted that several of their patients were receiving immunosuppressive drugs prior to the development of LYG, and LYG has been reported in renal transplant recipients.[7,18-20] A necrotizing lymphoid vasculitis with features of LYG was also reported in a family with X-linked lymphoproliferative syndrome.[21] Jaffe and associates described a hemophagocytic syndrome in several patients with a T-cell lymphoproliferative process characteristic of LYG–AIL.[22] A hemophagocytic syndrome represents a marked benign but extensive histiocytic proliferation throughout the reticuloendothelial system, which frequently occurs in the setting of immunodeficiency, either iatrogenic, such as in the setting of organ transplant recipients, or endogenous, as in congenital immunodeficiency disorders.[23] Hemophagocytic syndromes also occur in patients with malignant lymphoproliferative disorders undergoing chemotherapy, most commonly of the T-cell system, such as T-cell acute lymphoblastic leukemia and peripheral T-cell lymphoma. The syndrome often appears precipitated by an infectious episode, most commonly a viral infection, and Epstein-Barr virus (EBV) frequently has been implicated.[24] What remains to be determined is whether immunosuppression is a predisposing factor for LYG–AIL, or whether it is a consequence of the disease itself, perhaps because of involvement of the T-cell arm of the immune system.

A recent report suggests a close relationship between EBV and LYG–AIL.[25] Using the sensitive polymerase chain reaction technique Katzenstein and Peiper reported EBV viral genomes in the involved tissues of 72% of cases. EBV could be causally implicated in the development of the disease, or alternatively, these patients might demonstrate expanded populations of EBV-infected cells because of their underlying immunodeficiency. The vast majority of normal adults have been exposed to EBV and harbor small numbers of immortalized EBV-infected lymphocytes. In trying to integrate current knowledge regarding the phenotypic and genotypic characteristics of LYG–AIL, one could speculate that these diseases represent an unusual host response to disseminated EBV infection. The T-cell response to EBV is known to be exuberant, and monoclonality would not be expected in such a reaction. If LYG–AIL did represent an abnormal immune response to EBV, it is not clear why chemotherapy would be of value in treating this disorder, as it clearly is.

The therapy of LYG–AIL has undergone considerable evolution. In early series most patients had undergone a trial of antibiotic therapy, not surprisingly without response. In the series of 152 patients reported by Katzenstein and associates, the therapy ranged from no initial therapy, or antibiotics alone, to corticosteroids, with or without chemotherapy and radiation therapy.[7] Treatment was extremely heterogeneous, and in this series, no conclusions could be reached regarding an optimal therapeutic approach.

Subsequently, Fauci and associates demonstrated the efficacy of cyclophosphamide (2 mg/kg body weight/day) and prednisone (1 mg/kg on alternate days).[26] Seven of the 13 patients in their series sustained complete remissions. Malignant lymphoma supervened in the 7 of 8 patients who ultimately died of their disease. This study suggested that more aggressive chemotherapeutic intervention might be of value. At the National Cancer Institute 5 patients diagnosed with grade III AIL (angiocentric lymphoma) were treated with aggressive combination chemotherapy: C-MOPP in two, ProMACE/MOPP in one, and ProMACE/CytaBOM in two.[9] One patient received radiation therapy to residual disease following completion of chemotherapy. All 5 patients are currently in continuous complete remission. The value of radiation therapy in treating localized disease had been demonstrated previously in patients with "polymorphic reticulosis." At the Mayo Clinic a regimen of doxorubicin 25 mg/m^2, bleomycin 2 mg/m^2 IM, vinblastine 6 mg/m^2 IV, and dacarbazine 250–350 ml/m^2 IV has been employed.[27] Their protocol avoids corticosteroids because of the potential danger of masking pulmonary infection. Preliminary studies demonstrate success with this regimen as well.

A consensus appears to have emerged that aggressive combination chemotherapy is required for patients with grade II and grade III AIL. For patients with grade I AIL lacking any cytologic atypia, the correct approach is less apparent. Some of these patients do well with limited chemotherapy employing cyclophosphamide and prednisone. Nevertheless, if they fail to respond to the initial therapeutic intervention, the prognosis becomes poor. If one is going to treat grade I AIL with aggressive therapy, it is essential to rule out a benign lymphoproliferative disorder. In this regard the relationship of benign lymphocytic angiitis and granulomatosis (BLAG) to grade I AIL must be clarified.[28] In contrast to grade I AIL, BLAG is usually limited to the lung. Histologically it is characterized by a diffuse cellular infiltrate that infiltrates vessels but also obliterates alveolar architecture and invades peripheral airways. The predominant cellular component is a small mature lymphocyte with lesser numbers of plasma cells. Occasionally there is vascular compromise leading to necrosis, but this is rare. According to Saldana and Israel, chlorambucil and prednisone or even prednisone alone are adequate therapy.[29] The differential diagnosis should also include small lymphocytic B-cell lymphoproliferative disorders such as small lymphocytic lymphoma and Waldenstrom's macroglobulinemia.

Angioimmunoblastic Lymphadenopathy (AILD)

Angioimmunoblastic lymphadenopathy (AILD) is another disorder that represents an interface between an abnormal immune response and malignant lymphoma. AILD as described by Frizzera, Moran and Rappaport[30] and immunoblastic-lymphadenopathy (IBL) of Lukes and Tindle[31] are a part of a single clinicopathologic entity characterized by constitutional symptoms, generalized lymphadenopathy, hepatosplenomegaly, skin rash, hypergammaglobulinemia, and immunodeficiency. In both series the process was considered to be benign, although progression to lymphoma was ultimately reported in one-third to one-half of patients.[32] Subsequently it was questioned whether AILD might itself represent a form of peripheral T-cell lymphoma.[33] The relationship of AILD to IBL-like T-cell lymphoma has been the subject of extensive discussion and debate.

Histologically, AILD is characterized by architectural effacement of involved lymph nodes and a polymorphous cellular infiltrate lacking cytologic atypia. The cellular composition includes lymphocytes, plasma cells, and immunoblasts. Many of the immunoblasts have abundant clear cytoplasm. Prognosis can be related to the extent of the immunoblastic proliferation, and when immunoblasts are present in large clusters, islands, or sheets, the prognosis is poor, with a median survival of less than 1 year.[32] Another characteristic feature of AILD is an arborizing vascular pattern with prominence of postcapillary venules.

Immunophenotypic studies have demonstrated a predominance of activated T cells in AILD.[34] The large immunoblasts appear to be of T-cell origin. The plasma cells are polyclonal and mature B lymphocytes are relatively rare. In most cases when malignant lymphoma supervenes it has a T-cell phenotype, although B-cell lymphomas have been reported as well.[35] Utilizing molecular genetic techniques a number of cases have demonstrated clonal T-cell proliferations in lymph nodes involved by AILD, suggesting that the process might be a variant of T-cell lymphoma.[36] However, other studies have failed to show evidence of clonality, have shown both T and B-cell clones, or have demonstrated that the clones are transient, not necessarily stable from one biopsy to the next.[37,38] These latter observations have suggested that AILD might represent an immunoregulatory disorder with a propensity for emergence of either T-cell or B-cell clones with subsequent evolution to malignant lymphoma. Notably, clonal cytogenetic abnormalities have been reported in a large number of patients with AILD, lending support to the hypothesis that AILD might represent a form of T-cell lymphoma.[39,40]

AILD is a systemic disorder that presents with generalized lymphadenopathy, hepatosplenomegaly, bone marrow involvement, and skin rash. Pulmonary infiltrates are not uncommon and may reflect direct infiltration by the lymphoproliferative process or secondary infection.[41–47] In the lung AILD is characterized by a perivascular and interstitial infiltrate that mimics that seen in lymph nodes. More commonly, however, pulmonary infiltrates in AILD are secondary to infectious complications.[48] Supervening infection with penumonia is the cause of death in nearly half of reported cases. Infections include bacterial or fungal pneumonia and cytomegalovirus and pneumocystis infection.

Therapeutic regimens attempted for AILD have included corticosteroid agents alone or in combination with chemotherapy, most commonly cyclophosphamide.[48,49]

TABLE 11-1. Classification of Post-thymic T-cell Malignancies

  I. T-cell chronic lymphocytic leukemia
     helper subtype
     suppressor or T-γ lymphoproliferative disease
 II. T-cell prolymphocytic leukemia
III. Mycosis fungoides/Sézary syndrome
 IV. Peripheral T-cell lymphomas
     Morphologic variants include:
     Node-based T-cell lymphoma
     T-zone lymphoma
     AILD-like T-cell lymphoma
     Lymphoepithelioid cell (Lennert's) lymphoma
     Multilobated T-cell lymphoma
  V. Large cell anaplastic lymphoma (Ki-1+)
 VI. Adult T-cell leukemia/lymphoma
     (HTLV-1–associated disease)
VII. AIL including angiocentric lymphomas
     (Lymphomatoid granulomatosis)
     (Polymorphic reticulosis)

Patients treated with chemotherapy do better than untreated patients. However, results with intensive chemotherapeutic regimens have not been rewarding, most commonly because severe opportunistic infections supervene. The current approach is usually an initial trial with cyclophosphamide and prednisone. If malignant lymphoma supervenes or there is evidence of progression, a more aggressive chemotherapeutic approach is warranted.

Peripheral T-Cell Lymphomas and Adult T-Cell Leukemia/Lymphoma

The term "peripheral T-cell lymphoma" was coined by Waldron and colleagues to describe six cases of non-Hodgkin's lymphomas that were postulated to be of peripheral or mature T-cell origin rather than of central or thymic origin.[50] Subsequently, the term peripheral T-cell lymphoma has been applied to those non-Hodgkin's lymphomas with a mature T-cell phenotype not belonging to one of the other distinct clinicopathologic entities such as mycosis fungoides/Sézary syndrome, angiocentric lymphoma, or adult T-cell leukemia/lymphoma (Table 11-1).[4] Peripheral T-cell lymphomas are all diffuse and represent a spectrum of cytologic subtypes. In the Working Formulation most cases are classified as either diffuse mixed cell or large cell immunoblastic type. Those cases classified as diffuse mixed often have an inflammatory background of lymphocytes, plasma cells, and eosinophils and may be difficult to differentiate from Hodgkin's disease. Those classified as large cell immunoblastic lack an inflammatory background but demonstrate marked pleomorphism of the malignant lymphoid cells. In many instances lymphoepithelioid cell lymphoma or Lennert's lymphoma is a form of peripheral T-cell lymphoma. An arborizing vascular pattern is another feature sometimes noted in peripheral T-cell lymphoma. Thus, given the prominent vascularity and polymorphous cellular composition, the differential diagnosis with AILD is often difficult. In contrast to AILD, the background lymphocytes should show clear-cut cytologic atypia.

Clinically, peripheral T-cell lymphoma is associated with stage III or IV disease at presentation with generalized lymphadenopathy and, often, with hepatosplenomegaly. Other common sites of involvement are skin, mucosal sites, and liver.[4] In the initial series reported by Waldron and co-workers four of six patients had either lung or pleural involvement by lymphoma at presentation.[50] Subsequent studies have not borne out this high frequency. For example at the NCI and at the University of Southern California, 20% and 14% of patients, respectively, presented with pulmonary or pleural disease.[4,51] Documentation of pulmonary involvement can be based on examination of pleural fluid or biopsy material.

Peripheral T-cell lymphomas should be approached as diffuse aggressive non-Hodgkin's lymphomas and treated with combination chemotherapeutic regimens. Although the natural history is aggressive, complete remissions can be obtained. At the NCI, survival of T-cell lymphoma patients treated with the ProMACE/MOPP protocol was equivalent to that of patients with diffuse aggressive B-cell lymphomas, a result that was confirmed by Horning and colleagues using comparable aggressive regimens.[52,53]

Adult T-cell Leukemia/Lymphoma (ATLL)

ATLL is a distinct clinicopathologic syndrome, originally described in southwestern Japan, that is associated with the human retrovirus HTLV-1.[54,55] It has also been identified in other parts of the world, including the southeastern United States and the Caribbean, where it is much more common in blacks than whites.[56] The usual clinical presentation includes lymphadenopathy, hepatosplenomegaly, hypercalcemia with or without lytic bone lesions, and skin disease. Peripheral blood involvement is exceedingly common and most patients develop a leukemic phase at some time during the clinical course. Epidermal infiltration is frequently observed in the skin, making a histologic distinction from mycosis fungoides/Sézary syndrome difficult.[57] Clinically, however, these disorders are quite distinctive, and in the appropriate clinical context differentiation from classic mycosis fungoides is usually not difficult.

Pulmonary infiltrates are common. Bilateral diffuse interstitial pulmonary infiltrates were initially present in nearly 50% of cases.[58] In three of five patients the infiltrates were assumed to be secondary to tumor infiltration and responded to chemotherapy. A positive diagnosis of tumor involvement was established by either cytologic examination of a pleural effusion or a transbronchial biopsy in two cases. Opportunistic infections are also extremely common in this patient population. Before therapy biopsy-confirmed *Pneumocystis carinii* pneumonia (PCP) was documented in 2 of 11 patients. Another patient had clinically suspected PCP pneumonia and one had cryptococcal meningitis. Infectious complications are also common following treatment, and include candidiasis, cytomegaloviral infections, and bacterial sepsis. Notably, these infectious complications may develop in the absence of granulocytopenia and are presumably related to the involvement of the T-cell system by the neoplastic process. Indeed, it was these observations that prompted Gallo and colleagues to speculate that another virus, similar to HTLV-1, might be involved as the etiologic agent of the acquired immunodeficiency syndrome.

ATLL is usually associated with an aggressive clinical course and a median survival of less than 1 year, despite the use of aggressive combination chemotherapy. In some patients a chronic or smoldering form of the disease may be manifested. This form is characterized by skin rash and small numbers of atypical cells in the peripheral blood without other organ system involvement.[59] Because of the lack of success with conventional combination chemotherapy and the frequent infectious complications, more recently tumor-directed immunotherapy has been attempted using the anti-TAC monoclonal antibody.[60] ATLL cells express large numbers of IL2 receptors. TAC represents one of the two IL2 binding peptides expressed on activated T lymphocytes. Anti-TAC recognizes the IL2 binding site of the 55 kDa peptide and thus blocks the binding of IL2 to its receptor, thereby preventing T-cell proliferation. In a recent series three of nine patients treated with anti-TAC had transient mixed partial or complete remissions lasting from 1 to more than 8 months after TAC therapy. Notably, these patients did not develop severe immunodeficiency although PCP pneumonia occurred in one and Kaposi's sarcoma in a second.

HODGKIN'S DISEASE

Hodgkin's disease constitutes approximately 40% of all malignant lymphomas. Although the treatment of Hodgkin's disease represents a major success for modern oncology, the nature of the malignant cell in Hodgkin's disease, the Reed-Sternberg cell and its mononuclear variants, represents a persistent enigma.[61] Most recent evidence favors a lymphoid origin for the malignant cell, most likely a B-cell. A characteristic feature of Hodgkin's disease is that the malignant cells, the Reed-Sternberg cells and variants, represent a minority of the cells present and are associated with an inflammatory background of lymphocytes, histiocytes, plasma cells, and eosinophils. Most of the background lymphocytes are of T-cell origin. The Lukes-Butler classification of Hodgkin's disease as modified at the Rye Conference remains in widespread clinical use.[62]

In the United States, nodular sclerosing Hodgkin's disease (NSHD) is the most common subtype, representing 75% to 85% of cases in many series. NSHD often presents with stage II disease, a mediastinal mass and supraclavicular or cervical adenopathy.[63] Although disseminated pulmonary disease is relatively rare, direct extension to the lung from bulky mediastinal disease is common. Bulky or massive mediastinal disease is defined as a mediastinal mass greater than one-third the chest diameter. In such cases direct extension into the pulmonary parenchyma is common. In current staging schemes, such patients are considered to have not stage IV disease, but "E" stage disease, indicating direct extension. In this setting pulmonary involvement does not imply hematogenous dissemination. Patients with bulky mediastinal disease are usually approached with combined modality therapy employing both combination chemotherapy and radiation therapy.[64] Combination chemotherapy is usually employed first to shrink the mass lesion. Following three or four cycles of the selected combination (MOPP or ABVD), conventional tumoricidal doses of radiotherapy may be delivered as a mantle or subtotal nodal radiotherapy. In other instances the inverse sequence may be followed, and radiotherapy to the bulk mass lesion is followed by six cycles of MOPP chemotherapy.

By contrast, disseminated pulmonary disease implies dissemination and is considered stage IV. In such patients MOPP or ABVD or a combination is the treatment of choice. Pulmonary involvement can be documented by fine-needle aspirate or open lung biopsy.[65,66] Bronchoscopy and endobronchial brush biopsies are rarely successful in documenting involvement because the lesions do not usually invade the bronchial mucosa.[67]

Radiation pneumonitis represents a significant complication of the treatment of Hodgkin's disease and may occur as early as 1 to 3 months following completion of therapy. It is characterized by a nonproductive cough, low-grade fever, and dyspnea. The incidence of serious or symptomatic pneumonitis is relatively low, usually less than 10%. The differential diagnosis of pulmonary infiltrates in a patient with Hodgkin's disease also includes bacterial, fungal, or viral infection as well as recurrent Hodgkin's disease involving the lungs.[64,65]

PROLIFERATIVE DISORDERS OF B-CELLS

Epstein-Barr Virus–Associated Lymphoproliferative Disorder (EBV-LPD)

EBV is a B-cell lymphotrophic virus capable of immortalizing normal B lymphocytes.[68] It is implicated as the etiologic agent of infectious mononucleosis and in the absence of an intact immune system can be associated with a fatal B-cell lymphoproliferative disorder and malignant lymphoma.[69] EBV-LPD is especially common in immunosuppressed transplant recipients receiving cyclosporine-A. Although it may present in any site, the lung is frequently affected.[70–72] A high incidence was reported in heart-lung transplantation recipients (9.4%).[73] Lung involvement was common, and was associated with bronchiolitis obliterans and opportunistic infections.

Pathologically, EBV-LPD is almost indistinguishable from an immunoblastic lymphoma and is composed of large, atypical lymphoid cells with an immunoblastic appearance.[70] Evidence of plasmacytoid differentiation favors a reactive process, whereas a more monomorphic infiltrate composed uniformly of large immunoblastic cells suggests lymphoma. It is thought that EBV-LPD starts out as a polyclonal B-cell process. In time one clone achieves dominance and monoclonality can ultimately be demonstrated.[74] If many sites are biopsied, a different clone may be demonstrated in each site, suggesting that the process does not necessarily disseminate. Thus, although the process may be clonal, it may not be truly malignant. It is postulated that the evolution to true malignant lymphoma is a multi-step phenomenon and that clonal expansion is followed by a second hit, such as a cytogenetic translocation. This second hit will result in true conversion to malignancy. However, in earlier stages EBV-LPD may respond to withdrawal of immunosuppression and antiviral therapy with acyclovir.[75]

Reactive Lymphoid Hyperplasia

Hyperplasia of the bronchial-mucosal associated lymphoid tissue (BALT or MALT) is a potential cause of interstitial lung disease.[76–79] Under the term follicular bronchitis/bronchiolitis it has been reported in patients with collagen vascular diseases (especially rheumatoid arthritis and Sjögren's syndrome), immunodeficiency syndromes (severe combined immunodeficiency, acquired immunodeficiency, Wiskott-Aldrich syndrome) and in a poorly defined group of patients with associated eosinophilia.[80] The radiographic and gross pathologic appearance is characterized by multiple millimeter-sized nodules scattered throughout the lung parenchyma. Histologically, it consists of hyperplastic lymphoid aggregates most commonly situated in a peribronchiolar or perivascular location and sometimes seen along the pleura or interlobular septa. Hyperplastic lymphoid follicles are commonly seen as a secondary component of other pulmonary processes such as idiopathic pulmonary fibrosis or localized inflammatory lesions. Rarely is lymphoid hyperplasia the dominant pathologic finding; only in such cases should the term follicular bronchiolitis/bronchitis be used for the primary diagnosis.

Intrapulmonary lymph nodes represent another form of pulmonary lymphoid tissue that may become hyperplastic.[79] The hyperplastic nodes may present as pulmonary coin nodules[81,82] or as enlarging pulmonary masses.[83] Intrapulmonary lymph nodes are sometimes excised as suspected metastases in patients with cancer.[84] They may be found away from the pulmonary hilum in up to 7% of autopsied lungs.[85] Histologically, these lymph nodes appear as encapsulated nodules of lymphoid tissue, which often contain sclerotic nodules and anthracosilicotic dust pigment.[79]

Pseudolymphoma

Pseudolymphoma of the lung, as its name implies, is a benign lymphoid lesion that can mimic malignant lymphoma.[2,79,86–98] It usually consists of a solitary, localized mass.[79,88,92,95] Rarely, multiple pulmonary masses may occur.[98] The majority of patients are 50 to 60 years old.[88,92] Most cases are discovered as an incidental mass seen on a routine chest radiograph in an asymptomatic patient. One case has been reported in a patient with systemic lupus erythematosus.[98] Hilar and mediastinal lymphadenopathy are characteristically absent. The etiology of pseudolymphoma is not known; however, it appears to be an inflammatory lesion that could be postinfectious or allergic in origin.[87] Radiographically and pathologically, pseudolymphoma of the lung is characterized by a localized parenchymal nodule that ranges from several centimeters up to 10 centimeters in size.[92,95] Histologically, pseudolymphomas are composed of a circumscribed mass of lymphoid tissue, often with infiltrative borders and a central fibrotic scar. The tumor consists of a variable mixture of cytologically mature lymphocytes, plasma cells, and histiocytes; germinal centers are often present. Dutcher bodies are rarely found.[79] Amyloid may be present but is usually scant compared to the amount seen with lymphoma.[79] Pseudolymphoma does not involve the hilar lymph nodes. Plaque-like involvement of the pleura and erosion of bronchial cartilage are features usually associated with malignant lymphoma rather than pseudolymphoma.[94,95]

A major difficulty in histopathologic diagnosis is distinction from small lymphocytic (SL) lymphoma.[86–98] SL lymphoma in the lung usually demonstrates a distinctive pattern of infiltration characterized by infiltration or "tracking" along lymphatic routes (that is, along the pleura, interlobular septa, and bronchovascular bundles).[2] Lymph node involvement supports a diagnosis of lymphoma; however, since only a minority of SL lymphomas involve hilar lymph nodes, this feature cannot be relied upon very often.[2,94]

In contrast to SL lymphomas, which are monoclonal, the lymphoid cells in pseudolymphomas demonstrate a polyclonal immunophenotype by immunohistochemistry for immunoglobulin light chains.[2,89,94] Immunohistochemistry performed on sections from paraffin-embedded tissue will only detect cytoplasmic immunoglobulins; therefore only cases with substantial numbers of plasma cells or plasmacytoid lymphocytes can be evaluated for clonality by this method. If plasma cell differentiation is not prominent, frozen sections are necessary to detect surface immunoglobulins on small lymphocytes.[89] In interpreting immunohistochemical stains one has to keep in mind that a polyclonal reactive inflammatory infiltrate may occur at the edges of a lymphoma.[2] Cell suspensions can be helpful if a monoclonal lymphoid population is demonstrated,[87,91] but a polyclonal result could be misleading since a reactive inflammatory infiltrate adjacent to a tumor could cause a lymphoma to appear polyclonal.

Most patients with pulmonary pseudolymphoma have an excellent prognosis and surgical removal of the lesion is curative. Recurrence is infrequent[95] and rare examples of progression to malignant lymphoma have been reported.[90,92,95]

Lymphocytic Interstitial Pneumonitis

Shortness of breath and cough are the most frequent presenting symptoms of patients with lymphocytic interstitial pneumonia (LIP).[99–102] Patients may also present with fever and joint stiffness.[99–102] LIP may be idiopathic, but it also occurs with a variety of associated conditions (Table 11-2).[103–124] Rare cases of familial LIP have been reported.[125] In patients infected with the human immunodeficiency virus (HIV), LIP occurs most commonly in children; it is less common in adults and seems to occur more often in Haitians.[118–120] Chest radiographs may demonstrate a spectrum of fine to coarse, reticular or nodular interstitial infiltrates.[99–101] A restrictive defect is found by pulmonary function tests.[99–100] Serum laboratory tests frequently show hypergammaglobulinemia or hypogammaglobulinemia. If the patients have Sjögren's syndrome, a positive rheumatoid factor or other immunologic abnormalities may be found.[99,100]

Histologically, LIP is characterized by a diffuse lymphoplasmacytic interstitial infiltrate with a variable percentage of lymphocytes and plasma cells (Fig. 11-3). In some cases, plasma cells may predominate.[103–108] Atypical lymphoid cells are characteristically absent. Epithelioid granulomas or multinucleated giant cells may be present. Occasionally amyloid may be present.[112] Immunohistochemical studies demonstrate polyclonal staining for immunoglobulin light chains.

Although the cellular composition of LIP is similar to pseudolymphoma, LIP consists of a diffuse interstitial infiltrate rather than a discrete mass.[79,99] As with pseudolymphoma, the major differential diagnostic problem is separation from SL lymphoma. Histologically, lymphomas tend to have a more patchy distribution and show a distinctive "tracking" pattern of infiltration along lymphatic routes (along the pleura, septa, and around bronchovascular bundles). Other inflammatory interstitial lesions, such as hypersensitivity pneumonitis, sarcoidosis, and nonspecific chronic interstitial pneumonitis, may also enter into the differential diagnosis.

In general, patients with LIP have a good prognosis. Steroid therapy is effective in some patients. Others may progress to end-stage interstitial fibrosis. Malignant lym-

TABLE 11-2. Lymphocytic Interstitial Pneumonia: Associated Conditions

CONDITION	REFERENCE
Idiopathic	100
Dysproteinemia	99,103,104
Monoclonal gammopathy	105
Polyclonal gammopathy	106,107
Macroglobulinemia	108
Hypogammaglobulinemia	109
Pernicious anemia/agammaglobulinemia	110
Autoerythrocyte sensitization syndrome	111
Collagen Vascular Disease	
Sjögren's syndrome	112–114,*127
Systemic lupus erythematosus	115
Immunodeficiency	
Common variable immunodeficiency	116
Immunodeficiency, unclassified	117
Viral Infection	
HIV infection	118–120
Epstein-Barr virus infection	121
Chronic active hepatitis	122
Drug or Therapy-Induced	
Dilantin	123
Bone marrow transplantation	124

*Although this case was reported as an example of pseudolymphoma, it actually represents a case of LIP, because the patient had a diffuse rather than nodular infiltrate according to the radiographic and pathologic description (114).

phoma has developed in a few reported cases.[126–129] Due to the difficulty in distinguishing LIP from SL lymphoma, it is possible that some of these cases actually represented SL lymphoma from the beginning. However, in at least one case, immuno-histochemical studies suggested that the initial lesion was a polyclonal B-cell proliferation.[129]

Low-Grade Lymphoma

In the lung, the majority of low-grade lymphomas (Table 11-3) are small lymphocytic (SL) lymphomas.[130–136] In fact, SL lymphoma (including SL lymphoma with plasmacy-toid features) is the most common histologic type of primary pulmonary malignant lymphoma; it comprises 50% to 60% of cases in most large series.[93,94,130] The remaining types of low-grade lymphomas are uncommon; these include SL lymphomas of intermediate differentiation, follicular small cleaved cell lymphomas, and follicular mixed small and large cleaved cell lymphomas.[136–138] Patients with Sjögren's syndrome are prone to develop pulmonary malignant lymphomas, the majority of which are low-grade lymphomas.[133]

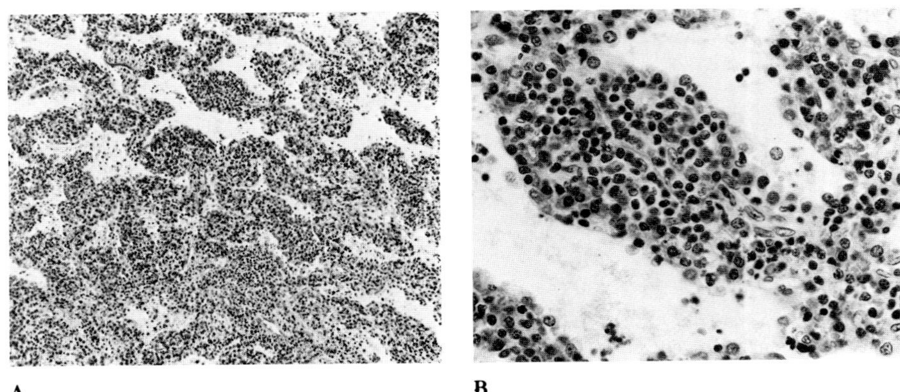

Figure 11-3. Lymphocytic interstitial pneumonitis. (*A*) The diffuse interstitial infiltrate is characteristic (H&E, × 125). (*B*) Higher power reveals that the infiltrate is composed of a heterogeneous population of small round lymphocytes and plasma cells. Immunohistochemistry revealed polyclonal staining for immunoglobulin light chains (H&E, × 500).

In recent years, the criteria for the diagnosis of SL lymphoma in the lung have been redefined.[131] As a result, many cases of pulmonary pseudolymphoma and LIP have been reclassified as low-grade malignant lymphomas. Terms such as "localized lymphoid nodule"[79] and "small lymphocytic proliferation"[93] have been proposed to encompass SL lymphoma, pseudolymphoma, and LIP, since a clearcut distinction is not always possible. The concept of mucosa- or bronchi-associated lymphoid tissue (MALT or BALT) has also been applied to lymphomas arising in the lung.[91,132]

SL lymphoma presents in patients 30 to 85 years.[93,134] The sex predominance slightly favored females in one study[134] and males in another.[93] Most cases are detected as an incidental chest radiographic finding in an asymptomatic patient. Cough and dyspnea are the most common symptoms. Hemoptysis and weight loss are uncommon. A monoclonal gammopathy may be found in up to 22% of cases.[93]

The major gross pathologic and radiologic features from a large series reported by Kennedy and colleagues are summarized in Figure 11-4A.[93] According to another large series of pulmonary SL lymphoma reported by Turner and associates, chest radiographs most often demonstrate a solitary noncavitating pulmonary mass (36%), followed by multiple nodules (25%), a dense localized infiltrate (14%), a mass combined with a localized infiltrate (11%), diffuse bilateral infiltrates (9%), or pleural effusions (5%).[134] The majority of lung nodules caused by SL lymphoma measure less than 5 cm,[93] but tumors up to 13 cm in diameter may occur.[135] Histologically, SL lymphoma consists of an infiltrate of small round lymphocytes without cytologic atypia (Fig. 11-5); variable numbers of plasma cells or plasmacytoid lymphocytes may also be present. The histologic features observed in the study by Kennedy and colleagues are summarized in Figure 11-4B.[93]

Immunohistochemical demonstration of a monoclonal immunophenotype is diagnostic of malignant lymphoma. However, much emphasis has been placed on establishing histologic criteria for the diagnosis of SL lymphoma, since immunohistochemistry

TABLE 11-3. Working Formulation of Non-Hodgkin's Malignant Lymphomas (ML)[136]

Low Grade

ML, small lymphocytic

   Consistent with chronic lymphocytic leukemia

   Plasmacytoid

ML, lymphocytic, of intermediate differentiation*

ML, follicular, predominantly small cleaved cell

ML, follicular mixed (small cleaved and large cell)

Intermediate Grade

ML, follicular, predominantly large cell

ML, diffuse, small cleaved cell

ML, diffuse, mixed (small and large cell)

ML, diffuse, large cell

High Grade

ML, large cell, immunoblastic

ML, lymphoblastic

ML, small noncleaved cell

   Burkitt's

Miscellaneous

Histiocytic

Extramedullary plasmacytoma

---

* The working formulation has been modified to include the category of ML, lymphocytic, of intermediate differentiation, in the group of low-grade lymphomas (refs 136–138).

may not always be available. The major diagnostic criteria proposed by Salzstein in 1967 to separate SL lymphoma from pseudolymphoma were: (1) "immature lymphocytes"; (2) absence of germinal centers; and (3) involvement of hilar lymph nodes.[97] However, several recent studies have demonstrated that germinal centers can be found in up to 45% of pulmonary SL lymphomas.[94,134] Saltzstein's criteria were revised by Turner and co-workers, who proposed that a lymphangitic pattern and a monomorphous small lymphocytic or homogeneous lymphoplasmacytic infiltrate were the most important criteria for the diagnosis of pulmonary SL lymphoma.[134] The presence of extrapulmonary lymph node involvement is still diagnostic of SL lymphoma. However, this is found only in the minority of cases. When a patient with chronic lymphocytic leukemia (CLL) develops lung involvement, the histologic picture is identical to that of SL lymphoma.[139] Rarely, the infiltrates of CLL may be predominantly centered around airways, giving a bronchiolocentric distribution.[140]

Open lung biopsy provides the best opportunity to establish the diagnosis of low-grade pulmonary lymphomas; in some cases, even with an open biopsy, the separation of SL lymphoma from pseudolymphoma or LIP may be difficult. A generous and well-preserved transbronchial biopsy specimen may, occasionally, be sufficient for the diagnosis of SL lymphoma. Rarely, the diagnosis may be established by transthoracic fine-needle aspiration biopsy.[141] However, both transbronchial biopsies and fine-needle

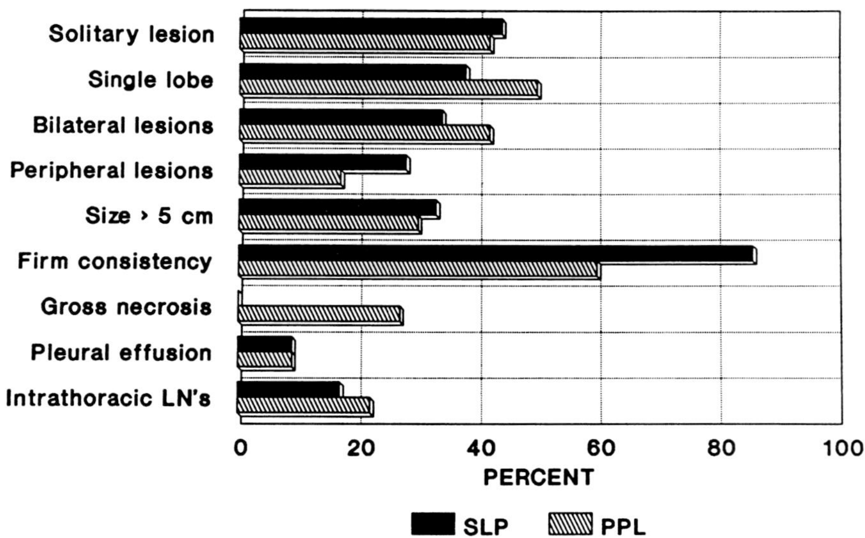

A

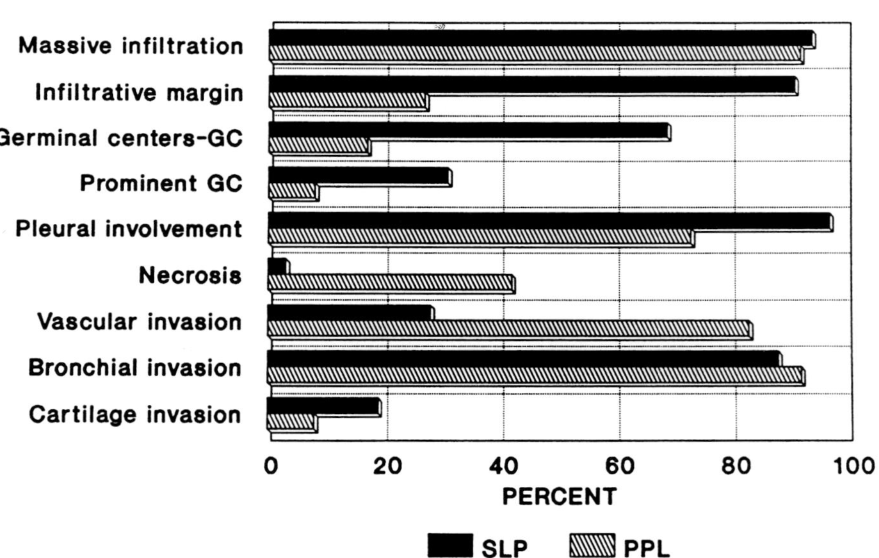

B

Figure 11-4. Comparison of small lymphocytic proliferations (SLP) and primary pulmonary lymphoma (PPL), as reported by Kennedy and associates.[93] SLP includes a heterogeneous group of 32 patients with SL lymphoma, lymphocytic interstitial pneumonitis, or pseudolymphoma. PPL represents 12 patients presenting with lymphoma of histologic subtypes other than SL. (*A*) Radiographic and gross pathologic features. (*B*) Histologic features.

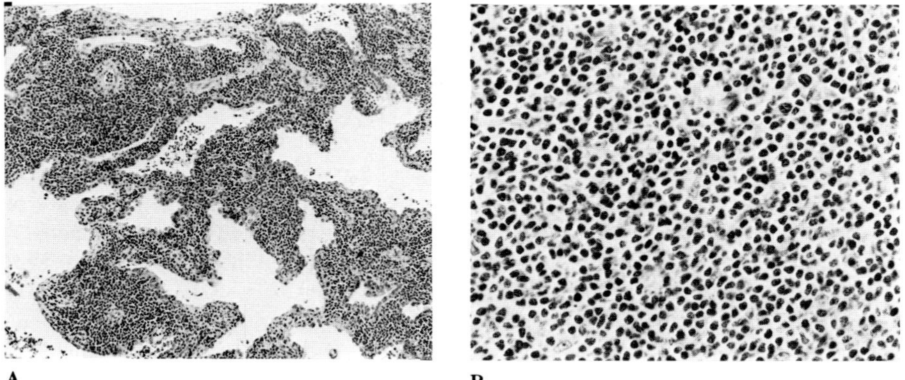

A   B

Figure 11-5. SL lymphoma. (*A*) A diffuse interstitial infiltrate is apparent (H&E, × 125). (*B*) The infiltrate consists of a homogeneous population of small lymphocytes (H&E, × 500).

aspiration biopsies for the diagnosis of malignant lymphoma should be interpreted with caution and correlated carefully with clinical, radiographic, and immunohistochemical information.

Secondary histologic changes are frequently seen in pulmonary SL lymphoma and may obscure the lymphomatous infiltrate.[2,131] These include germinal centers; focal polymorphous infiltrate, especially at the edge of the tumor; sclerosis; amyloid; obstructive pneumonia with intra-alveolar foamy macrophages; hyperplastic type II pneumocytes; interstitial infiltrates of lymphocytes and plasma cells; bronchiolitis obliterans with or without organizing pneumonia; intra-alveolar macrophage accumulation; and alveolar exudate unassociated with obstruction.[2,131]

The key histopathologic and immunohistologic criteria for separating SL lymphoma from pseudolymphoma and LIP have already been discussed. In cases where the histopathologic differential diagnosis is uncertain, several extrapulmonary tests may be of assistance. Serum protein electrophoresis can be helpful, since a monoclonal gammopathy is likely to be found in a patient with a lymphoma. Other potential helpful investigations include bone marrow biopsy, examination of the peripheral blood for evidence of CLL, and a search for lymphadenopathy by careful physical examination or computed tomography of the chest and abdomen.

The majority of patients presenting with primary pulmonary SL lymphoma have an excellent prognosis; surgical excision may be curative in patients with localized lesions.[134] Adjuvant radiotherapy or chemotherapy is necessary only in patients who have progressive disease; it may not always be effective.[2,131,134] The presence of multiple pulmonary lesions[134] or a monoclonal gammopathy[93] have been identified as poor prognostic factors. About 25% of patients with pulmonary SL lymphoma as the major presenting manifestation will prove to have extrapulmonary lymphoma at initial staging or with subsequent follow-up. Extrapulmonary spread is more likely to occur in patients with multiple pulmonary lesions at presentation. In one series recurrence or dissemination occurred in 33% of cases.[130] All of these recurrences occurred at least

38 months after initial diagnosis, indicating that long-term follow-up is necessary to determine clinical outcome.[130] A small number of patients may progress to a high-grade lymphoma.[2,131]

Plasmacytoma

Extramedullary plasmacytoma presenting in the lung is extremely rare; less than 30 cases have been reported.[142–148] It occurs most often in patients 60 to 70 years of age[142,145] but may rarely occur in children.[143] Although it may present as an incidental finding in an asymptomatic patient,[145] a significant percentage of patients present with symptoms such as fever, weight loss, chest or shoulder pain, dyspnea, cough, and hemoptysis.[142–144] Plasmacytomas may be localized to the lung, but they may also occur in association with plasmacytomas in other extramedullary sites.[142,146] Lung involvement occurs in fewer than 1% of patients with multiple myeloma, according to one study of 958 patients; the lung lesions in this study consisted of plasmacytomas in 6 patients and diffuse pulmonary infiltrates in 4.[149]

Plasmacytomas are discrete nodular lung lesions that are usually solitary. Histologically, plasmacytomas are composed entirely of plasma cells with varying degrees of atypia. By definition, they demonstrate monoclonal staining for immunoglobulin light chains.[142,144] Amyloid[148] or amorphous deposits that appear to represent nodular accumulations of immunoglobulin may be present.[144]

The differential diagnosis includes plasma cell granuloma (inflammatory pseudotumor), SL lymphoma with plasmacytoid features, LIP with plasmacytoid features, and plasma cell granuloma. If polyclonal staining is encountered in a plasmacytic tumor, it should be called a plasma cell granuloma.[145,150] The term "plasma cell granuloma" is favored over "inflammatory pseudotumor," since the latter term has been applied to a number of entities, including pseudolymphoma.[151,152] Plasma cell granulomas consist of a nodular mass of chronic inflammatory and fibroblastic tissue.[150–152] The inflammatory component is composed of a variable mixture of polyclonal plasma cells and lymphocytes; foamy histiocytes are sometimes prominent, giving the appearance of a xanthoma or fibroxanthoma. Plasmacytomas differ from cases of pulmonary SL lymphoma with plasmacytoid features in that they consist of a pure population of plasma cells. Plasmacytomas also must be separated from cases of plasma-cell–rich LIP, which by definition is polyclonal and is characterized by diffuse rather than nodular lung infiltrate.[103,108]

The finding of a plasmacytoma in the lung should prompt a workup for multiple myeloma. A bone marrow biopsy sample with less than 10% plasma cells, the absence of anemia, and a normal radiographic skeletal survey suggest that myeloma is not present.[142] A monoclonal gammopathy in serum or urine can occur with or without systemic myeloma. However, if the M-protein does not resolve after surgical removal of the lung tumor[143,147] or if the level is markedly elevated, the presence of extrapulmonary disease should be suspected.[142]

The clinical course of plasmacytomas of the lung is somewhat variable. Approximately 30% of extramedullary plasmacytomas evolve into multiple myeloma.[142] Plasmacytomas are generally radiosensitive tumors; however, dissemination may occur despite an initial response to surgery and radiation.[142]

Aggressive B-Cell Malignant Lymphoma

To simplify the rest of this discussion, we have grouped the remainder of the pulmonary lymphomas as "aggressive B-cell malignant lymphomas." These lymphomas comprise the remainder of the histologic subtypes of malignant lymphoma, which are classified under the intermediate and high-grade categories in the Working Formulation (Table 11-3).

Most patients presenting with aggressive B-cell lymphomas in the lung are between 30 and 80 years of age; the mean age is 60 years.[93] A significantly greater number of patients with aggressive B-cell lymphomas are symptomatic at presentation compared with patients with low-grade lymphomas.[93] Symptomatic patients often presented with dyspnea, cough, chest pain, and weight loss.[93] In Japan, but not in Western countries, pleural malignant lymphomas have been reported in patients after a long history (20–30 years) of tuberculosis-associated pyothorax.[153,154] Von Willebrand's syndrome has been reported in one patient with a pulmonary lymphoma.[155] This patient's factor VIII–von Willebrand factor complex levels returned to normal following surgical removal of the lung tumor.

The presenting radiographic and gross pathologic features from one large series are summarized in Figure 11-4A.[93] The cellular composition of pulmonary aggressive B-cell lymphomas will vary depending on the histologic subtype. The tumor may consist of a pure or mixed population of small or large cleaved cells, or large noncleaved cells. The lymphoma may have either a diffuse or a follicular growth pattern; sometimes both patterns may be present in a single tumor. As with SL lymphoma, a variety of secondary histologic changes may occur and can obscure the tumor.[2,131] A variety of histologic features have been described by Kennedy and associates (see Fig. 11-4B).

In contrast to SL lymphomas, most large cell lymphomas are easily recognizable as a malignant process, owing to the atypical cytologic features of the lymphoid cells. Occasionally, distinction from a poorly differentiated carcinoma may be difficult, especially in small or crushed biopsy specimens. In such cases immunohistochemistry for cytokeratin (a marker for epithelial differentiation) and common leukocyte antigen (a marker for lympoid differentiation) may be very helpful.[156–158] Small cleaved cell lymphomas can be distinguished from reactive lymphoid lesions by the presence of a homogeneous cell population and the convoluted shape of the lymphocyte nuclei. Lymphomas consisting of a mixed population of large and small cleaved cells may raise the question of a T-cell lymphoma or lymphomatoid granulomatosis, which have already been discussed. Rarely, true histiocytic lymphomas may primarily affect the lung.[159–161] These tumors have distinctive histochemical and immunologic features.[162]

The prognosis for aggressive B-cell lymphomas as a whole is worse than that for small lymphocytic lymphomas. L'Hoste and colleagues found that 88% of patients with small lymphocytic lymphomas were alive at 5 years, compared with 47% of patients with other histologic types of lymphomas.[130] Some patients with localized lesions may be cured by surgery alone.[2,131] Koss and associates found that a pleural effusion and systemic symptoms were predictors of poor survival.[94] Several studies have shown a lack of correlation between survival and tumor size or stage.[94,130] Part of the difficulty in establishing statistically significant predictors of survival is that these tumors are relatively uncommon; therefore most studies have small numbers of patients.

Furthermore, most affected patients have not received uniform therapy, making it difficult to compare the clinical outcome.

Intravascular Lymphomatosis (Malignant Angioendotheliomatosis)

Intravascular lymphomatosis (IVL) is a rare form of malignant lymphoma that is characterized by intravascular growth.[163,164] Before immunohistochemical studies revealed its lymphoid nature, this entity was considered to be an endothelial-derived process and was often referred to as "malignant angioendotheliomatosis."[163] The most common presentation for IVL is neurologic; IVL can also present primarily with cutaneous, renal, nasal, and hepatic symptoms. The first case of IVL presenting primarily in the lung was reported by Remberger and associates in 1987,[165] and another case was reported by Tan and colleagues in 1988.[166] Yousem and associates recently reported four additional patients presenting with pulmonary IVL, two of whom had associated neurologic symptoms.[167] Pulmonary hypertension is another recently reported presentation of IVL in the lung.[168]

Thus, pulmonary IVL may present clinically, radiologically, and pathologically as a form of interstitial lung disease.[165–168] Dyspnea and fever are common symptoms. Chest radiographs may show bilateral reticular or nodular interstitial infiltrates. Histologically, at low-power magnification, the lungs may show patchy thickening of the interstitium; high-power examination of blood vessels reveals intravascular growth of atypical lymphoid cells within arterioles, venules, capillaries, and lymphatics.[165–168] The intravascular lymphoid cells stain immunohistochemically for lymphoid markers. The histologic differential diagnosis includes malignant lymphoma (especially angiocentric lymphoma), metastatic carcinoma, leukemic infiltration, and vascular sarcomas.[165–168] IVL is fatal in most cases, but several patients with pulmonary IVL have shown a response to chemotherapy.[167]

REFERENCES

1. Turner RR, Colby TV, Doggett RS. Well differentiated lymphocytic lymphoma: A study of 47 patients with primary manifestation in the lung. Cancer 1984;54:2088.
2. Colby TV, Yousem SA. Pulmonary lymphoid neoplasms. Semin Diagn Pathol 1985;2:183.
3. Liebow AA, Carrington CRB, Friedman PJ. Lymphomatoid granulomatosis. Hum Pathol 1972;3:457.
4. Jaffe ES. Pathologic and clinical spectrum of post-thymic T-cell malignancies. Cancer Invest 1984;2:413.
5. Eichel BS, Harrison EG Jr, Devine KD, Scanlon PW, Brown HA. Primary lymphomas of the nose including a relationship to lethal midline granuloma. Am J Surg 1966;112:597.
6. DeRemee RA, Weiland LH, McDonald TJ. Polymorphic reticulosis, lymphomatoid granulomatosis (two diseases or one?). Mayo Clin Proc 1978;53:634.
7. Katzenstein A, Carrington CB, Liebow AA. Lymphomatoid granulomatosis: A clinicopathologic study of 152 cases. Cancer 1979;43:360.
8. Colby TV, Carrington CB. Malignant lymphoma of the lung simulating lymphomatoid granulomatosis: A series of 20 cases. Am J Surg Pathol 1982;6:19.

9. Lipford EH Jr, Margolick JB, Longo DL, Fauci AS, Jaffe ES. Angiocentric immunoproliferative lesions: A clinicopathologic spectrum of post-thymic T-cell proliferations. Blood 1988;72:1674.

10. Nichols PW, Koss M, Levine AM, Lukes RJ. Lymphomatoid granulomatosis: A T-cell disorder. Am J Med 1982;72:467.

11. Chan JKC, Ng CS, Lau WH, Lo STH. Most nasal/nasopharyngeal lymphomas are peripheral T-cell neoplasms. Am J Surg Pathol 1987;11:418.

12. Jaffe ES, Lipford EH Jr, Margolick JB, Longo DL, Fauci AS. Lymphomatoid granulomatosis and angiocentric lymphoma: A spectrum of post-thymic T-cell proliferations. Semin Respir Med 1989;10:167.

13. Jaffe ES. Relationship of classification to biologic behavior of non-Hodgkin's lymphomas. Semin Oncol 1986;13:3.

14. Hubbard SM, Chabner BA, DeVita VT, et al. Histologic progression in non-Hodgkin's lymphoma. Blood 1982;59:258.

15. Jaffe ES, Andrade R, Elwood LJ, Medeiros LJ, Cossman J, Raffeld M. Peripheral T-cell lymphomas and the spectrum of their clinicopathologic presentation. In: Dammacco F, ed. Immunological aspects of malignant lymphomas and cryglobulinemia. Milan: Edi-ermes, 1990: 17–27.

16. Ferry JA, Jacobson JO, Zukerberg LR, Sklar J, Harris NL. Angiocentric lymphoma: A study of 6 cases with immunophenotypic and genotypic analysis. Mod Pathol 1990;3:33A.

17. Weiss LM, Picker LJ, Grogan TM, Warnke RA, Sklar J. Absence of clonal beta and gamma T-cell receptor gene rearrangements in a subset of peripheral T-cell lymphomas. Am J Pathol 1988;130:436.

18. Hammar S, Mennemeyer R. Lymphoid granulomatosis in a renal transplant recipient. Hum Pathol 1976;7:111.

19. Michaud J, Banerjee D, Kaufmann JCE, et al. Lymphomatoid granulomatosis involving the central nervous system: Complication of a renal transplant with terminal monoclonal B-cell proliferation. Acta Neuropathol 1983;61:141.

20. Walter M, Thomson NM, Dowling J, et al. Lymphomatoid granulomatosis in a renal transplant recipient. Aust NZ J Med 1979;9:434.

21. Loeffel S, Chang CH, Heyn R, et al. Necrotizing lymphoid vasculitis in X-linked lymphoproliferative syndrome. Arch Pathol Lab Med 1985;109:546.

22. Jaffe ES, Costa JC, Fauci A, et al. Malignant lymphoma and erythrophagocytosis simulating malignant histiocytosis. Am J Med 1983;75:741.

23. Risdall RJ, McKenna RW, Nesbit ME, et al. Virus-associated hemophagocytic syndrome: A benign histiocytic proliferation distinct from malignant histiocytosis. Cancer 1979;44:993.

24. Jaffe ES. Histiocytoses of lymph nodes: Biology and differential diagnosis. Semin Diagn Pathol 1988;5:376.

25. Katzenstein ALA, Peiper SC. Detection of Epstein-Barr virus genomes in lymphomatoid granulomatosis: Analysis of 29 cases by the polymerase chain reaction technique. Mod Pathol 1990;3:435.

26. Fauci AS, Haynes BF, Costa J, et al. Lymphomatoid granulomatosis, prospective clinical and therapeutic experience over ten years. N Engl J Med 1982;306:68.

27. Letendre L. Treatment of lymphomatoid granulomatosis: Old and new perspectives. Semin Respir Med 1989;10:178.

28. Saldana MJ, Patchefsky AS, Israel HL, Atkinson GW. Pulmonary angiitis and granulomatosis: The relationship between histological features, organ involvement, and response to treatment. Hum Pathol 1977;8:391.

29. Saldana MJ, Israel HL. Necrotizing sarcoid granulomatosis, benign lymphocytic angiitis, and granulomatosis: Do they exist? Semin Respir Med 1989;10:182.

30. Frizzera G, Moran EM, Rappaport H. Angio-immunoblastic lymphadenopathy with dysproteinemia. Lancet 1974;i:1070.

31. Lukes RJ, Tindle BH. Immunoblastic lymphadenopathy: A hyperimmune entity resembling Hodgkin's disease. N Engl J Med 1975;292:1.
32. Nathwani BN, Rappaport H, Moran EM, Pangalis GA, Kim H. Malignant lymphoma arising in angioimmunoblastic lymphadenopathy. Cancer 1978;4:578.
33. Watanabe S, Shimosato Y, Shimoyama M, et al. Adult T-cell lymphoma with hypergammaglobulinemia. Cancer 1980;46:2472.
34. Jaffe ES. Morphologic features and immunoarchitecture. In: Steinberg AD, mod. Angioimmunoblastic lymphadenopathy with dysproteinemia. Ann Intern Med 1988;108:575.
35. Frizzera G, Kaneko Y, Sakurai M. Angioimmunoblastic lymphadenopathy and related disorders: A retrospective look in search of definitions. Leukemia 1989;3:1.
36. Weiss LM, Strickler JG, Dorfman RF, et al. Clonal T-cell populations in angioimmunoblastic lymphadenopathy and angioimmunoblastic lymphadenopathy-like lymphoma. Am J Pathol 1986;122:392.
37. Lipford EH, Smith HR, Pittaluga S, Jaffe ES, Steinberg AD, Cossman J. Clonality of angioimmunoblastic lymphadenopathy and implications for its evolution to malignant lymphoma. J Clin Invest 1987;79:637.
38. Feller AC, Griesser H, Schilling CV, et al. Clonal gene rearrangement patterns correlate with immunophenotype and clinical parameters in patients with angioimmunoblastic lymphadenopathy. Am J Pathol 1988;133:549.
39. Kaneko Y, Larson RA, Variakojis D, et al. Nonrandom chromosome abnormalities in angioimmunoblastic lymphadenopathy. Blood 1982;60:877.
40. Godde-Salz E, Feller AC, Lennert K. Chromosomal abnormalities in lymphogranulomatosis X (LgrX)/angioimmunoblastic lymphadenopathy (AILD). Leuk Res 1987;11:181.
41. Zylak CJ, Banerjee R, Galbraith PA, McCarthy DS. Lung involvement in angioimmunoblastic lymphadenopathy (AIL). Radiology 1976;121:513.
42. Myers TJ, Cole SR, Pastuszak WT. Angioimmunoblastic lymphadenopathy: Pleural-pulmonary disease. Cancer 1978;40:266.
43. Bradley SL, Dines DE, Banks PM, Hill RW. The lung in immunoblastic lymphadenopathy. Chest 1981;80(3);312.
44. Trenchard PM, Whittaker JA, Gough J, Parry H. Rapidly fatal respiratory failure and angioimmunoblastic lymphadenopathy: Possible contributions of immunoblastic leukaemia, chemotherapy, and multiple antibodies directed against mature blood cells. J Clin Pathol 1981; 34(5):486.
45. Kuijpers TJ, Shaw MP, Croonen AM. Pulmonary involvement in angioimmunoblastic lymphadenopathy (AILD): Case report and review of literature. Eur J Radiol 1983;3(2):155.
46. Starke ID, Elkon KB, Harmer CL, Hughes GR, Wiltshaw E. Pulmonary involvement in angioimmunoblastic lymphadenopathy following autoimmune disease. Respiration 1983;44(2):136.
47. Siegler D, Winner S. Pulmonary and pleural involvement in angioimmunoblastic lymphadenopathy. Br J Dis Chest 1980;74(3):296.
48. Cullen MH, Stansfeld AG, Oliver RTD, Lister TA, Malpas JS. Angioimmunoblastic lymphadenopathy: Report of 10 cases and review of the literature. Q J Med 1979;189:151.
49. Steinberg AD, Seldin MF, Jaffe ES, et al. Angioimmunoblastic lymphadenopathy with dysproteinemia. Ann Intern Med 1988;108:575.
50. Waldron JA, Leech JH, Glick AD, Flexner JM, Collins RD. Malignant lymphoma of peripheral T-lymphocyte origin. Cancer 1977;40:1604.
51. Levine AM, Taylor CR, Schneider DR, et al. Immunoblastic sarcoma of T-cell versus B-cell origin: I. Clinical features. Blood 1981;58:52.
52. Cossman J, Jaffe ES, Fisher RI. Immunologic phenotypes of diffuse, aggressive, non-Hodgkin's lymphomas: Correlation with clinical features. Cancer 1984;54:1310.
53. Horning SJ, Doggett RS, Warnke RA, et al. Clinical relevance of immunologic phenotype in diffuse large cell lymphoma. Blood 1984;63:1209.

54. Uchiyama T, Yodoi J, Sagawa K, Takatsuki K, Uchino H. Adult T-cell leukemia: Clinical and hematologic features of 16 cases. Blood 1977;50:481.
55. Poiesz BJ, Ruscetti FW, Gazdar AF, Bunn PA, Minna JD, Gallo RC. Detection and isolation of Type-C retrovirus particles from fresh and cultured lymphocytes of a patient with cutaneous T-cell lymphoma. Proc Natl Acad Sci USA 1980;77:7415.
56. Blayney DW, Jaffe ES, Blattner WA, et al. The human T-cell leukemia/lymphoma virus (HTLV) associated with American adult T-cell leukemia/lymphoma (ATL). Blood 1983;62:401.
57. Jaffe ES, Blattner WA, Blayney DW, et al. The pathologic spectrum of adult T-cell leukemia/lymphoma in the United States. Am J Surg Pathol 1984;8:263.
58. Bunn PA, Schecter GP, Jaffe ES, et al. Retrovirus-associated adult T-cell lymphoma in the United States: Staging, evaluation, and management. N Engl J Med 1983;309:257.
59. Kawano F, Yamaguchi K, Nishimura H, Tsuda H, Takatsuki K. Variation in the clinical courses of adult T-cell leukemia. Cancer 1985;55:851.
60. Waldmann TA, Goldman CK, Bongiovanni KF, et al. Therapy of patients with human T-cell lymphotrophic virus I–induced adult T-cell leukemia with anti-Tac, a monoclonal antibody to the receptor for interleukin-2. Blood 1988;72;1805.
61. Jaffe ES. The elusive Reed-Sternberg cell. N Engl J Med 1989;320:529.
62. Lukes RJ, Butler JJ. The pathology and nomenclature of Hodgkin's disease. Cancer Res 1971;31:1755.
63. Kaplan HS. Hodgkin's disease, 2nd ed. Cambridge, MA: Harvard University Press, 1980.
64. Hellman S, Jaffe ES, DeVita VT. Hodgkin's disease. In: DeVita VT, Hellman S, Rosenberg SA, eds. Cancer: Principles and practice of oncology. 3rd ed. Philadelphia: JB Lippincott, 1989:1696.
65. Catterall JR, McCabe RE, Brooks RG, Remington JS. Open lung biopsy in patients with Hodgkin's disease and pulmonary infiltrates. Am Rev Respir Dis 1989;139(5):1274.
66. Flint A, Kumar NB, Naylor B. Pulmonary Hodgkin's disease: Diagnosis by fine needle aspiration. Acta Cytol 1988;32(2):221.
67. Rubin AH, Ben-Shachar M, Malberger E. Cytologic diagnosis of pulmonary Hodgkin's disease via endobronchial brush preparation. Chest 1989;96(4):948.
68. Klein G. The Epstein-Barr virus and neoplasia. N Engl J Med 1975;293:1353.
69. Purtilo DT. Defective immune surveillance in viral carcinogenesis. Lab Invest 1984;51:373.
70. Frizzera G, Hanto DW, Gajl-Peczalska KJ, et al. Polymorphic diffuse B-cell hyperplasias and lymphomas in renal transplant recipients. Cancer Res 1981;41:4262.
71. Nalesnik MA, Jaffe R, Starzl TE, et al. The pathology of posttransplant lymphoproliferative disorders occurring in the setting of cyclosporin A-prednisone immunosuppression. Am J Pathol 1988;133:173.
72. Rappaport DC, Weisbrod GL, Herman SJ. Cyclosporine-induced lymphoma following a unilateral lung transplant. The Toronto Lung Transplant Group. Can Assoc Radiol J 1989;40(2);110.
73. Yousem SA, Randhawa P, Locker J, et al. Posttransplant lymphoproliferative disorders in heart-lung transplant recipients: Primary presentation in the allograft. Hum Pathol 1989;20(4):361.
74. Cleary ML, Warnke R, Sklar J. Monoclonality of lymphoproliferative lesions in cardiac-transplant recipients. N Engl J Med 1984;310:477.
75. Starzl TE, Porter KA, Iwatsuki S, et al. Reversibility of lymphoma and lymphoproliferative lesions developing under cyclosporine-steroid therapy. Lancet 1984;i:583.
76. Bienenstock J, Johnston N, Perey DYE. Bronchial lymphoid tissue. I. Morphologic characteristics. Lab Invest 1973;28:686.
77. Bienenstock J, Johnston N, Perey DYE. Bronchial lymphoid tissue. II. Functional characteristics. Lab Invest 1973;28:693.
78. Bienenstock J, Befus D. Gut- and bronchus-associated lymphoid tissue. Am J Anat 1984;170:437.

79. Kradin RL, Mark EJ. Benign lymphoid disorders of the lung, with a theory regarding their development. Hum Pathol 1983;14:857.

80. Yousem SA, Colby TV, Carrington CB. Follicular bronchitis/bronchiolitis. Hum Pathol 1985;16:700.

81. Rogers PM, Ayres SM, Ribaudo CA. Intrafissural mid-zonal anthracotic lymph node presenting as a coin lesion. Chest 1972;61:501.

82. Rosenthal DS, Weg JG. Intrapulmonary lymph node presenting as a solitary pulmonary nodule. Dis Chest 1967;51:336.

83. Ehrenstein FI. Pulmonary lymph node presenting as an enlarging coin lesion. Am Rev Respir Dis 1970;101:595.

84. Travis WD, Roth D. Histopathologic evaluation of lung biopsies in the immunosuppressed host. In: Shelhamer JH, Pizzo PA, Parrillo JE, Masur H, eds. Respiratory disease in the immunocompromised host. Philadelphia: JB Lippincott, 1990.

85. Trapnell EH. Recognition and incidence of intrapulmonary lymph nodes. Thorax 1964;19:44.

86. Addis BJ, Hyjek E, Isaacson PG. Primary pulmonary lymphoma: A reappraisal of its histogenesis and its relationship to pseudolymphoma and lymphoid interstitial pneumonia. Histopathology 1988;13:1.

87. Feoli F, Carbone A, Dina MA, Lauriola L, Musiani P, Piantelli M. Pseudolymphoma of the lung: Lymphoid subsets in the lung mass and in peripheral blood. Cancer 1981;48:2218.

88. Fisher C, Grubb C, Kenning B, Lincoln JCR, Peters JL. Pseudolymphoma of the lung: A rare cause of a solitary nodule. J Thorac Cardiovasc Surg 1980;80:11.

89. Gephardt GN, Tubbs RR, Liu AC, Petras RE, Ahmad M, Golish JA, Tomashefski JF. Pulmonary lymphoid neoplasms: Role of immunohistology in the study of cellular immunotypes and in differential diagnosis. Chest 1986;89:545.

90. Greenberg SD, Heisler JG, Gyorkey F, Jenkins DE. Pulmonary lymphoma versus pseudolymphoma: A perplexing problem. Southern Med J 1972;65:775.

91. Hebert A, Wright DH, Isaacson PG, Smith JL. Primary malignant lymphoma of the lung: Histopathologic and immunologic evaluation of nine cases. Hum Pathol 1984;15:415.

92. Julsrud PR, Brown LR, Li C-Y, Rosenow EC, Crowe JK. Pulmonary processes of mature-appearing lymphocytes: Pseudolymphoma, well-differentiated lymphocytic lymphoma, and lymphocytic interstitial pneumonitis. Radiology 1978;127:289.

93. Kennedy JL, Nathwani BN, Burke JS, Hill LR, Rappaport H. Pulmonary lymphomas and other pulmonary lymphoid lesions: A clinicopathologic and immunologic study of 64 patients. Cancer 1985;56:539.

94. Koss MN, Hochholzer L, Nichols PW, Wehunt WK, Lazarus AA. Primary non-Hodgkin's lymphoma and pseudolymphoma of lung: A study of 161 patients. Hum Pathol 1983;14:1024.

95. Marchevsky A, Padilla M, Kaneko M, Kleinerman J. Localized lymphoid nodules of lung: A reappraisal of the lymphoma versus pseudolymphoma dilemma. Cancer 1983;51:2070.

96. Reich NE, McCormack LJ, Van Ordstrand HS. Pseudolymphoma of the lung. Chest 1974;65:424.

97. Saltzstein SL. Pulmonary malignant lymphomas and pseudolymphomas: Classification, therapy, and prognosis. Cancer 1963;16:928.

98. Yum MN, Ziegler JR, Walker PD, Ridolfo AS, Brashear RE. Pseudolymphoma of the lung in a patient with systemic lupus erythematosus. Am J Med 1979;66:172.

99. Liebow AA, Carrington CB. Diffuse pulmonary lymphoreticular infiltrations associated with dysproteinemia. Med Clin North Am 1973;57:809.

100. Strimlan CV, Rosenow EC, Weiland LH, Brown LR. Lymphocytic interstitial pneumonitis: Review of 13 cases. Ann Intern Med 1978;88:616.

101. Koss MN, Hochholzer L, Langloss JM, Wehunt WD, Lazarus AA. Lymphoid interstitial pneumonia: Clinicopathological and immunopathological findings in 18 cases. Pathology 1987;19:178.

102. Glickstein M, Kornstein MJ, Pietra GG, Aronchick JM, Gefter WB, Epstein DM, Miller W. Non-lymphomatous lymphoid disorders of the lung. AJR 1986;147:227.
103. Moran TJ, Totten RS. Lymphoid interstitial pneumonia with dysproteinemia: Report of two cases with plasma cell predominance. Am J Clin Pathol 1970;54:747.
104. Greenberg SD, Haley MD, Jenkins DE, Fischer SP. Lymphoplasmacytic pneumonia with accompanying dysproteinemia. Arch Pathol 1973;96:73.
105. Montes M, Tomasi TB, Noehren TH, Culver GJ. Lymphoid interstitial pneumonia with monoclonal gammopathy. Am Rev Respir Dis 1968;98:277.
106. Young RC, Tillman L, Burton AF, et al. Lymphoid interstitial pneumonia with polyclonal gammopathy. J Nat Med Assoc 1969;61:310.
107. Yoshizawa Y, Ohdama S, Ikeda A, Ohtsuka M, Masuda S, Tanaka M. Lymphoid interstitial pneumonia with depressed cellular immunity and polyclonal gammopathy. Am Rev Respir Dis 1984;130:507.
108. Essig LJ, Timms ES, Hancock DE, Sharp GC. Plasma cell interstitial pneumonia and macroglobulinemia: A response to corticosteroid and cyclophosphamide therapy. Am J Med 1974;56:398.
109. Church JA, Isaacs H, Saxon A, Keens TG, Richards W. Lymphoid interstitial pneumonitis and hypogammaglobulinemia in children. Am Rev Respir Dis 1981;124:491.
110. Levinson AI, Hopewell PC, Stites DP, Spitler LE, Fudenberg HH. Coexistent lymphoid interstitial pneumonia, pernicious anemia, and agammaglobulinemia. Arch Intern Med 1976;136:213.
111. DeCoteau WE, Tourville D, Ambrus JL, Montes M, Adler R, Tomasi TB. Lymphoid interstitial pneumonia and autoerythrocyte sensitization syndrome: A case with deposition of immunoglobulins on the alveolar basement membrane. Arch Intern Med 1974;134:519.
112. Bonner H, Ennis RS, Geelhoed GW, Tarpley TM. Lymphoid infiltration and amyloidosis of lung in Sjögren's syndrome. Arch Pathol Lab Med 1973;95:42.
113. Case Records of the Massachusetts Hospital, Case 38-1977. New Engl J Med 1977;297:652.
114. Faguet GB, Webb HH, Agee JF, Ricks WB, Sharbausgh AH. Immunologically diagnosed malignancy in Sjögren's pseudolymphoma. Am J Med 1978;65:424.
115. Benisch B, Peison B. The association of lymphocytic interstitial pneumonia and systemic lupus erythematosus. Mt Sinai J Med 1979;46:398.
116. Popa V. Lymphocytic interstitial pneumonia of common variable immunodeficiency. Ann Allergy 1988;60:203.
117. Richmond JM, Dawkins RL, Henderson DW, Tan NTS. Immunodeficiency, pulmonary lymphoreticular infiltration, paraproteinemia, and terminal lymphoma. Cancer 1981;47:2641.
118. Teirstein AS, Rosen MJ. Lymphocytic interstitial pneumonia. Clin Chest Med 1988;9:467.
119. Oldham SAA, Castillo M, Jacobson FL, Mones JM, Saldana MJ. HIV-associated lymphocytic interstitial pneumonia: Radiologic manifestations and pathologic correlation. Radiology 1989;170:83.
120. Travis WD, Lack EE, Ognibene FP, Suffrediini AF, Shelhamer J. Lung biopsy interpretation in the acquired immunodeficiency syndrome: Experience of the National Institutes of Health with literature review. Progress in AIDS Pathology 1989;1:51.
121. Myers JL, Peiper SC, Katzenstein A-LA. Pulmonary involvement in infectious mononucleosis: Histopathologic features and detection of Epstein-Barr virus-related DNA sequences. Mod Pathol 1989;2:444.
122. Helman CA, Keeton GR, Benatar SR. Lymphoid interstitial pneumonia with associated chronic active hepatitis and renal tubular acidosis. Am Rev Respir Dis 1977;115:161.
123. Chamberlain DW, Hyland RH, Ross DJ. Diphenylhydantoin-induced lymphocytic interstitial pneumonia. Chest 1986;90:458.
124. Perreault C, Cousineau S, D'Angelo G, et al. Lymphoid interstitial pneumonia after allogeneic bone marrow transplantation: A possible manifestation of chronic graft-versus-host disease. Cancer 1985;55:1.

125. O'Brodovich HM, Moser MM, Lawrence L: Familial lymphoid interstitial pneumonia: A long term follow-up. Pediatrics 1980;65:523.

126. Kradin RL, Young RH, Kradin LA, Mark EJ. Immunoblastic lymphoma arising in chronic lymphoid hyperplasia of the pulmonary interstitium. Cancer 1982;50:1339.

127. Schuurman H-J, Gooszen HC, Tan IWN, Kluin PM, Wagenaar SS, Unnik JAMV. Low-grade lymphoma of immature T-cell phenotype in a case of lymphocytic interstitial pneumonia and Sjögren's syndrome. Histopathology 1987;11:1193.

128. Case Records of the Massachusetts General Hospital, Case 13-1980. N Engl J Med 1980;302:795.

129. Banerjee D, Ahmad D. Malignant lymphoma complicating lymphocytic interstitial pneumonia: A monoclonal B-cell neoplasm arising in a polyclonal lymphoproliferative disorder. Hum Pathol 1982;13:780.

130. L'Hoste RJ, Filippa DA, Lieberman PH, Bretsky S. Primary pulmonary lymphomas: A clinico-pathologic analysis of 36 cases. Cancer 1984;54:1397.

131. Colby TV, Carrington CB. Pulmonary lymphomas: Current concepts. Hum Pathol 1983;14:884.

132. Isaacson P, Wright DH. Extranodal malignant lymphoma arising from mucosa-associated lymphoid tissue. Cancer 1984;53:2515.

133. Hansen LA, Prakash UBS, Colby TV. Pulmonary lymphoma in Sjögren's syndrome. Mayo Clin Proc 1989;64:920.

134. Turner RR, Colby TV, Doggett RS. Well-differentiated lymphocytic lymphoma: A study of 47 patients with primary manifestation in the lung. Cancer 1984;54:2088.

135. Peterson H, Snider HL, Yam LT, Bowlds CF, Arnn EH, Li C-Y. Primary pulmonary lymphoma: A clinical and immunohistochemical study of six cases. Cancer 1985;56:805.

136. Non-Hodgkin's Lymphoma Pathologic Classification Project: National Cancer Institute sponsored study of classifications of non-Hodgkin's lymphoma: Summary and description of a working formulation for clinical usage. Cancer 1982;49:2112.

137. Weisenburger DD, Nathwani BN, Diamond LW, Winberg CD, Rappaport H. Malignant lymphoma, intermediate lymphocytic type: A clinicopathologic study of 42 cases. Cancer 1981;48:1415.

138. Jaffe ES, Bookman MA, Longo DL. Lymphocytic lymphoma of intermediate differentiation-mantle zone lymphoma: A distinct subtype of B-cell lymphoma. Hum Pathol 1987;18:877.

139. Rollins SD, Colby TV. Lung biopsy in chronic lymphocytic leukemia. Arch Pathol Lab Med 1988;112:607.

140. Palosaari DE, Colby TV. Bronchiolocentric chronic lymphocytic leukemia. Cancer 1986;58:1695.

141. Sprague RI, deBlois GG. Small-lymphocytic pulmonary lymphoma: Diagnosis by transthoracic fine needle aspiration. Chest 1989;96:929.

142. Amin R. Extramedullary plasmacytoma of the lung. Cancer 1985;56:152.

143. Baroni CD, Mineo TC, Ricci C, Guarino S, Mandelli F. Solitary secretory plasmacytoma of the lung in a 14-year-old boy. Cancer 1977;40:2329.

144. Morinaga S, Watanabe H, Gemma A, et al. Plasmacytoma of the lung associated with nodular deposits of immunoglobulin. Am J Surg Pathol 1987;11:989.

145. Roikjaer O, Thomsen JK. Plasmacytoma of the lung: A case report describing two tumors of different immunologic type in a single patient. Cancer 1986;58:2671.

146. Tenholder MF, Scialla SJ, Weisbaum G. Endobronchial metastatic plasmacytoma. Cancer 1982;49:1465.

147. Wile A, Olinger G, Peter JB, Dornfeld L. Solitary intraparenchymal pulmonary plasmacytoma associated with production of an M-protein: Report of a case. Cancer 1976;37:2338.

148. Hinz W. Polypoeses Plasmocytom des linken Hauptbronchus mit oertlicher Amyloidablagerung. Frankfurt Z Pathol 1941;55:509.

149. Kintzer JS, Rosenow EC, Kyle RA. Thoracic and pulmonary abnormalities in multiple myeloma: A review of 958 cases. Arch Intern Med 1978;138:727.
150. Warter A, Satge D, Roeslin N. Angioinvasive plasma cell granulomas of the lung. Cancer 1987;59:435.
151. Titus JL, Harrison EG, Clagett OT, Anderson MW, Knaff LJ. Xanthomatous and inflammatory pseudotumors of the lung. Cancer 1962;15:522.
152. Spencer H. The pulmonary plasma cell/histiocytoma complex. Histopathology 1984;8:903.
153. Iuchi K, Aozasa K, Yamamoto S, et al. Non-Hodgkin's lymphoma of the pleural cavity developing from long-standing pyothorax: Summary of clinical and pathological findings in thirty-seven cases. Jpn J Clin Oncol 1989;19:249.
154. Iuchi K, Ichimiya A, Akashi A, et al. Non-Hodgkin's lymphoma of the pleural cavity developing from long-standing pyothorax. Cancer 1987;60:1771.
155. Rao KPPP, Kizer J, Jones TJ, Anunciado A, Pepkowitz SH, Lazarchick J. Acquired von Willebrand's syndrome associated with an extranodal pulmonary lymphoma. Arch Pathol Lab Med 1988;112:47.
156. Thomas P, Battifora H. Keratins versus epithelial membrane antigen in tumor diagnosis: An immunohistochemical comparison of five monoclonal antibodies. Hum Pathol 1987;18:728.
157. Michels S, Swanson PE, Frizzera G, Wick MR. Immunostaining for leukocyte common antigen using an amplified avidin-biotin-peroxidase complex method and paraffin sections. Arch Pathol Lab Med 1987;111:1035.
158. Weiss LM, Yousem SA, Warnke RA. Non-Hodgkin's lymphomas of the lung: A study of 19 cases emphasizing the utility of frozen section immunologic studies in differential diagnosis. Am J Surg Pathol 1985;9:480.
159. Aozasa K, Tsujimoto M, Inoue A. Malignant histiocytosis: Report of twenty-five cases with pulmonary, renal and/or gastro-intestinal involvement. Histopathology 1985;9:39.
160. Colby TV, Carrington CB, Mark GJ. Pulmonary involvement in malignant histiocytosis: A clinicopathologic spectrum. Am J Surg Pathol 1981;5:61.
161. Wongchaowart B, Kennealy JA, Crissman J, Hawkins H. Respiratory failure in malignant histiocytosis. Am Rev Respir Dis 1981;124:640.
162. Turner RR, Wood GS, Beckstead JH, Colby TV, Horning SJ, Warnke RA. Histiocytic malignancies: Morphologic, immunologic, and enzymatic heterogeneity. Am J Surg Pathol 1984;8:485.
163. Wick MR, Mills SE, Scheithauer BW, Cooper PH, Davitz MA, Parkinson K. Reassessment of malignant "angioendotheliomatosis": Evidence in favor of its reclassification as "intravascular lymphomatosis." Am J Surg Pathol 1986;10:112.
164. Ferry JA, Harris NL, Picker LJ, et al. Intravascular lymphomatosis (malignant angioendotheliomatosis), a B-cell neoplasm expressing surface homing receptors. Mod Pathol 1988;1:444.
165. Remberber K, Nawrath-Koll I, Bokel JM, Haider M. Systemic angioendotheliomatosis of the lung. Pathol Res Pract 1987;182:265.
166. Tan TB, Spaander PJ, Blaisse M, Gerritzen FM. Angiotropic large cell lymphoma presenting as interstitial lung disease. Thorax 1988;43:578.
167. Yousem SA, Colby TV. Intravascular lymphomatosis presenting in the lung. Cancer 1990;65:349.
168. Snyder LS, Harmon KR, Estensen RD. Intravascular lymphomatosis (malignant angioendotheliomatosis) presenting as pulmonary hypertension. Chest 1989;96:1199.

12

Other Pulmonary Granulomatous Vasculitic Syndromes

Joseph P. Lynch III
Joseph C. Fantone III

Vasculitis is a rare and poorly understood condition characterized by inflammation of vascular walls in which the dominant clinical manifestations relate to ischemia and infarction of affected organs.[1–9] Several distinct vasculitic syndromes have been recognized that display differences in clinical and histopathologic features, prognosis, and therapy. [1–9] Distinguishing the various subtypes may be difficult, however, as clinical and histopathologic features overlap. The pathogenesis of these vasculitides remains obscure, and laboratory studies do not reliably differentiate the various entities. Thus, as discussed in Chapter 10, systems categorizing vasculitides according to histologic features (such as vessel size, type of inflammatory cell infiltrate, and the presence or absence of granulomas) and clinical features (such as type and extent of organ involvement) have emerged.[1–9] Notwithstanding the limitations of these classification systems, the attempt to stratify vasculitic disorders on the basis of differences in clinical and histologic features has merit, because such schemes provide a framework upon which clinicians may base prognostic and therapeutic judgments.

It is well recognized that pulmonary manifestations rarely complicate the nongranulomatous vasculitides, such as classic polyarteritis nodosa,[1,3,5,10] Behçet's disease,[3,5,11] mixed essential cryoglobulinemia,[3,5,6,12] Henoch-Schönlein purpura, [3,5,6,13] or hypersensitivity vasculitis.[1,3,5,6] However, pulmonary hemorrhage or other manifestations may occur commonly in the overlap syndrome[5] or in vasculitis complicating connective tissue disorders.[1,3,5,6] Clinically significant pulmonary symptoms have rarely been reported among patients with Takayasu's arteritis,[3,5,14,15] but involvement of pulmonary arteries has been documented in up to 50% of cases when carefully looked for.[14] Nevertheless, clinically or radiographically evident pulmonary involvement is rare in the above conditions, and a discussion of the pulmonary manifestations of these disorders is beyond the scope of this chapter.

The focus of this chapter will be the pulmonary granulomatous vasculitides, a group of disorders that share not only a striking propensity to affect the lung, but also a pronounced granulomatous character and a tendency to cause extensive necrosis.[1-9] Owing to their rarity and the fact that specific diagnostic tests differentiating them have not been available, attempts to provide a conceptual framework for these diseases have been based primarily on histopathologic criteria. In 1973, Liebow proposed a classification scheme recognizing five types of pulmonary granulomatoses: Wegener's granulomatosis (WG), limited WG, bronchocentric granulomatosis (BCG), necrotizing sarcoid angiitis (NSG), and lymphomatoid granulomatosis (LYG).[8] Allergic angiitis and granulomatosis (Churg-Strauss syndrome), a systemic vasculitis with a propensity to involve the lung, had been previously recognized in 1951[16] and was not included in this schema. Two of the disorders in Liebow's classification schema, BCG and NSG, had not been previously described. However, it was thought that the histopathologic material of the 9 and 11 cases, respectively, were sufficiently distinctive to warrant classification as disease entities. Although such a schema appeared to provide organization to an otherwise chaotic group of disorders, very little was understood about the pathogenesis of the disease processes. Further studies also recognized that histologic features compatible with WG or BCG may be seen in specific granulomatous inflammatory or infectious processes.[4,17] Thus, it became apparent that diagnosis of these disorders involves interpretation of the histopathologic changes in the context of the patient's clinical presentation and laboratory findings.

The lung has a limited number of stereotypic host responses to antigen or foreign substances, and granuloma formation appears to be a particularly common response to inhaled antigens. Inhaled antigens may deposit in the lower respiratory tract, where they are phagocytosed by alveolar macrophages, one of the early and critical arms of immune defense in the lower respiratory tract.[18] Immunoglobulin production in response to the foreign antigens may then lead to immune complex formation, which may further stimulate alveolar macrophages, leading to cytokine release and a series of cell-cell interactions that may result in granulomatous response. This sequence, in which antigen stimulation in the respiratory tract may lead to a pulmonary granulomatous response, often involving the vasculature, appears to have an important role in the pathogenesis of several of these pulmonary granulomatoses. We now know that the development of a granulomatous response involves the complex interaction of soluble cell-derived mediators (e.g., cytokines) and plasma mediator systems with both inflammatory and parenchymal cells, including monocytes/macrophages, lymphoctyes, neutrophils, fibroblasts, endothelial cells, and epithelial cells.[18] Although the precise mechanisms responsible for the initiation of these vasculitic conditions have not been clarified, human data and animal models suggest that immune complexes are involved in the pathogenesis of polyarteritis nodosa (see discussion in Chapter 10). With further investigation, including the application of sophisticated cell and molecular biological techniques to human tissues, the pathogenesis of these unusual host responses may be appreciated in the near future.

A historical perspective illustrates the difficulties of defining disease entities on the basis of criteria in the absence of clinical information and an understanding of disease pathogenesis. For example, as more insight was gained into the pathogenesis of the pulmonary granulomatoses, it has become apparent that at least three of these entities (bronchocentric granulomatosis, necrotizing sarcoid angiitis, and lymphomatoid granulomatosis) may be expressions of unusual host responses to underlying disease[7,19-22] or neoplasm.[23,24] For example, lymphomatoid granulomatosis (LYG), originally described in 1972 by Liebow as a novel type of granulomatous necrotizing vasculitis with a pronounced tendency to involve the lung whose clinical features overlapped with WG,[25] is a clinical-pathologic syndrome rather than a distinct disease. As discussed in Chapter 11, subsequent investigations have determined that LYG represents an unusual host response to a spectrum of lymphoproliferative disorders, including malignant lymphoma. Similar considerations apply for both BCG and NSG, disorders that were first described in Liebow's classic article in 1973.[8] As will be discussed, it is now recognized that BCG represents a histologic response to specific antigens (primarily aspergillus species) and is not a distinct entity. Although NSG remains more controversial, it has been suggested that NSG most likely represents an unusual variant of sarcoidosis and does not deserve recognition as a distinct disorder. Benign lymphocytic angiitis and granulomatosis (BLAG) is another disorder the existence of which is highly controversial. BLAG was originally described by Saldana and colleagues in 1977[26] as a vasculitic disorder resembling WG and LYG but exhibiting histologic and prognostic features that distinguished it from either of those conditions. In this chapter, we will review the granulomatous angiitides initially defined and categorized by Liebow[8] and by Saldana and co-workers[26] but will also include as part of the spectrum of granulomatous vasculitis the entity allergic angiitis and granulomatosis, or Churg-Strauss syndrome, which also exhibits a granulomatous character and has a striking predilection for pulmonary involvement.[1,27,28]

BENIGN LYMPHOCYTIC ANGIITIS AND GRANULOMATOSIS (BLAG)

Benign lymphocytic angiitis and granulomatosis (BLAG) was originally described in 1977 by Saldana and colleagues as a pulmonary granulomatous vasculitic process that shared some histologic features with WG and LYG but was largely limited to the lungs and was remarkably responsive to therapy with chlorambucil.[26] Histologically, BLAG was characterized by richly cellular nodules composed of mature lymphocytes, plasma cells, histiocytes, and occasional multinucleated giant cells.[26] Infiltration or compression of respiratory bronchioles by the mononuclear cell infiltrate, clusters of foam-filled macrophages, and foci of bronchiolitis obliterans were common associated features. Several histologic features differentiated BLAG from WG and LYG. The extent of angiitis and necrosis was mild in BLAG compared with either of these conditions. Mature lymphocytes predominated in the cellular infiltrate in BLAG, whereas lymphocytes were much less numerous in WG. More importantly, the mononuclear cells composing the infiltrate in BLAG were cytologically benign and mitoses were rare, which contrasted with the extreme cytologic atypia and high degree of proliferation characteristic of LYG. Although a granulomatous component existed in BLAG, it was less pronounced than in most of the other pulmonary granulomatoses, and only small numbers of giant cells were evident scattered throughout the lesion. Well-formed sarcoid-like granulomas were identified in only one of the 14 cases originally described. Clinically, BLAG was much less aggressive than either WG or LYG, diseases in which extrapulmonary dissemination is typical. Only one of 14 patients with BLAG exhibited extrapulmonary features and none had upper airway or glomerular pathology. Six were asymptomatic, with incidental pulmonary lesions being noted on routine chest radiographs. Chest radiographs revealed multiple nodular infiltrates in 11 of 14 cases, with the remaining three demonstrating single pulmonary nodules. Cavitation was noted in four cases. A remarkable feature of BLAG was its overall excellent prognosis and exquisite sensitivity to cytotoxic therapy. Remission was achieved in only one of three patients treated with corticosteroids alone, but in all seven patients treated with chlorambucil (in combination with corticosteroids). The response to chlorambucil was often dramatic, with complete resolution of radiographic abnormalities within one month of initiation of therapy in some cases.[26] Remissions were also achieved in one patient treated with cyclophosphamide and in one of two patients treated with azathioprine. Surgical resection of pulmonary lesions without ancillary therapy was curative in four of seven cases. At long-term follow-up, three of 14 patients had died (one of infectious complications of azathioprine therapy and two of unrelated causes).

Israel, Patchefsky, and Saldana rediscussed the clinical and histologic features of BLAG, WG, and LYG in a subsequent publication[29] and emphasized that the differentiation between LYG and BLAG was imprecise. Two cases originally diagnosed as BLAG evolved into lymphomatoid granulomatosis several years later.[29] Since these two seminal reports, a few case reports have been published,[30–33] but no large series has been reported, and BLAG has not been accepted as a distinct disorder in several reviews.[1,3,5,6] Tukianinen and colleagues described a case in which left lower lobe lobectomy was performed for a persistent pulmonary parenchymal mass.[33] A mass lesion infiltrating into the visceral pleura was resected. Microscopic examination revealed a prominent vasculitis, with infiltration of the vascular walls by lymphocytes, plasma cells, occasional histiocytes, and giant cells. No necrosis was evident. The diagnosis of BLAG was suspected, but no additional therapy was administered. At 2-year follow-up, the patient was well without evidence of recurrence or additional lesions. Although the authors believed that their case represented BLAG, it is important to recognize that pseudolymphoma or well-differentiated pulmonary lymphomas may present in precisely this fashion. Pulmonary lymphomas often manifest as single or multiple nodular mass lesions on chest radiographs and may be asymptomatic.[24] Prominent vascular invasion by lymphoid cells, associated with polymorphous mononuclear inflammatory cell infiltrates and a granulomatous reaction, may be observed with pulmonary lymphomas.[24] In addition, the course of primary pulmonary lymphomas may be indolent, and surgical resection alone may be curative if the tumor mass can be completely resected.[24]

Levy and associates[32] described a patient with diffuse reticulonodular infiltrates on chest radiograph with hemoptysis and fever in whom initial transbronchial lung biopsy demonstrated nonspecific features of alveolar hemorrhage and interstitial fibrosis. Subsequent open lung biopsy demonstrated a dense pleomorphic interstitial infiltrate with lymphocytes, plasma cells, histiocytes, and multinucleated giant cells in which foci of necrosis were also observed. Moderate mononuclear cell infiltrates were noted in the walls of both arteries and veins, and a few vessels were obliterated by the inflammatory cell infiltrate. The histologic features were believed to be compatible with the diagnosis of BLAG, and therapy with chlorambucil and prednisone was initiated. Although the patient exhibited improvement while receiving immunosuppresive therapy, subsequent cultures of bronchial washings demonstrated *Mycobacterium tuberculosis* and antituberculous chemotherapy was added to the regimen. Despite the histologic resemblances to BLAG on lung biopsy, the isolation of *M. tuberculosis* from bronchial washings strongly suggests that the pronounced lymphoid vasculitic infiltrate in this case represented an exuberant tissue reaction to tuberculous infection rather than an independent and distinct disease process. The favorable response to immunosuppressive therapy prior to initiation of antituberculous medications does not contradict this, as corticosteroids have often been associated with improvement in the local or systemic reaction to tuberculosis in patients with overwhelming infection or an exuberant inflammatory component.

Weiss and colleagues[30] described a patient with BLAG with lung, kidney, and prostatic involvement and suggested that BLAG may represent an early phase of LYG. Investigators at the Mayo Clinic[31] recently described three patients with dense pulmonary infiltrates on chest radiographs who exhibited histologic features consistent with BLAG on open lung biopsy. Microscopic examination revealed dense nodular lymphoid infiltrates composed of mature lymphocytes, plasma cells, and histiocytes within the pulmonary parenchyma and extending into the pulmonary vasculature. Necrosis was never prominent. Transformed lymphoid cells and mild cellular atypia were occasionally observed, but severe atypia was never seen and mitoses were infrequent. These bland cytologic features were in sharp contrast to the more malignant features characteristic of lymphomatoid granulomatosis. Immunostaining for light chains was negative in the one case examined, but immunologic studies were not performed in the remaining two cases. Consistent with previous reports, none had extrapulmonary features and the clinical course was benign. Two patients were treated with chlorambucil, which resulted in complete resolution of the disease in both cases; the remaining case remitted spontaneously following surgical biopsy and removal of coexistent spindle cell thymoma.

It is difficult to formulate the salient clinical and histopathologic features of a disease on the basis of scattered case reports. Churg and associates[7] emphasized that BLAG probably is not a distinct disease entity and suggested that some cases represent LYG whereas others may encompass a diverse group of pulmonary vasculitic and lymphoproliferative disorders. Until additional cellular and molecular characterization occurs, it is difficult to accept BLAG as a distinct disease entity. It is not possible to exclude unequivocally the possibility that individual cases of BLAG represent a host response to underlying disorders such as infection, neoplasm, or variants of WG or LYG. The classification scheme applied by Jaffe and investigators at the NCI for lymphoproliferative disorders with a vasculitic component may also encompass lesions resembling BLAG.[23,34] In this classification, the term angiocentric immunoproliferative lesion (AIL) was coined to refer to a spectrum of lesions that included LYG and angiocentric lymphomas. Three histologic grades, based on the degree of cytologic atypia in the lymphoid cells and the extent of the inflammatory background, are recognized. Grade I lesions are composed of a polymorphous cellular infiltrate without any cytologic atypia and often respond to therapy with cyclophosphamide and prednisone.[23] Pulmonary lesions with histologic features of grade I AIL resemble BLAG in many respects but several differences between grade I AIL and BLAG appear to exist.[23,35] Among the nine patients with grade I AIL in the NCI series, only six presented with pulmonary lesions and three had extrapulmonary involvement, features not characteristic of BLAG. In addition, three developed malignant lymphomas within 3 to 48 months that were refractory to therapy.[23] As immunophenotypic analysis has been performed on very few cases of either grade I AIL or BLAG, the relationship (if any) between these disorders remains unclear. The use of modern immunologic techniques to include B- and T-cell markers and clonal rearrangements of T-cell receptor genes may better clarify the relationship between AIL, BLAG, lymphomatoid granulomatosis, and other pulmonary lymphoproliferative disorders.[23,35]

BRONCHOCENTRIC GRANULOMATOSIS (BCG)

Liebow first described bronchocentric granulomatosis in 1973 on the basis of nine patients who exhibited a striking granulomatous response centered within bronchi and bronchioles, resulting in destruction and obliteration of affected airways.[8] In the original histologic description of this entity, bronchiolar walls were infiltrated with large numbers of inflammatory cells (predominantly eosinophils, lymphocytes, and mononuclear cells), and the bronchial lumens were filled with necrotic exudate, with both intact and fragmented eosinophils, neutrophils, and other inflammatory cells.[8] Epithelioid cells, palisading histiocytes, and multinucleated giant cells were a prominent feature within the bronchial mucosa and necrotic exudate, imparting a granulomatous character to the inflammatory process. Necrosis was often extensive. In some cases, the inflammatory process resulted in loss of cartilage with collapse and stenosis of the larger bronchi; in others, necrosis of bronchioles resulted in bronchiectasis.[8] The distal lung parenchyma demonstrated foam-filled macrophages, mononuclear cell infiltration, and eosinophils within alveolar spaces and interstitium.[8] Mild perivascular infiltrates were occasionally identified within pulmonary vessels contiguous to the primary granulomatous process, but these vascular changes were rarely prominent and appeared to be incidental to the airways involvement.[8] Fever, cough, malaise, dyspnea, and wheezing were the dominant clinical manifestations. No patient had extrapulmonary involvement, and three were asymptomatic.[8] Chest radiographic abnormalities, ranging from patchy pneumonic infiltrates to segmental or lobar atelectasis, were present in all cases.[8] A history of severe asthma since childhood was elicited in two patients, a point that later became appreciated as a possible clue to pathogenesis. Although limited follow-up was available at the time of the initial report, most patients did well with surgical resection either alone or in combination with corticosteroids.[8]

Following the original description, several case reports[36-43] and a few small series by individuals with specific expertise in pulmonary pathology and access to cases from multiple referring institutions expanded the knowledge base of this disease.[7,19,20,44,45] In contrast to most primary pulmonary vasculitides, extrapulmonary involvement is rare in BCG. Among approximately 80 cases of BCG reported, only two cases of glomerulonephritis [20,42] and one case of scleritis[43] have been described; a few cases have had concomitant sinusitis or nonspecific skin rash,[19,41,45] and the remaining cases exhibited only pulmonary manifestations. Early insights into the pathogenesis of BCG were gained in a study by Katzenstein and co-workers,[20] who re-reviewed the original cases of Liebow[8] and added 14 new cases obtained from several centers.

Consistent with the previous reports, symptoms were nonspecific and usually included cough, wheezing, fever, and malaise. Chest radiographs revealed atelectasis or consolidation of a segment or lobe in 21 of 22 cases, 70% of which involved the upper lobes. Large nodular or mass densities (2 cm) were present in five cases, and smaller nodular or linear patterns were found at some point in the course of the disease in five cases. Areas of cavitation were demonstrable in six patients, usually in the context of markedly dilated bronchi consistent with fluid-filled bronchiectatic cavities. Two demonstrated the classic finger-and-glove pattern of mucoid impaction.[20] These radiographic patterns were highly compatible with the features seen in allergic bronchopulmonary aspergillosis (ABPA) and suggested that at least some cases of BCG represented the histologic expression of ABPA rather than a distinct disease process. This hypothesis was supported by the finding that 10 of the 23 cases of BCG had a history of asthma, and 9 of these 10 had peripheral blood eosinophilia (a cardinal feature of ABPA) and noninvasive fungal hyphae (primarily aspergillus) within the bronchial lumen or bronchial tissue.[20] Further, dense aggregates of intact and fragmented eosinophils, with occasional Charcot-Leyden crystals, predominated in the inflammatory cell infiltrate in the asthmatics, and two exhibited features consistent with eosinophilic pneumonia distal to the involved bronchi. These findings pointed to the eosinophil as a critical cell in the pathogenesis of the BCG lesion in this subset of asthmatics. However, a different pathogenic mechanism appeared to be operative among the 13 nonasthmatics with BCG, as only two had blood eosinophilia (never exceeding 9%), none had aspergillus hyphae identified in tissue, and only occasional eosinophils were detected in the bronchial infiltrate. In the nonasthmatics, neutrophils, plasma cells, and other mononuclear inflammatory cells predominated.[20] Two of the 13 nonasthmatics with BCG had severe rheumatoid arthritis (an association that has since been noted by others[36,41,45] and four had a history of exposure to potentially toxic inhalants. Although the pathogenesis of BCG was not clear, the authors noted that histologic features similar to BCG could be seen in tuberculosis, coccidioidomycosis, and other infectious disorders, and speculated that BCG may represent an unusual host response to inhaled or intrabronchial antigens.

Several subsequent studies have corroborated that two subsets of BCG appear to exist, only one of which is associated with chronic asthma and eosinophilia. Saldana and associates described 17 patients with BCG, three of whom had bronchial asthma.[45] Robinson and co-workers noted that 3 of 15 cases of BCG extracted from the pathology files of the Armed Forces Institute of Pathology (A.F.I.P.) had chronic asthma, two of whom exhibited peripheral blood eosinophilia.[44] By contrast, none of the 12 nonasthmatic patients had blood eosinophilia. Chest radiographs were abnormal in all 15 cases; nine exhibited solitary or multiple mass lesions and the remainder demonstrated alveolar or diffuse reticulonodular infiltrates. Consistent with previous reports, an upper lobe predominance was noted and cavitation was rare. Analysis of the histopathologic features of these 15 cases demonstrated a necrotizing granulomatous process within small bronchi and bronchioles in all cases, which often extended into the lung parenchyma as an organizing pneumonia.[19] Pulmonary arteritis was mild in all cases and appeared to be an extension of the airways lesion rather than a primary vasculitis. Distinct clinicopathologic subgroups could be defined according to the relative number of eosinophils within the inflammatory infiltrate. Among five patients exhibiting striking eosinophilic infiltration within the granulomatous process, three had chronic asthma and two had blood eosinophilia. Fragments of degenerating aspergilli were identified within the necrotizing granulomas in one case.[19] Polymorphonuclear leukocytes predominated within the necrotic granulomas in the remaining 10 cases, and few eosinophils were visualized. None of these 10 patients had asthma and only one had blood eosinophilia.

More recent investigations have suggested that BCG may represent the histopathologic expression of ABPA in at least some cases. Several cases of BCG developing in chronic asthmatics with ABPA have been described.[7,37,39,40,46] The association of BCG with ABPA was demonstrated in one recent study that reviewed the pathologic features of resected lung specimens from 18 patients with ABPA.[46] Among the gross pathologic features were bronchiectasis and dilated bronchi filled with thick mucous plugs or purulent material. Microscopically, a necrotizing granulomatous process invading the bronchiolar wall, consistent with BCG, was present in 15 patients. Palisading histiocytes, admixed with lymphocytes, plasma cells, and necrotic debris within the center of the granulomatous lesions, were characteristic. Eosinophils were prominent in the inflammatory infiltrate in 11 cases, often mixed with clumps of eosinophilic granular material and necrotic debris. A mild vasculitis was often present in surrounding vessels but necrosis was not a prominent feature. A distinctive exudative bronchiolitis, in which bronchiolar lumens were filled with necrotic neutrophils and eosinophils in a basophilic mucinous exudate, was present distal to the BCG in 72% of cases. Most cases exhibited severe chronic bronchiolitis, characterized by dense peribronchiolar infiltrates of lymphocytes and plasma cells with variable number of eosinophils and foreign body giant cells. In some cases the bronchiolar epithelium was entirely destroyed and the bronchocentric distribution of the granulomatous process was inferred by virtue of its location adjacent to a pulmonary artery. Foci of bronchiolitis obliterans and eosinophilic pneumonia were present in eight cases, and fungal hyphae were identified in 14.

These data strongly suggest that BCG represents a hypersensitivity response to a variety of intrabronchial antigens rather than a distinct disease entity. In asthmatics, a reaction to aspergillus or fungal hyphae appears plausible as a pathogenic mechanism, whereas in nonasthmatics, BCG may reflect an unusual host response to specific inflammatory or infectious granulomatous processes, such as tuberculosis,[17,22] echinococcal pulmonary infection,[38] histoplasmosis,[17,22], coccidioidomycosis,[20] or rheumatoid arthritis.[36,41,45] Specific therapy directed against the responsible organism or underlying disease may be curative.[17,22,36]

Owing to the rarity of BCG, few data regarding therapy are available. The diagnosis of BCG has usually been established by evaluation of surgically resected lung tissue, and additional therapy has not usually been necessary. However, it should be emphasized that biopsy or resection of infiltrates in patients with ABPA is rarely necessary or appropriate since the diagnosis can usually be established by ancillary tests (such as serum IgE assay, eosinophil count, skin test reactivity to aspergillus and so on) and corticosteroid therapy is usually highly efficacious. Both surgical and corticosteroid therapy have been associated with high cure rates for BCG, and fatalities have been rare.[7,19,20,45] Occasional spontaneous remissions have also been described.[19,20] Among 10 asthmatics with BCG reported by Katzenstein and associates,[20] surgical resection of the involved lobe was carried out in eight (three of whom also received corticosteroids), and all did well. Cures were achieved with corticosteroids in the two remaining patients who had biopsy without resection. Among the 13 nonasthmatics with BCG, the involved lobe was resected in eight. In this group, three were cured without additional therapy; one improved with corticosteroids; one died while receiving cyclophosphamide and prednisone and showed no evidence of active disease at necropsy. No follow-up was available in the remaining three cases. Five patients had biopsy without resection, two of whom remained well without further therapy. One improved with azathioprine and two cases were lost to follow-up. Among 12 cases from the A.F.I.P. in whom follow-up data was available, surgical resection alone was curative in five patients and corticosteroids were effective in all four cases in whom they were tried.[19] One patient remitted with cyclophosphamide and corticosteroids; two clearly spontaneously. Saldana and co-workers reported that surgical excision was curative in six of seven patients with localized disease, and corticosteroids were effective in all five patients in whom they were tried.[45] Chlorambucil was ineffective in one patient, and the only death occurred in a patient treated with cyclophosphamide.[45] Immunosuppressive or cytotoxic agents have been used in BCG with occasional favorable responses,[19,20,43] as well as fatalities due to complications of therapy.[20,45] In view of the localized nature of BCG and the excellent response rate with corticosteroids or surgical resection,[7,19,20,36,37,45] there is little role for cytotoxic agents except in rare instances of progressive disease refractory to corticosteroids or surgical resection. More importantly, the histopathologic changes of BCG occur in response to various pathologic insults, including infection, rheumatoid arthritis, and ABPA, and should stimulate search for a causative antigen. Cultures and special stains for acid-fast bacilli, fungi, and nocardia should always be done. As BCG appears to represent a hypersensitivity reaction to specific underlying immunologic or infectious disease processes, therapy should be directed against the underlying antigen or stimulus. For example, treatment with mebendazole (an antiparasitic agent) in combination with corticosteroids was curative in a case of BCG associated with echinococcosis[36] and treatment with antituberculous or antimycotic agents has been efficacious in granulomatous infectious due to mycobacteria or fungi.[7,17] When BCG is seen in association with ABPA, corticosteroid therapy is warranted and surgical resection should be avoided. Serial serum IgE assays and blood eosinophil counts may guide therapy in ABPA because these parameters often correlate with disease activity. In cases where the diagnosis of BCG has been established on histopathologic material but no specific etiologic agent has been identified, surgical resection without additional therapy has usually been adequate.

NECROTIZING SARCOID ANGIITIS AND GRANULOMATOSIS (NSG)

Necrotizing sarcoid angiitis and granulomatosis (NSG) was first described by Liebow in 1973 on the basis of characteristic histopathology from 11 patients who exhibited a pulmonary necrotizing granulomatous vasculitis with a sarcoid-like reaction.[8] Histologically, confluent noncaseating granulomas involving bronchi, bronchioles, and pulmonary parenchyma were noted, consistent with sarcoidosis. However, the presence of a small vessel granulomatous vasculitis, often associated with necrosis of vessel walls and

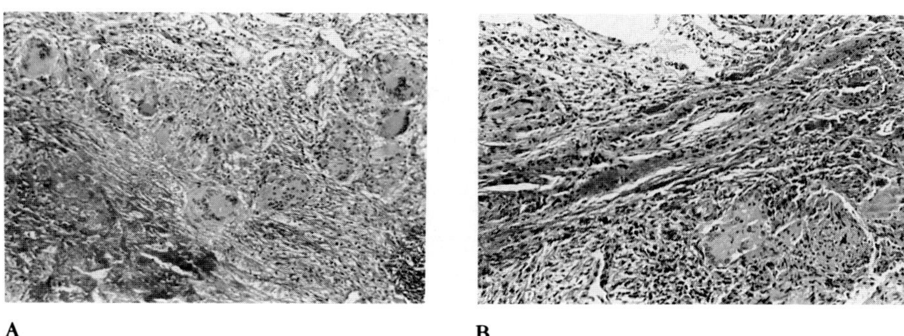

A   B

Figure 12-1. Necrotizing sarcoid granulomatosis. (*A*) In this photomicrograph of lung tissue from a patient with necrotizing sarcoid granulomatosis, well-formed multinucleated giant cells and chronic inflammatory cells are apparent adjacent to a large region of parenchymal necrosis. (H&E, ×165). (*B*) This photomicrograph from the same patient demonstrates granulomatous vasculitis with destruction of the vessel wall and occlusion of the lumen. Noncaseating granulomas with multinucleated giant cells are present in the pulmonary parenchyma. (H&E, ×330).

parenchyma, distinguished the condition from ordinary sarcoidosis. Vascular walls and lumens were infiltrated and in some cases obliterated by lymphocytes, plasma cells, histiocytes, and multinucleated giant cells (Fig. 12-1). The granulomatous inflammatory process commonly involved bronchi and bronchioles, but extension of the process into the lung with areas of consolidation and foci of bronchiolitis obliterans was common. Clinical features were nonspecific. Physical findings were minimal. Hepatosplenomegaly was noted in only one patient, and none had lymphadenopathy, uveitis, salivary gland enlargement, or skin lesions to suggest disseminated sarcoidosis. Fever, sweats, malaise, fatigue, or cough were the most common symptoms; two patients were asymptomatic. Chest radiographs demonstrated unilateral nodular densities in two cases; nine patients had multiple, bilateral pulmonary nodules (Fig. 12-2). Hilar lymphadenopathy was present in only one patient, and this was transient. The clinical course was benign. All four patients treated with corticosteroids responded favorably, with one asymptomatic relapse 3 years later; the remaining seven patients did well and there were no deaths or serious sequelae.[8]

In 1979, Churg and co-workers[47] reviewed 12 cases of NSG from the pathology files of Stanford University. Histologic features included large masses of confluent granulomas, variable amounts of necrosis and hyalinization, and a prominent granulomatous vasculitis involving both arteries and veins, sometimes associated with destruction of vascular walls. The distribution of granulomas followed the lymphatics, as in sarcoidosis. Chest radiographs demonstrated bilateral nodules in seven patients, solitary nodules in four, and a diffuse miliary pattern in one. Concomitant hilar adenopathy was present in six cases. Cough, dyspnea, chest pain, fever, and malaise were the most common symptoms, but three patients were asymptomatic. The course was benign. No patient had glomerulonephritis or systemic vasculitis and extrapulmonary involvement was rare. Five patients received no additional therapy following surgical resection of one or more nodules, and all remained well without recurrence of disease. Chest radiographs

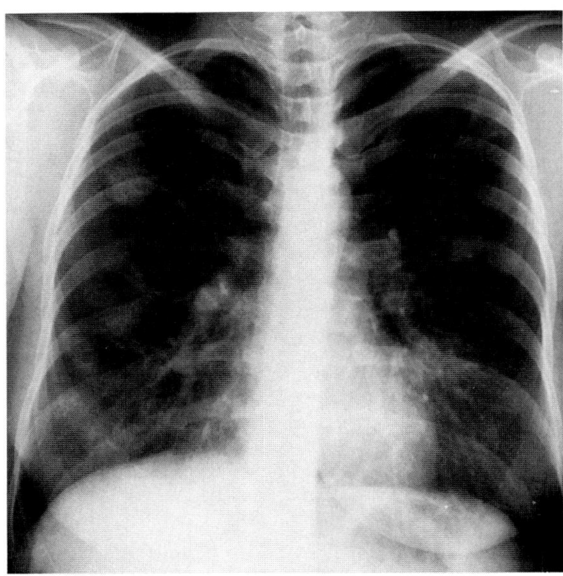

Figure 12-2. Chest radiograph from a patient with necrotizing sarcoid angiitis demonstrating multiple nodular pulmonary infiltrates.

improved or stabilized in three of four patients treated with corticosteroids and in both patients treated with cyclophosphamide. Overall, 10 of 12 patients were asymptomatic at follow-up 6 months to 11 years after diagnosis. The only death occurred in a patient treated with cyclophosphamide and was due to streptococcal pneumonia.

Koss and co-workers reviewed 13 cases of NSG from the pathology files of the A.F.I.P.[21] Histologic features resembled those previously described, with a granulomatous vasculitis and pneumonitis, a background of confluent, sarcoid-like granulomas, and variable degrees of parenchymal necrosis. Pulmonary symptoms of cough, chest pain, or dyspnea were present in 10 patients. Systemic symptoms, such as fever, malaise, weight loss, or fatigue were noted in seven patients. Two patients were entirely asymptomatic. The most characteristic feature on chest radiography was the presence of solitary or multiple pulmonary nodules, but diffuse infiltrates were also observed; cavitation was noted in three cases. Hilar adenopathy was present in only one of 13 cases. Five patients with localized pulmonary lesions were treated by surgical resection and remained disease-free at short-term follow-up. Six patients with diffuse infiltrates were treated with corticosteroids, and all showed radiographic improvement; however, two patients relapsed after corticosteroids were discontinued. In one of these cases, chlorambucil was introduced and the disease remitted. Two patients had no specific therapy and did well, exhibiting stabilization or spontaneous improvement in the chest radiograph.

In 1983, Churg[7] reviewed 32 cases displaying typical histopathologic features of NSC. Invariably, a pulmonary vasculitis involving both arteries and veins was present, often with intramural granulomas and multinucleated giant cells, but systemic vasculitis was never seen. Most patients had nonspecific pulmonary symptoms; 25% were asymptomatic. Four had extrapulmonary features, including uveitis in three and hypothalamic insufficiency in one. Chest radiographs were available for review in 29 cases and exhibited multiple nodules in 21 and solitary nodules in seven. Hilar adenopathy, a rare finding in prior reports,[8,21] was detected in 11 of 17 cases when this was specifically assessed. Churg concluded that NSG resembles ordinary sarcoidosis in most respects and probably represents a variant of pulmonary sarcoidosis rather than a distinct disease entity. This hypothesis is supported by previous findings that areas of pulmonary angiitis may be seen in 42% to 89% of open lung biopsy samples in patients with sarcoidosis[48,49] and may occasionally lead to vascular obliteration and infarct-like necrosis.[49] In addition, a granulomatous vasculitis involving both arteries and veins, often with areas of necrosis and infarction, has been a common feature in sarcoidosis involving the central nervous system (CNS).[50,57] Caplan and associates[50] described a severe granulomatous vasculitis with multiple CNS infarcts at necropsy in two patients dying of CNS sarcoidosis. In another case,[51] a child with multiple neurologic lesions resulting in paraplegia later developed multiple pulmonary nodular infiltrates: open lung biopsy demonstrated a florid vasculitis with areas of necrosis and confluent sarcoid granulomas. Spiteri and colleagues[52] described a 26-year-old patient with fever, sweats, dry cough, and patchy nodular pulmonary infiltrates in whom open lung biopsy demonstrated virtually complete effacement of the normal pulmonary architecture by confluent sarcoidal granulomas. Multiple foci of necrosis, surrounded by granulomas and inflammatory cells, were noted throughout the biopsy tissue and pulmonary vessels demonstrated a similar inflammatory cell infiltrate, occasionally with obliteration of the lumen. The extensive granuloma formation, foci of necrosis, and granulomatous vasculitis were consistent with Liebow's description of NSG. Marked increases in T4/T8 (helper/suppressor) ratio on lung biopsy and increases in serum angiotensin converting enzyme (ACE) were also demonstrated, features commonly ascribed to sarcoidosis.[52] A dramatic response to corticosteroids was noted. The authors suggested that sarcoidosis and NSG appear to have similar underlying immune mechanisms.

Stephen and co-workers[53] described a patient with a localized pulmonary mass lesion that exhibited histologic features compatible with NSG. Abundant granulation tissue, areas of hyalinization and fibrosis, epithelioid and Langhans-type giant cells forming granulomas, and a vasculitic response involving all layers of the vessel wall suggested the diagnosis of NSG. The patient recovered without specific therapy, but presented 6 months later with worsening dyspnea and respiratory insufficiency. At that time a left hilar mass was evident, and biopsy of an enlarged cervical lymph node revealed oat cell carcinoma. Although the authors speculate that the NSG and the oat cell carcinoma were unrelated and independent processes, it is possible that NSG represented in this instance an exuberant reaction to intrabronchial tumor antigens.

Rolfes and colleagues[54] described a 26-year-old black female with hilar adenopathy and a 3-cm nodule on the right upper lobe. Open lung biopsy demonstrated typical changes of NSG: confluent granulomas effacing the pulmonary architecture and extensive vasculitis with large areas of bland necrosis. Corticosteroids were associated with initial improvement. One year later, bilateral hilar adenopathy and diffuse reticulonodular infiltrates developed and repeat open lung biopsy demonstrated confluent granulomas with suppurative necrosis (associated with neutrophils) and vasculitis. Corticosteroids were again associated with improvement. These authors argued that the presence of a suppurative (neutrophilic) component, a normal level of ACE in the serum, and the absence of ACE within granulomas in the lung biopsy tissue by immunofluorescence suggested that NSG was an entity distinct from sarcoidosis. However, the other clinical and radiographic features are indistinguishable from ordinary sarcoidosis.

Thus, it is likely that most cases of NSG represent variants of sarcoidosis[3,7,9] that may resemble "nodular sarcoid."[56,57] Additional cases with histologic features consistent with NSG could reflect an exaggerated immune response to antigens, as described by Stephen and co-workers.[53] In view of the overall excellent prognosis of NSG, specific therapy is usually not required. However, corticosteroids are warranted in patients with severe or progressive pulmonary disease or central nervous system involvement. Immunosuppressive or cytotoxic agents could be considered in patients with progressive disease refractory to corticosteroid therapy or with intolerable corticosteroid side effects, but experience with these agents is limited.

ALLERGIC ANGIITIS AND GRANULOMATOSIS (CHURG-STRAUSS SYNDROME)

Allergic angiitis and granulomatosis (AG) was first described by Churg and Strauss who in 1951 reported 13 patients with a syndrome of severe asthma, peripheral eosinophilia, and a systemic necrotizing vasculitis with both eosinophilic and granulomatous components.[16] Abdominal pain, hypertension, and involvement of the skin, heart, pulmonary arteries, and peripheral and central nervous systems were common associated features. The salient histopathologic features included a necrotizing eosinophilic and granulomatous vasculitis involving small and medium-sized arteries, capillaries, and veins. Vascular walls were intensely infiltrated by eosinophils and by lesser numbers of plasma cells, lymphocytes, and polymorphonuclear leukocytes. There was also a pronounced granulomatous component, with palisading histiocytes and multinucleated giant cells (Fig. 12-3). Varying degrees of necrosis, hemorrhage, and fibrosis were also present. In involved extravascular tissues, granulomatous lesions with macrophages and giant cells surrounding a central eosinophilic core were characteristic. The prominent eosinophilic and granulomatous components and the striking predilection for the pulmonary vasculature distinguished AG from classic polyarteritis nodosa, a disorder in which lung involvement is rare.[1,3,5]

In 1957, Rose and Spencer reviewed autopsy data from 111 patients with polyarteritis nodosa and noted that 32 patients manifested pulmonary symptoms and 14 had histologic evidence for vasculitis involving the pulmonary arteries.[10] In this subset of patients with pulmonary vasculitis, many had a prior history of severe asthma and 70% exhibited peripheral eosinophilia. In contrast to classic polyarteritis nodosa, in which neither eosinophils nor granulomas are typically observed, the vascular lesions in the patients with pulmonary involvement displayed a striking eosinophilic infiltration in the acute stages and a granulomatous reaction with giant cells during the later healing phases. The authors concluded that this subset of "polyarteritis nodosa" with pulmonary involvement and an eosinophilic, granulomatous vasculitis probably represented Churg-Strauss angiitis.[10]

Apart from scattered case reports,[58,59] little additional information was available on this disorder until 1977, when Chumbley and co-workers reviewed 30 cases of AG seen

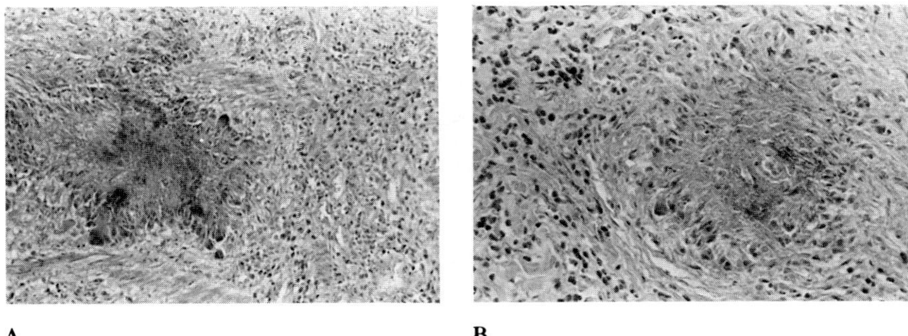

A   B

Figure 12-3. Allergic angiitis and granulomatosis (Churg-Strauss syndrome). (*A*) This photomicrograph of lung tissue from a patient with allergic angiitis and granulomatosis (Churg-Strauss syndrome) demonstrates necrotic lung tissue surrounded by a chronic inflammatory cell infiltrate, occasional giant cells, palisading histiocytes, and eosinophils. (H&E, × 165). (*B*) A higher magnification view from the same patient shows a necrotic region with palisading histiocytes. (H&E, × 330).

at the Mayo Clinic during a 24-year period.[27] All 30 cases exhibited a necrotizing vasculitis with prominent eosinophilic infiltration of vessels associated with asthma and blood eosinophilia.[27] However, only 22 of the 30 demonstrated the typical extravascular granulomas with necrosis. Fever and multisystemic involvement were characteristic. Allergic rhinitis was present in 21 patients, an association that will be discussed later. Neurologic manifestations, most commonly mononeuritis multiplex, were present in 19 patients. Twenty patients had cutaneous lesions, varying from subcutaneous nodules to petechial or purpuric rashes. Abdominal pain was a feature in five cases, three of whom underwent laparotomy. Renal failure was present in only one patient. Corticosteroid therapy was administered in 27 patients, and appeared to favorably influence survival. One patient with fulminating vasculitis received cyclophosphamide but died in spite of therapy. Azathioprine successfully induced remission in the one patient in whom it was tried. Although 15 patients died during long-term follow-up (often of cardiac or unrelated causes), only three died within 1 year of the onset of vasculitis. The 5-year survival rate was 62% and the median survival time was greater than 9 years.[27]

Because of the rarity of Churg-Strauss syndrome, clinical experience with this disorder is limited. A review of the files of the A.F.I.P. in 1981 disclosed only four cases of AG.[60] As of 1982, only 138 cases of AG had been published.[28] In 1984, Lanham and co-workers reported 16 cases of AG seen at a large referral hospital in England over a 6-year period and suggested that the apparent rarity of AG may in part reflect the stringent criteria used for the diagnosis.[28] In this series, only eight patients had histologic confirmation of vasculitis and only a minority of cases exhibited all three of the cardinal histologic features of the syndrome: that is, necrotizing vasculitis, eosinophilic infiltration of tissue, and extravascular granulomas.[28] However, these authors suggested that the definition of AG could be liberalized to include patients with systemic vasculitis, asthma, blood eosinophila, and some (but not necessarily all) histopathologic criteria. They also emphasized that in many cases the fully developed vasculitic syndrome represented a late phase of an allergic or hypersensitivity diathesis, which had usually been present for several years. A history of hay fever or atopy prior to the development of vasculitis could be elicited in up to 75% of cases.[1,28] In the earliest phase of the disorder, allergic rhinitis, sinusitis, and nasal polyposis may be the dominant clinical features. Later in the course of the illness, clinical asthma and blood eosinophilia occur.[27,28] Although systemic vasculitis may occur simultaneously with the onset of asthma, typically the vasculitic phase occurs as a late event, 10 or more years after the onset of allergic rhinitis and 3 to 5 years after the onset of asthma.[1,27,28,60] Characteristically, increasingly severe and more frequent attacks of asthma precede the development of the systemic vasculitis phase.[1,28] A shorter duration from the onset of asthma to the development of vasculitis has been associated with a worse prognosis.[27,28]

The characteristic clinical, radiographic, and histopathologic features of AG have been well delineated.[16,27,28,60] As has been discussed, pulmonary involvement, primarily presenting as progressive asthma, is virtually always present.[5,27,28,60,61] Abnormalities on chest radiograph are present in 20% to 70% of cases.[1,27,28,60] Transient fluffy pulmonary infiltrates, often in a peripheral distribution consistent with chronic eosinophilic pneumonia, are characteristic.[27,28,60] In contrast to other pulmonary granulomatous vasculitides, nodular densities are uncommon in AG, and cavitation virtually never occurs. The histologic features of AG in the lung may mimic chronic eosinophilic pneumonia, as intense infiltration of the pulmonary interstitium and alveolar spaces by eosinophils, macrophages, and giant cells may be evident[27,28,60]; however, the vasculitic component and parenchymal necrosis characteristic of AG are not seen in chronic eosinophilic pneumonia.

Constitutional symptoms such as fatigue, malaise, and weight loss are common in AG, and fever is present in over 90% of cases.[1,27,28] Arthralgias and myalgias occur in up to 20% to 40% of cases.[1,27,28] Peripheral or central nervous system manifestations have been described in 40% to 60% of cases.[1,27,28] Mononeuritis multiplex or peripheral neuropathy are the most common clinical manifestations, but more severe complications of CNS vasculitis such as cerebral infarction or hemorrhage occur in 5% to 10% of cases.[1,27,28] Cardiac involvement has been demonstrated in 30% to 50% of cases.[1,27,28] Any part of the myocardium, pericardium, or epicardium may be affected, and involvement may result in cardiac conduction defects, arrythmias, cardiomyopathy, or infarction from coronary vasculitis.[1,27,28] Approximately 50% of deaths in AG have been attributed to congestive heart failure or myocardial infarction, although in some cases the relationship between the cardiac lesion and AG has not been clear.[1,28] Systemic hypertension occurs in 50% of cases [1,27,28] and is an important cause of long-term sequelae. Renal failure occurs in less than 5% of cases, but microscopic hematuria or proteinuria has been described in 20% to 30% of cases in recent studies.[27,28] Owing to the rarity of clinically significant renal involvement in AG, few renal biopsies have been carried out in this disorder. However, granulomatous or eosinophilic infiltrates within the renal parenchyma or vessels have been noted in up to 40% of patients at necropsy.[1] Gastrointestinal symptoms (typically, abdominal pain due to vasculitis of the mesentery, bowel, stomach, liver, or spleen) are present in 20% to 40% of cases.[1,27,28,62] Severe visceral ischemia, gastrointestinal bleeding, or perforation may be catastrophic and have accounted for 5% to 10% of deaths.[1,27,28,62] Skin lesions, including petechiae, purpura, ulcerations, urticaria, maculopapular rash, or nodules, occur in two-thirds of patients.[1,27,28]

Although laboratory findings in AG are nonspecific, they may be helpful in monitoring the course of the disease. Elevations in blood eosinophils and Westergren sedimentation rate occur in 80% to 90% of cases, and both parameters usually correlate with disease activity.[1,2,5,27,28] Serum complement, immune complexes, and collagen vascular studies are usually normal or negative.[1,5,28] Although serum IgE determinations have been performed in only a few cases, several investigators have reported increases in serum IgE in patients with AG.[1,27,28,60,63] Lanham and colleagues[28] and Chumbley and associates[27] detected elevations in serum IgE in five of five and two of two cases of AG, respectively, in whom levels were obtained, suggesting this is a frequent and probably important association. Although additional data are needed to confirm this hypothesis, serial determinations of serum IgE may be helpful in monitoring the course of the disease.[27,63,64] Elevations of IgE have also been described in other allergic states, such as asthma, ABPA, and chronic eosinophilic pneumonia. It is thus intriguing to speculate that sustained antigen stimulation and IgE formation may have a pathogenic role in AG, particularly in light of reports of AG developing in patients with a prior history of ABPA[65] or chronic eosinophilic pneumonia.[66]

Early studies suggested that the mortality of AG approached 90% in the absence of therapy[10,16]; however, recent studies suggest that survival exceeds 90% with the early use of corticosteroids.[28] The course is usually indolent, and fulminant vasculitis or renal failure are rarely seen. In one review of 138 cases of AG, renal failure was the proximate cause of death in only nine cases, none of whom received corticosteroids.[28] In three recent studies, significant impairment in renal function was demonstrated in only 3 of 50 cases.[27,28,60] Most deaths have resulted from congestive heart failure, myocardial infarction, cerebral hemorrhage, or renal failure but have been due to long-term sequelae of vasculitis or the underlying vasculopathy rather than an acute vasculitic process.[1,5,27,28] With early initiation of corticosteroid therapy, most of these late complications can be avoided and remissions can be achieved in over 90% of cases.[28] Response to corticosteroids is often dramatic, with remissions sometimes occurring within a few days of initiation of therapy.[27,28,63,64] Although the optimal dose and duration of corticosteroids have not been clarified, 40 to 80 mg prednisone or equivalent for the first few weeks is usually required to control the acute vasculitic process and prevent late sequelae. The dose can then be tapered gradually according to the clinical response and laboratory parameters. Once the disease is under control, converting to an alternate day regimen is reasonable, in order to minimize long-term side effects from corticosteroids. Serum IgE levels, total blood eosinophil count, and Westergren sedimentation rate should be measured when therapy is initiated. If elevated, serial measurements of one or more of these parameters should be done, as changes in these parameters may reflect disease activity more accurately than clinical findings. Once the vasculitic phase has been controlled, late relapse (beyond 12 months) has been uncommon, and corticosteroids may sometimes be discontinued altogether.[1,5,28] Long-term therapy (often for years or indefinitely) may be required, however, in some cases. Experience with immunosuppressive or cytotoxic agents is limited, but occasional favorable responses have been achieved with these agents in

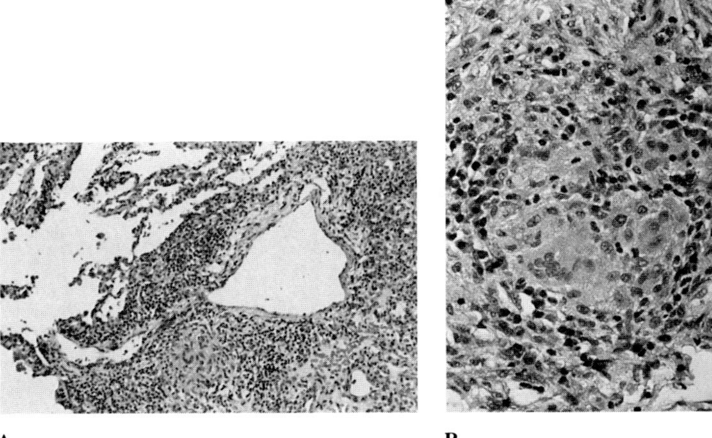

A   B

Figure 12-4. Pulmonary histoplasmosis. (*A*) This photomicrograph of lung tissue from a patient with pulmonary histoplasmosis demonstrates an interstitial granulomatous inflammatory process with infiltration of blood vessel walls by chronic inflammatory cells. (H&E, ×165). (*B*) This photomicrograph from the same patient demonstrates a noncaseating granuloma with multinucleated giant cells and chronic inflammatory cells. (H&E, ×528).

patients failing on steroids.[1,27,28,61] In view of the excellent response rate to corticosteroids alone, we believe that these agents should be reserved for patients who fail to respond to corticosteroids or who suffer serious corticosteroid side effects.

PULMONARY VASCULITIS COMPLICATING SPECIFIC GRANULOMATOUS INFECTIONS

From the preceding discussion, it is evident that the clinical presentation and histopathologic changes associated with this group of pulmonary granulomatous vasculitic syndromes may occur in response to pulmonary insults by specific pathologic agents. For example, specific pulmonary infections due to mycobacteria or fungi may manifest histologic features indistinguishable from Wegener's and bronchocentric granulomatosis.[4,17,22,46] In one series that evaluated the histopathologic characteristics of surgically resected solitary pulmonary nodules, vasculitis with fibrinoid necrosis and destruction of the vascular wall was demonstrated in over 50% of tuberculous granulomas and in 30% of fungal granulomas (Fig. 12-4).[17] The differentiation of primary granulomatous vasculitis from infectious granulomas may be difficult, and special staining and cultures for fungi and acid-fast bacilli should be performed on all pathology specimens where primary vasculitis is a consideration. The sensitivity of cultures in infectious granulomas may be only 20% to 30%, but a microbiologic diagnosis can be established in 70% to 90% of cases by the application of special stains for AFB and fungi, particularly if areas within the necrotic center of the granuloma are examined and two or more blocks are reviewed.[4,7,17,20,46] In view of the prominent overlapping histologic features of infectious and noninfectious pulmonary granulomatoses, one should be particularly cautious about making the diagnosis of a primary vasculitis in the absence of extrapulmonary manifestations. In a study of 86 consecutive resected solitary pulmonary nodules that exhibited a caseating granulomatous process (several of which were initially diagnosed as Wegener's granulomatosis), a specific infectious etiology was documented in 71% of cases.[17] In addition, even when no specific diagnosis was established, the course was benign even without specific therapy apart from surgical resection.[17] Thus, even when areas of granulomatous vasculitis are detected within a solitary lung nodule, systemic vasculitis is unlikely unless additional extrapulmonary manifestations can be demonstrated.

REFERENCES

1. Cupps TR, Fauci AS. The vasculitides. Philadelphia: W. B. Saunders, 1981.
2. DeRemee RA, Weiland LH, McDonald TJ. Respiratory vasculitis. Mayo Clin Proc 1980:55; 492–498.
3. Dreisen RB. Pulmonary vasculitis. Clin Chest Med 1982:3;607–618.
4. Katzenstein AL. Necrotizing granulomas of the lung. Hum Pathol 1980:11;596–597.
5. Leavitt RY, Fauci AS. Pulmonary vasculitis. Am Rev Respir Dis 1986:134;140–166.
6. McCluskey RT, Feinberg R. Vasculitis in primary vasculitides, granulomatoses, and connective tissue diseases. Hum Pathol 1983:14;305–315.
7. Churg A. Pulmonary angiitis and granulomatosis revisited. Hum Pathol 1983:14;868–883.
8. Liebow AA. Pulmonary angiitis and granulomatosis. Am Rev Respir Dis 1973:108;1–18.
9. Lie JT. Classification of pulmonary angiitis and granulomatosis: Histopathologic perspectives. Semin Respir Med 1989:10;111–121.
10. Rose GA, Spencer H. Polyarteritis nodosa. Q J Med 1957:26;43–81.
11. Slavin RF, de Groot WG. Pathology of the lung in Behçet's disease: Case report and review of the literature. Am J Surg Pathol 1981:5;779–788.
12. Bombardieri S, Paoletti P, Ferri C, DiMunno O, Fornai E, Giuntini C. Lung involvement in essential mixed cryoglobulinemia. Am J Med 1979:66;748–756.
13. Kathuria S, Cheifec G. Fatal pulmonary Henoch-Schönlein syndrome. Chest 1982:82;654–656.
14. Hall S, Barr W, Lie JT. Takayasu arteritis: A study of 32 North American patients. Medicine (Baltimore) 1985:64;89–99.
15. Lupi-Herrera E, Sanchez-Torres G, Horwitz S. Pulmonary artery involvement in Takayasu's arteritis. Chest 1975:67;69–74.
16. Churg J, Strauss L. Allergic granulomatosis, allergic angiitis, and periarteritis nodosa. Am J Pathol 1951:27;277–301.
17. Ulbright TM, Katzenstein AL. Solitary necrotizing granulomas of the lung: Differentiating features and etiology. Am J Surg Pathol 1980:4;13–28.
18. Kunkel SL, Chensue SW, Strieter RM, Lynch JP, Remick DG. Cellular and molecular aspects of pulmonary granuloma formation. Am J Resp Cell Mol Biol 1989:1(6);439–448.
19. Koss MN, Robinson RG, Hochholzer L. Bronchocentric granulomatosis. Hum Pathol 1981:12;632–638.
20. Katzenstein AL, Liebow AA, Friedman PJ. Bronchocentric granulomatosis, mucoid impaction, and hypersensitivity reactions to fungi. Am Rev Respir Dis 1975:111;497–537.
21. Koss MN, Hochholzer L, Geigin DS, Garancis JC, Ward PA. Necrotizing sarcoid-like granulomatosis. Hum Pathol 1980:11(suppl);510–519.

22. Katzenstein AL, Myers JL. Granulomatous infection mimicking bronchocentric granulomatosis. Am J Surg Pathol 1986:10;317–322.
23. Jaffe ES, Lifford EH Jr, Margolick JB, Longo DL, Fauci AS. Lymphomatoid granulomatosis and angiocentric lymphoma: A spectrum of post-thymic T-cell proliferations. Semin Respir Med 1989:10;167–172.
24. Colby TV, Carrington CB. Pulmonary lymphomas: Current concepts. Hum Pathol 1983:14; 884–887.
25. Liebow AA. Lymphomatoid granulomatosis. Hum Pathol 1972:3;457–558.
26. Saldana MJ, Patchefsky AS, Israel HI, Atkinson GW. Pulmonary angiitis and granulomatosis: The relationship between histological features, organ involvement, and response to treatment. Hum Pathol 1977:8;391–409.
27. Chumbley LC, Harrison EG, DeRemee RA. Allergic granulomatosis and angiitis (Churg-Strauss syndrome): Report and analysis of 30 cases. Mayo Clin Proc 1977:52;477–484.
28. Lanham JG, Elkon KB, Pusey CD, Hughes GR. Systemic vasculitis with asthma and eosinophilia: A clinical approach to the Churg-Strauss syndrome. Medicine (Baltimore) 1984:63;65–81.
29. Israel HL, Patchefsky AS, Saldana MJ. Wegener's granulomatosis, lymphomatoid granulomatosis, and benign lymphocytic angiitis and granulomatosis of lung: Recognition and treatment. Ann Intern Med 1977:87;691–699.
30. Weiss MA, Rolfes DB, Alvira MA, Cohen LJ. Benign lymphocytic angiitis and granulomatosis: A case report with evidence of an autoimmune etiology. Am J Clin Pathol 1984:81;110–116.
31. Gracey DR, DeRemee RA, Colby TV, Unni KK, Weiland LH. Benign lymphocytic angiitis and granulomatosis: Experience with three cases. Mayo Clin Proc 1988:63;323–331.
32. Levy A, Avidor I, Spitzer S, et al. Massive hemoptysis as a presenting sign of benign lymphocytic angiitis and granulomatosis. Eur J Respir Dis 1984:65;311–314.
33. Tukiainen H, Terho E, Syrjanen K, Sutinen S. Benign lymphocytic angiitis and granulomatosis. Thorax 1988:43;649–650.
34. Jaffe ES. Pathological and clinical spectrum of post-thymic T-cell malignancies. Cancer Invest 1984:2;413–426.
35. Jaffe ES. Pulmonary lymphocytic angiitis: A nosologic quandary. Mayo Clin Proc 1988:63;411–413.
36. Berendsen HH, Hofstee N, Kapsenberg PD, van Reesema DR, Klein JJ. Bronchocentric granulomatosis associated with seropositive polyarthritis. Thorax 1985:40;396–397.
37. Clee MD, Lamb D, Urbaniak SJ, Clark RA. Progressive bronchocentric granulomatosis: Case report. Thorax 1982:37;947–949.
38. Den Hertog RW, Wagenaar SS, Westermann CJJ. Bronchocentric granulomatosis and pulmonary echinococcosis. Am Rev Respir Dis 1982:126;344–347.
39. Goodman DH, Sacca JD. Pulmonary cavitation, allergic aspergillosis, asthma, and bronchocentric granulomatosis. Chest 1977:72;368–369.
40. Hanson G, Flor N, Wells I, Novey H, Galant S. Bronchocentric granulomatosis: A complication of allergic bronchopulmonary aspergillosis. J Allergy Clin Immunol 1977:59;83–90.
41. Hellems SO, Kanner RE, Renzetti AD. Bronchocentric granulomatosis associated with rheumatoid arthritis. Chest 1983:5;831–832.
42. Warren J, Pitchenik AE, Saldana MJ. Bronchocentric granulomatosis with glomerulonephritis. Chest 1985;87;832–834.
43. Wiedemann HP, Bensinger RE, Hudson LD. Bronchocentric granulomatosis with eye involvement. Am Rev Respir Dis 1982: 126;347–350.
44. Robinson RG, Wehunt WD, Tsou E, Koss MN, Hochholzer L. Bronchocentric granulomatosis: Roentgenographic manifestations. Am Rev Respir Dis 1982:125;751–756.
45. Saldana MJ. Bronchocentric granulomatosis: Clinicopathologic observations in 17 patients. Lab Invest 1979;40:281–282.
46. Bosken CH, Myers JL, Greenberger PA, Katzenstein AL. Pathologic features of allergic bronchopulmonary aspergillosis. Am J Surg Pathol 1988:12(3);216–222.

47. Churg A, Carrington CB, Gupta R. Necrotizing sarcoid granulomatosis. Chest 1979:76;406–413.
48. Carrington CB, Gaensler EA, Mikus JP, Schaechter AW, Burke GW, Goff AM. Structure and function in sarcoidosis. Ann NY Acad Sci 1976:278;265–282.
49. Rosen Y, Moon S, Huang C, Gourin A, Lyons HA. Granulomatous pulmonary arteritis in sarcoidosis. Arch Pathol Lab Med 1977:101;170–174.
50. Caplan L, Corbett J, Goodwin J, Thomas C, Shenker D, Schatz N. Neuro-ophthalmologic signs in the angiitic form of neurosarcoidosis. Neurology 1983:33;1130–1135.
51. Beach RC, Corrin B, Scopes JW, Graham E. Necrotizing sarcoid granulomatosis with neurologic lesions in a child. J Pediatr 1980:97;950–953.
52. Spiteri MA, Gledhill A, Campbell D, Clarke SW. Necrotizing sarcoid granulomatosis. Br J Dis Chest 1987:81;70–75.
53. Stephen JG, Braimbridge MV, Corrin B, Wilkinson SP, Day D, Whimster WF. Necrotizing "sarcoidal" angiitis and granulomatosis of the lung. Thorax 1976:31;356–360.
54. Rolfes DB, Weiss MA, Sanders MA. Necrotizing sarcoid granulomatosis with suppurative features. Am J Clin Pathol 1984:82;602–607.
55. Saldana MJ, Israel HL. Necotizing sarcoid granulomatosis, benign lymphocytic angiitis, and granulomatosis: Do they exist?. Semin Respir Med 1989:10;182–188.
56. Sharma OP, Hewlett R, Gordonson J. Nodular sarcoidosis: An unusual radiographic appearance. Chest 1973:64;189–192.
57. Tellis CJ, Putnam JS. Cavitation in large multinodular pulmonary disease: A rare manifestation of sarcoidosis. Chest 1977:71;792–793.
58. Sokolov RA, Rachmaninoff N, Kaine HD. Allergic granulomatosis. Am J Med 1962:32;131–141.
59. Varriale P, Minogue WF, Alfenito JC. Allergic granulomatosis: Case report and review of the literature. Arch Intern Med 1964:113;235–240.
60. Koss MN, Antonovych T, Hochholzer L. Allergic granulomatosis (Churg-Strauss syndrome): Pulmonary and renal morphologic findings. Am J Surg Pathol 1981:5;21–28.
61. Cooper BJ, Bacal E, Patterson R. Allergic angiitis and granulomatosis: Prolonged remission induced by combined prednisone-azathioprine therapy. Arch Intern Med 1978:138;367–371.
62. Suen KC, Burton JD. The spectrum of eosinophilic infiltration of the gastrointestinal tract and its relationship to other disorders of angiitis and granulomatosis. Hum Pathol 1979:10;31–43.
63. Sale S, Patterson R. Recurrent Churg-Strauss vasculitis: With exophthalmos, hearing loss, nasal obstruction, amyloid deposits, hyperimmunoglobulinemia E, and circulating immune complexes. Arch Intern Med 1981:141;1363–1365.
64. Kus J, Bergin C, Miller R, Ongley R, Churg A, Enarson D. Lymphocyte subpopulations in allergic granulomatosis and angiitis (Churg-Strauss syndrome). Chest 1985:87;826–827.
65. Stephens M, Reynolds S, Gibbs AR, Davies B. Allergic bronchopulmonary aspergillosis progressing to allergic granulomatosis and angiitis (Churg-Strauss syndrome). Am Rev Respir Dis 1988:137;1226–1228.
66. Cogan FC, Mayock RL, Zweiman B. Chronic eosinophilic pneumonia followed by polyarteritis nodosa complicating the course of bronchial asthma: Report of a case. J Allergy Clin Immunol 1977:60;377–382.

13

Asthma: Chronic Desquamating Eosinophilic Bronchitis

Charles E. Reed

In all of medicine asthmatic patients may well be the most difficult and complex for physicians to understand and treat. Current knowledge about the epidemiology, natural history, pathogenesis, and response to treatment does not allow simple unifying concepts about its nature or universally applicable treatment plans. Students of asthma do not even agree about whether it is a single disease with a single as yet unidentified molecular biological defect or a syndrome that represents a final similar result brought about by a variety of causes, although they do agree that it is a recognizable entity. Complexity of disease manifestations does not necessarily exclude a single basic molecular defect. Consider, for example, cystic fibrosis. On the other hand, nothing now known about asthma promises much hope that a hypothetical molecular defect will be uncovered soon. Rather, emphasis in current asthma research centers on mechanisms of its various manifestations and on empirical evaluation of various modes of therapy that might alter these mechanisms.

DEFINITION

Asthma has proved extraordinarily difficult to define, as the persisting popularity of ambiguous synonyms such as "asthmatic bronchitis," "wheezy baby," "reversible airway obstruction," and "bronchospastic disease" attests. Different disciplines use different definitions. Epidemiologists define asthma as a pattern of answers to a standardized questionnaire, although other parameters such as allergy skin tests or bronchial hyperresponsiveness may be included in their surveys. Physiologists using spirometry define it as generalized narrowing of the airways that changes in severity over short periods, either spontaneously or with treatment, or as hyperresponsiveness to bronchoconstrictive stimuli. Pathologists define it histologically as a variety of bronchitis characterized

322

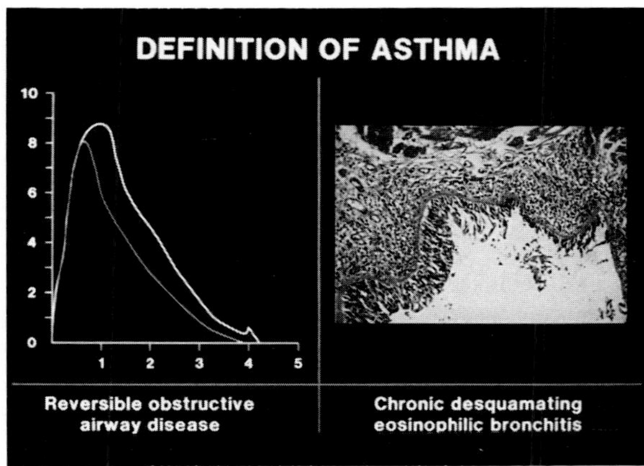

Figure 13-1. Clinical definition of asthma emphasizing both reversible airway reactivity and airway inflammation.

by a distinctive exudate in the lumen containing plasma proteins, eosinophils, and degenerate respiratory columnar epithelial cells.

Immunologists' definition has in the past focused on the release of anaphylactic mast cell mediators that occurs when an allergen reacts with mast cell–bound IgE antibody. Recent emphasis has been on the late inflammatory phase that follows 3 to 12 hours after an IgE-initiated asthmatic response, and on the relationship between the inflammation of the late phase and bronchial hyperresponsiveness. Not all patients have definable allergy to airborne allergens. It has long been useful to classify asthma into *extrinsic* (or allergic) and *intrinsic* (or idiopathic or infectious). Many patients have both and are classified as *mixed.* Indeed, there is some rationale for considering all asthma as mixed, for most patients allergic to ragweed or cats, for example, do not have asthma; they have only allergic rhinitis. And patients who for the most part have asthma only after exposure to an allergen wheeze when they exercise in cold air. Ignorance about why some individuals develop asthma in addition to rhinitis is hidden under the old concept of "tissue factors." Although the histopathology of bronchial inflammation is indistinguishable in "extrinsic" IgE-mediated asthma and "intrinsic" non–IgE-mediated asthma, there is as yet no immunologic explanation for this characteristic type of inflammation in intrinsic cases.

Clinicians must integrate all of these definitions into useful methods for diagnosing and treating patients with asthma. An important development in the past few years is the growing realization that the once popular concept of asthma as "bronchospasm" has failed the clinician. Not that it is wrong; it is merely incomplete (Fig. 13-1). Although in the United States prescriptions for effective bronchodilators have increased almost tenfold since 1960, hospital admissions have also increased at about the same rate (Fig. 13-2).[1] Mortality has either stayed the same or has also increased.[2] This change in frequency or severity of asthma appears to be worldwide, for other Western countries have experienced similar trends.[3,4] It is obvious that liberal treatment with modern, effective bronchodilators has not solved the problem. The best explanation for their inadequacy is that asthma is not so much "bronchospasm" or airway

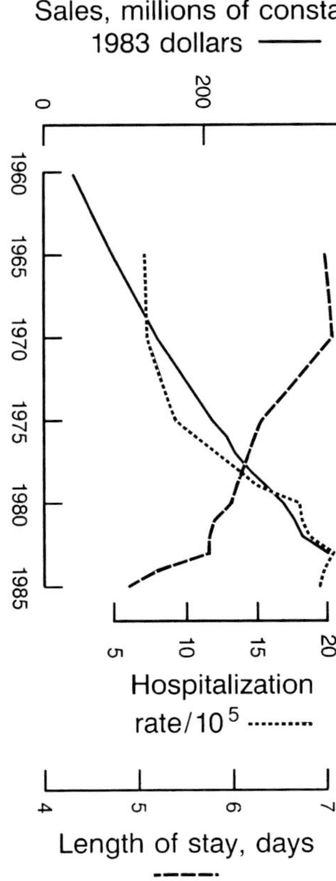

Figure 13-2. Change in sales of bronchodilator medications for asthma in the United States since 1960 compared with rates of hospitalization. Most of the increase in hospitalization has occurred in children and the elderly. Similar changes have occurred in other Western countries. (Redrawn from Reed CE. New therapeutic approaches in asthma. J Allergy Clin Immunol 1986, 77:537.)

hyperresponsiveness as it is "chronic desquamating eosinophilic bronchitis." Important as it is in causing the day-to-day variability in symptoms, hyperresponsiveness is mainly secondary to inflammation. The inescapable conclusion follows that treatment needs to be directed at the inflammation.

EPIDEMIOLOGY AND NATURAL HISTORY

Asthma affects all ages, all races, and both sexes. For unknown reasons boys are more often affected than girls, but by the third decade the prevalence becomes equal and subsequently more women than men are affected. Prevalence varies in different geographical locations. In developing countries it is rare in people living in tribal cultures but occurs as they become westernized.[5] In the United Kingdom, it is more frequent among children born of immigrants from the Caribbean or Indian subcontinent.[6] In the United States, it is more frequent among blacks and hispanics living in the inner city.[7] Reasons for these differences are not known definitively but presumably are pri-

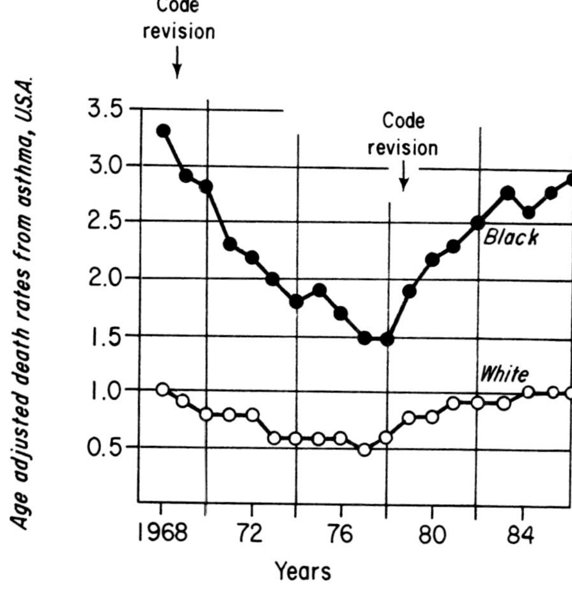

Figure 13-3. Age-adjusted rates of death from asthma per 100,000 general population by race, 1968–1986. (From Sly RM. J Allergy Clin Immunol 1989, 84:421–434).

marily socioeconomic, though a racial predisposition to an exuberant IgE immune response may also contribute. In prospective studies of children conducted in Australia, cumulative prevalence reaches 20% by the third decade.[8] A retrospective study in the United States found asthma to be the most common of the respiratory diseases. Prevalence in children was 7.6%. Prevalence among adults is less certain but is approximately 3% to 5%.[9] Asthma has changed in the last 20 years. It may be more prevalent; it certainly is more severe. Williams has reported that the increase in admissions to the Montifiore Hospital in the Bronx as well as the increase in patients needing assisted ventilation is not due to change in criteria for admission or intubation but to an increase in frequency of more severe disease.[10] In the United States, the age-corrected mortality rate has increased since 1975 and the hospitalization rate has increased tenfold since 1960 (Figs. 13-2, 13-3).[1,2] Reported asthma mortality rates are higher in Australia, New Zealand, and the United Kingdom than they are in North America, but rates have been increasing in all countries.[3,4] Asthma is now the most frequent discharge diagnosis for children.[11]

In the United States, increased mortality from asthma is concentrated among the indigent in large metropolitan areas.[2,12] Social reasons having to do with education, medical care expectations, and medical care availability obviously account in large part for this increase in metropolitan areas. Poor indoor air quality in city apartments is likely to be another key contributing factor to the excess morbidity and mortality in metropolitan areas. Urban Americans now spend more than 95% of their time indoors. Outdoor air quality has improved in the past 20 years in most cities, but indoor air quality has not. It may be worse, because in an attempt to conserve energy ventilation has been reduced. Respirable particulates, chiefly from tobacco smoke, and irritant gas concentrations, especially oxides of nitrogen from combustion of gas cooking stoves or kerosene heaters, can reach very high levels. Poor sanitary conditions lead to high indoor concentrations of cockroach, mite, mouse, and possibly mold allergens.[13]

Available information about the natural history of asthma indicates that the course of the disease in individual patients is highly variable.[8] Overall, asthma in children tends to improve, especially in boys without major allergic factors. Severe disease, onset before age 2 years, coexisting atopic dermatitis, and high levels of IgE are features that lead to poor prognosis. Many children who had a remission in their teens have a recurrence in their third decade.

There is much less information available about the natural history of asthma in adults, either those whose asthma began in childhood or those with asthma beginning in later years. Although some adults enjoy a remission, others progress and some at least develop irreversible airway obstruction.[14,15] Levels of IgE decline with age and mild allergic disease often improves after the age of 40 or 50 years. Development of allergy to aeroallergens is uncommon before age 2 and virtually unknown after age 40, except for individuals who are exposed to allergens they have never previously encountered. Examples are Asians who come to North America and are exposed to ragweed or individuals who encounter a new occupational allergen at work. There is, however, an association between asthma and IgE levels whether or not the skin tests are positive.[16]

PATHOLOGY

The concept that asthma is a particular kind of bronchial inflammation is not a contemporary one. Curshmann coined the term "bronchiolitis exudativa" in 1883 and Dunnill had fully described the histopathology by 1960.[17,18] More recently, Kleineman has extended these studies quantifying the changes.[19] Pathologically, as Curshmann said, asthma is a variety of bronchitis characterized by a distinctive exudate into the lumen. The inflammation extends into the lung parenchyma surrounding the airway (Fig. 13-4). This exudate contains plasma proteins, lymphocytes, neutrophils, eosinophils, and degenerated respiratory columnar epithelial cells. The bronchial mucous membrane shows mucosal edema with vacuolization, and shedding of the normal ciliated epithelium. Mitosis may be present in the remaining basal cells. In places, even the basal cell layer has been desquamated leaving a naked basement membrane. Proteins of eosinophil granules, particularly major basic protein,[20] are prominent both in the bronchial secretions and in the areas of damaged epithelium. Beneath the epithelial basement lies an abnormal zone of thickened collagen. The submucosa shows dilated capillaries, edema, and a mononuclear cell infiltrate containing lymphocytes and plasma cells. Mast cells, both intact and degranulated, are present in increased numbers. Either intact eosinophils or deposits of eosinophil major basic protein are especially abundant near areas of epithelial damage, but neutrophils are usually conspicuously absent in the tissues. Bronchial mucous glands are enlarged and bronchial smooth muscle is hypertrophied (Fig. 13-5). The obstruction is uneven (Fig. 13-6). Although the bulk of this information about histopathology comes from autopsies, both biopsies

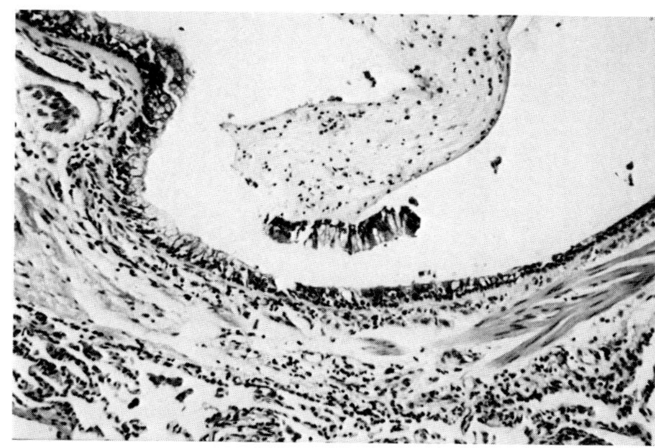

Figure 13-4. Photomicrograph of bronchus of patient who died of asthma. Note loss of cilia, vacuolization of the epithelium, inflammatory cells in the submucosa, and extension of the inflammation beyond the muscularis toward the parenchyma of the lung. Note also the plug of mucus and inflammation cells in the lumen. Attached to the mucus is a piece of epithelium that has been detached from some other area of the lung.

and studies of bronchial secretions have confirmed that similar inflammatory changes are present in the airways even when the disease is mild.[21–23] The term "chronic desquamating eosinophilic bronchitis" summarizes and emphasizes these abnormalities and distinguishes asthma from airway obstruction associated with emphysema or the chronic neutrophilic metaplastic bronchitis of cigarette smoking or other causes.

There is no satisfactory description of the histologic changes that account for the progression of asthma from a fully reversible process to a phase where complete reversal of the obstruction can no longer be achieved. Emphysema does not explain the irreversibility, for patients with asthma do not lose lung parenchyma. There is need for prospective study correlating ante mortem clinical status with postmortem pathology using quantitative morphometric techniques to define the dimensions of the various components of the airways. It is also possible, of course, that this irreversibility when the obstruction no longer responds fully to glucocorticoids has a biochemical rather than anatomic explanation.[24] Perhaps for unknown reasons the cells responsible for the inflammation and epithelial desquamation with resulting mucus plugs become resistant to the antiinflammatory action of glucocorticoids.

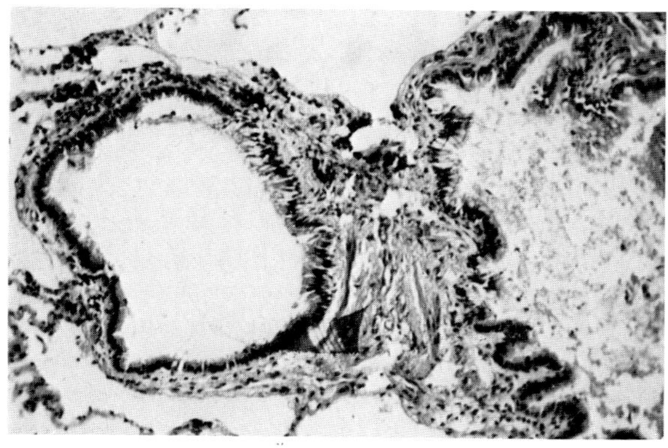

Figure 13-5. Uneven distribution of the mucus plugs. Twin bronchioles are evident, one patent and the other occluded by mucus.

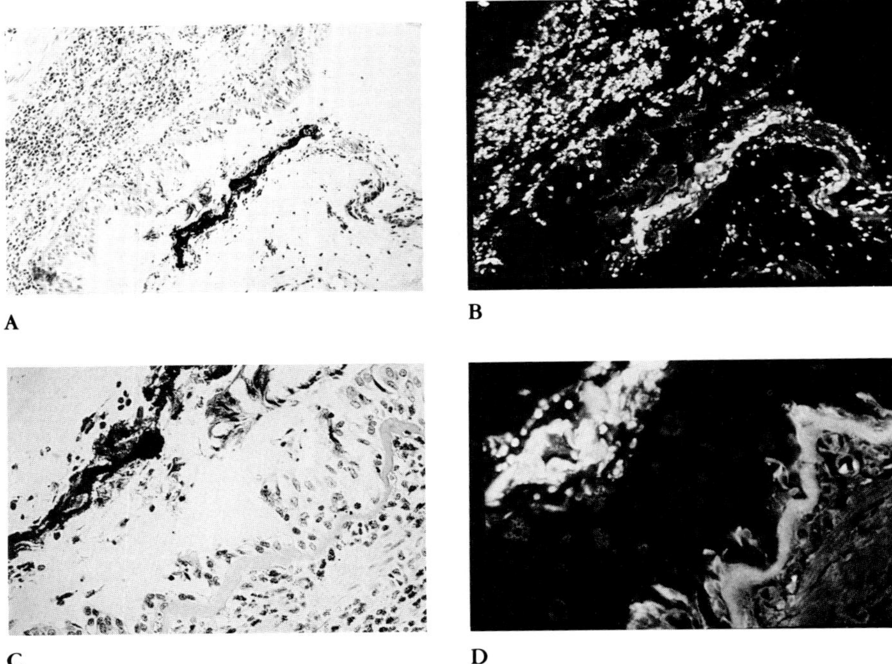

Figure 13-6. Photomicrographs illustrating localization of major basic protein (MBP) in lung epithelium of a patient dying of asthma. (*A*) Hematoxylin and eosin-stained respiratory epithelium shows striking submucosal eosinophil infiltration and a cluster of desquamated epithelial cells in the bronchial lumen next to a "stringy" deposit of a black-appearing substance, presumably soot. (Original magnification ×160). (*B*) Section stained for MBP by immunofluorescence illustrates bright staining of eosinophils in the submucosa. There is also MBP staining of the epithelial cells on their luminal surfaces. (Original magnification ×160). (*C*) Higher-power view of *A* illustrates areas of mainly intact epithelium (*left*) and desquamated epithelium (*top center*). Note the thickened basement membrane zone and the cluster of desquamated epithelial cells. (Original magnification ×400). (*D*) Higher-power view of *B* illustrates MBP deposition on the desquamated epithelial cells. Note the deposition of MBP on the luminal surfaces and outlining the more superficial epithelial cells. (Original magnification ×400). (From Gleich GJ, Flavahan NA, Fujisawa T, Vanhoutte PM. J Allergy Clin Immunol 1988, 81:776–781).

PATHOPHYSIOLOGY

Asthma affects all aspects of pulmonary function, especially during the acute attacks.[25] The increase in airway resistance results in decreased forced expiratory volumes (FEV_1) and reduced flow rates, premature airway closure, hyperinflation of the lungs, increased work of breathing, and changes in the elastic recoil and frequency-dependent behavior of the lungs. Gas exchange is also affected, causing a reduced arterial oxygen tension (Fig. 13-7). The primary reason for the reduced arterial oxygen retention is abnormal distribution of ventilation. Airway obstruction is quite patchy, some airways being completely occluded. The regional airway obstruction is accompanied by a partial compensatory vasoconstrictor decrease in perfusion, but even so, a rather severely mismatched ventilation-perfusion ratio results. Widely diverse time constants in different parts of the lung also contribute to the abnormal ventilation-perfusion ratio. In all but the most severe episodes of asthma there is compensatory hyperventilation. This results in a reduced arterial carbon dioxide tension, and usually during acute episodes of asthma there is a respiratory alkalosis (Fig. 13-7). Alveolar hypoventilation with hypercapnia occurs only when there is overwhelming obstruction. Alveolar hypoventilation can also occur if there is a secondary abnormality in control of ventilation. The most common reason for this is administration of sedatives, but there appear to be occasional patients with asthma whose hypoxic ventilatory drive is reduced. During severe asthmatic episodes cardiac function is altered. There is sinus tachycardia. The electrocardiogram may show right axis deviation and electrical evidence of right ventricular strain and cor pulmonale. Many patients have pulsus paradoxus and the severity of the fall in systolic pressure with respiration correlates with the severity of an attack. Because of the increased intrathoracic pressure, there is decreased venous return and a compensatory increase in antidiuretic hormone secretion, which can result in several liters of fluid accumulation and hyponatremia.[26]

The severity of the symptoms often correlates poorly with the measured physiological abnormalities. Some patients who are unusually anxious may overreport the severity of the obstruction. More important, however, is the observation that many patients with asthma have much more severe physiological impairment than their symptoms suggest.[27] As patients recover from an acute episode, the symptom of breathlessness disappears at about the time the use of accessory muscles and pulsus paradoxus remit. Rhonchi and wheezing take longer to resolve. When the patient considers the attack to be over, the FEV_1 may frequently be quite abnormal. Diminished forced expiratory flow rates (FEF_{25-75}) persist still longer. It has been estimated that even when asthma has become asymptomatic, as many as 50% of the alveoli lie behind occluded airways.[28]

PATHOGENESIS

Immunopathology and Inflammation

The identification of the human skin sensitizing antibody as IgE and discovery of high-affinity IgE receptors on mast cells and basophils has emphasized the importance of the IgE–mast cell system in the pathogenesis of allergic asthma.[29] Mast cell numbers are increased in asthmatic airways. They develop in the mucosa from bone marrow precursors under the influence of lymphokines produced by T lymphocytes, particularly interleukin-3. Factors from epithelial cells also influence their proliferation and differentiation. Furthermore, studies of allergen-induced skin reactions indicated that IgE antibody was both necessary and sufficient for the late phase of the immediate hypersensitivity reaction.[30] By extension, it was assumed that IgE and mast cells were central to the initiation of allergic asthma. Study of the pathogenesis of the inflammation of asthma, therefore, has focused on the late phase and the recruitment of basophils, neutrophils, eosinophils, platelets, lymphocytes, and macrophages into the arena

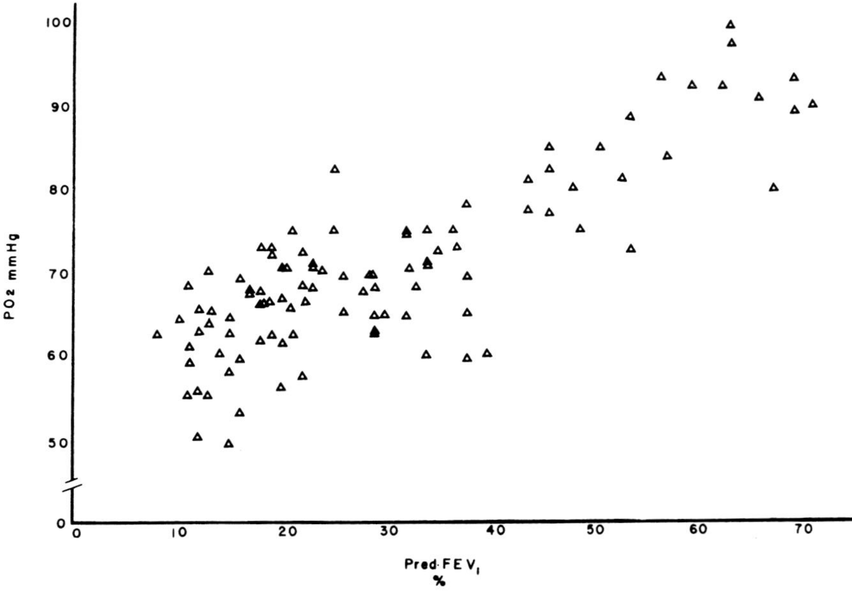

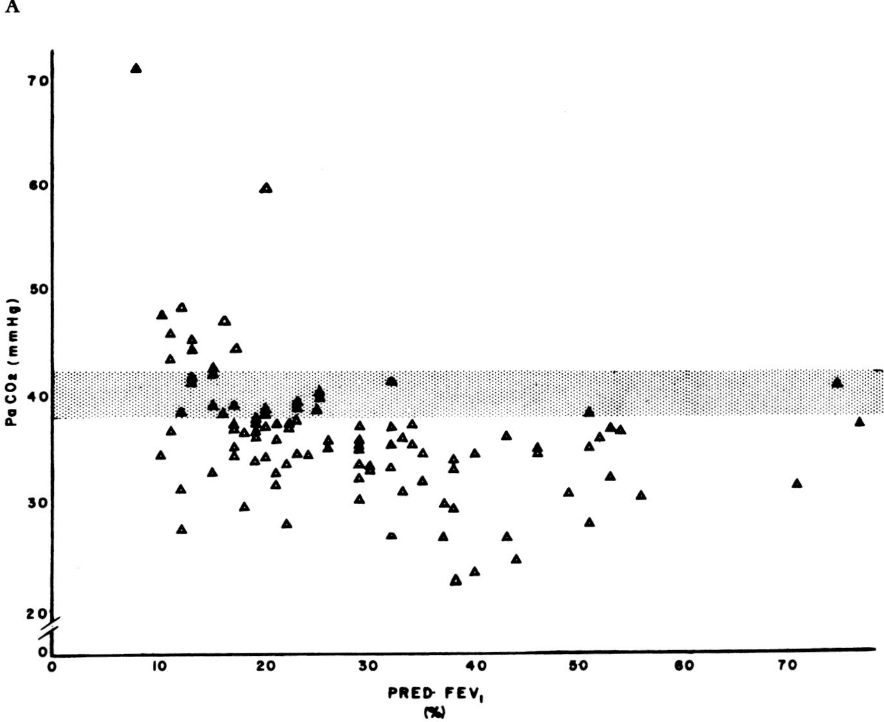

Figure 13-7. Relationship between PaO_2 and $PaCo_2$ and the degree of airway obstruction as measured by FEV_1 during acute episodes of asthma. (From McFadden ER Jr and Lyons H. N Engl J Med 1968, 278:1027).

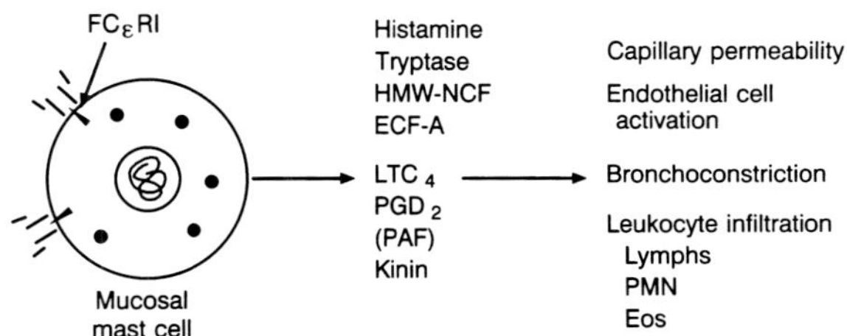

Figure 13-8. Hypothetical role of mast cell in asthma. Mast cells bearing IgE bound to high affinity receptors (FC$_\varepsilon$R1) in their surface membranes react with allergen. This reaction triggers the release of preformed mediators like histamine from granules and the synthesis of lipid mediators like prostaglandin D$_2$ (PGD$_2$) and leukotriene (LTC$_4$). These mediators act not only to contract bronchial smooth muscle but, equally importantly, to cause capillary permeability and edema. They stimulate endothelial cells to produce leukocyte binding factors that localize inflammatory cells at the site. Chemotactic activity of the mediators then attracts inflammatory cells across the endothelium into the extravascular arena of the reaction.

by various low-molecular-weight and macromolecular chemotactic factors released or newly synthesized by mast cells. Early studies on these mediators emphasized bronchoconstriction, vasodilatation, and increased vascular permeability. More recent studies disclose that they have other actions, including leukocyte chemotaxis and activation of endothelial cells to promote leukocyte adherence, both essential steps in localization of leukocytes at the site of inflammation (Fig. 13-8).[31] Elucidation of the action of a mediator depends not only upon having ample supplies of it but also upon having specific antagonists. Some antihistamines, for example, prevent accumulation of eosinophils during the late phase, although intradermal injection of histamine itself cannot evoke a late phase and does not elicit accumulation of eosinophils in tissues.[32] Whether this "antihistamine" effect depends upon a direct effect on histamine receptors of eosinophils or—as seems more likely—an effect on capillary endothelial cells is not yet clear. Since this effect appears to be limited to only some antihistamine compounds, another explanation is some other unknown action of the drugs. Clarification of the role in asthma of other mediators, especially prostaglandins, leukotrienes, and platelet activation factor, has been hampered by lack of potent specific antagonists that can be used in human research.

Mast cells, traditionally the star performers in the production of IgE-mediated asthma, have lately been upstaged by lymphocytes, macrophages, eosinophils, and platelets, which bear low-affinity receptors for IgE (see Fig. 13-8). The various arguments against a solo unsupported role of mast cells in the continuing (and apparently self-perpetuating) drama of the inflammation of asthma include not only the fact that drugs that are potent mast cell inhibitors and block many animal and human models of allergenic disease have proved disappointing therapy for asthma, but also the fact that mast cells are increased in other, very different lung diseases, such as sarcoidosis and idiopathic interstitial fibrosis, and also that mast cell degranulation is not inhibited by glucocorticoids. Mast cells are poor producers of platelet activating factor, currently the most potent known eosinophil chemotactic factor and a substance capable of inducing long-lasting airway hyperresponsiveness after a single aerosol dose.[33] The processes that evoke the lymphocytic eosinophilic inflammation and the processes that perpetuate this inflammation year after year are still very obscure indeed. IgE-mediated reactions often initiate the inflammation and sometimes continued allergen exposure may maintain it, but we must look elsewhere to explain adequately the chronicity of asthma and especially to account for the disease in patients who are not allergic.

Lymphocytes have moved into the spotlight for a number of reasons. First of all, they are there in large numbers. There has as yet not been a full description of the phenotypes of these resident lymphocytes by appropriate histochemical studies of bronchial biopsies, but it is known that helper CD4+ lymphocytes are abundant in bronchoalveolar lavage fluid during the late phase and both helper and suppressor cells are resident in the nasal mucosa in patients with nasal polyps.[34,35] Second, acting through lymphokines, helper CD4+ lymphocytes have profound effects on B cells and other bone-marrow–derived leukocytes. It is now known that in mice two kinds of helper T cells exist, T_{h1} and T_{h2}. T_{h1} cells stimulate B cells to produce IgM and IgG. T_{h2} cells stimulate IgE and IgA. T_{h1} cells produce interleukin-2 (IL2), interferon-gamma and tumor necrosis factor, while T_{h2} cells produce IL4 and IL5.[36] Interferon-gamma inhibits IgE production. In humans, separate clones of lymphocytes analogous to T_{h1} and T_{h2} have not been identified, but the two separate functions do exist and human IL4 and IL5 have been cloned. Recombinant products are available. The actions of IL4 and IL5 are of particular interest in the context of allergic inflammation: IL4 enhances IgE production and expression of CD23 molecules, the low-affinity receptors for IgE. IL5 enhances IgA production and, with granulocyte-macrophage colony stimulating factor (GM CSF), the growth of eosinophils.[37] Activated lymphoctyes and CD23 appear in the circulation during severe asthma episodes.[38] Asthma, whether allergic or not, is associated with elevated levels of IgE in the plasma. Burrows has recently suggested that this indicates that intrinsic asthma is the result of allergy to as yet unidentified allergens.[39] Another plausible explanation is that the elevated IgE is not specific antibody but is the result of increased production of IL4—a result of the disease, not its cause. It seems as if asthma is a disease of increased activity of T_{h2}-like CD4+ cells with sustained and copious production of IL4 and IL5. It is likely that there are two

Figure 13-9. Hypothetical role of macrophages, lymphocytes, and other cells in asthma. Macrophages may interact with allergen through low affinity receptors for IgE FC$_\epsilon$RII to become activated. In turn, they activate helper CD4 lymphocytes to produce lymphokines. IL3 promotes growth of mast cells. IL4 induces differentiation of B lymphocytes to produce IgA and IgE. Cytokines

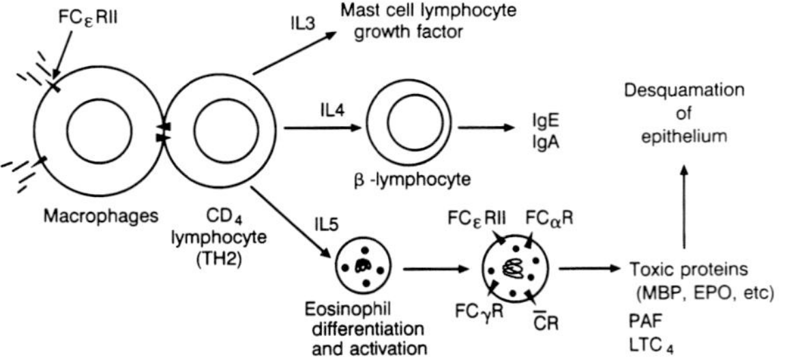

from macrophages or lymphocytes stimulate mast cell histamine release. IL5, with other growth factors, promotes eosinophil differentiation and activation. Interaction between antigen-antibody complexes and eosinophil surface receptors stimulates eosinophil degranulation and release of toxic granule proteins and production of mediators such as platelet activating factor and leukotriene C$_4$.

analogous types of suppressor lymphocytes, and there are some hints of defective function of the suppressor cells acting on T_{h2}-like helper cell function. For example, pertussis toxin and castor bean ricin enhance IgE production, perhaps acting by selective toxicity on this subclass of suppressor cells. Another interleukin from CD4 + cells, IL3, is a widely acting cell stimulating factor amplifying the more specific effects of interferon-gamma and IL4. It also promotes the growth of mast cells and can be produced by epithelial and other cells.[36] Interleukin-3 and another lymphokine, histamine releasing factor, activate mast cells and promote mediator release.[40] Recently, it has been found that a clone of murine mast cells can produce IL3, IL4, and IL5 in response to activation of IgE receptors.[41] Whether human mast cells produce these interleukins is not yet known, but if they do, interesting feedback amplification networks could be operating between lymphocytes, mast cells, and eosinophils. This meager but tantalizing information raises many questions for future research.

EOSINOPHILS

Eosinophils, increased not only in the lumen and bronchial mucosa but also in the circulation and marrow, play a key role in the damage to ciliated respiratory epithelium.[42] Eosinophil granule proteins, especially the major basic protein and eosinophil peroxidase, are toxic to respiratory epithelium (and other cells) in vitro at concentrations that occur in the sputum of asthmatics. The lesions of asthma contain abundant major basic protein deposits even in areas where intact eosinophils are not evident (Fig. 13-9). The eosinophils in the lumen either spontaneously or after bronchial challenge show morphologic and functional indications of activation. Much has been learned about the biology of eosinophils.[43,44] They arise in the bone marrow, circulate through the blood to the bronchi, adhere to capillary endothelium, pass into the airways (having become activated somewhere along the way), and finally degranulate in the mucosa, where they cause the epithelial desquamation.

There are a number of eosinophil growth factors including macrophage-granulocyte colony stimulating factor, IL3, and IL5. To reach the bronchial mucosa eosinophils pass through two capillary beds. The first step of diapedesis is binding of the leukocyte by endothelial cells, which accounts for the specific regional localization. The second step is chemotaxis. Several chemotactic factors are known, including eosinophil chemotactic factor of anaphylaxis, leukotriene, and platelet activating factor. The last is particularly interesting because after injection into the skin it evokes a local eosinophil infiltration, because after inhalation it causes a prolonged airway hyperresponsiveness, and because eosinophils themselves produce it copiously. Perhaps platelet activating factor is involved in the feedback loop that accounts for the persistence of asthma or airway hyperresponsiveness after a single allergen exposure.

Two kinds of eosinophils can be separated by their density.[45] The eosinophils in the circulation of normal persons are denser than the eosinophils that account for eosinophilia of disease, including the eosinophilia of asthma. These low-density eosinophils have been reported to bear low-affinity IgE receptors and are in an activated state. It is not known whether some are already activated before they enter the circulation, but it is known that eosinophils recovered from bronchoalveolar lavage are the low-density, activated type. Platelet activating factor activates eosinophils, and other mechanisms for eosinophil activation exist, such as IL5 and endothelial factors. Since incubation of normal-density eosinophils with endothelial monolayers converts them to the activated, low-density phenotype, it seems plausible that activation occurs during the process of tissue localization.

After eosinophils arrive in the airways, they degranulate and their toxic granules injure tissues, particularly epithelium. Eosinophil killing of parasites is antibody dependent. Although activated eosinophils have been reported to have low-affinity IgE receptors, the most potent immunologic stimulus for degranulation described to date is secretory IgA. The mechanism of degranulation, like the mechanisms of the preceding steps, are as yet poorly understood.

OTHER INFLAMMATORY CELLS

During the late phase of skin, nasal, or bronchial challenge the other two granulocytes, basophils and neutrophils, are also recruited into the arena. Once there, basophils continue to secrete histamine, and presumably other mediators, thus contributing to the late phase of IgE-initiated inflammation. During the late phase reaction neutrophils appear in blister fluid in the skin, or in bronchoalveolar lavage fluid in the lung, but are rare in the tissues of either chronic urticaria, nasal polyps, or asthma. Whether neutrophils contribute significantly to chronic asthma is doubtful. Macrophages are the major cell in bronchoalveolar lavage fluid of asthmatics as well as normal and may play an important role in inflammation.[46] The role of platelets in inflammation is also receiving considerable attention.[46,47]

ALLERGY

The antigens that cause asthma are airborne except for the rare case when asthma is part of a systemic anaphylactic reaction. The more abundant the allergen, the more likely it is to provoke asthma and the more severe the response becomes. But not all abundant airborne immunogens evoke an IgE response, and not all individuals respond to the same components in a mixture of allergens. What is the molecular basis for these particular specificities?

Those allergens that have been characterized do share some common properties. They are relatively small, highly soluble glycopeptides. Many are either enzymes or recognition proteins that function for their parent organism as extracellular ligands. They seem particularly well adapted to penetrate tissues. Many can even pass through intact skin to cause contact urticaria. The properties of these particular molecules that evoke an IgE but not an IgG antibody response are not known. Immune response genes can explain the differences in response of different individuals exposed to the same mixture of allergens, but continued study of the molecular structure of purified allergens will be needed to explain why these particular molecules evoke such a selective IgE rather than an IgG antibody response.[48]

VIRAL RESPIRATORY INFECTIONS

Respiratory infections often provoke episodes of asthma that account for many hospitalizations and emergency room visits. In infants and young children, respiratory syncytial virus is the most frequent agent.[49] In older children and adults most infections are caused by rhinoviruses.[50] Influenza, parainfluenza, and occasionally other viruses also cause asthmatic attacks. Bacteria, such as streptococcus, do not. Postulated mechanisms of virus-induced attacks include IgE antibody production (particularly in the case of respiratory syncytial virus),[49,51,52] increased release of asthma-causing substances such as lipid mediators and cytokines from epithelial cells or inflammatory cells acting upon other inflammatory cells and endothelium. These cytokines include but are probably not limited to IL5, interferon gamma, and histamine releasing factor.[53] Respiratory viruses, of course, also directly damage respiratory epithelium. Viral infections also cause defects in adenylate cyclase in stimulus-response coupling in peripheral blood leukocytes.[54] Study of the mechanisms of virus-induced attacks is a promising means of elucidating the mechanisms of the inflammation of asthma, for these attacks last for many days and increase bronchial hyperresponsiveness.[55]

AIRWAY HYPERRESPONSIVENESS

Airway hyperresponsiveness is a hallmark of asthma. The severity of the hyperresponsiveness correlates with the degree of inflammation and the eosinophilia. Research into the role of inflammation has stressed the late phase of the IgE-initiated allergic reaction of specific allergen challenge. Hyperresponsiveness exists not only during the late phase, 2 to 8 hours after exposure but may persist for weeks.[56] It also persists after a respiratory viral infection. Inflammation causes airway hyperresponsiveness in several ways. The first is mechanical and geometric.[57] Airway resistance varies with the fourth power of the diameter. The inflamed thickened airway wall encroaches on the lumen so that the same shortening of bronchial smooth muscle that has little effect on the caliber of the lumen of a normal airway causes an exaggerated effect on the lumen of an inflamed airway. The second is the interrelationship between the chemical mediators of inflammation and neurotransmitters. Desquamation of the epithelium lays bare and sensitizes the irritant receptors of the afferent limb of reflex bronchoconstriction. In addition, antidromic stimulation of sensory neurons liberates substance P, a potent pro-inflammatory neuropeptide.[58] Many of these mediators amplify the smooth muscle response to neurotransmitters—and neurotransmitters, particularly neuropeptides, evoke release of mast cell mediators and dilate blood vessels. The third way in which inflammation causes hyperactivity stems from the fact that respiratory epithelium inhibits bronchial smooth muscle tone; denuded airways therefore become hyperresponsive.[59] Knowledge is still accumulating about the role of the nonadrenergic-noncholinergic-peptidergic nervous system in bronchial smooth muscle physiology in health and disease.[60] Here, too, progress has been hampered by lack of selective antagonists.

Airway hyperresponsiveness is the basis for the increased bronchoconstriction in the early morning after 4 to 6 hours of sleep, the "morning dip."[61] The mechanism for these diurnal changes characteristic of asthma is imperfectly understood. Circulating levels of epinephrine and cortisol are at low ebb and histamine is at high tide, but the physiological rhythms that drive these changes are still largely undefined.

It is important not to lose sight of the fact that inflammation is not the only basis for hyperresponsiveness, which has a multifactorial origin.[62] Also, epidemiologic studies have shown that nonspecific hyperresponsiveness to methacholine is only one mechanism underlying airflow limitation in asthma, and that its relationship to the clinical state of asthma is not close enough to be of practical diagnostic use in epidemiologic research.[63] For example, there is good correlation between the responses to histamine and to methacholine but poor correlation between the responses to methacholine and to adenosine. Exercise-induced bronchoconstriction, a common phenomenon, has as its basis evaporative cooling of the central airways and is considered to act through the release of mediators from mast cells or by reactive hyperemia of the bronchial mucosa.[64]

There is considerable circumstantial evidence for an abnormality in stimulus-response coupling in smooth muscle. Healthy first-degree relatives of asthmatics respond excessively to inhaled methacholine.[65] Patients with asthma or other atopic diseases have abnormal autonomic stimulus-response coupling in many tissues besides the airways, including liver (glycogenolysis), skin (blood vessels, epidermal mitosis, and sweat glands), pupils, and leukocytes.[66,67]

In this regard peripheral blood leukocytes, both neutrophils and lymphocytes, have been studied extensively as an accessible cell to explore Szentivanyi's hypothesis that airway hyperresponsiveness is the result of decreased response of the airways to beta-adrenergic stimulation. As a result of these studies, several points have been clarified: (1) Leukocytes of asthmatics respond less than normal to beta-adrenergic agonists and other agonists linked to adenylate cyclase.[68] (2) Beta-adrenergic receptor numbers and affinity are normal in mild untreated asthmatics.[69] (3) Treatment with beta-adrenergic agonists decreases the numbers of beta receptors.[69] (4) Lymphocyte adenylate cyclase becomes less responsive after allergen challenge.[70] Thus, the molecular basis for abnormal response to beta-adrenergic agonists in untreated asthmatics remains to be explained. Hanafin has suggested that the molecular basis is increased activity of phosphodiesterase.[71] Or perhaps there is an abnormality in the G proteins that link the receptors to adenylate cyclase. At this point it is not certain whether these observed changes in stimulus-response coupling are fundamental to the disease process or are a result of it.

DIAGNOSIS

The objectives of clinical evaluation and diagnostic testing are (1) to identify the disease; (2) to identify specific provocative factors; (3) to evaluate the severity of the airway obstruction and its reversibility; and (4) to evaluate the patient's understanding of the disease and his ability to cope with it, to accept responsibility for his own management, and to identify barriers in the family, school, or workplace that would interfere with implementing the management program. Generally, the diagnosis of asthma is a straightforward matter of pattern recognition. A patient of any age recounts repeated episodes of dyspnea, cough, chest tightness, and wheezing—usually under consistent circumstances, such as a respiratory infection, exercise in cold air, or exposure to a cat or other allergen or to airborne irritants. If the symptoms are chronic, they are characteristically worse at night and almost all patients with asthma are awakened at times by cough and chest tightness. Sputum varies from none at all, through scanty amounts of thick, tenacious, clear material, to yellow to green mucopurulent sputum, and to copious amounts of watery mucus (bronchorrhea). Physical examination between episodes yields normal findings but during an episode shows overinflation of the lungs, prolonged expiration, increased breath sounds, and high-pitched musical wheezes. The wheeze arises from a segmental or subsegmental bronchus that is virtually completely occluded. The musical tone develops when this airway wall vibrates from open to shut like an oboe reed as a small current of air passes through it.[72] Thus, a wheeze signifies quite severe localized obstruction. If more than one airway becomes so affected, there will be wheezes of various pitches and at various times during the respiratory cycle. When airways are simply concentrically narrowed the result is increased velocity of flow with increased turbulence, which generates "white noise" heard as increased breath sounds. As airway obstruction progresses to respiratory failure both wheezes and breath sounds become less intense. Beware.

Infants have pronounced sternal and lower rib cage retraction, and chronic obstruction in children may permanently deform the chest in a characteristic way. Examination of the nose shows nasal polyps or edema of the turbinates and increased secretions.

Objective confirmation of airflow obstruction is essential not only to establish the diagnosis but to evaluate the severity of the obstruction. Simple economical equipment and methods are readily available for any physician's office.[73] Spirometry before and after a beta-adrenergic agonist bronchodilator is inhaled measures the reversibility of the smooth muscle contraction component. Further reversibility after several days' treatment with systemically administered glucocorticoids establishes reversibility of the inflammatory component. When the history suggests asthma but spirometry measurements are normal, a provocative test with methacholine is useful to identify the presence of hyperresponsiveness. Histamine, exercise, or hyperventilation of cold dry air can be used for the same purpose. Recent epidemiologic studies have indicated that the specificity and sensitivity of the methacholine test may be less than once thought.[63] Relative of asthmatics, normal subjects recovering from an acute respiratory infection, and hay fever sufferers may react, whereas some asthmatics do not. An alternative approach that has as yet to be fully validated is monitoring of peak flow at home, morning and evening. A variation of 20% or more indicates hyperresponsiveness. Chest radiographs serve to disclose complications such as pneumothorax, atelectasis, bronchiectasis, pneumonia, or other coexisting lung diseases.

Examination of blood or sputum for eosinophilia is at present time the most practical means of testing for the characteristic inflammatory component of asthma.[74] Unfortunately, demonstration of sputum or peripheral blood eosinophilia is neither sensitive nor specific enough to serve as an absolutely reliable diagnostic criterion. In cases severe enough to require hospital treatment, sputum stained by the Papanicolaou technique usually shows creola bodies (bits of desquamated bronchial epithelium).[75] Although it is highly specific, this test lacks sufficient sensitivity to be a useful clinical diagnostic procedure. Much the same thing applies to measurement of serum IgE levels. As a group, asthmatics have elevated IgE levels, but the range of overlap with non-asthmatics is too great for the test to be considered positive unless the level is high.[16]

Tests for specific IgE antibody to aeroallergens in the patient's environment are indicated in most, if not all, cases. When positive they provide guidance for avoiding exposure or for immunotherapy, and when negative they reassure the patient and physician that such treatment is unnecessary. As with all diagnostic procedures, quality control is necessary for reliable results.[76] Skin testing can be performed in a manner that achieves very high sensitivity but with such a loss of specificity that the procedure becomes misleading. The preferred technique is to use prick or puncture tests with standardized glycerinated extracts of allergens that are abundant in the patient's environment. Histamine for a positive control and saline for a negative control should be included. A positive reaction consists of a wheal and erythema developing after 20 minutes. Reactions that develop after several hours are of doubtful significance. Intradermal testing is more sensitive but less specific. Radioallergosorbent tests (RAST) serve as a reliable alternative but are more expensive, somewhat less sensitive, and entail a delay in reporting. On the other hand, RAST lends itself well to standard laboratory quality control procedures and is particularly useful for patients with widespread dermatitis or dermographism that interferes with skin testing. Aeroallergens can be classified into those that are outdoors and community-wide, those that are indoors in the home, and those that are occupational.[77] The important community-wide allergens are tree, grass, and weed pollens; mold spores; and insect debris. They vary greatly in different climates. Indoor allergens vary between homes and include house dust mites, pets, cockroaches, and occasionally molds. Occupational allergens will be considered in a separate chapter. Interpretation of allergy tests requires information about the abundance of the allergen in the patient's environment. Severity of the asthmatic reaction is a combined function of the amount of exposure, of the amount of IgE antibody, and of the degree of bronchial hyperresponsiveness. Allergens, like all stimuli, have a dose-response relationship, though this relationship is difficult to quantify and varies from patient to patient. There is clearly, however, a level below which an allergen will not elicit a response even in a sensitive person, and so allergens that elicit a positive skin test but are present in the air in only trace amounts are best discounted.

To cause asthma, allergenic particles must be respirable. Pollen grains, for example, lodge in the nose and do not penetrate the lung. Asthma due to pollen allergy comes from amorphous particles that are less than 5 μm mean mass aerodynamic diameter and arise from parts of the plant other than pollen grains, chiefly the male flower or leaves. The most common molds that cause asthma are alternaria and cladosporium, which are the common saprophytic fungi imperfecti responsible for decaying leaves and similar dead vegetation. The variety and amount of mold spores, particularly basidiomycetes, in the air is very large. Unfortunately, the unavailability of reproducible testing reagents has hampered evaluation of their importance as a cause of allergy.[78] In sharply restricted regions like lake shores or river banks, allergens from mayflies and caddis flies cause localized outbreaks of asthma. An epidemic of asthma in Barcelona, Spain, was traced to allergens from soybeans when clouds of grain dust from the harbor drifted over the city.[79]

House dust mites are the main cause of asthma in homes.[80] These pyroglyphid mites live in such microhabitats as carpets, mattresses, pillows, and upholstered furniture where humidity is high and a food source abundant. Mites are more abundant in mild humid climates, but changes in construction and reduced ventilation in contemporary energy-efficient homes have raised indoor humidity in colder, drier climates to the point that mite allergy is a worldwide problem. Indoor molds are important only when they are obviously growing in a spot where there is water damage or moisture accumulation. Molds growing on house plants are rarely abundant enough to be significant. Cockroach allergy is particularly important in lower socioeconomic level homes where cockroach infestation is heavy.[81] It is a common, possibly the major, cause of asthma in children of these families.

Testing for food allergy is rarely useful. When asthma results from food allergy, it is usually only a part of a severe systemic anaphylactic reaction.

Bronchial provocation testing with allergens is a research procedure and not needed for clinical management decisions.

Now and then patients develop allergy to exotic, previously unrecognized allergens. In my experience with these cases it is the patient, not the physician, who makes the diagnosis.

There are patients who experience acute severe attacks that may progress in minutes from near-normal airflow to life-threatening respiratory failure. A few of these attacks come from sudden overwhelming exposure to an allergen, but more have a pharmacologic basis. Aspirin and other cyclooxygenase-inhibiting nonsteroidal antiinflammatory agents are the most common cause. These patients typically develop asthma as adults, have nasal polyps, and do not have allergy to common allergens. The biochemical basis for the reaction is not yet known.[82] Food additives—most often sulfite preservatives in wine, beer, dried fruit, restaurant salads, and shrimp—can cause similar reactions.[83] Monosodium glutamate and benzoic acid have been reported in a few cases to cause similar reactions. Anticholinesterase insecticide exposure can provoke an asthmatic attack and very occasionally pilocarpine eye drops increase its severity. Beta-adrenergic blocking agents are the most common prescription drugs responsible for asthma attacks. Even the more selective beta-1-antagonists, and even eye drops, can do so. Angiotensin converting enzyme inhibitors often cause cough in nonasthmatic persons. They have been suspected of aggravating asthma, but the association has not been proved. Calcium channel blocking agents are well tolerated. They have been reported to reduce exercise-induced bronchoconstriction but have not proved to be useful therapy for asthma. Challenge tests with these agents have been invaluable in research but are dangerous and should be performed only in centers experienced in these procedures.

Concomitant Diseases

A number of coexisting conditions may make asthma worse. Gastroesophageal reflux with or without esophagitis (which may be aggravated by theophylline), sinusitis, and hyperthyroidism should be considered when asthma fails to respond to treatment as expected.

Also, asthma in the sense of eosinophilic bronchitis with hyperresponsiveness may occasionally coexist with other lung diseases such as cystic fibrosis, alpha-1-antitrypsin deficiency, or sarcoidosis. Optimal patient management requires treatment of asthma as well as the other disease.

DIFFERENTIAL DIAGNOSIS OF ADULTS

Extrathoracic Obstruction

Tracheal narrowing after intubation or neck surgery rarely generates serious diagnostic confusion, but the syndrome of vocal cord adductor spasm does.[84] Affected patients have acute episodes of severe airway obstruction with a stridor that can be easily mistaken for a wheeze. Because of the severity of the episode and the patients' anxiety, prednisone is often prescribed both to treat the episode and to prevent others, so these patients become cushingoid. Between episodes spirometry is normal. Eosinophilia is not present. Diagnosis is made during an episode either by spirometry, which shows the characteristic pattern of extrathoracic obstruction, or better, by direct visualization of the vocal cords. Treatment is speech therapy. Occasionally vocal cord paralysis may mimic asthma.[85]

Pulmonary Disease Other Than COPD

Mediastinal lymph nodes or other tumors may encroach on the bronchi to cause cough and wheeze, and endobronchial lesions such as carcinoid or even cancer may, for a time, mimic asthma.

Bronchiolitis obliterans occasionally needs to be considered in differential diagnosis of asthma. This distinction is made by the history; by presence of other diseases, such as rheumatoid arthritis; and by lack of response of airflow obstruction to treatment.

Chronic cough may be the only symptom of asthma—but, of course, cough may have many other causes as well.[86] Features that suggest that a chronic cough may represent asthma are (1) its tonal characteristics (an asthmatic cough sounds as different from a habit cough as a trumpet from a violin); (2) cough is worse during sleep and wakes the patient at night; (3) eosinophilia in blood, sputum or bronchial washings; (4) demonstration of bronchial hyperresponsiveness to methacholine. Cough with eosinophilia but without airway hyperresponsiveness may respond to aerosol glucocorticoid treatment.[87]

Chronic Obstructive Pulmonary Diseases

In adults over the age of 40 years, the most difficult differential diagnosis lies among the chronic obstructive pulmonary diseases. A large part of this difficulty is conceptual. We rely on physiological tests to distinguish among different histopathologic entities (e.g., asthma, emphysema, chronic metaplastic bronchitis of cigarette smoking) because more specific diagnostic criteria of the histopathology are not available.

Furthermore, some patients may have more than one histopathologic process. A patient with asthma since youth may be a heavy smoker, or a patient with alpha-1-antitrypsin deficiency may become allergic.[88] Severe chronic asthmatics who have never smoked may progress to a state in which the obstruction no longer can be fully reversed. In the absence of reliable criteria for distinguishing among the obstructive pulmonary diseases, it is often necessary to accept diagnostic uncertainty and to take a pragmatic approach. If the obstruction reverses substantially a few minutes after a bronchodilator is administered, the diagnosis is asthma and treatment proceeds accordingly. In this context, the term "substantially" means achieving an FEV_1 of 70% to 100% of the predicted value rather than just a 15% improvement over the baseline value. If the obstruction does not reverse, a similar test of reversibility with prednisone can be considered. This test of reversibility employs an adequate dose (40–60 mg) and adequate time (7–21 days) for the hypothetical inflammation to respond. Eosinophilia is a clue predicting a response. Conversely, a response is unlikely if diffusing capacity is reduced or there is radiographic evidence of bullous or diffuse emphysema. Early collapse of airways with a sharp reduction in flow rates after the air in the dead space has been expelled and disproportionate obstruction of expiratory compared to inspiratory flow are spirometric features of emphysema.

There will remain a number of patients who do not reverse "substantially" but do reverse "significantly" and in whom a nonspecific diagnosis of "COPD with a reversible component" is appropriate. In such patients a judgment of whether or not treatment can usefully include bronchodilators or glucocorticoids depends on factors other than spirometry.

Heart Disease

Mitral stenosis and left ventricular failure can cause cough and paroxysmal dyspnea and are an occasional source of diagnostic confusion, particularly since left ventricular failure can cause bronchial hyperresponsiveness.[89]

DIFFERENTIAL DIAGNOSIS IN CHILDREN

In infants and toddlers, bronchiolitis caused by respiratory syncytial virus or other respiratory viruses is common and has led to much diagnostic confusion. A single episode does not constitute asthma, but recurrent episodes do. Some children, boys more often than girls, have asthma only with respiratory viral infections; others have asthma at other times as well. These episodes of viral infection–induced asthma may have much the same immunopathogenesis as severe allergic reactions, but as yet IgE antibody has been demonstrated only to respiratory syncytial virus and parainfluenza virus.[90] In children, congenital malformations of the heart and great vessels can cause symptoms that resemble asthma. Aspirated foreign bodies and airway obstruction from mediastinal masses or laryngotracheal malacia occasionally cause wheezing.

TREATMENT

In response to the increased morbidity and mortality of asthma and the perception that the traditional approach emphasizing bronchodilators has been inadequate there has been a substantial change in thinking about asthma therapy among students of asthma

TABLE 13-1. Definition of Control of Asthma

Major Criteria

1. Minimal symptoms, ideally none.
2. No restriction of activities of daily living (work, school, recreational exercise). Not waking at night because of asthma.
3. Inhaled adrenergic agonist needed not more than twice daily, ideally none.

Minor Criteria

1. Minimal side effects from medications.
2. Airflow rates normal or near normal at rest.
3. Airflow rates normal after inhaled adrenergic agonist.
4. Daily variation of PEFR <20%, ideally <10%.

PEFR = peak expiratory flow rate

in many countries. In May of 1989, a conference of experts from Europe, North America, and Australasia was held to seek consensus and to develop a practical guide to assessment and treatment of asthma. The plan of management outlined in this chapter draws heavily on the report of that conference.[91]

Office Treatment

Goals of Therapy

The primary objective of treatment of asthma is to achieve and maintain control of the disease—that is, to achieve the outcomes defined in Table 13-1. Not only should the physician have these outcomes clearly in mind, but more importantly, so should the patient and the family. It is astounding how many people with asthma accept as "normal" waking up several times at night to inhale a bronchodilator, or needing emergency room treatment for an attack every few weeks.

Control is achievable for most patients with asthma, though it may not be possible for a few when the disease is severe. In such patients vigorous initial treatment is needed to achieve and define "best result" as the fewest symptoms and best airflow that can be achieved without unacceptable side effects. Then the management goal becomes maintaining and improving upon this "best result."

Principles of Treatment

The principles guiding treatment are as follows:

1. Treatment is outcome oriented. Achieve and maintain control or best result and modify treatment whenever control becomes inadequate.

2. Avoid harmful factors: allergens, occupational chemical sensitizers, cigarette smoke, viral respiratory infections, sulfites and other food additives, drugs (beta-adrenergic blockers, including eye drops for glaucoma, nonsteroidal antiinflammatory agents, and possibly angiotensin converting enzyme inhibitors), and gastroesophageal reflux. Other less harmful but common factors, such as cold air, exercise, air pollution, and emotional stress, deserve consideration. These factors are considered less harmful because they cause symptoms by stimulating hyperreactive airways

rather than by causing inflammation. These factors usually become of less importance when control is achieved, and if symptoms frequently follow exposure to them, control is less than ideal.

3. Control of disease (inflammation) is superior to control of symptoms (bronchospasm). Control of disease is accomplished by avoiding harmful factors that cause inflammation and by use of inhaled glucocorticoids or cromolyn, or in severe cases by oral glucocorticoids. Bronchodilators, including theophylline, do not improve the inflammation or bronchial hyperresponsiveness.[92]

4. Steps in implementing the management plan are as follows:
   a. Make the diagnosis and identify harmful factors (see preceding section).
   b. Provide initial treatment to achieve control or best result.
   c. Determine the smallest amount of medication needed to maintain control or best result.
   d. Educate the patient about the nature of the disease, specific harmful factors in his case, the goals of management, the actions of the drugs, and how to use the drugs to achieve control. Often it is also important to enlist appropriate cooperation of the family, teachers, school nurses, or employers. *Careful coaching in proper inhalation techniques for aerosol medications is a key part of patient education:* many patients have difficulty mastering the hand–lung coordination necessary for effective aerosol treatment.
   e. Provide a written action plan for early management of exacerbations individualized to the patient.
   f. Review the case at appropriate intervals to ensure that control or best result is maintained.

Initial Treatment to Establish Control or Best Result

The diagnostic procedures of history and allergy testing are directed toward identifying potential harmful factors that can contribute to smoldering airway inflammation or trigger sudden, severe, potentially fatal airflow limitation. Detailed avoidance instructions should be available as handouts with feasible plans for avoiding house dust mite or molds and, in unusual cases, a list of sources of exposure to aspirin, sulfites, or food allergens. Although avoiding sensitizing agents, particularly occupational ones, is exceedingly important, it is equally important that disruptive advice such as moving or quitting a job be based on a confirmed diagnosis. Unnecessary restrictions should not become an adverse social or economic side effect of the treatment. Exercise is a cause of airway constriction that ordinarily does not need to be avoided. Generally, optimal day-to-day maintenance treatment prevents it. If not, inhalation of adrenergic aerosols or cromolyn or both just before exercise is useful.[93] Occasionally, epinephrine aerosol is more effective for this purpose than a selective beta agonist. Similarly, symptoms provoked by minor exposures to irritant dusts or gases in the course of normal daily activities should be considered an indication that control has not been achieved.

Since avoidance of potentially harmful factors may not yield immediate results and often is not sufficient by itself, medications are generally required as well. Inhaled medications are preferred because they have fewer side effects. The level of initial treatment with medications obviously depends on the severity of asthma at the time

TABLE 13-2. Symptoms/Ventilatory Function Criteria of the Level of Severity of Asthma at a Particular Time[1,2]

LEVEL	FUNCTIONAL LEVEL
1	The asthma is controlled (see Table 13-1).
2	Symptoms are slightly more than when controlled or are elicited more readily in response to mild provocation.
	Inhaled adrenergic agonist is needed slightly more often (three or four times daily).
	PEFR or FEV_1 is about 85% of predicted or known best result.
	PEFR variability during the day of 20% to 30%.
3	Symptoms of breathlessness or chest tightness occur repeatedly during the day, disturb sleep, or are present on waking.
	Inhaled adrenergic agonist is required more than four times daily. (A refill can lasts less than a month).
	PEFR or FEV_1 is 60% to 85% of predicted or known best result.
	PEFR variability >30%.
4	Symptoms at rest, not completely reversed by inhaled adrenergic agonist.
	PEFR or FEV_1 is <60% of predicted value, deficit is not completely reversed by inhaled adrenergic agonist.

1. The allocation of particular symptom or flow rate criteria to particular levels of severity is based upon limited information. The levels should be taken only as a rough guide with the recognition that there may be discordance among criteria. In general, criteria indicating the highest level should be heeded.

2. The assessment of the severity of asthma, in the longer term, requires a consideration of symptoms and ventilatory function criteria in addition to the minimum level of treatment with medications required to maintain control or best result.

and the level of treatment with medication already being used. The severity of asthma is judged both by the symptoms and by objective measurement of airflow. Neither alone is sufficient. The severity of symptoms does not always correlate with the magnitude of reduction of flow rates. In some patients, symptoms are the more sensitive indicator; in others, who seem to perceive or communicate airflow limitation poorly, the reduction in flow rates is more sensitive. Measurement of peak expiratory flow rate (PEFR) or FEV_1 in the office during the day may underestimate the severity of an exacerbation because of the usual improvement of flow rates during the daytime. The daily variability of PEFR monitored at home is closely related to airway hyperresponsiveness measured by histamine or methacholine sensitivity, and is also related to other findings such as frequency of symptoms and dosing with beta-agonist aerosols.

The levels of severity are outlined in Table 13-2. The level of medication (Table 13-3) is chosen to match the severity. In patients not on any medications whose severity is Level 1, initial treatment at Level 1 is usually appropriate. For example, two inhalations of adrenergic agonist or cromolyn before occasional stimuli such as exercise or visiting a house with a cat may prevent symptoms entirely, and if symptoms do occur an adrenergic agonist may relieve them entirely. When symptoms increase in severity, occur daily, interfere with sleep or daytime activities, or lead to more frequent inhalations, control has not been maintained and progression to Level 2 therapy is required. For a patient already taking a higher level of treatment for control who develops an exacerbation, the level of treatment needed to regain control is usually greater than

TABLE 13-3. Treatment with Medications According to Level of Severity[1-4]

LEVEL	TREATMENT
1	Inhaled adrenergic agonist, as needed, ± cromoglycate (before provocation only)
2	Level 1 treatment + trial of regular cromoglycate (favored in children by some specialists) or + low-dose inhaled steroid or low-dose sustained-released theophylline with supper.
3	Level 2 treatment + higher dose inhaled steroid ± trial of additional sustained-release theophylline ± trial of sustained-release adrenergic agonist tablet ± inhaled ipratropium bromide
4	Level 3 treatment + ingested prednisone

1. When the patient is seen, the level of treatment will be determined by the level of severity of asthma and the medications and their doses already being used (see Table 13-2 and sections on medications in text).

2. Once control or the best result is achieved, the medications should be reduced to the minimum that will maintain this result.

3. Special considerations for young children and infants are discussed in the text.

4. All levels of treatment should be regarded as a trial of therapy. If the desired outcome is not achieved, the therapy should be changed.

symptoms might indicate. Recommended adrenergic agonists available in metered dose inhalers include metaproterenol, albuterol, terbutaline, and pirbuterol. Albuterol is also available as a powder (Rotohaler®). Metaproterenol and albuterol are available as solutions for nebulization.

Many pediatricians prefer an initial 3- to 6-week trial of cromolyn to low-dose aerosol glucocorticoids; this regimen may also occasionally be useful in adults. The dose of cromolyn is 2 mg by metered dose inhaler or 20 mg by Spinhaler® four times daily. Cromolyn is also available as a solution for nebulization. When inhaled glucocorticoid is used, the usual starting dose would be beclomethasone 200 to 400 μg/day, budesonide 200 to 400 μg/day (not available in the United States), flunisolide 1,000 μg/day, or triamicinolone acetonide 400 to 800 μ/day in two divided doses.

It is also important to treat concomitant allergic disease in the nose and sinuses. Restoration of normal nasal functions of humidification and filtration protects the airways from the stimuli of evaporative water loss and allergenic particle deposition[94] and treatment of sinusitis is accompanied by improvement of asthma.[95] Treatment of gastroesophageal reflux should also be considered.[96]

When asthma is more severe, or has not been controlled by 1 to 2 weeks of Level 2 treatment, the dose of aerosol glucocorticoid should be doubled or increased fourfold, or oral prednisone should be added. In countries other than the United States where more potent glucocorticoid formulations are available, administration of adequate aerosol doses is greatly simplified. Budesonide or beclomethasone can be increased to 1000 μg or more per day and should be administered with an add-on spacer device to maximize intrathoracic deposition and minimize side effects from oral and laryngeal deposition.[97] A four times a day schedule is more effective than a twice a day schedule.[98] High-dose aerosol glucocorticoids cause a dose-related suppression of endogenous cortisol production and other systemic glucocorticoid actions, but these systemic actions are substantially less than those accompanying equivalently effective doses of prednisone. Local side effects of aerosol glucocorticoids include thrush and dysphonia. They are reduced by add-on spacer devices. Thrush may require topical antifungal treatment. Both thrush and dysphonia improve when the dose is reduced and may not recur when larger doses are resumed.

At Level 2 when nocturnal symptoms are particularly troublesome, sustained-release theophylline administered at a time calculated to provide peak blood levels 5 to 8 hours after going to sleep may be useful.[99] The target theophylline blood level is low—5 to 10 μg/ml at 8 A.M.—and modest doses usually suffice to control the nocturnal symptoms. Sustained-release albuterol tablets can be used in the same way.

At Level 3, to take advantage of their longer, steadier effect, sustained-release theophylline or adrenergic agonist tablets can be used during the day as well. Theophylline administration needs to be managed carefully taking into account blood levels and changing conditions that change dose requirements.[100] It is rarely desirable to have blood levels over 10 to 15 μg/ml. Higher levels increase toxicity more than benefit. Ipratropium is an effective bronchodilator in some but not all asthmatics and may be considered for patients who do not tolerate beta-agonist aerosols. It is wise to confirm by spirometry that the patient does not respond to it. If attainable doses of aerosol glucocorticoids do not achieve control promptly, prednisone should be added. A common schedule is to start with a dosage of 25 to 50 mg/day in one or two doses until control is reached and then quickly reduce the dose while continuing inhalant treatment.

Virtually all patients at Level 4 severity will require oral prednisone.[101] Doses of 40 to 80 mg/day are usually required to achieve best result and the dose is then reduced to the lowest amount that will maintain best result. There are few adverse effects from treatment lasting less than 3 weeks, even if such treatment is necessary several times a year. Unfortunately, there are no proven effective means of preventing the adverse effects of long-term continuous prednisone administration. These effects are generally related to dose and duration of treatment. Depressed hypophyseal pituitary adrenal function is to be expected but is minimized by giving the dose on alternate days. Growth suppression is the major adverse effect in children. Insomnia, increased appetite, hyperglycemia, and weight gain with central obesity, skin atrophy, and cataracts occur at all ages. Osteoporosis and myopathy become more important with increasing age. Exercise may help osteoporosis. Also, supplemental calcium or estrogens in women are often prescribed. Aseptic necrosis of the femoral head and severe psychiatric reactions are uncommon but, unlike the above complications, may occur early during a course of treatment. Despite these adverse effects of prednisone, overtreatment with prednisone is virtually never fatal. But undertreatment is. Patients with asthma die of too little, too late. In contrast, overdosage with bronchodilators, particularly the combination of theophylline and adrenergic agonists, is a common mode of death in elderly asthmatics. Theophylline toxicity kills many more asthmatics than prednisone.

Peak Expiratory Flow Rate (PEFR) Measurements at Home

In difficult cases home monitoring of peak flow rates has become a valuable tool to control asthma, analogous to home monitoring of blood glucose in controlling diabetes. The method of using a peak flow meter is as follows:

1. A full inspiration is followed by a maximal expiratory effort with the lips closed tightly around the mouthpiece.
2. The best of three readings on each occasion is recorded.
3. The times of measurement will depend on the objectives. Best post-inhaled beta-agonist values and daily variation can be obtained from twice daily measurements, on waking and before bed, before and after inhalation of an adrenergic agonist. Variability can be calculated from the mean highest and mean lowest values recorded for 1 or 2 weeks:
   Variability $(\%) = [(\text{highest} - \text{lowest}) \text{ highest}] \times 100.$

Home monitoring is useful for the following purposes:

1. To find the "best" airway function during intensive treatment.
2. To measure the daily variability of PEFR readings as an indicator of the degree of airway responsiveness.
3. To educate the patient about managing asthma.
4. To keep airway function close to "best" at all times.
5. To determine the severity of an exacerbation and to detect this early when the patient perceives symptoms poorly.
6. To allow the patient to adjust drug dosages to maintain normal function with minimal doses.
7. To identify unknown or suspected trigger factors.

Peak flow monitoring is indicated for:

1. Patients who get severe attacks with little warning.
2. Patients requiring Level 2 treatment who have special circumstances, such as living a long distance from medical attention.
3. Patients who require Level 3 or 4 maintenance treatment.
4. Patients with known marked diurnal variation of PEFR ($>20\%$).
5. Patients in whom the history seems to provide an unsatisfactory guide to treatment.

Lowest Level of Treatment to Maintain Control or Best Result

Once symptoms have been minimized and highest flow rates have been achieved, the level of treatment with medications can be gradually reduced to the lowest level that will maintain control. Regular treatment that maintains control or best result and prevents severe exacerbations may, over time, produce improvement in best results, allow a reduction in regular medications, and prevent deterioration in airflow. Home peak flow monitoring is invaluable in following the response to treatment.

An antibiotic is not a treatment for asthma, including episodes of asthma associated with viral upper respiratory infections. Prescription of an antibiotic should be reserved for patients with pneumonia, acute bacterial sinusitis, or other intercurrent bacterial illness. Antihistamines and calcium channel blockers have not proved particularly useful for management of asthma, but their administration to asthmatics for other indications is not contraindicated.[102,103] Iodides or mucolytics are of no value. A number of experimental drugs for asthma, including ketotifen, methotrexate, auronofin, troleandomycin, and nedocromil are under investigation, but their place has not been established.

Written Action Plan for Managing Exacerbations

It is useful for each patient who requires more than Level 1 treatment to have an individualized written management plan that includes symptom and PEFR criteria for introducing or increasing the glucocorticoid aerosol and specifying the dose, and also includes criteria for introducing or increasing prednisone and specifying the dose. Patients who are likely to need prednisone should have a supply at home. A home nebulizer compressor system may be useful for delivering aerosols to small children or to older children and adults who have difficulty using a metered dose inhaler effectively, especially during an acute severe episode. Add-on spacer devices with a valve, such as Aerochamber® or Inspirease®, can often substitute for the compressor. It is important to emphasize that aerosol glucocorticoids are not effective during severe exacerbations but that prednisone is required. It is also important to emphasize that although during acute exacerbation, the dose of adrenergic agonist aerosols can and should be increased, the patient needs to understand that it is inappropriate to rely on extra doses of adrenergic aerosols alone. *Prednisone is required.*

An example of an action plan for a patient on a program of regular inhaled beclomethasone 200 µg twice daily who usually needs an adrenergic aerosol twice daily is as follows:

1. If cough, wheeze, or breathlessness begin to occur with milder provocation or if you need an inhaled adrenergic aerosol more often, increase the dose of inhaled beclomethasone two or fourfold.

2. If cough, wheeze, or breathlessness cause nighttime or early morning symptoms two nights in a row, or if you need inhaled adrenergic aerosol more than four times daily for more than 1 day, begin prednisone 20 mg twice a day until symptoms are fully controlled.

3. If symptoms persist at rest or if the adrenergic aerosol provides relief for less than 4 hours, go for medical treatment to a specified facility.

An example of an action plan based on PEFR that could be given to an adult patient on a program of inhaled beclomethasone with a best PEFR of 500 L/min is as follows:

If, for 24 hours, PEFR after inhaled adrenergic aerosol is less than:

1. 425 (85% of best result): Increase the dose of inhaled beclomethasone two- or fourfold until readings are within 10% of the best result.
2. 300 (60% of best result): Take prednisone, 20 mg twice a day until readings are again within 10% of the best result.
3. 250 (50% of best result): Take an additional 40 mg prednisone and go to a specified medical facility.

Provision at home for extra treatment can include:

1. Prednisone tablets for patients who might require prednisone for the treatment of exacerbations and who fully understand the indications for its use.
2. Epinephrine for subcutaneous injection, for the very few patients who have a history of unusually severe sudden attacks of asthma with or without anaphylaxis.
3. A home nebulizer-compressor system. This may have been introduced as a consequence of the inefficient use of the metered dose inhaler.
4. A home oxygen supply, particularly for patients who develop sudden severe attacks and do not have easy access to a medical facility for emergency treatment.

Written Action Plan for Emergency Treatment for High-Risk Patients

Patients who have a history of severe exacerbations requiring emergency room treatment and particularly patients identified as being at risk of death from an exacerbation should have written instructions in addition to the above action plan that include criteria for an immediate call to the physician or an immediate visit to a specified emergency room. These instructions should include emergency telephone numbers, methods of transportation, and information identifying the patient to the emergency room staff as being unusually vulnerable.

Factors that have been identified to increase the risk of death from asthma are:

1. Previous episode of respiratory failure, especially one requiring intubation.
2. Hospitalization for status asthmaticus within the past year.
3. More than one emergency room visit for acute asthma in the past year.
4. Need for high-dose prednisone treatment with recent reduction in dose.
5. Treatment with three or more drugs.
6. Psychiatric diseases, including psychosis, depression, and severe personality disorders, that lead to noncompliance or inability to communicate severity of symptoms.
7. History of seizures.
8. Wide diurnal swing in PEFR (more than 50%).

Follow-Up Visits

Regular follow-up visits are essential and should address the following points:

1. Determination of the current level of symptoms.
2. Objective determination of airflow by spirometry or at least PEFR.
3. Review of present treatment and side effects of medications.

4. Review of exacerbations since last visit for severity and duration, probable causes, and appropriateness of treatment by previous action plan.
5. Reconsideration of harmful causal factors and the possibility of changes to avoid them.
6. Consideration of additional investigations such as allergy tests, evaluation of importance of occupational exposure, and chest, sinus, or stomach radiographs.
7. Repeat coaching in the technique of aerosol inhalation and use of the peak flow meter.
8. Review of the patient's understanding of the causes and nature of the disease, its severity, the objectives of treatment (control or best result), the purpose, action and side effects of medications.
9. A decision on new level of treatment and a review of the action plan.
10. Scheduling of the return appointment.

Immunotherapy

Immunotherapy has proved to be effective in reducing airway response to inhaled allergens and improving symptoms in patients allergic to pollens, cats, and house dust mites. It can be considered for patients who have positive skin or RAST tests and who have symptoms on exposure to an allergen that cannot be avoided. It is greatly preferable to remove the cat from the home, for example, than to embark on a 3-year program of cat immunotherapy. Immunotherapy should be supervised by a physician experienced in the technique because it carries a risk of systemic allergic reactions and a fatality of approximately 1:1,000,000. To be effective, the dose of allergen must be as large as tolerated by the patient's degree of sensitivity. Injections are given in increasing doses weekly for about 20 weeks, and monthly maintenance doses are given for 3 to 5 years. Improvement is usually evident within a year.

Emergency Care

Severe, life-threatening asthma can develop very quickly following ingestion of certain foods (e.g., peanuts), aspirin or other nonsteroid antiinflammatory drug, a beta-blocker, or sulphite, after exposure to a high dose of aeroallergen or chemical sensitizer, or occasionally for unknown reasons. However, the usual case is an exacerbation in which there is progressive deterioration for days or weeks. Early recognition by the patient or physician and early adequate glucocorticoid treatment can usually prevent it from becoming severe. Thus, severe life-threatening asthma and asthma mortality should be regarded as almost always preventable. Many emergency room visits represent a failure to implement effectively the management plan outlined in the preceding section. An important special concern is asthma care in the large metropolitan city hospitals where socioeconomic barriers pose a very different and difficult set of management problems. Asthmatic patients living in the inner city often adopt a crisis-oriented rather than a preventive approach and depend on the emergency room for their primary care. Presumably, this is an important factor contributing to the higher morbidity and mortality rates in this segment of the population.

Surveys of emergency care of acute exacerbations of asthma have highlighted the following deficiencies in assessment and treatment:

1. Failure to measure the severity of airflow limitation by spirometry or PEFR and to determine the amount of improvement after treatment.
2. Failure to treat early with adequate doses of glucocorticoid.
3. Failure to arrange adequate follow-up for long-term treatment to achieve control and prevent subsequent severe exacerbations.

Assessment

The history should elicit the severity and duration of symptoms, the amount of inhaled beta-agonist, theophylline, prednisone, and other drugs taken recently, and the severity and medication requirements during previous exacerbations. The physical examination should focus on the state of exhaustion, level of consciousness, use of accessory muscles, pulsus paradoxus, and cyanosis. Complications of severe asthma, such as atelectasis, pneumothorax, and pneumonia, should be excluded.

Spirometry or PEFR measurements must be made before an adequate dose of inhaled beta-agonist is given unless the patient is too ill to permit it. Certainly, such measurement should be made after this treatment. It cannot be overemphasized that attempting to manage asthma without objective measurement of airflow and its response to treatment is like attempting to manage acute chest pain without an electrocardiogram, or diabetic acidosis without blood chemistry assessment. Estimation of severity and response to treatment by symptoms alone is unreliable. Measurement of blood gases is indicated if the FEV_1 or PEFR remains below 40% of predicted values after initial treatment, or if the patient appears fatigued and responds poorly to treatment. A chest radiograph is not required in all cases but should be performed for suspected pneumothorax, atelectasis, or pneumonia, and in patients who fail to respond to initial treatment.

Treatment in the Emergency Room

The immediate objective of emergency room treatment are as follows:

1. To relieve hypoxemia.
2. To relieve airflow limitation to the degree that is possible.
3. To initiate treatment designed to reverse inflammation.
4. To avoid overdosage with bronchodilators, particularly theophylline.

Treatment should begin at once and takes precedence over investigations (e.g. spirometry) unless these can be done within minutes of arrival and the episode does not appear to be life-threatening.

Priorities of treatment are as follows:

1. Oxygen should be administered by mask in concentrations high enough to relieve the expected hypoxemia. In patients with asthma, in contrast to patients with chronic respiratory failure, the $F_{I_{O_2}}$ is not limited by the potential for CO_2 retention. In elderly patients where there is a possibility of chronic respiratory insufficiency, the initial $F_{I_{O_2}}$ should be limited and the effect on blood gases monitored. PaO_2 should be maintained at 60 mm Hg or higher.

2. An inhaled adrenergic agonist should be administered immediately by nebulizer or a metered dose inhaler with a valved add-on device in a dose larger than the usual outpatient dose. In severe asthma, the dose actually deposited in the airways bears little relationship to the amount aerosolized. Most of it is wasted. Usually the adrenergic agonist is delivered with a nebulizer powered by oxygen. Recommended dose of albuterol is 2.5 mg, of terbutaline 2.5 mg, and of metaproterenol 10 to 15 mg. If a metered dose inhaler with an add-on device is used (this may be more convenient and less expensive) the dose should be four puffs over a 2-minute period and then one puff each minute until there are side effects such as tremor, or until breathlessness decreases and flow rates improve. The aerosol treatment should be repeated in 15 to 30 minutes and then hourly as long as severe obstruction persists.

3. Glucocorticoids administered orally or by injection are imperative and should not be deferred in severe asthma even if there is an initial positive response to bronchodilator, as this response may be temporary.[104,105] Appropriate doses of prednisone or methylprednisolone are 30 to 40 mg immediately, repeated two or three times a day (up to 2 mg/kg/24 hours) and continued for 7 to 21 days until control is achieved. An alternative for patients with a very severe exacerbation is intravenous methylprednisolone, 125 mg (or hydrocortisone, 500 mg), in a single dose followed by prednisone or methylprednisolone orally as above.[103,104] The risk of side effects from a few days of treatment with glucocorticoids is very much less than the risk of death and disability from asthma. Acute psychiatric reactions occasionally occur, but it is often difficult to determine how much of these reactions to attribute to the glucocorticoid and how much to the patient's premorbid personality. Past experience of response to prednisone, current high maintenance prednisone dose, or poor initial response can be indications for increasing the above recommended doses in selected patients. The dose of glucocorticoid should be sufficient to eradicate eosinophils from the circulation.

4. Spirometry or at least peak flow measurement is required to follow the response to treatment and guide decisions about ongoing therapy. Blood gas measurements may need to be repeated if the initial $PaCO_2$ is elevated or the PaO_2 is below 50 mm Hg, or if there is subsequent deterioration.

5. Intubation and assisted ventilation are used if necessary. Obviously, respiratory arrest and disturbed consciousness require immediate intubation. Intubation and assisted ventilation are also indicated if $PaCO_2$ persists above 65 mm Hg after initial treatment. Intubation should be considered when severe obstruction persists, use of accessory muscles continues, or the patient becomes exhausted.

6. Other medications that can be considered are anticholinergic aerosols, intravenous aminophylline or beta-adrenergic agonists, and subcutaneous or intramuscular epinephrine. Atropine by aerosol is less effective than beta-adrenergic agonist aerosols when given alone and adds no further benefit to an adequate dose of the adrenergic drug.[106] It is fully absorbed and can cause systemic toxicity. Ipratroprium is available in some countries for use in a nebulizer and has an advantage over atropine in having much less systemic effects. Its benefit, however, is debatable except for occasional patients who cannot tolerate the more effective beta-

adrenergic agonists.[107] Aminophylline intravenously has traditionally been the mainstay of treatment for severe asthma but because of its potential toxicity and because it is a less effective bronchodilator than aerosol beta-adrenergic agonists, its place in therapy has become controversial.[108] It should be reemphasized that failure of severe airway obstruction to reverse during an asthma episode is not due to failure of administered medications to relax smooth muscle, but is due to occlusion of airways by an inflammation exudate. Adding a second bronchodilator may increase toxicity without increasing benefit.[109] With theophylline, particularly, this becomes an important issue because the combination of theophylline and beta-adrenergic agonists increases myocardial damage, especially in elderly patients and patients with heart disease. Hypokalemia from glucocorticoids and beta-adrenergic agonists combined with hypoxemia amplify the risk. In asthmatics, the potential value of theophylline in stimulating respiratory drive or relieving respiratory muscle fatigue is not a consideration. If aminophylline is used, the loading dose is 5 mg/kg over 20 minutes (this should be reduced if the patient has previously been taking theophylline) and the maintenance dose is usually 0.1 to 0.2 mg/kg/minute. The maintenance dose must be individualized, taking into account the patient's age, smoking history, concomitant medications, and other factors that alter theophylline metabolism.[100] Heart failure and liver disease greatly reduce theophylline metabolism.

In exceptional cases, intravenous beta-adrenergic agonists can be used, but the intravenous route has not been shown to be superior to aerosol treatment. Epinephrine, subcutaneously, intramuscularly, or in extraordinary circumstances intravenously or intratracheally, may be given for acute severe attacks of asthma accompanying anaphylaxis or angioedema. Such asthmatics should also carry kits for self-administered epinephrine to use for future sudden severe attacks while they are going to the emergency room.

Criteria for Admission to the Hospital or Discharge Home

There are no absolute criteria for these decisions. Admission to the hospital is mandatory if there is any concern about an inadequate response to emergency treatment or there is persisting severe airflow obstruction. If aerosol or parenteral treatment needs to be repeated frequently, if the patient has a past history of respiratory arrest or needs frequent monitoring for other reasons, admission should be arranged. Additional reasons for admission include the patient's inability to care for himself at home and severe social or emotional difficulties.[110,111] Generally if the patient feels the need for admission for safety, admission should be arranged. Treatment in the hospital consists of continuing the treatment initiated in the emergency room. Monitoring peak flow rates at least twice daily is necessary to evaluate adequacy of treatment and to choose an appropriate time to reduce doses of medication. Discharge from the hospital can be considered when peak flows have improved to 50% to 70% of predicted or best known previous values. It is wise to err on the side of a few more days of hospital care than to discharge the patient too soon.

Discharge from the emergency room can be considered if the symptoms have greatly improved and if the FEV_1 or PEFR has improved to at least 50% of predicted (or

50% of known previous best value) and if the improvement is likely to be sustained. Reliance on symptoms alone can overestimate the degree of improvement. Unless the FEV_1 or peak flow has returned to normal (or previous best value), the patient must understand the need to continue prednisone for several days until the exacerbation has fully resolved. If compliance with this advice is questionable, an injection of a long-acting glucocorticoid is a reasonable alternative. Before the patient is discharged from the hospital emergency room arrangements must be made for follow-up, and if the patient is not following the management plan to control asthma, he should be referred to a specialist for implementation of the plan.

YOUNG CHILDREN AND INFANTS

The objectives and principles of treatment are the same for all ages. Methods of measuring ventilating function are not generally available for young children and infants, and assessment depends on the unaided history and physical examination. Respiratory rate is a useful guide to the severity during an episode, and sternal or lower rib cage retraction indicates quite severe obstruction.

Underdiagnosis of asthma remains a common problem. More than 50% of children with asthma develop it during the first year of life, and there is still commonly a mislabeling of young asthmatics whose episodes occur with viral respiratory infections as wheezy bronchitis, asthmatic bronchitis, or recurrent bronchiolitis. Another cause for underdiagnosis is the failure to recognize that asthma may accompany other chronic respiratory diseases that dominate the picture, such as bronchopulmonary dysplasia or cystic fibrosis.

Harmful factors (indoor allergens, cigarette smoke, air pollutants such as fumes from gas stoves or open fires) are of major importance and can often be controlled. Such control involves the entire family. Parents, teachers, and school nurses need to be educated how to participate in the management plan. Continuity of care and compliance with instructions is a major requirement for successful control.

Choice of medications is similar in children and adults, and the aerosol route is preferred. In treating infants, a compressor nebulizer system is generally used for adrenergic agonists; doses are similar to those for adults. For Level 2 therapy, many pediatricians prefer cromolyn to glucocorticoids and, indeed, glucocorticoids are not licensed for use in a nebulizer. Some children can inhale from powder devices more efficiently than from metered dose inhalers. Valved add-on devices with either a mouthpiece or a face mask can be used to expedite a child's use of the inhalers. Sustained-release theophylline preparations formulated for infants and a liquid prednisone preparation are available for children too young to swallow tablets or capsules.

As a general rule, chronic or severe asthma in infancy should be treated by a specialist with experience of managing asthma in children.

REFERENCES

1. Reed CE. New therapeutic approaches in asthma. J Allergy Clin Immunol 1986;77:537–542.
2. Sly RM. Mortality from asthma. J Allergy Clin Immunol 1989;84:421–434.

3. Sheffer AL, Buist AS (eds): Workshop: Asthma mortality. J Allergy Clin Immunol 1987;80: 361–514.

4. Buist AS, Sears MR, Reid LM, Bouchey HA, Spector SL, Sheffer AL. Asthma mortality, trends and determinants. Am Rev Resp Dis 1987;136:1037–1039.

5. Cookson JB. Prevalence rate of asthma in developing countries and their comparison with those of Europe and North America. Chest 1987;91:97S–103S.

6. Smith JM. Studies on the prevalence of asthma in childhood. Allergol Immunopathol 1975;3:127–132.

7. Gergen PJ, Mullally DI, Evans R. National survey of prevalence of asthma among children in the United States, 1976–1980. Pediatrics 1988;81:1–7.

8. Anderson HR, Bland JM, Patel S, Peckham S. The natural history of asthma in childhood. J Epidemiol Community Health 1986;40:121–126.

9. Dodge RR, Burrows B. The prevalence and incidence of asthma and asthma-like symptoms in a general population sample. Am Rev Respir Dis 1980;122:567–575.

10. Perrin JM, Homer J, Berwick DM, Wolf AD, Freeman JL, Wennberg JE. Variation in rates of hospitalization of children in three urban communities. N Engl J Med 1988;320:1183–1187.

11. Williams MH Jr. Increasing severity of asthma from 1960 to 1987. N Engl J Med 1989;320:1015.

12. Malveaux FJ. Asthma care for the indigent. J Allergy Clin Immunol 1989;83:1027–1029.

13. Reed CE, Swanson MC. Indoor allergens: Identification and quantification. Environment Internat 1986;12:115–120.

14. Burrows B. The natural history of asthma. J Allergy Clin Immunol 1987;80:373–377.

15. Burrows B, Bloom JW, Trover GA, Cline MS. The course and prognosis of different forms of airway obstruction in a sample from the general population. N Engl J Med 1987;317:1309–1314.

16. Burrows B, Martinez FD, Halonen M, Barbee RA, Cline MG. Association of asthma with serum IgE levels and skin-test reactivity to allergens. N Engl J Med 1989;320:271–277.

17. Curshman H. Über bronchiolitis exudativa und ihr verhaltim's zum asthma nervosum. Deutsch Arch Klin Med 1883;32:1–20.

18. Dunnill MS. The pathology of asthma with special reference to changes in the bronchial mucosa. J Clin Pathol 1966;13:27–33.

19. Kleinerman J, Adelson L. A study of asthma deaths in a coroner's population. J Allergy Clin Immunol 1987;80:406–409.

20. Filley WV, Holley KE, Kephart GM, Gleich GJ. Identification by immunofluorescence of eosinophil granule major basic protein in lung tissues of patients with bronchial asthma. Lancet 1982;ii:11–16.

21. Laitinen LA, Heino M, Laitinen A, Kava T, Haahtela T. Damage of the airway epithelium and bronchial reactivity in patients with asthma. Am Rev Respir Dis 1985;131:599–606.

22. Laitinen LA, Laitinen A. Mucosal inflammation and bronchial hyperreactivity. Eur J Respir Dis 1988;5:488–489.

23. Wardlaw AJ, Dunnette S, Gleich GJ, Collins JV, Kay AB. Eosinophil and mast cells in bronchoalveolar lavage in subjects with mild asthma. Relationship to bronchial hyperreactivity. Am Rev Respir Dis 1988;137:62–69.

24. Poznansky MC, Gordon ACH, Douglas JG, Krajewski AS, Wyllie AH, Grant IWB. Resistance to methylprednisolone in cultures of blood mononuclear cells from glucocorticoid resistant asthmatic patients. Clin Sci 1984;67:639–645.

25. McFadden ER. Asthma, airway dynamics, cardiac function and clinical correlates. In: Middleton ER Jr, Reed CE, Ellis EF, Adkinson NF, Yunginger JW, eds. Allergy principles and practice. St. Louis: CV Mosby, 1988:1018–1036.

26. Baker JW, Yerger S, Segar WE. Elevated plasma antidiuretic hormone levels in status asthmaticus. Mayo Clin Proc 1976;51(1):31–34.

27. Shim CS, Williams MH Jr. Evaluation of the severity of asthma: Patients versus physicians. Am J Med 1980;68:11–13.

28. Wagner PD, Dantzker DR, Iacovoni VE, Tomilin WC, West JB. Ventilation-perfusion inequality in asymptomatic asthma. Am Rev Respir Dis 1978;118(3):511–524.
29. Kaliner M. Asthma and mast cell activation. J Allergy Clin Immunol 1989;83:510–520.
30. Solley GD, Gleich GJ, Jordon RE, Schroeter AL. The late phase of the immediate wheal and flare reaction: Its dependence upon IgE antibodies. J Clin Invest 1976;58:408–420.
31. Kimani G, Tonnesen MC, Henson PM. Stimulation of eosinophil adherence to human vascular endothelial cells *in vitro* by platelet activating factor. J Immunol 1988;140:3161–3164.
32. Leprevost C, Capron M, deVos C, Tomassini M, Capron A. Inhibition of eosinophil chemotaxis by a new antiallergic compound (cetirizine). Int Arch Allergy Appl Immunol 1988;87:9–13.
33. Townley RG, Hopp RJ, Agrawal D, Bewtra AK. Platelet activating factor and airway hyperreactivity. J Allergy Clin Immunol 1989;83:997–1010.
34. Gerblich AA, Campbel AE, Schuyler MR. Changes in T-lymphocyte subpopulation in asthmatics. N Engl J Med 1989;310:1349–1352.
35. Stoop AE, Homeleers DMH, Run PEM, Biewengar, vander Baan S. Lymphocytes and nonlymphoid cells in the nasal mucosa of patients with nasal polyps and of healthy subjects. J Allergy Clin Immunol 1988;84:734–741.
36. Denberg JA, Dolovich J, Harnish D. Basophil mast cell and eosinophil growth and differentiation factors in human allergic disease. Clin Exp Allergy 1989;19:249–254.
37. Miyajima A, Miyatake S, Schreurs J, de Vries J, Arai N, Yokota T, Arai K. Coordinate regulation of immune and inflammatory responses by T derived lymphokines. FASEB J 1988;2:2462–2473.
38. Corrigan CJ, Hartnell A, Kay AB. T lymphocyte activation in acute severe asthma. Lancet 1988;i:1129–1132.
39. Burrows B, Martinez ED, Halonen M, Barbee RA, Cline MG. Association of asthma with serum IgE levels and skin test reactivity to allergens. N Engl J Med 1989;320:271–277.
40. Lichtenstein L. Histamine releasing factors and IgE heterogeneity. J Allergy Clin Immunol 1988;81:814–820.
41. Plaut M, Pierce JH, Nielson CJ, Hanley-Hyde J, Nordan RP, Paul WE. Mast cell lines produce lymphokines in response to cross linkage of Fc_eR1 or to calcium ionophores. Nature 1989;339:64–67.
42. Gleich GJ, Flavahan NA, Fujisawa T, Vanhoutte PM. The eosinophil as a mediator of damage to respiratory epithelium: A model for bronchial hyperreactivity. J Allergy Clin Immunol 1988;81:778–781.
43. Slifman NR, Adolphson CR, Gleich GJ. Eosinophils: Biochemical and cellular aspects. In: Middleton ER Jr, Reed CE, Ellis EF, Adkinson NF, Yunginger JW, eds. Allergy principles and practice, 3rd ed. St. Louis: CV Mosby, 1988;179–205.
44. Gleich GJ, Abu-Ghazaleh R. Update on eosinophils. Allergy Proc 1989;10:71–72.
45. Fukada T, Gleich GJ. Heterogeneity of human eosinophils. J Allergy Clin Immunol 1989;83:369–373.
46. Roakin JA. The contribution of alveolar macrophage to hyperreactive airway disease. J Allergy Clin Immunol 1989;83:722–729.
47. Page CP. Platelets as inflammatory cells. Immunopharmacology 1989;17:51–59.
48. Marsh DG. Immunogenetics of allergic disease. In: Middleton ER Jr, Reed CE, Ellis EF, Adkinson WF, Yunginger JW, eds. Allergy principles and practice, 3rd ed. St. Louis: CV Mosby, 1988;99–105.
49. McIntosh K, Ellis EF, Hoffman LS, Lybass TG, Eller JJ, Fulginit VA. The association of viral and bacterial respiratory infections with exacerbations of wheezing in young asthmatic children. J Pediatr 1973;82:578–590.
50. Minor TE, Dick EC, Baker JW, Ouellette JJ, Cohen M, Reed CE. Rhinovirus and influenza Type A infections as precipitants of asthma. Am Rev Respir Dis 1976;113:149–153.
51. Welliver RC, Wong DT, Sun M, Middleton E Jr, Vaughan RS, Ogra PL. The development of respiratory syncytial virus–specific IgE and the release of histamine in nasopharyngeal secretions after infection. N Engl J Med 1981;305:841–846.

52. Welliver RC, Wong DT, Middleton E Jr, Sun M, McCarthy N, Ogra PL. Role of parainfluenza virus–specific IgE in pathogenesis of croup and wheezing subsequent to infection. J Pediatr 1982;101:889–896.

53. Ida S, Hooks JJ, Siraganian RP, Notkins AL. Enhancement of IgE-mediated histamine release from human basophils by viruses: Role of interferon. J Exp Med 1977;145:892–896.

54. Busse WW. Decreased granulocyte response to isoproterenol in asthma during upper respiratory infections. Am Rev Respir Dis 1977;115:783–791.

55. Lemansky RF Jr, Dick EL, Swenson CA, Vrlis RF, Busse WW. Rhinovirus upper respiratory infection increases airway hyperreactivity and late asthmatic reactions. J Clin Invest 1989;83:1–10.

56. Dolovich J, Hargreave FE, Jordana M, Denberg J. Late phase airway reaction and inflammation. J Allergy Clin Immunol 1989;83:521–524.

57. Jines A, Pare P, Hogg J. The mechanics of airway narrowing in asthma. Am Rev Respir Dis 1989;139:242–246.

58. Barnes PJ. Asthma as an axon reflex. Lancet 1986;i:242–245.

59. Wanner A, Nadel J (eds). Conference on interaction between inflammatory response and smooth muscle. Am Rev Respir Dis 1987;135:S1–S75.

60. Barnes PJ. Neural control of human airways in health and disease. Am Rev Respir Dis 1986;134:1289–1314.

61. Barnes PJ. Circadian variation in airway function. Am J Med 1985;79(suppl 6A):5–9.

62. Pauwels R, Joos R, vander Straeten M. Bronchial hyperresponsiveness is not bronchial asthma. Clin Allergy 1988;18:317–321.

63. Josephs LK, Gregg I, Mullee MA, Holgate ST. Nonspecific bronchial reactivity and its relationship to the clinical expression of asthma: A longitudinal study. Am Rev Respir Dis 1989;140:350–357.

64. Anderson SD. Exercise induced asthma. In: Middleton ER Jr, Reed CE, Ellis EF, Adkinson WF, Yunginger JW, eds. Allergy principles and practice, 3rd ed. St. Louis: CV Mosby, 1988;1156–1175.

65. Townley RG, Bewtra A, Nilson FF, Hopp RJ, Elston RC, Nair N, Watt GD. Segregation analysis of bronchial response to methacholine inhalation challenge in families with and without asthma. J Allergy Clin Immunol 1986;77:101–107.

66. Shelhamer, J, Metcalfe D, Smith L, Kaliner M. Abnormal beta adrenergic responsiveness in allergic subjects: Analysis of isoproterenol-induced cardiovascular and plasma cyclic AMP responses. J Allergy Clin Immunol 1980;66:52–58.

67. Smith JJ, Shelhamer JH, Kaliner M. The cholinergic nervous system and immediate hypersensitivity. II. An analysis of pupillary responses. J Allergy Clin Immunol 1980;66:374–382.

68. Parker CW, Smith JW. Alteration in cyclic adenosine monophosphate metabolism in human bronchial asthma. I. Leukocyte responsiveness to beta-adrenergic agents. J Clin Invest 1973;52:48–60.

69. Conolly ME, Greenacre JK. The lymphocyte beta-adreno-receptor in normal subjects and patients with asthma: The effect of different forms of treatment on receptor function. J Clin Invest 1976;58:1307–1314.

70. Meurs H, Kauffman HF, Koeter GH, Timmermans A, de Vries K. Regulation of the beta-receptor-adenylate cyclase system in patients with asthma: Possible role for protein kinase C in allergen-induced nonspecific refractiveness of adenylate cyclase. J Allergy Clin Immunol 1989;80:326–339.

71. Grew SR, Chan SC, Hanafin JM. Elevated leukocyte cyclic AMP phosphodiesterase in atopic disease: A possible mechanism for cAMP agonist hyporesponsiveness. J Allergy Clin Immunol 1982;70:452–458.

72. Gaoriely N, Palti Y, Alroy G, Grotberg JB. Measurement and theory of wheezing breath sounds. J Appl Physiol 1989;57:481–492.

73. Enright PL, Hyatt RE. Office spirometry: A practical guide to selection and use of spirometers. Philadelphia: Lea & Febiger, 1987.

74. Gibson PG, Girgis-Gabardo A, Morris MM, Maltoli S, Kay JM, Dolovich J, Denberg J, Hargreave FE. Cellular characteristics of sputum from patients with asthma and chronic bronchitis. Thorax 1989;44:693–699.

75. Naylor B. The shedding of the mucosa of the bronchial tree in asthma. Thorax 1962;17:69–78.

76. Bernstein IL, ed. Proceedings of the task force on guidelines for standardizing old and new technologies used for the diagnosis and treatment of allergic diseases. J Allergy Clin Immunol 1988;82:487–526.

77. Reed CE, Swanson MC. Antigens and allergic asthma. Chest 1987;91:161S–165S.

78. Reed CE. What we do and do not know about mold allergy and asthma. J Allergy Clin Immunol 1985;76:773–775.

79. Anto JM, Sunyer J, Rodriguez M, Roisin R, Suarey M, Vazguy L. Asthma epidemics associated with soybean dust released during harbor unloading activities. N Engl J Med 1989;320:1097–1102.

80. Platts-Mills TAE, de Weck AL. Dust mite allergens and asthma: A worldwide problem. J Allergy Clin Immunol 1989;83:416–427.

81. Stankus RP, O'Neil CE. Antigenic/allergenic characterization of American and German cockroach extracts. J Allergy Clin Immunol 1988;81:563–570.

82. Stevenson DD. Diagnosis, prevention, and treatment of adverse reactions to aspirin and nonsteroidal anti-inflammatory drugs. J Allergy Clin Immunol 1984;74:617–622.

83. Taylor SL, Bush RK, Selner JC, Nordlee BS, Weiner MB, Holden K, Koepke SW, Busse WW. Sensitivity to sulfited foods among sulfite sensitive subjects with asthma. J Allergy Clin Immunol 1988;81:1159–1167.

84. Christopher KL, Wood RP, Eckert RC, Blager FB, Raney RA, Souhrada JF. Vocal cord dysfunction presenting as asthma. N Engl J Med 1983;308:1566–1570.

85. Randolph C, Lapey A, Shannon DC. Bilateral vocal cord paralysis masquerading as asthma. J Allergy Clin Immunol 1988;81:1122–1125.

86. Irwin RS, Corrao WM, Prater MR. Chronic cough: The spectrum of frequency of causes and successful outcomes of specific therapy. Am Rev Respir Dis 1981;123:413–417.

87. Gibson PG, Dolovich J, Denburg J, Ramsdale EH, Hargreave FE. Chronic cough: Eosinophilic bronchitis without asthma. Lancet 1989;i:1346–1348.

88. Silverman EK, Pierce JA, Province MA, Roo DC, Campbell EJ. Variability of pulmonary function in alpha-1-antitrypsin deficiency: Clinical correlates. Ann Intern Med 1989;982–991.

89. Siefert AF, Allison RC, Bryars CH, Kirkpatrick MB. Normal airway responsiveness to methacholine in cardiac asthma. Am Rev Respir Dis 1989;140:1805–1806.

90. Lemanske RF, Dick EG, Swenson CA, Vritis RF, Busse WW. Rhinovirus upper respiratory infection increases airway hyperreactivity and late asthmatic reactions. J Clin Invest 1989;83:1–10.

91. Hargreave FE, Dolovich J, Newhouse MD, eds. The assessment and treatment of asthma: A conference report. J Allergy Clin Immunol 1990;85:1098–1111.

92. Dutoit JI, Salome CM, Woolcock AJ. Inhaled corticosteroids reduce the severity of bronchial hyperresponsivenes in asthma but oral theophylline does not. Am Rev Respir Dis 1987;136:1174–1178.

93. Latimer KM, O'Byrne PM, Morris MM, Roberts R, Hargreave FE. Bronchoconstriction stimulated by airway cooling: Better protection with combined inhalation of terbutaline sulphate and cromolyn sodium than with either alone. Am Rev Respir Dis 1983;128:440–443.

94. Welsh PW, Stricker WE, Chu CP, Naessens JM, Reese ME, Reed CE, Marcoux JP. Efficacy of beclomethasone nasal solution, flunisolide and cromolyn in relieving symptoms of ragweed allergy. Mayo Clin Proc 1987;62(2):125–134.

95. Rachelefsky GS, Katz RM, Siegel SC. Chronic sinus disease with associated reactive airway disease in children. Pediatrics 1984;73(4):526–529.

96. Boyle JT, Tuchman DN, Altschuler SM, Nixon TE, Pack AI, Cohen S. Mechanisms for the association of gastroesophageal reflux and bronchospasm. Am Rev Respir Dis 1985;131:S16–S20.

97. Konig P. Spacer devices used with metered-dose inhalers. Breakthrough or gimmick? Chest 1985;88:276–284.

98. Toogood JH, Baskerville JC, Jennings B, Lefcoe NM, Johansson SA. Influence of dosing frequency and schedule on the response of chronic asthmatics to the aerosol steroid budesonide. J Allergy Clin Immunol 1982;70:288–298.

99. Li JTC, Reed CE. Nocturnal asthma and timing of treatment. Am J Med 1985;79(6A):10–15.

100. Hendeles L, Massanari M, Weinberger M. Theophylline. In: Middleton ER Jr, Reed CE, Ellis EF, Adkinson NF Jr, Yunginger JW, eds. Allergy principles and practice, 3rd ed. St. Louis: CV Mosby, 1988; Chapter 30:673–714.

101. Woolcock A. Use of corticosteroids in patients with asthma. J Allergy Clin Immunol 1989;84:975–978.

102. Sly RM, Kemp JP. The use of antihistamines in patients with asthma. J Allergy Clin Immunol 1988;82:481–482.

103. Simons FE. H_1-receptor antagonists: Clinical pharmacology and therapeutics. J Allergy Clin Immunol 1989;84:845–861.

104. Littenberg B, Gluck EH. A controlled trial of methylprednisolone in the emergency treatment of acute asthma. N Engl J Med 1986;314:150–152.

105. Ratto D, Alfaro C, Sipsey J, Glovsky MM, Sharma OP. Are intravenous corticosteroids required in status asthmaticus? JAMA 1988;260:527–529.

106. Rebuck AS, Chapman KR, Abboud R, Pare PD, Kreisman H, Wolkove N, Vickerson F. Nebulized anticholinergic and sympathomimetic treatment of asthma and chronic obstructive airways disease in the emergency room. Am J Med 1987;82:59–64.

107. Higgins RM, Straddling JR, Lane DJ. Should ipratropium bromide be added to beta agonists in treatment of acute severe asthma? Chest 1988;94:718–722.

108. Littenberg B. Aminophylline treatment in severe, acute asthma. JAMA 1988;259:1678–1684.

109. Siegel D, Sheppard D, Gelb A, Weinberg PF. Aminophylline increases the toxicity but not the efficacy of an inhaled beta-adrenergic agonist in the treatment of acute exacerbations of asthma. Am Rev Respir Dis 1985;132:283-286.

110. Corre KA, Rothstein RJ. Assessing severity of adult asthma and need for hospitalization. Ann Emerg Med 1985;14:103–110.

111. Verbeek PR, Chapman KR. Asthma: Whom to send home, when to hospitalize. J Respir Dis 1986;7(12):15–31.

14

Occupational Asthma

Moira Chan-Yeung

Occupational asthma is defined as variable airflow obstruction caused by a specific agent in the workplace. There is considerable controversy over the definition. Whereas many investigators regard occupational asthma as a condition characterized by variable airflow obstruction caused by either an immunologic or a nonimmunologic mechanism, others recognize only those caused by an immunologic mechanism. In this chapter both immunologically and nonimmunologically induced variable airflow obstruction will be discussed.

PREVALENCE

A large number of agents in the workplace have been shown to cause occupational asthma. With the rapid introduction of new compounds into industries, it is likely that the prevalence of occupational asthma will continue to increase.

The overall prevalence of occupational asthma is unknown. In Japan, it has been estimated that 15% of asthma in males is due to occupational exposure.[1] In general, the prevalence of occupational asthma depends largely on the industrial agent, the degree of exposure, and the susceptibility of the host. For example, in the cotton industry, the prevalence of byssinosis varies from 25% to 29% among workers exposed in the carding process and from 10% to 29% among those exposed in the spinning process.[2] In some villages in Egypt, 90% of all workers exposed to cotton dust developed byssinosis because they were exposed to very high concentrations of the dust.[1] In one study, about 6% of animal handlers developed clinical symptoms due to allergy to animal protein.[3] The prevalence of asthma among workers exposed to proteolytic enzymes has been estimated to be between 10% and 45%.[4] Approximately 5% of workers exposed to volatile isocyanates developed asthma.[5] Similarly, approximately 5% of the workers exposed to western red cedar (*Thuja plicata*) dust had occupational asthma.[6]

360

In certain instances, very high percentages of subjects exposed to an occupational inhalant develop asthma. For example, it has been reported that almost every worker in the power plants along the Mississippi River eventually becomes sensitized to river flies.[7]

Cross-sectional studies of the prevalence of occupational asthma usually underestimate the problem because affected workers leave the industry. Moreover, it is difficult to establish an accurate figure for prevalence because of the problems in the identification of asthma. Most epidemiologic studies have relied on questionnaires rather than on objective tests. Some studies have included the use of histamine or methacholine challenge tests to identify individuals with airway hyperresponsiveness; very few included specific challenge tests, the "gold standard" in the diagnosis of occupational asthma.

PATHOGENESIS

Gandevia[8] introduced the classification of occupational asthma according to pathophysiological mechanisms: reflex, acute inflammatory, pharmacologic, and immunologic. In many instances of occupational asthma, the pathogenetic mechanism is not known and at times more than one mechanism may be involved for a single agent.

Reflex Bronchoconstriction

Cold air, exercise, and exposure to low levels of noxious gases and fumes cause bronchoconstriction by directly affecting irritant receptors in the airways.[9–11] Reflex bronchoconstriction in patients with pre-existing asthma should not be considered as a cause of occupational asthma.

Inflammatory Bronchoconstriction

Gandevia[8] described acute inflammatory bronchoconstriction caused by accidental exposure to high concentrations of irritant gases and vapors such as hydrogen sulphide, diethylene diamine, fume from overheated plastics, or smoke and fume from combustion of a variety of materials. The airflow obstruction usually developed within hours, reached a maximum in a week, and stabilized or resolved within 3 to 4 months.[12–17] Pathologic studies of patients who died after exposure showed extensive damage and sloughing of the mucosa of the large and small airways along with hemorrhagic pulmonary edema.[12] Dense inflammatory cell infiltration, hyperplasia of the bronchial submucosal glands, and terminal bronchiolar fibrosis in addition to destruction of the bronchial epithelium were also observed in one study.[18] Lung function studies of patients after acute inhalation injury revealed reversible airflow obstruction or airway hyperresponsiveness in some patients.[13,14]

Brooks and associates[19] described "reactive airways dysfunction syndrome" in 10 subjects after a single accidental exposure to high levels of irritating vapor, fume, or smoke. In all cases, symptoms of cough, wheeze, and shortness of breath developed within a few hours and often minutes after exposure and all subjects had evidence of airway hyperresponsiveness compatible with asthma. The respiratory symptoms and airway hyperresponsiveness persisted for several years after the incident in most of the subjects. In addition to bronchial/bronchiolar epithelial desquamation and mucus cell hyperplasia, inflammatory changes with infiltration of lymphocyte and plasma cells were found. A nonimmunologic mechanism is the likely pathogenesis in this syndrome. Many investigators do not regard this syndrome as occupational asthma because there is no previous history of exposure, and re-exposure of these subjects to low levels of the gas or irritant did not induce bronchoconstriction.[20] This syndrome is an excellent example of an acute inflammatory process inducing airway hyperresponsiveness. Further research in this area may yield insights into the mechanism of airway hyperresponsiveness.

Pharmacologic Bronchoconstriction

Some of the agents in the workplace induce variable airflow obstruction similar to that induced by pharmacologic agents. There is a dose relationship between exposure and response. Eosinophilia and airway hyperresponsiveness are not associated with the airflow obstruction. Again, many investigators do not regard airflow obstruction due to these agents as occupational asthma.

Cotton Dust

The best example of an agent causing pharmacologic bronchoconstriction is cotton dust. Exposure to cotton dust gives rise to byssinosis.[21] Typically, the worker complains of "Monday" chest tightness, which tends to improve or disappear by the second working day. The chest tightness is sometimes associated with a fall in forced expiratory volume (FEV_1) within a few hours of beginning work on Mondays.[22,23] Chest tightness and acute airflow obstruction also occur in some healthy naive subjects exposed to cotton dust in the laboratory, indicating that previous exposure is not necessary for the development of symptoms.[24] Nonasthmatic responders to cotton dust do not demonstrate an increase in airway hyperresponsiveness to histamine.[25,26]

The pathogenesis of byssinosis and cross-shift (pre and post) changes in FEV_1 in cotton workers is not clear. Cross-shift changes in FEV_1 in cotton workers have been studied by many investigators.[27–29] Imbus and Suh,[28] in a study of over 10,000 workers, found that cross-shift decrease in FEV_1 was associated with bronchitis as well as byssinosis. Smoking, although associated with a lower overall FEV_1, was not associated with a greater decrement in FEV_1 during the working day.[28] Atopic (as defined by positive immediate skin test reactivity) subjects were found to have a greater cross-shift decline in FEV_1 than nonatopic subjects.[27] The level of dust exposure was found to be the most important determinant of the cross-shift change in FEV_1 in all studies[27–29]; the higher the dust level, the greater the decline in FEV_1.

One hypothesis for byssinosis is that cotton dust extracts contain histamine-releasing substances that act on the lungs.[30] However, cotton dust extracts were also found to contain histamine.[31] Plasma histamine levels were found to be elevated in cotton and flax workers, being significantly higher on Mondays.[32]

The other etiologic theory for byssinosis is that an endotoxin in cotton dust causes the clinical syndrome of byssinosis. Rylander and co-workers[33] reported that acute FEV_1 decrements on Monday among cardroom workers correlated better with an exposure index that took into consideration the number of gram-negative bacteria contaminating bale cotton than with the levels of vertical elutriated cotton dust alone. In a study of human volunteers exposed to cotton dust in a laboratory,[24] the levels of endotoxin in the dust were highly correlated with acute changes in FEV_1. When endotoxins were given to laboratory animals by aerosol, fever and dyspnea occurred after inhalation. When endotoxins were given on the second day, no symptoms were induced.[34] These findings simulate the "Monday tightness" characteristic of byssinosis. On the other hand, Buck and associates[35] found that the acute decline in lung function in normal volunteers after exposure to cotton bract extracts persisted even when endotoxin was virtually removed. The role of endotoxin in byssinosis is still uncertain.

Grain Dust

Grain dust is another organic dust that gives rise to cross-shift changes in FEV_1 greater than 10% in about 5% to 11% of exposed workers.[36] As with cotton dust, the cross-shift change in flow rates was less on Wednesdays than on Mondays.[37] The cross-shift in FEV_1 depended on the dust level and was not influenced by smoking or atopy.[37] Grain workers who demonstrated a cross-shift change in FEV_1 did not necessarily have airway hyperresponsiveness.[38] Grain extracts, in vitro, were found to release histamine and leukotrienes from human lung fragments directly and to activate both the alternative and the classical complement pathways.[40]

Both grain and cotton dusts have many components and are often contaminated by a number of bacteria and fungi. Studies showed that extracts of these two organic dusts share similar fungal antigens.[41] It is not unexpected, then, that they give rise to similar clinical syndromes of acute airway reaction.

Unlike cotton dust, grain dust induces asthma in only a small proportion of exposed workers.[42] The prevalence of grain dust asthma is low because those affected tend to leave the industry.[42] In these patients, specific immediate or late asthmatic reactions occur on inhalation challenge with an extract of grain dust.[43] They have increased airway hyperresponsiveness and eosinophilia, suggesting that they are asthmatics.[43]

Organophosphate Insecticides

Acute asthma has been described in farm workers spraying crops with organophosphate insecticides, which act as an anticholinesterase in causing acute airflow obstruction.[44]

Isocyanates and Plicatic Acid

The pathogenesis of occupational asthma caused by exposure to isocyanates and western red cedar (*Thuja plicata*) is not entirely clear. Both isocyanates and plicatic acid (the compound responsible for red cedar asthma) have pharmacologic properties that affect the airways. Toluene diisocyanate (TDI) competes with isoproterenol-induced production of intracellular cyclic AMP in peripheral blood lymphocytes.[45] Plicatic acid activates the classical complement pathway, generating mediators of anaphylaxis.[46] It is unlikely, however, that these properties account for the pathogenetic mechanism of occupational asthma due to these two compounds since only 5% to 10% of exposed individuals are affected.

Allergic Bronchoconstriction

The majority of occupational agents cause asthma through allergic bronchoconstriction. Comprehensive lists of such agents have been published elsewhere.[47,48] In general, these agents can be divided into two major categories: high molecular weight compounds

TABLE 14-1. Clinical Features of Patients with Occupational Asthma Due to High Molecular Weight Compounds

AGEN T	n	% ATOPIC SUBJECTS[1]	% SKIN TEST	POSITIVE SPECIFIC IgE	INHALATION IIR[2]	ILR[3]	REACTION (%) Biphasic	REFERENCE
Animal dander	12	80	86	NA[4]	40	0	60	49
Flour	20	83	91	80	100	0	0	50
	7	75	100	100	100	0	0	51
Detergent enzyme	9	63	88	NA	0	0	100	52
Proteolytic enzyme	8	67	100	78	33	0	67	53
Snow crab	33	18	61	NA	3	27	70	54

1. Atopy is a state characterized by immediate skin test reactions to one or more common allergens.

2. IIR: Isolated immediate reaction.

3. ILR: Isolated late reaction.

4. NA: Not available.

TABLE 14-2. Clinical Features of Patients with Occupational Asthma Due to Low Molecular Weight Compounds

AGENT	n	% ATOPIC SUBJECTS[1]	% POSITIVE TO SKIN TEST	HAPTEN-CONJUGATE RAST	INHALATION REACTION (%)			REFERENCE
					IIR^2	ILR^3	Biphasic	
Toluene diisocyanate	28	25	0	27	32	43	25	61
	14	NA[4]	NA	0	50	50	0	62
	30	56	NA	NA	20	40	40	63
Western red cedar	44	25	0	30	7	44	49	64
Platinum salt	10	6	63	NA	70	20	10	60
Tetrachlorophthalic anhydride	7	14	100	100	0	50	50	59

1. Atopy is a state characterized by immediate skin test reactions to one or more common allergens.

2. IIR: Isolated immediate asthmatic reaction.

3. ILR: Isolated late asthmatic reaction.

4. NA: Not available.

and low molecular weight compounds (MW<1000 daltons). There are good reasons for such a division because of the differences in clinical presentation and predisposing host factors.

High Molecular Weight Compounds

High molecular weight occupational agents such as proteins, polysaccharides, and peptides induce allergic responses by producing specific IgE antibodies and sometimes specific IgG antibodies (Table 14-1).[49–54] In most instances, positive immediate skin test reactions can be elicited with extracts of the offending agents, and specific IgE antibodies to these antigens can be detected. Clinically, the patients are usually atopic subjects with a history of allergic rhinitis or eczema. Moreover, they usually complain of asthma symptoms within a few minutes of exposure. Inhalation challenge tests with high molecular weight occupational allergens induce an isolated immediate asthmatic reaction or a biphasic reaction (immediate and late) and seldom an isolated late asthmatic reaction. Asthma due to occupational allergens has the same pathogenetic mechanism as asthma due to common inhalant allergens such as house dust or pollens.

Low Molecular Weight Compounds

Many low molecular weight compounds (MW<1000 daltons) have been shown to cause occupational asthma in industries.[55–64] Some examples are shown in Table 14-2. In some instances, the compound acts as a hapten and combines with a carrier protein molecule to form an allergen. The acid anhydrides, such as phthalic anhydride,[55] trimellitic an- hydride,[56–58] and tetrachlorophthalic anhydride,[59] and platinum salts[60] are good examples of occupational haptens. However, in the case of isocyanates[61–63] and plicatic acid,[64] specific IgE antibodies are found in only a small proportion of affected subjects.

Occupational asthma due to isocyanate exposure and that due to western red cedar exposure are similar in many respects: in the 5% to 10% prevalence of affected subjects in the industry, in the clinical picture, in the predominant occurrence of a late asthmatic reaction (isolated or late component of biphasic) on inhalation challenge test, in the persistence of asthma despite removal from exposure in a large proportion of sensitized subjects, and in the lack of predilection for atopic subjects. Despite the low prevalence of specific IgE antibodies to the hapten-conjugates in affected subjects, the clinical features of isocyanate-induced and plicatic acid–induced asthma are those of an allergic disease. In addition, both isocyanate and plicatic acid have been shown to sensitize animals.[65,66] Chen and Bernstein[65] sensitized guinea pigs parenterally using bifunctional isocyanate conjugated to protein and were able to demonstrate diisocyanate-specific precipitating and IgE antibodies. Further analysis showed that the immune response mounted by these guinea pigs to diisocyanate protein conjugates was heterogeneous and involved multiple specificities for hapten, carrier protein, and new antigenic determinants. Since toluene diisocyanate (TDI) is a highly reactive material, it is difficult to know what type of conjugate it might form in the airways when it is inhaled. The inability to detect antibodies is likely to reflect the inability to produce an appropriate antigen. Using a plicatic acid–human serum albumin conjugate, Chan and associates[66] were also able to sensitize rabbits parenterally; high titers of antibodies specific for the hapten were found. Challenge with the hapten led to the development of cyanosis, rapid shallow breathing, and an increase in pulmonary resistance. There is sufficient evidence to suggest that both isocyanates and plicatic acid act as haptens.

Mechanism of Immediate and Late Asthmatic Reaction in Occupational Asthma

Inhalation challenge tests with occupational agents may induce different patterns of asthmatic reactions in the laboratory: isolated immediate, isolated late, and biphasic asthmatic reactions.

In patients with specific IgE antibodies or an immediate wheal and flare reaction to the offending agent, the immediate asthmatic reaction is likely to be mediated by IgE antibodies. When an antigen-IgE reaction takes place on the surface of mast cells, it causes the release of a number of preformed mediators, such as histamine, eosinophil chemotactic factor (ECF-A), and neutrophil chemotactic factor (NCF-A), and induces newly formed mediators, such as the metabolites of arachidonic acid. It has been postulated that histamine and perhaps the metabolites of arachidonic acid are responsible for the bronchospasm during the immediate asthmatic reaction.[67] There are now several studies confirming the release of mediators in the bronchoalveolar lavage (BAL) fluid during an immediate asthmatic reaction induced by allergens in patients with asthma.[68-71]

The mechanism of the late asthmatic reaction has been the object of intensive study during the last two decades. The current hypothesis is that the late asthmatic reaction is merely the late phase of the IgE-mediated allergic reaction[67] and is characterized by airway inflammation.[67] The ECF-A, NCF-A, and leukotriene B_4 (LTB_4) released from the mast cells during the immediate asthmatic reaction are potent chemotactic factors for recruiting cells into the airways. Several studies of the late asthmatic reaction induced by occupational agents confirmed that it is associated with airway inflammation.

The sequence of cellular and protein changes after a late asthmatic reaction induced by plicatic acid was studied in 44 patients with red cedar asthma by BAL, and the results were compared with 31 healthy subjects.[72] The late asthmatic reaction was found to be associated with an increase in eosinophils in the lavage fluid, an increase in sloughing of bronchial epithelial cells, and an increase in albumin in the lavage fluid. Although there was a slight but significant increase in neutrophils 48 hours after challenge, neutrophil infiltration was not a prominent feature earlier. Multiple bronchial biopsies were performed in three of the patients 24 hours after inhalation challenge. Biopsy tissue showed denudation of the bronchial epithelium, a thickened basement membrane, and infiltration of eosinophils in the bronchial epithelium and submucosa (Fig. 14-1).

Patients with isocyanate-induced asthma were studied by Fabbri and associates.[73-75] They measured airway hyperresponsiveness and determined the degree of airway inflammation by BAL during the late asthmatic reaction and compared the results with those from patients who developed an isolated immediate asthmatic reaction induced by TDI challenge. In subjects with a late asthmatic reaction, neutrophils were increased at both 2 and 8 hours after challenge, and eosinophils and airway hyperresponsiveness were increased only at 8 hours. Neutrophils, eosinophils, and airway hyperresponsiveness were not increased at 8 hours after TDI challenge in subjects with an isolated

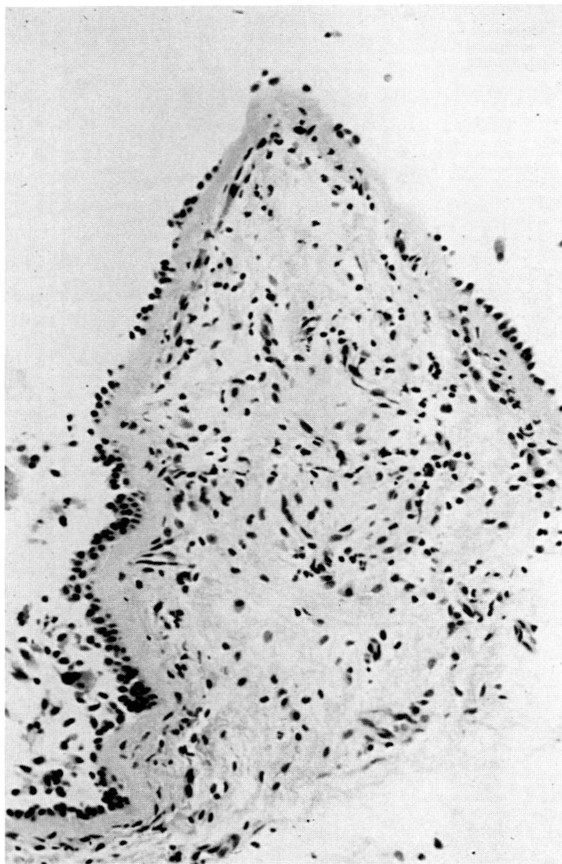

Figure 14-1. Bronchial biopsy sample from a patient with red cedar asthma. In this late asthmatic reaction denudation of the epithelium, thickening of the basement membrane, and cellular infiltration are apparent. (Reproduced from J Allergy Clin Immunol, 1987;80:47.)

immediate asthmatic reaction.[73] These results again suggest that late asthmatic reactions to TDI and the associated airway hyperresponsiveness may be caused by airway inflammation. Further evidence of the importance of airway inflammation was provided by another study by the same group of investigators.[74,75] They found that prednisone inhibited both the late asthmatic reaction and the associated increase in airway hyperresponsiveness induced by TDI in sensitized subjects. The inhibition by prednisone was accompanied by the absence of neutrophilia and an increase in albumin in BAL fluid after inhalation challenge with TDI.[75] In a more recent study of patients with red cedar asthma, inflammatory mediators—predominantly histamine, PGD_2, PGE_2, and LTE_4— were found in the BAL fluid during immediate asthmatic reactions induced by plicatic acid challenge[76]; BAL during late asthmatic reactions also showed an increase in inflammatory mediators (unpublished preliminary observation). These findings of airway inflammation and the release of inflammatory mediators during bronchoconstriction induced by occupational agents resemble the findings in bronchoconstriction induced by nonoccupational allergens.

RISK FACTORS

Environment

Many patients with isocyanate-induced asthma develop symptoms after accidental exposure to high levels of TDI.[77] There appears to be a relationship between the degree of exposure and the prevalence of sensitization and development of asthma. The studies on the prevalence of red cedar asthma in sawmills provide excellent examples.[78,79] Once sensitized, however, subjects develop symptoms on exposure to very low levels of the sensitizing agent. Patients with TDI-induced asthma often react to 0.001 or 0.005 ppm TDI on inhalation challenge tests, levels much lower than the permissible limit of 0.02 ppm.[63]

Host Factors

Given the same levels of exposure, only a proportion of subjects developed occupational asthma, suggesting that host factors are important. Very little is known about the predisposing host factors. The few important ones will be discussed.

Atopy

In general, atopy appears to be an important risk factor for occupational asthma due to high molecular weight compounds. Most epidemiologic studies confirm this observation. Newhouse and co-workers[80] studied 103 workers exposed to enzyme detergent and found a strong association between atopy, as defined by either personal or family history of allergy or skin test positivity to common inhalant allergens, and specific sensitization. Mitchell and Gandevia[81] found that atopy correlated strongly with specific skin test response to enzyme detergent but not with work-related symptoms. Among laboratory workers exposed to animals, Slovak and Hill[82] and Cockcroft and co-workers[83] demonstrated an association between atopy and work-related asthma.

Atopy, however, is not an important risk factor in asthma due to low molecular weight compounds. Chan-Yeung and co-workers[84] found the prevalence of airway hyperresponsiveness to be higher in workers exposed to western red cedar than in a control group of civic workers. The increase in airway hyperresponsiveness was entirely limited to the nonatopic group. However, in a group of workers exposed to tetrachlorophthalic anhydride, another low molecular weight compound, Venables and associates[85] found an association between atopy and sensitization to the anhydride (presence of specific IgE antibodies to conjugate of the anhydride). The relationship between atopy and occupational asthma appears to be dependent on the specific agent responsible for the asthma.

Smoking

The role of cigarette smoking in the development of occupational sensitization and asthma is not known. It has been postulated that there is an increase in epithelial permeability among smokers, thus allowing greater penetration of antigens.[86] Cigarette smoking was not associated with work-related symptoms among workers exposed to detergent enzymes,[81] laboratory animals,[82] and colophony[87]. However, Venables and colleagues[85] found an interaction between cigarette smoking and atopy in workers exposed to tetrachlorophthalic anhydride. Atopic smokers had the highest prevalence of sensitization (16%) and nonatopic nonsmokers the lowest (0%). This study was confined to the prevalence of sensitization and did not consider work-related symptoms.

Most patients with red cedar asthma[88] and isocyanate-induced asthma[89] were found to be life-long nonsmokers; only a small proportion were current smokers. This suggests that nonsmokers are more susceptible. Moreover, among workers exposed to red cedar dust, the prevalence of airway hyperresponsiveness was not related to smoking.[84]

Airway Hyperresponsiveness

The majority of patients with symptomatic occupational asthma had demonstrable airway hyperresponsiveness.[90] There is no good evidence to suggest that airway hyperresponsiveness is a risk factor for the development of occupational asthma. In fact, most of the evidence suggests airway hyperresponsiveness is acquired as a result of exposure. Lam and co-workers[90] found a progressive decrease in airway hyperresponsiveness among patients with red cedar asthma who recovered after the cessation of exposure. They also found an increase in airway hyperresponsiveness after development of a late asthmatic reaction induced by inhalation test in the same group of patients. Longitudinal studies with sufficient power to test whether pre-existing airway hyperresponsiveness predisposes to eventual development of occupational asthma following exposure are needed.

MANAGEMENT APPROACH

In approaching a patient suspected to be suffering from occupational asthma, it is necessary first to establish the diagnosis of asthma and then to establish that the asthma is due to occupational exposure. The diagnosis of asthma has been covered in Chapter 13.

To establish that the patient's asthma is due to occupational exposure, it is essential to take a careful and detailed history of the patient's working environment. Careful inquiry is necessary concerning not only the materials the patient is working with but also those being used by his co-workers. There are certain clues in the history that are useful. There is usually a latent period between the patient's first exposure to the offending agent and the onset of asthma. This may vary from a few weeks to over 20 years. A patient who develops symptoms immediately every time he or she works with the same substance usually recognizes the causal relationship. However, a large number of substances, particularly low molecular weight compounds, give rise to late asthmatic reactions. The patient usually complains of chest symptoms after working hours, in the evenings, and at night but not during the working hours initially. In these instances, the causal relationship between exposure and symptoms is less easily recognized. Symptoms that are worse on work days and better on weekends and holidays suggest a work relationship.

It is important to document objectively that the patient's asthmatic symptoms are related to occupational exposure. Specific inhalation challenge tests or occupational exposure tests are often considered as the "gold standard" for the diagnosis of occupational asthma. There are very few centers where inhalation tests are regularly carried out for the investigation of such patients. For clinicians without access to such facilities, the following methods are often used to establish a causal relationship:

1. Measurement of lung function before and after a work shift. This test is not very helpful in establishing a causal relationship between symptoms and work exposure. Burge and associates[91] found that only 20% of patients with occupational asthma due to colophony showed a significant drop in FEV_1 ($>10\%$) over one work shift, while 10% of the subjects without occupational asthma also showed a similar degree of fall in FEV_1 after a shift.

2. Prolonged recording of the peak expiratory flow rate (PEFR) by the patient at work and at home. This has been found by several investigators[91–93] to be a good method of establishing a causal relationship between work exposure and asthma, since serial measurements of lung function give a better assessment of the patient than only one or two measurements. The patient is asked to do readings every 2 hours from waking to sleep; the record should be kept for at least 2 to 3 weeks at work followed by 10 days off work. Improvement in symptoms and peak expiratory flow rates when away from work and recurrence of symptoms and deterioration in peak expiratory flow rates on return to work confirm that the symptoms are due to an adverse work environment. Serial measurements of airway hyperresponsiveness when away from work and on return to work provide further evidence of sensitization if there is an increase in airway hyperresponsiveness on return to work.[92]

Inhalation challenge tests in a laboratory with the suspected substance and an appropriate control substance will demonstrate asthma due to sensitization. These tests are time consuming and are not devoid of danger. They should be performed by experienced personnel in hospital settings where resuscitation facilities are available and frequent observations can be made. The methods of specific challenge test and the types of asthmatic reaction induced have been described in detail by Pepys and Hutchcroft[94] and will not be described here (Fig. 14-2).

Is specific challenge testing the "gold standard" for confirming occupational asthma? In subjects who develop an asthmatic reaction with a greater than 15% fall in FEV_1 following an exposure to a subirritant level of the offending agent, the diagnosis of occupational asthma can be firmly established. However, absence of a reaction to challenge testing does not exclude the diagnosis of occupational asthma with certainty. First, the patient may have left the workplace for a long time and lost the sensitivity to the offending agent. This has been shown in patients with isocyanate-induced asthma.[95] It is therefore important to assess the patient as early as possible when occupational asthma is suspected. The patient should not be told to resign from the job until the diagnosis has been confirmed. Second, there may be other chemicals or substances in the workplace that can cause sensitization and have not been tested. It is not uncommon to find formaldehyde, isocyanate, and furanes present together in a work environment.[96] Third, the testing method may not be correct for the offending agent. In the laboratory it is often difficult to reproduce exactly the process in the workplace; this was examplified by a study of workers with occupational asthma due to oil mist.[97]

Skin tests and tests for specific IgE antibodies in vitro are available for only a few causes of occupational asthma. It should be remembered that a positive test result only indicates sensitization to a particular agent. When a worker is found to be sensitized

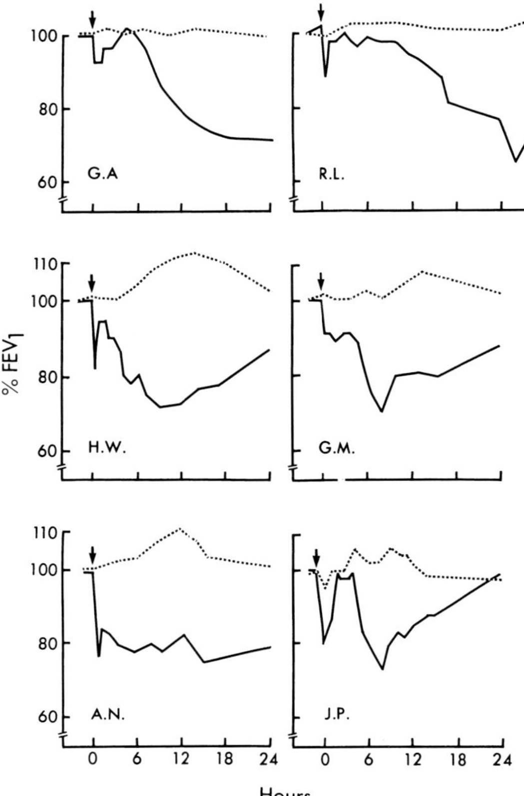

Figure 14-2. Patterns of asthmatic reaction to diphenylmethane diisocyanate (MDI) challenge in six subjects: formaldehyde challenge (---), MDI challenge (—). Arrow indicates time of challenge. (Reprinted with permission of the American Review of Respiratory Disease 1983;128:226–230.)

but has no asthma, there is no justification for recommending a change of job. On the other hand, a negative test result in a patient with occupational asthma does not exclude the diagnosis.

PROGNOSIS

There are now many studies confirming that most patients with occupational asthma do not recover after the removal from exposure.[89,95,98–102] The most important prognostic factor for a favorable outcome is early diagnosis and early removal from exposure.[98,102] The majority of patients who opted to remain in the same job deteriorated.[89,103] Attempts to reduce the degree of exposure by a transfer to a less dusty job or by the use of respirators were not found to be helpful in preventing the worsening of symptoms in patients with red cedar asthma.[103]

One fatal case has been reported in the medical literature[104] of a patient with documented isocyanate-induced asthma who continued to work using a respirator after the diagnosis was made. Another death was reported in an industrial journal[105] of a worker in a garage after he had used a two-pack polyurethane paint.

THERAPY

Since most occupational agents have "sensitizing" properties, it is logical to assume that exposure to minute quantities of these agents can induce an attack of asthma in "sensitized" subjects. The report of fatal cases despite respiratory protection should leave no doubt that patients with occupational asthma must be advised to avoid exposure to the offending agent. Drug treatment of occupational asthma is not different from that offered to patients with nonoccupational asthma.

REFERENCES

1. Karr RM, Davis RJ, Butcher BT, Lehrer SB, Wilson MR, Dharmarajan V, Salvaggio JE. Occupational asthma. J Allergy Clin Immunol, 1978;61:54–64.
2. Zuskin E, Wolfson RL, Harpel G, et al. Byssinosis in carding and spinning workers. Arch Environ Health, 1979;19:666–675.
3. Newman-Taylor A, Longbottom JL, Pepys J. Respiratory allergy to urine proteins of rats and mice. Lancet, 1977;ii:847–849.
4. Brooks SM. Bronchial asthma of occupational origin. Scand J Work Environ Health, 1977;3: 53–72.
5. NIOSH Criteria for a Recommended Standard: Occupational exposure to diisocyanates. U.S. Dept of Health, Education, and Welfare. PHS CDC Publication, No. 78-215, September 1978.
6. Chan-Yeung M, Ashley MJ, Corey P, Willson G, Dorken E, Grzybowski S. A respiratory survey of cedar mill workers: I. Prevalence of symptoms and lung function abnormalities. J Occup Med, 1978;20:328–332.
7. Figley KD. Mayfly (*Ephemerida*) hypersensitivity. J Allergy, 1940;11:376–387.
8. Gandevia B. Occupational asthma I. Med J Aust, 1970;2:332–335.
9. Horton DJ, Chen WY. Effects of breathing warm humidified air on bronchoconstriction induced by body cooling and by inhalation of methacholine. Chest, 1979;75:24–28.
10. Widdicombe JT, Kent DC, Nadel JA. Mechanisms of bronchoconstriction during inhalation of dust. J Appl Physiol, 1962;17:613–616.
11. Frank NR, Amdur MO, Worcester J, Whitenberger JL. Effects of acute controlled exposure to SO_2 on respiratory mechanics in healthy male adults. J Appi Physiol, 1962;17:252–258.
12. Charan NB, Myers CG, Lakshminarayan S, Spencer TM. Pulmonary injuries associated with acute sulphur dioxide inhalation. Am Rev Respir Dis, 1979;119:555–560.
13. Harkonen H, Nordman H, Korhonen O, Winblad I. Long term effects of exposure to sulphur dioxide: Lung function four years after a pyrite dust explosion. Am Rev Respir Dis, 1983;128:890–893.
14. Flury KE, Dines DE, Rodarte JR, Rodgers R. Airway obstruction due to inhalation of ammonia. Mayo Clin Proc, 1983;58:389–393.
15. Hasan FM, Gehshan A, Fulechan FJD. Resolution of pulmonary dysfunction following acute chlorine exposure. Arch Environ Health, 1983;38:76–80.
16. Kaufman J, Burkons D. Clinical roentgenologic and physiologic effects of acute chlorine exposure. Arch Environ Health, 1971;23:29–34.
17. Whitener DR, Whitener LM, Robertson KG, Baxter CR, Pierce AK. Pulmonary function measurements in patients with thermal injury and smoke inhalation. Am Rev Respir Dis, 1980;122:731–739.
18. Galea M. Fatal sulfur dioxide inhalation. Can Med Assoc J, 1964;91:345.
19. Brooks SM, Weiss MA, Bernstein IL. Reactive airways dysfunction syndrome (RADS): Persistent airways hyperreactivity after high level irritant exposure. Chest, 1985;88:376–384.

20. Boulet LP. Increases in airway responsiveness following acute exposure to respiratory irritants. Chest, 1988;94:476–481.
21. Schilling RSF. Byssinosis in cotton and other textile workers. Lancet, 1956;ii:261–265.
22. Berry G, McKerrow CB, Molyneux MKB, Rossiter CE, Tombleson JBL. A study of acute and chronic changes in ventilatory capacity of workers in Lancashire cotton mills. Br J Ind Med, 1974;31:18–27.
23. Merchant JA, Lumsden JL, Kilburn KH, et al. Dose response studies in cotton textile workers. J Occup Med, 1973;15:220–230.
24. Castellan RM, Olenchock SA, Hankinson J, et al. Acute bronchoconstriction induced by cotton dust: Dose-related response to endotoxin and other dust factors. Ann Intern Med, 1984;101:157–163.
25. Massoud AAW, Altounyan RS, Howell JBL, Lane RE. Effect of histamine aerosol in byssinotic subjects. Br J Ind Med, 1967;24:38–40.
26. Schacter NE, Brown S, Zuskin E, Buck E, Kolack B, Bouhuys A. Airway reactivity in cotton bract–induced bronchospasm. Am Rev Respir Dis, 1981;123:273–276.
27. Jones RN, Butcher BT, Hammad YY, et al. Interaction of atopy and exposure to cotton dust in the bronchoconstrictor response. Br J Ind Med, 1980;37:141–146.
28. Imbus HR, Suh MW. Byssinosis. Arch Environ Health, 1973;26:183–191.
29. Jones RN, Diem JE, Glindmeyer H, Dharmarajan V, Hammad YY, Carr J, Weill H. Mill effect and dose-response relationship in byssinosis. Br J Ind Med, 1979;36:305–313.
30. Bouhuys A, Londell SE. Release of histamine by cotton dust extract from human lung tissues in vitro. Experientia, 1961;17:211–215.
31. Butcher BT, O'Neill CE, Jones RN. The respiratory effects of cotton dust. In: Salvaggio JE, Stankus RP, eds. Clinics in chest medicine, vol. 4.1. Philadelphia: W. B. Saunders, 1983;63–70.
32. Noweir MH. Highlights of broad spectrum industrial-hygiene research activities in a developing country—Egypt. Am Ind Hyg Assoc J, 1979;40:839–859.
33. Rylander RK, Imbus HR, Suh MW. Bacterial contamination of cotton as an indicator of respiratory effects among cardroom workers. Br J Ind Med, 1979;36:299–304.
34. Pernis B, Vigliani EC, Cavagna C, Finulli M. The role of bacterial endotoxins in occupational diseases caused by inhaling vegetable dusts. Br J Ind Med, 1961;18:120–129.
35. Buck MG, Schachter EN, Wall JH. Partial composition of a low molecular weight cotton bract extract which induces acute airway constriction in humans. In: Wakekyn PE, ed. Proceedings of the Sixth Cotton Dust Research Conference. Memphis, Tenn: National Cotton Council, 1982;19–23.
36. Chan-Yeung M, Enarson D, Grzybowski S. Grain dust and respiratory health. Can Med Assoc J, 1985;133:969–973.
37. Corey P, Hutcheon M, Broder I, Mintz S. Grain elevator workers show work-related pulmonary function changes and dose-effect relationship with dust exposure. Br J Ind Med, 1982;39:330–337.
38. Enarson D, Vedal S, Chan-Yeung M. Fate of grainhandlers with bronchial hyperreactivity. Clin Invest Med, 1988;11:193–197.
39. Chan-Yeung M, Chan H, Salari H, Walls R, Tse KS. Grain dust–induced release of chemical mediators. J Allergy Clin Immunol, 1987;80:279–284.
40. Olenchock SA, Mull JC, Major P. Extracts of airborne grain dust activate alternative and classical complement pathway. Ann Allergy, 1980;44:23–28.
41. O'Neil C, Butcher B, Chan H. Chan-Yeung M. Comparison of aqueous grain dust, cotton dust, mold extracts by cross-immunoelectrophoretic technique. Int Arch Allergy Immunol, 1988;85:116–118.
42. Chan-Yeung M. Grain dust asthma: Does it exist? In: Dosman JA, Cockcroft DW, eds: Handbook of health and safety in agriculture. Boca Raton, FL: CRC Press, 1989;169–171.

43. Chan-Yeung M, Wong R, MacLean L. Respiratory abnormalities among grain elevator workers. Chest, 1979;75:461–467.
44. Weiner A. Bronchial asthma due to organic phosphate insecticide. Ann Allergy, 1961;19:397–401.
45. Davies RJ, Butcher BT, O'Neil CE, Salvaggio JE. The in vitro effect of toluene diisocyanate on lymphocyte cyclic adenosine monophosphate production by isoproterenol, prostaglandin, and histamine: A possible mode of action. J Allergy Clin Immunol, 1977;60:223–229.
46. Chan-Yeung M, Giclas P, Henson P. Activation of the complement system by plicatic acid: The chemical compound responsible for asthma due to western red cedar (*Thuja plicata*). J Allergy Clin Immunol, 1980;65:333–337.
47. Chan-Yeung M, Lam S. State of the art: Occupational asthma. Am Rev Respir Dis, 1986;133:686–703.
48. Parkes WR. Occupational asthma (including byssinosis). In: Occupational lung disorders, 2nd ed. Butterworth, London, 1982;415–453.
49. Gross NJ. Allergy to laboratory animals: Epidemiologic, clinical, and physiologic aspects and a trial of cromolyn in its management. J Allergy Clin Immunol, 1980;66:158–166.
50. Thiel H, Ulmer WNT. Baker's asthma: Development and possibility of treatment. Chest, 1986;133:686–703.
51. Block G, Tse KS, Kijek K, Chan H, Chan-Yeung M. Baker's asthma: Clinical and immunological studies. Clin Allergy, 1983;13:359–370.
52. Granz T, McMurrain KD, Brooks S, Bernstein IL. Clinical, immunologic, and physiologic observations in factory workers exposed to *B subtilis* enzyme dust. J Allergy, 1971;42:170–180.
53. Baur X, Konig G, Bencze K, Fruhmann G. Clinical symptoms and results of skin test, RAST and bronchial provocation test in thirty-three papain workers: Evidence for strong immunogenic potency and clinically relevant "proteolytic effects of airborne papain." Clin Allergy, 1983;12:9–17.
54. Cartier A, Malo JL, Forest F, Lafrance M, et al. Occupational asthma in snow crab processing worker. J Allergy Clin Immunol, 1984;74:261–269.
55. Maccia CA, Bernstein IL, Emmett EA, Brooks SM. In vitro demonstration of specific IgE in phthalic anhydride hypersensitivity. Am Rev Respir Dis, 1976;113:701–704.
56. Zeiss CR, Patterson R, Pruzansky JJ, Miller M, Rosenberg M, Levitz D. Trimellitic anhydride–induced airway syndromes: Clinical and immunologic studies. J Allergy Clin Immunol, 1977;60:96–103.
57. Patterson R, Addington W, Banner A, et al. Anti-hapten antibodies in workers exposed to trimellitic anhydride fumes: A potential immunopathogenetic mechanism for the trimellitic anhydride pulmonary disease-anemia syndrome. Am Rev Respir Dis, 1979;120:1259–1267.
58. Patterson R, Zeiss CR, Roberts M, Pruzansky JJ, Wolkonsky P, Chacon R. Human antihapten antibodies in trimellitic anhydride inhalation reactions: Immunoglobulin classes of anti-trimellitic anhydride antibodies and hapten inhibition studies. J Clin Invest, 1979;62:971–978.
59. Howe W, Venables KM, Topping MD, et al. Tetrachlorophthalic anhydride asthma: Evidence for specific IgE antibodies. J Allergy Clin Immunol, 1983;71:5–11.
60. Pepys J, Pickering CAC, Hughes EG. Asthma due to inhaled chemical agents: Complex salts of platinum. Clin Allergy, 1972;2:391–396.
61. Pezzini A, Riviera A, Paggiaro P, et al. Specific IgE antibodies in twenty-eight workers with diisocyanate-induced asthma. Clin Allergy, 1984;14:453–461.
62. Danks JM, Cromwell O, Buckingham JA, Newman-Taylor AJ, Davies RJ. Toluene-diisocyanate induced asthma: Evaluation of antibodies in the serum of affected workers against a tolyl mono-isocyanate protein conjugate. Clin Allergy, 1981;11:161–168.
63. Banks DE, Sastre J, Butcher B, Ellis E, Rando R, Barkman HW, Hammad YY, Glindmeyer HW, Weill H. Role of inhalation challenge testing in the diagnosis of isocyanate-induced asthma. Chest, 1989;95:414–423.

64. Chan-Yeung M. Immunologic and nonimmunologic mechanisms in asthma due to western red cedar (*Thuja plicata*). J Allergy Clin Immunol, 1983;70:32–37.

65. Chen SE, Bernstein IL. The guinea pig model of diisocyanate sensitization. I: Immunological studies. J Allergy Clin Immunol, 1983;70:383–392.

66. Chan H, Tse H, Oostdam J, Moreno R, Pare P, Chan-Yeung M. A rabbit model of hypersensitivity to plicatic acid, the agent responsible for red cedar asthma. J Allergy Clin Immunol, 1987;79:762–767.

67. Kaliner M. Hypothesis on the contribution of late-phase allergic responses to the understanding and treatment of allergic diseases. J Allergy Clin Immunol, 1984;73:311–315.

68. Gravelyn TR, Pan PM, Eschenbacker WL. Mediator release in an isolated airway segment in subjects with asthma. Am Rev Respir Dis, 1988;137:641–646.

69. Wenzel SE, Westcott JY, Smith HR, Larsen GL. Spectrum of prostanoid release after bronchoalveolar allergen challenge in atopic asthmatics and in control groups. Am Rev Respir Dis, 1989;139:450–457.

70. Diaz P, Gonzalez MC, Galleguillos FR, Ancic P, Cromwell O, Shepherd D, Durham SR, Gleich GJ, Kay AB. Leukocytes and mediators in bronchoalvolar lavage during allergen-induced late-phase asthmatic reactions. Am Rev Respir Dis, 1989;139:1383–1389.

71. Lam S, Al-Majed S, Chan H, Salari H, Tse K, LeRiche JC, Chan-Yeung M. Factors which determine the occurrence of asthma in atopic subjects. J Allergy Clin Immunol, 1990 (in press).

72. Lam S, LeRiche J, Phillips D, Chan-Yeung M. Cellular and protein changes in bronchial lavage fluid after late asthmatic reaction in patients with red cedar asthma. J Allergy Clin Immunol, 1987;80:44–50.

73. Fabbri LM, Boschetto P, Zocca E, Milani G, Pivirotto F, Plebani M, Burlina A, Licata B, Mapp CE. Bronchoalveolar neutrophilia during late asthmatic reactions induced by toluene diisocyanate. Am Rev Respir Dis, 1987;136:36–42.

74. Fabbri LM, Chiesure-Corona P, DalVecchio L, DiGiacoma GR, Zocca E, DeMarzo N, Maestrelli P, Mapp CE. Prednisone inhibits late asthmatic reactions and the associated increase in airway hyperresponsiveness induced by toluene-diisocyanate in sensitized subjects. Am Rev Respir Dis, 1985;132:1010–1014.

75. Boschetto P, Fabbri LM, Zocca E, Milani G, Pivirotto F, DalVecchio A, Plebani M, Mapp C. Prednisone inhibits late asthmatic reactions and airway inflammation induced by toluene diisocyanate in sensitized subjects. J Allergy Clin Immunol, 1987;80:261–267.

76. Chan-Yeung M, Chan H, Salari H, Lam S. Histamine, leukotrienes and prostaglandins release in bronchial fluid during plicatic acid-induced bronchoconstriction. J Allergy Clin Immunol, 1989;84:762–768.

77. Karol M. Survey of industrial workers for antibodies to toluene diisocyanate. J Occup Med, 1981;23:741–747.

78. Vedal S, Enarson D, Kus J, McCormack G, MacLean L, Chan-Yeung M. Symptoms and pulmonary function in western red cedar workers related to duration of employment and dust exposure. Arch Environ Health, 1986;41:179–184.

79. Brooks SM, Edwards JJ, Agol A, Edwards FH. An epidemiologic study of workers exposed to western red cedar and other wood dusts. Chest, 1981;80:30–32S.

80. Newhouse ML, Tagg B, Pocock SJ, McEwan AC. An epidemiology study of workers producing enzyme washing powder. Lancet, 1970;i:689–692.

81. Mitchell CA, Gandevia B. Respiratory symptoms and skin reactivity in workers exposed to proteolytic enzymes in the detergent industry. Am Rev Respir Dis, 1971;104:1–12.

82. Slovak AJM, Hill RN. Laboratory animal allergy: A clinical survey of an exposed population. Br J Ind Med, 1981;38:38–41.

83. Cockcroft A, McCarthy P, Edwards J, Andersson N. Allergy in laboratory animal workers. Lancet, 1981;i:825–830.

84. Chan-Yeung M, Vedal S, Kus J, MacLean J, Enarson DA, Tse KS. Symptoms, pulmonary function, and bronchial hyperreactivity in western red cedar workers compared with those in office workers. Am Rev Respir Dis, 1984;40:53–57.

85. Venables KM, Topping MD, Howe W, Luczynski CM, Hawkins R, Newman-Taylor AJ. Interaction of smoking and atopy in producing specific IgE antibody against a hapten protein conjugate. Br Med J, 1985;290:201–204.

86. Leskowitz S, Salvaggio JE, Schwarz HJ. An hypothesis for the development of atopic allergy in man. Clin Allergy, 1972;2;237–246.

87. Burge PS, Perks WH, O'Brien IM, et al. Occupational asthma in an electronics factory: A case control study to evaluate aetiological factors. Thorax, 1979;34:300–307.

88. Chan-Yeung M, Lam S, Kerner S. Clinical features and natural history of occupational asthma due to western red cedar (*Thuja plicata*). Am J Med, 1982;72:411–415.

89. Paggiaro PL, Loi AM, Rosso O, et al. Follow up study of patients with respiratory disease due to toluene diisocyanate (TDI). Clin Allergy, 1984;14:463–469.

90. Lam S, Wong, Chan-Yeung M. Nonspecific bronchial reactivity in occupational asthma. J Allergy Clin Immunol, 1979;63:28–34.

91. Burge PS. Single and serial measurements of lung function in the diagnosis of occupational asthma. Eur J Respir Dis, 1982;63 (suppl 123):47–59.

92. Cartier A, Pineau L, Malo JL. Monitoring of maximum peak expiratory flow rates and histamine inhalation tests in the investigation of occupational asthma. Clin Allergy, 1984;14:193–196.

93. Cote J, Kennedy S, Chan-Yeung M. Sensitivity and specificity of pCO_2 and PEFR in cedar asthma. J Allergy Clin Immunol, 1990;85:592–598.

94. Pepys J, Hutchcroft BJ. Bronchial provocation tests in etiologic diagnosis and analysis of asthma. Am Rev Respir Dis, 1975;112:829–859.

95. Mapp CE, Corona PC, DeMarzo N, Fabbri L. A follow-up study of subjects with occupational asthma due to toluene diisocyanate (TDI). Am Rev Respir Dis, 1988;137:1326–1329.

96. Burge PS, Harries MG, Lam WK, O'Brien IM, Patchett PA. Occupational asthma due to formaldehyde. Thorax, 1985;40:255–260.

97. Robertson AS, Weir DC, Burge PS. Occupational asthma due to oil mists. Thorax, 1988;43:200–205.

98. Chan-Yeung M, MacLean L, Paggiaro PL. A follow-up of 232 patients with occupational asthma due to western red cedar (*Thuja plicata*). J Allergy Clin Immunol, 1987;79:792–796.

99. Moller DR, McKay RT, Bernstein IL, Brooks S. Long term follow up of workers with TDI asthma. Am Rev Respir Dis, 1984;129:A159.

100. Lozewicz S, Assoufi BK, Hawkins R, Newman-Taylor AJ. Outcome of asthma induced by isocyanates. Br J Dis Chest, 1987;81:14–22.

101. Burge PS. Occupational asthma in electronic workers caused by colophony fumes: Follow-up of affected workers. Thorax, 1982;37:348–353.

102. Hudson P, Cartier A, Pineau L, Lafrance M, St. Aubin JJ, Dubois JY, Malo JL. Follow-up of occupational asthma caused by crab and various agents. J Allergy Clin Immunol, 1985;76:262–268.

103. Cote J, Kennedy SM, Chan-Yeung M. Outcome of patients with cedar asthma with continuous exposure. Am Rev Respir Dis, 1990;141:373–376.

104. Fabbri LM, Danieli D, Crescioli S, Bevilacqua P, Meli S, Saetta M, Mapp CE. Fatal asthma in a subject sensitized to toluene diisocyanate. Am Rev Respir Dis, 1988;137:1494–1498.

105. Incident reports: Car paint death. Toxic Substances Bulletin, December 1985;4:7.

15

Allergic Bronchopulmonary Aspergillosis

Paul F. Detjen
Paul A. Greenberger
Roy Patterson

Allergic bronchopulmonary aspergillosis (ABPA) is an immunologically mediated lung disease that occurs predominantly but not exclusively in atopic patients with asthma and that can be superimposed on a wide clinical spectrum ranging from mild to severe corticosteroid-dependent asthma. First described in 1952 by Hinson and associates[1] and initially thought to be a rare disease, ABPA is now recognized internationally to be an emerging and important disease in which the immunologic, radiologic, and pathologic findings and clinical sequelae range from minimal symptoms to fatal pulmonary fibrosis.

BACKGROUND

Hinson, Moon, and Plummer's classic 1952 paper described three adult patients aged 37, 45, and 55 years with severe asthma who, for periods ranging from months to years, had suffered from "pyrexial attacks" associated with severe cough, purulent "stained" sputum, dyspnea, and vague chest discomfort.[1] One patient was a farmer's wife who handled and fed chickens; another was a schoolmistress who just prior to her first attack had used "hop manure" in her garden (from which *Aspergillus fumigatus* was later cultured). The third patient, a 37-year-old male, had worked in a flour mill and subsequently developed asthma. One of the patients died in status asthmaticus. In all three, chest roentgenograms demonstrated episodic lobar and segmental collapse, with consolidation, that persisted from 4 to 6 weeks or longer and left residual scars after gradually resolving. Sputum was purulent and showed white or brownish flecks barely visible to the naked eye. Microscopic studies of the sputum showed plugs of mycelia aggregated with Charcot-Leyden crystals (lysophospholipase), Curschmann's spirals, mucus, and eosinophils. The blood eosinophil counts in these patients were always greater than 1000 per mm^3 and ranged from 2000 to 4200 per mm^3 during attacks.

Bronchoscopy identified mucus plugs within bronchi leading to affected segments, from which A. *fumigatus* was cultured. Histologic sections of bronchial biopsy specimens did not show invasion of the organism. The diagnostic criteria suggested by Hinson and colleagues were recurrent pyrexial attacks with pulmonary infiltrates, eosinophilia, and purulent sputum containing A. *fumigatus*. They found bronchiectasis in two of the three patients but did not require it for diagnosis. They postulated hypersensitivity to A. *fumigatus* as the cause.[1] Many of these findings have come to typify ABPA, although more specific diagnostic criteria are now available and additional immunopathologic data have come to light.

In 1968, the first North American case of ABPA was described in a 27-year-old botanist with asthma, episodic bilateral pulmonary infiltrates, eosinophilia, positive immediate and late (Arthus-type) skin reactivity to *Aspergillus* mix, and positive results on precipitin testing.[2] In addition, passive serum transfer from human to primate gave a positive immediate reaction on cutaneous *Aspergillus* antigen challenge, consistent with passive transfer of IgE.[2] Treatment with prednisone resulted in improvement in the patient's condition, attenuation of immediate skin reactivity, and loss of precipitating antibody to *Aspergillus*.[2] Thus, at least two immunologic mechanisms were implicated in the pathogenesis of the lung destruction seen with ABPA: reaginic and precipitating antibodies, now known as IgE and IgG, respectively. In 1971, McCarthy and Pepys showed that 111 of 143 patients with "pulmonary eosinophilia" fulfilled some of the criteria for ABPA, thus bringing to the forefront the potential magnitude of this disease.[3]

THE ORGANISM

Aspergillus species are ubiquitous, commonly being found in potting soil, decaying organic matter, compost heaps, spoiled hay and grain, and rotting wood. They were originally described by an Italian priest, Micheli, in 1729.[4] He was the first to describe the separate stalk (conidiophore) and spore head (vesicle) from which the conidia (spores) are borne.[5] This pattern resembled in structure the aspergillium used for sprinkling holy water, which gave the fungus its name.[5]

The spores are widely disseminated in the environment, and in fact sometimes contaminate laboratory cultures. Consequently, absolute avoidance is not possible. Most species are thermotolerant and are capable of growing at temperatures from 15°C to 53°C. Aspergilli may represent the dominant fungus in high-temperature compost heaps—up to 70% of the total, according to some authors.[5] *Aspergillus* species can be cultured on Sabouraud's dextrose agar slants when incubated at 37°C to 40°C. Earlier substrates for culture media included brewery wort, white bean extract, potato or carrot plugs, licorice root, string beans, and manure preparations. Hyphae are 7 to 10 μm in diameter and septate. They branch at a 45-degree angle. Individual spores are 2 to 3.5 μm in diameter.[5] *Aspergillus* species are the only molds used as fermentation starters for soybean.[5,6]

Aspergillus long has been known as a major respiratory pathogen for domesticated fowl. Outbreaks of "brooder pneumonia" in newly hatched chicks have in the past caused up to 90% mortality in chickens, 50% in turkeys.[7,8] The economic effects in the agricultural industry continue to be significant: 5% to 10% of turkey poults die of avian aspergillosis. Spontaneous abortions are also known to result from *Aspergillus* infections in sheep. *A. fumigatus* is the species that infects humans most frequently. Great quantities of spores are released from disturbed moldy hay, compost piles, and other sources of decaying organic matter, and in some locales small numbers of spores have been identified in the atmosphere year-round.[9] There have been correlations between seasonal elevations in atmospheric mold counts and exacerbations of ABPA in the United States and England.[10]

ASPERGILLUS-ASSOCIATED RESPIRATORY DISEASES

The *Aspergillus* organism can interact with the human host in several ways other than ABPA, depending on the genetic and immunologic status of the patient. All of the respiratory diseases noted below occur in the setting of an altered or hypersensitive immune response, altered or damaged anatomy, or a general decline in the patient's level of immunologic competence.

IgE-Mediated Asthma

Patients with IgE-mediated asthma demonstrate immediate cutaneous reactivity to *Aspergillus* extract and have clinical symptoms of bronchospasm when exposed to the inhaled antigen. This is in contrast to many patients with asthma whose positive skin reactivity is not correlated with clinical symptoms or findings. IgE-mediated asthma does not fulfill the criteria for allergic bronchopulmonary aspergillosis.

Invasive Disseminated Aspergillosis

Immunocompromised or debilitated patients (e.g., those with AIDS or leukopenia) can have bronchial wall invasion by overgrowth of aspergilli resulting in pneumonia, abscesses, mycetoma, metastatic septic emboli, and, characteristically, central nervous system infections. The fungus is angioinvasive and can cause infarction of involved organs. This picture contrasts with aspergilloma, ABPA, and other conditions, in which bronchial wall invasion and septicemia do not occur.

Aspergilloma

Within damaged pulmonary parenchyma (caused by, for example, bronchiectasis, cavitary lung disease, previous tuberculosis, cystic fibrosis, or lung cancer) *Aspergillus* hyphae can grow into a complex tangled mass called a fungus ball or aspergilloma,[11] which can be identified by its dependent position on decubitus chest films. In contrast to ABPA, there is no hypersensitivity or systemic response to the aspergilli in this condition, and hemoptysis is the most common symptom.

Hypersensitivity Pneumonitis

Inhalation of a variety of organic dusts or environmental antigens by both atopic and nonatopic patients can cause hypersensitivity pneumonitis, the manifestations of which depend on the patients' immunologic responsiveness, the intensity of the exposure, and the antigenicity of the organic dust itself. There are acute, subacute, and chronic forms. Characteristically, precipitating antibodies can be identified in the patient's serum by gel diffusion techniques. For example, *A. fumigatus* and *A. clavatus* grow in germinating barley and cause malt-worker's disease. *A. fumigatus* may also be responsible for papermill-worker's lung. The predictable exposure history, diffuse chest radiographic abnormalities, demonstration of precipitating antibody to the putative agent, and response to avoidance help distinguish hypersensitivity pneumonitis from ABPA.

Chronic Necrotizing Pneumonia

Rarely, patients with mild immunosuppressive consequences of diabetes mellitus or ethanol abuse can develop an indolent cavitating pneumonia. This condition differs from aspergilloma and ABPA because it results in tissue invasion and necrosis, and patients present as with a pulmonary abscess—that is, with progressive cough, fever, purulent sputum, and cavitary pulmonary infiltrates.

Allergic Aspergillus Sinusitis

Allergic aspergillus sinusitis resembles ABPA in which there is hyphal growth within an eosinophilic mucoid impaction of sinuses. It primarily affects patients with chronic nasal polyps. Tissue invasion, septicemia, and proptosis do not occur.[12]

DIAGNOSTIC FEATURES OF ABPA

The initial report of ABPA in 1952 by Hinson and colleagues describes the clinical features as these are recognized today.[1] The age at onset is variable: children less than 1 year of age have been affected,[13,14] as have adolescents and young adults.[15,16] The most common clinical symptoms are poorly controlled asthma, cough, purulent sputum (with plugs containing *Aspergillus* hyphae), dyspnea, fever, chest pain, malaise, and/or hemoptysis.[3,15–17] Safirstein and co-workers showed in a large series that episodic flares of ABPA documented by serology, by pulmonary function tests, and with impressive chest roentgenographic findings could be associated with minimal symptomatology.[17] Thus, symptoms may bear little or no relation to the severity or chronicity of the disease. Attempts to control environmental exposure did not affect the incidence of ABPA exacerbations.[17] Scheduled serologic and roentgenographic evaluations are required, because in some patients clinically unsuspected mucoid impaction with associated pulmonary infiltrates and consolidation will be revealed on routine chest roentgenographs.[18]

Some patients proven to have ABPA do not present to the allergist or pulmonologist with symptoms of asthma. Grammer evaluated 62 consecutive patients with presenting complaints of seasonal allergic rhinitis, one-quarter of whom were diagnosed to have asthma with positive immediate cutaneous reactivity to *A. fumigatus* mix.[19] Three of these patients (5% of the total) were serologically proven to have quiescent ABPA, underscoring the need for heightened awareness of the clinical spectrum of this problem.[19] Similarly, ABPA has been diagnosed in a patient presenting with contact dermatitis.[20] At the other extreme, some patients are treated for years for severe corticosteroid-dependent asthma and progressive respiratory failure before a diagnosis of ABPA is made. Diagnostic criteria are presented in Table 15-1.

TABLE 15-1. Diagnostic Criteria for Allergic Bronchopulmonary Aspergillosis–CB (Central Bronchiectasis)

CLASSIC PRESENTATION	MINIMAL ESSENTIAL CRITERIA*
Asthma	Asthma
Immediate cutaneous reactivity to *A. fumigatus*	Immediate cutaneous reactivity to *A. fumigatus*
Elevated total serum IgE (>1000 ng/ml)	Elevated total serum IgE (>1000 ng/ml)
Precipitating antibodies to *A. fumigatus*	Precipitating antibodies to *A. fumigatus*
Proximal bronchiectasis	Proximal bronchiectasis
Chest roentgenographic infiltrates	
Peripheral blood eosinophilia at time of chest roentgenographic infiltrates	
Elevated serum IgE and IgG antibodies to *A. fumigatus*	

*Elevated serum IgE and IgG antibodies to *A. fumigatus* should be present. These assays provide additional support for the diagnosis in the absence of roentgenographic infiltrates.

Ricketti and associates examined 38 patients with ABPA and described the associated clinical allergic features.[21] There was a high (60–80%) incidence of concurrent or subsequent allergic rhinitis, allergic conjunctivitis, previous immunotherapy, or family history of allergic diseases. Food allergy, drug allergy, eczema, and urticaria were all significantly more common than in mold-sensitive patients with asthma who did not have ABPA. In addition, there was marked cutaneous reactivity to common inhalant antigens and molds, regardless of the age at onset of ABPA. These findings differ somewhat from those in ABPA patients described in England,[22] where late onset (>30 years) may be associated with a "low atopic state." Note that despite their universal cutaneous reactivity to *Aspergillus* antigen, many patients do not give a clinical history of rhinitis or asthma associated with moldy environments.[21]

Sputum production can be minimal or absent early in the disease or in cases of serologic ABPA (ABPA-S, defined as ABPA without roentgenographic evidence of bronchiectasis, even during an exacerbation).[17] If a productive cough is present, sputum eosinophilia can be demonstrated by the appropriate stain. This finding, however, can also be present in asthma without ABPA and therefore is not a specific diagnostic criterion. Oral corticosteroids can diminish eosinophilia both in peripheral blood and in sputum.[3] Further, they may reduce the concentration of total serum IgE and cause the disappearance of precipitating antibodies to *A. fumigatus*.

PHYSICAL EXAMINATION

Patients in stages II or IV ABPA (see below and Table 15-2) may have a normal appearance on physical examination. Exacerbations in stages I, III, or V may exhibit all the typical findings of pulmonary consolidation—that is, tachypnea, fever, rales, dullness, bronchial breath sounds, and egophony. End-stage fibrotic lung disease in stage V ABPA may be associated with clubbing, cyanosis, rales, and signs of cor pulmonale.

TABLE 15-2. Stages of ABPA

	I (ACUTE)	II (REMISSION)	III (EXACERBATION)	IV (CORTICOSTEROID- DEPENDENT ASTHMA)	V (FIBROSIS)
Total serum IgE	Markedly elevated	Above normal	Markedly elevated	Elevated	Variable, may be normal
Precipitins to *A. fumigatus*	Positive	Variable	Positive	Variable	May be negative
Specific IgE Specific IgG	Index elevated	Index elevated	Index elevated	May be normal	May be normal
Chest radiographs	May have infiltrates	Normal	May have infiltrates	Central bronchiectasis	Fibrosis
Blood eosinophilia	Positive	Negative	Positive	Variable	Negative

LABORATORY FINDINGS

Routine laboratory studies are generally not helpful with the exception of percent eosinophilia and total eosinophil count, although there may be leukocytosis as well. The earliest descriptions [1–3,15,22,23] include blood eosinophilia as a diagnostic criterion, often greater than 1000 cells per mm^3, with flare-associated rises. Most patients demonstrate positive immediate cutaneous reactivity to *Aspergillus* mix (1:10 w/v) by prick testing; however some patients require intradermal injection (1:1000 w/v) to manifest a response.[15,21] Rosenberg showed that 33% of patients studied also showed a late (6-hour, Arthus-type) reaction following prick testing.[15]

Repeated recovery of *A. fumigatus* from sputum cultures can help suggest the diagnosis, but neither the sensitivity nor the specificity of this finding is 100%.[3,15] McCarthy reported positive cultures in nearly 60% of cases, with the incidence diminishing with corticosteroid therapy.[3]

The diagnosis rests in large part on clinical suspicion and on the results of serologic tests, including total (nonspecific) serum IgE, immunodiffusion demonstration of precipitins to *A. fumigatus*, and elevated levels of serum IgE and IgG antibodies directed against *A. fumigatus* (IgE-Af, IgG-Af).[15,24,25] Patterson and colleagues showed that there was a marked increase in total (nonspecific) serum IgE during the acute phase of pneumonitis associated with ABPA and suggested it was of diagnostic value, especially in differentiating ABPA from hypersensitivity pneumonitis, vasculitis, aspergilloma, or asthma without ABPA.[24] The serum IgE level was above 20,000 ng/ml in ten samples and above 38,000 ng/ml in six (normal = 300 ng/ml). It has become apparent that most of the markedly increased serum IgE is not directed against measurable *Aspergillus* antigen; it therefore represents an elevation in nonspecific IgE, possibly stimulated by growth of *Aspergillus* in endobronchial mucus.[25] Removal of specific IgE-Af from ABPA serum with polystyrene tube absorption techniques caused a drop of only 8% in the total IgE level.[25] Corticosteroid therapy diminishes both total and specific IgE levels toward normal ranges. Reduction of the total IgE to less than 35% of its pretreatment value with corticosteroid therapy (usually within 2 months) can aid in confirming the diagnosis and in documenting therapeutic compliance.[26] Typically, the total serum IgE level does not return to normal values, but remains in the 2,000 to 4,000 ng/ml range. Precipitating antibodies against *A. fumigatus* (IgG-Af), as demonstrated by the double immunodiffusion technique of Ouchterlony,[27] were found in over 90% of sera from patients with asthma, eosinophilia, infiltrates, and sputum production, according to McCarthy and Pepys' early report.[3] Further evaluation has shown that neither serum precipitins themselves nor immediate cutaneous reactivity to *A. fumigatus* are diagnostically specific for ABPA. Both can be seen with asthma alone.[19] Conversely, the absence of precipitating antibody to *A. fumigatus* does not rule out ABPA.[24,28]

Wang and co-workers compared serum IgG and IgE antibody activity against *A. fumigatus* (IgG-Af, IgE-Af) in ABPA patients with antibody activity in mold-sensitive, non-ABPA patients with asthma and in healthy controls. Both precipitating antibody and total IgE levels lack specificity, but high serum levels of IgG-Af or IgE-Af are diagnostic for ABPA in the appropriate clinical setting.[28] These values were obtained using an ^{125}I-labeled antibody radioimmunoassay. Rosenberg and colleagues showed that a rise in total nonspecific serum IgE levels can predict an exacerbation of ABPA,[29] and elevated serum IgE-Af level can predict recurrence in an asymptomatic treated patient with the diagnosis of ABPA.[30] An index for serum IgG-Af and IgE-Af levels in patients with ABPA compared with serum from mold prick skin test–positive patients with asthma but without ABPA (controls) was established in 1983.[31] This index successfully identifies ABPA patients in Stages I and III and is also helpful in other stages, although values can be affected by corticosteroid therapy.[31] It has been shown by an enzyme immunoassay that *A. fumigatus*–specific IgA levels are elevated in ABPA, a finding that can be used similarly to distinguish patients in Stages I, III, and V (see below). The patients who are most difficult to differentiate from those with ABPA are *Aspergillus* prick skin test–positive patients with asthma who do not meet criteria for ABPA.[32] Using a highly sensitive biotin-avidin technique, it has been shown that ABPA is associated with a polyclonal specific antibody response: that is, all isotypes are elevated to some degree.[33] Thus, for a patient in whom ABPA is suspected either because of asthma, peripheral blood eosinophilia, and pulmonary infiltrates, or because of simply asthma and positive immediate cutaneous reactivity to *A. fumigatus* extract, the following laboratory studies should be obtained: (1) total serum IgE; (2) precipitating antibodies to *A. fumigatus*; (3) peripheral blood eosinophil count; (4) chest roentgenogram; (5) serum IgE and IgG to *A. fumigatus*, compared with sera from patients with asthma with immediate cutaneous reactivity to *Aspergillus* but without ABPA; and (6) a search for proximal bronchiectasis using anteroposterior (AP) hilar thin-layer tomography. Thin-layer computed tomography (CT) also can be of value.[16,26,28,31,34]

Patients who present with mucoid impactions of upper lobes usually have asthma, perhaps a history of prior abnormal chest roentgenographic infiltrates, peripheral blood eosinophilia, immediate skin reactivity to *Aspergillus fumigatus*, precipitating antibodies to *A. fumigatus*, elevated total serum IgE, proximal bronchiectasis, and, if tested, elevated serum IgE-Af and IgG-Af levels compared with sera from patients with asthma and immediate cutaneous reactivity to *A. fumigatus* but in whom additional criteria are not sufficient to secure a diagnosis of ABPA. The diagnosis in patients who fulfill these criteria is ABPA-CB (central bronchiectasis). The minimal essential criteria for this diagnosis are asthma, immediate skin reactivity to *A. fumigatus*, elevated total serum IgE levels, and central bronchiectasis. If tested, the sera should show elevated levels of isotypic antibodies to *A. fumigatus*. Should a patient fulfill the criteria for ABPA but not have identifiable central bronchiectasis, the diagnosis is ABPA-S (seropositive). Such patients may have future exacerbations of ABPA and develop bronchiectasis. ABPA-S is thought to reflect early recognition of ABPA before significant lung destruction has occurred.

IMMUNOPATHOGENESIS OF ABPA

The exact mechanism of lung destruction in ABPA is not known. *Aspergillus* spores are inhaled, colonize the excess mucus within large bronchi, and grow at body temperature. Antigenic exposure occurs, as evidenced by the development of multiple IgG, IgA, and IgE anti-*Aspergillus* antibodies.[33] ABPA has been characterized as a disease with Gell and Coombs types I, III, and IV immune reactions; however, it is not known whether the lung destruction is mediated predominantly by complement, by sensitized lymphocytes, or by a combination of humoral and cellular reactions. Investigation into the immunopathogenesis of parenchymal destruction has proceeded along several paths.

Aspergillus organisms growing in the respiratory tract are a potent stimulus to IgE production, most of which is not directed specifically at *A. fumigatus*.[25] It is not known which antigens most of the IgE is directed against, and the stimulus can occur without tissue invasion. Total IgE levels are not significantly elevated in bronchoalveolar lavage (BAL) fluid from ABPA patients, but levels of IgE and IgA directed against *A. fumigatus* are elevated, suggesting local production in the bronchoalveolar compartment.[35] BAL IgA levels against *A. fumigatus* remain elevated after corticosteroid therapy and clinical remission.[35] These data, therefore, provide evidence for local production of IgE-Af and IgA-Af in the bronchoalveolar compartment, with persistence of the latter during clinical remission. There are no such data for IgG although IgG-Af can be detected in BAL fluid. The source of the elevated total serum IgE that characterizes ABPA is not known. It is thought that IgE production requires T and B cell cognate interaction, macrophage–T cell interaction, and production of IL4, IL5, and IL6 by T cells. It remains to be established whether and how these steps occur in ABPA.

In 1970, passive transfer of serum from the first North American ABPA patient to rhesus monkey recipients followed by aerosol challenge with *Aspergillus* antigen resulted in the full spectrum of ABPA, including fever, cough, eosinophilia, and pulmonary infiltrates.[36] Pathologic studies showed no tissue invasion. Both IgG-Af and IgE-Af are essential for the development of pathologic lesions in primate models of ABPA.[36] These experiments support the hypothesis that fungus growing in the mucus of some patients with chronic asthma releases fungal antigens to which the host responds by producing polyclonal specific antibodies and in some cases by producing increased quantities of isotypic antibodies. Antigenic exposure may be increased by the release of proteolytic enzymes from *Aspergillus* spores. It is presumed that the host's exaggerated immunologic response then initiates a reactive cascade that may well involve immunoglobulin-mediated cytokine release, lymphocyte sensitization, cellular hyperreactivity, complement activation, and subsequent tissue injury.

In addition to antibody-mediated hypersensitivity, there is evidence that cellular interactions play a role. In vitro release of histamine by peripheral blood basophils in response to an *Aspergillus* mix and to anti-human IgE is greater in ABPA patients than in mold-sensitive patients with asthma.[37] This is especially notable in the later stages of ABPA, when large doses of corticosteroids are often required to control asthma and prevent recurrences. This increase in histamine release from basophils does not correlate with levels of total IgE, IgE-Af, or IgG-Af.[37] It remains to be seen whether bronchial mast cells yield similar findings. Cromwell and associates showed that IgG-Af immune complexes stimulated eosinophils to release the potent mediator leukotriene C_4 in a dose-dependent fashion and hypothesized that eosinophilic activity may contribute to the pathogenesis of *Aspergillus*-associated pulmonary disease.[38] Clearly, there are many potential mediators for the associated bronchospasm. The role of Gell and Coombs Type IV cell-mediated immunity by sensitized leukocytes is not yet clear, although pathologic studies show granulomas and mononuclear cell infiltration in the pulmonary lesions in ABPA. Patients with ABPA do not usually demonstrate delayed skin reactivity to *Aspergillus* antigen.[39] Lymphocyte transformation may be present in ABPA but is not common enough to be a diagnostic criterion.[15,40]

Geha reported that the early components of the classical complement pathway were depressed in acute ABPA[41] and that C3 split products and Clq precipitin bands were present in the serum. These changes, which resolved after corticosteroid therapy, suggest that the classical complement pathway is activated and that circulating immune complexes such as IgG-Af exist. *Aspergillus* antigen has also been shown to activate the alternate complement pathway directly.[42] Despite these findings ABPA is not felt to be primarily a manifestation of the effects of circulating immune complexes.

Serologic diagnostic techniques are important for distinguishing the various manifestations of aspergillosis in the lung; unfortunately, commercial extracts of *A. fumigatus* are notoriously impure and weakly antigenic.[43] Several investigators have attempted to isolate and purify relevant antigens associated with ABPA. Longbottom demonstrated two types of antigenic components of *A. fumigatus*: low molecular weight components with strong IgE-binding activity (major allergenic potential) that produce weak precipitin bands; and higher molecular weight components with weak IgE-binding activity (minor allergenic potential) that produce strong precipitin bands.[44] Comparing self-crossed immunoelectrophoresis and anti-IgE autoradiography, Longbottom showed that some IgG and IgE antibodies in ABPA patients' sera bind the same *A. fumigatus* antigens and that specific IgG-IgE immune complexes are formed.[45] Further work has resulted in partial characterization of the biochemical, electrophoretic, and physical properties of some of the major antigens.[46–51] Some antigens appear to be conidia-derived, whereas others are intracellular and are released during the terminal autolytic growth phase.[49] One study suggests that most major antigens are derived from mycelial extracts, not spore extracts.[51] In addition, a mouse myeloma monoclonal antibody to *A. fumigatus* developed using hybridoma techniques has both IgG and IgE binding activity.[52]

In summary, the pathogenesis of ABPA is not fully understood. It seems clear that the critical components are (1) chronic exposure to *A. fumigatus* antigens because of excessive colonization and growth of hyphae in mucus and (2) an exaggerated immune response. The combination results in a relapsing destructive inflammatory process within the bronchoalveolar compartment manifested by asthma, bronchiectasis, mucous plugging, and progressive pulmonary fibrosis. ABPA involves more distal regions of lung and should not be considered a condition limited to proximal bronchi.

PATHOLOGY OF ABPA

The diagnosis of ABPA is based on clinical, serologic, and radiographic findings. Lung biopsy findings are nonspecific and variable, and seem to represent the results of chronic noninvasive antigenic stimulation of tissue inflammatory cells. Multiple histologic findings may coexist in the same lobe. Surgical procedures for persistent pulmonary infiltrates may give diagnoses that are consistent with ABPA, such as mucoid impaction syndrome, bronchiolitis obliterans, granulomatous bronchiolitis, eosinophilic pneumonia, and pulmonary fibrosis. Bosken and associates reviewed 18 lung tissue specimens in patients with ABPA.[53] Gross and microscopic examination revealed dilated, predominantly upper lobe bronchi containing thick tenacious mucus, eosinophils, fungal hyphae (without tissue invasion), fibrin, Charcot-Leyden crystals, and Curschmann's spirals. In addition to generalized bronchiolar wall inflammation, either bronchocentric granulomatosis, mucoid impaction of bronchi, or both were universally present.[53] Bronchocentric granulomatosis is characterized by replacement of bronchiolar wall by necrotizing granulomatous inflammation. Palisading histocytes are surrounded by lymphocytes and plasma cells. There is central necrosis and tissue eosinophilia. Mucoid impaction of bronchi is characterized by the filling of bronchiectatic bronchi and bronchioles with the characteristic "allergic" mucin: concentric layers of cells (basophils, eosinophils, sloughed epithelial cells) and amorphous and granular debris within a pale pink to basophilic staining mucin. Charcot-Leyden crystals appearing as refractile orange-pink needles (or hexagons in cross section) are mixed with other elements.[53] Focal collections of chronic inflammatory cells and eosinophils, severe chronic bronchitis, and focal cartilagenous destruction are seen. Fungal hyphae may be present and are not invasive. Foreign body giant cell reactions and bronchiolitis obliterans with organizing pneumonia may also be seen. These pathologic findings in patients with asthma and persistent infiltrates should strongly suggest the diagnosis of ABPA.

STAGING OF ABPA

There are five stages of ABPA.[54] Two longitudinal studies[17,55] showed that patients can present after long histories of severe asthma, chronic bronchitis, and recurrent, apparently resolving pneumonias. These patients may have had extensive lung destruction from ongoing inflammation. Other patients demonstrated serologic evidence of hypersensitivity to *Aspergillus* but had normal conventional chest roentgenograms. Long-term evaluations of these patients suggested that management and prognosis could be aided by grouping patients into five stages (see Table 15-2).[54]

Stage I is characterized by the presence of the classic symptoms of asthma, eosinophilia, immediate cutaneous reactivity to *Aspergillus*, precipitins against *A. fumigatus*, elevated total serum IgE, elevated indices of serum IgE or IgG to *A. fumigatus*, and pulmonary infiltrates. Central bronchiectasis may or may not be present. Fibrosis is absent by chest roentgenogram or biopsy. Therapy with oral corticosteroids results in prompt resolution of symptoms, pulmonary infiltrates, and peripheral blood eosinophilia, and total serum IgE levels decline by at least 35%. The total serum IgE concentration frequently remains elevated but at a lower level than during the acute exacerbation.

Serum IgE-Af and IgG-Af concentrations may remain elevated. A reduction of total IgE to less than 35% of its pretreatment value can be an indicator of therapeutic compliance, as well as a diagnostic aid.[26] Therapy for Stage I ABPA consists of 0.5 mg prednisone/kg/day for 14 days followed by alternate-day therapy over 3 months.

Stage II is characterized by prolonged or permanent clinical remission after therapy for stage I ABPA. Serial total IgE levels are often greater than normal but do not demonstrate the striking fluctuations and increases characteristic of Stage I disease. Chest roentgenograms do not reveal new infiltrates. Exacerbations of the asthma may occur and are treated conventionally. If there has been no recurrence and the patient has been asymptomatic for several years, annual chest films and serum IgE assays may be done to check for the presence of subclinical exacerbations. Patients with a history of previous recurrent "pneumonia" may present with Stage II ABPA.[19,20]

Stage III (exacerbation) ABPA may mimic symptoms and serology of the acute stage. Exacerbations may occur, however, without prominent cough, sputum, dyspnea, or other symptoms. Thus, serial serologic and roentgenographic evaluations are required for all patients with ABPA in clinical remission.[17,30,55] More than a twofold rise in total serum IgE level with pulmonary infiltrates identifies an exacerbation.[54] Treatment is as for Stage I. Recurrence can occur even after years of remission.[56]

Stage IV (corticosteroid-dependent asthma) includes patients who regularly develop an exacerbation of asthma when tapering of corticosteroid therapy is attempted. Many patients fall into this category.[57] Results of most serologic studies remain abnormal. Symptoms can be controlled with modest doses of alternate-day prednisone (an average of 20 mg every other day in one study).[54] Differentiating a flare of asthma from ABPA requires obtaining both total serum IgE and IgE-Af and IgG-Af measurements. The fact that serum IgE-Af and IgG-Af levels are higher in patients with ABPA than in patients with asthma is a valuable diagnostic aid.

In all of the above patients, central bronchiectasis may be apparent on AP hilar pulmonary tomography or computed tomography; this is evidence of bronchial wall destruction. ABPA with central bronchiectasis is subcategorized ABPA-CB. Some patients, however, manifest only clinical and serologic evidence, without bronchiectasis; in this case the disease is labeled ABPA-S. In such patients the disease theoretically is in an earlier or milder phase.[57] It is clear that aggressive corticosteroid therapy in Stage IV ABPA can prevent progression to Stage V (pulmonary fibrosis).[57] It is not yet certain whether central bronchiectasis can be prevented in ABPA-S patients.

Repeated episodes of ABPA can cause end-stage fibrotic lung disease or Stage V ABPA. Such patients either manifest persistent pulmonary infiltrates consistent with fibrosis in the absence of exacerbations or have fibrosis on lung biopsy. These patients have significant irreversible lung disease by pulmonary function tests. They show no improvement with corticosteroids and require high daily or alternate-day doses of steroids to prevent exacerbations.[54,57,58] Complications can include bacterial pneumonia, colonization with nontuberculous ("atypical") mycobacteria, and iatrogenic Cushing's syndrome. Death may occur from respiratory failure or cor pulmonale. In one series of 17 patients with Stage V ABPA, Lee and associates found that although all patients fulfilled most of the criteria for ABPA, the total serum IgE concentration and precipitin levels to *A. fumigatus* lacked high sensitivity.[58] Diagnostic impressions before recognition of ABPA varied widely and included asthma, chronic bronchitis, Löffler's syndrome, and pulmonary tuberculosis.[58] The interval between the onset and the diagnosis of ABPA ranged from 5 months to 35 years. After diagnosis and therapy with moderate-dose alternate-day corticosteroids, patients with a forced expiratory volume in 1 second (FEV_1) greater than 0.8 L at diagnosis maintained an acceptable functional status. All patients with an FEV_1 at diagnosis of 0.8 L or less died within 7 years.[58]

PULMONARY FUNCTION TESTS

Pulmonary function tests (PFTs) may yield normal results or show severe restrictive or irreversible obstructive disease, or both, depending on the stage of ABPA. Acute exacerbations of ABPA cause reductions of lung volumes and diffusing capacity. In some cases, solely obstructive findings consistent with asthma return to normal values with therapy.[59] Many patients in remission (Stage II) have normal flow rates and lung volumes, even if roentgenographic studies show saccular bronchiectasis.[59] This observation suggests that pulmonary function tests are not a sensitive indicator of early lung damage in ABPA. A longitudinal study of Stage IV ABPA patients (i.e., patients with corticosteroid-dependent asthma) demonstrated that early intervention and therapy with prednisone appears to prevent loss of pulmonary function, despite progression through the first four stages of ABPA.[60] In patients presenting with Stage V ABPA, results of pulmonary function tests reflect the underlying parenchymal fibrosis: lung volumes are reduced and there is airflow obstruction without bronchodilator response (i.e., a mixed restrictive and obstructive pattern).[55] The diffusing capacity for carbon monoxide is also typically reduced, reflecting the abnormalities in gas exchange in these patients. Despite corticosteroid therapy, patients with an FEV_1 less than 0.8 L at diagnosis have a markedly worse prognosis than other patients with similar symptoms.[58]

RADIOLOGY OF ABPA

Although central bronchiectasis has been a cardinal diagnostic criterion for ABPA in the past, it has been shown that patients with clinical and serologic evidence of ABPA do not necessarily have proximal bronchiectasis on routine chest radiography.[18,57,61,62] Bronchograms were helpful in establishing the presence of dilated central bronchi in these patients.[61] Linear AP tomography to view the first few orders of bronchi has replaced bronchography as the test of choice because it is simple, noninvasive, and sensitive.[63] Thin-section CT has been used to identify bronchiectesis, but its sensitivity compared to conventional tomography has not been conclusively established in ABPA patients. Patients with ABPA-S manifest transient pulmonary infiltrates with exacerbations, but even CT scans do not reveal bronchiectatic change.[57,63] These patients should be considered to have ABPA, possibly in an earlier phase, prior to significant bronchial destruction.

The radiologic changes seen in ABPA preferentially affect the upper lobes and must be distinguished from those seen in other conditions with a similar distribution, such as cystic fibrosis, bronchiectasis due to immunoglobulin deficiency or ciliary dysfunction, and sarcoidosis.[61,63] These changes include both transient and permanent alterations, most of them secondary to mucus accumulation, mucus plugging with distal atelectasis, thickened bronchial walls, and (later) parenchymal fibrosis. None is pathognomonic of ABPA. Among the transient findings are nonspecific mucoid impaction, atelectasis, pulmonary infiltrates, and massive homogeneous consolidation, which resolve rapidly with corticosteroid therapy.[61] Thickening of a larger bronchus causes "tramline" shadows: two parallel hairline shadows extending from the hilus that approximate the width of a bronchus at that level. "Parallel line" shadows are dilated tramline shadows, indicating more pronounced bronchiectasis. Ring shadows are dilated bronchi seen en face and should be 1 cm in diameter.[61,62] When bronchiectatic segments become filled with mucus, "toothpaste shadows" can be detected (5–8 mm wide, up to 3 cm long). If bronchi are impacted and distally expanded, "gloved finger" shadows are visible. Both may clear with tussive episodes or oral corticosteroid

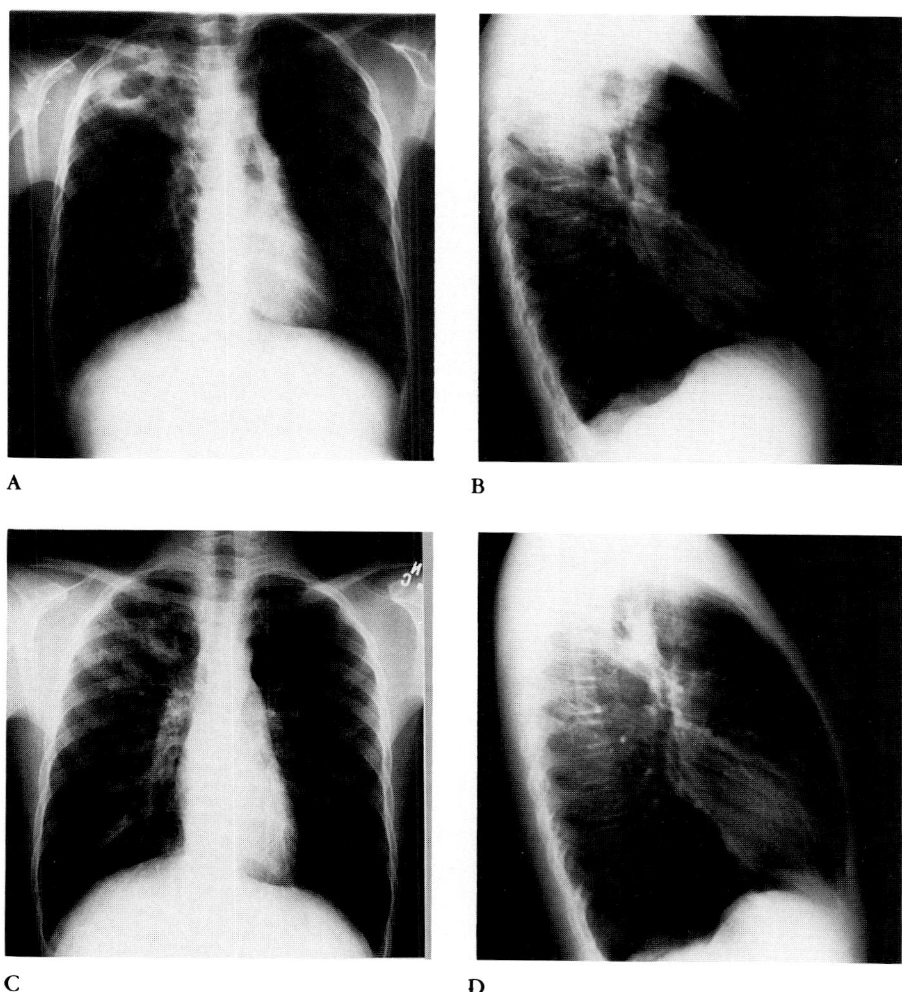

Figure 15-1. (*A*) Presentation posteroanterior radiograph of a 10-year-old boy with ABPA. A cavitary lesion of the left upper lobe is present. (*B*) Lateral view of the same patient. (*C*) An exacerbation of ABPA occurred 2 years later in the right upper lobe. (*D*) Lateral view of the right upper lobe from *C*.

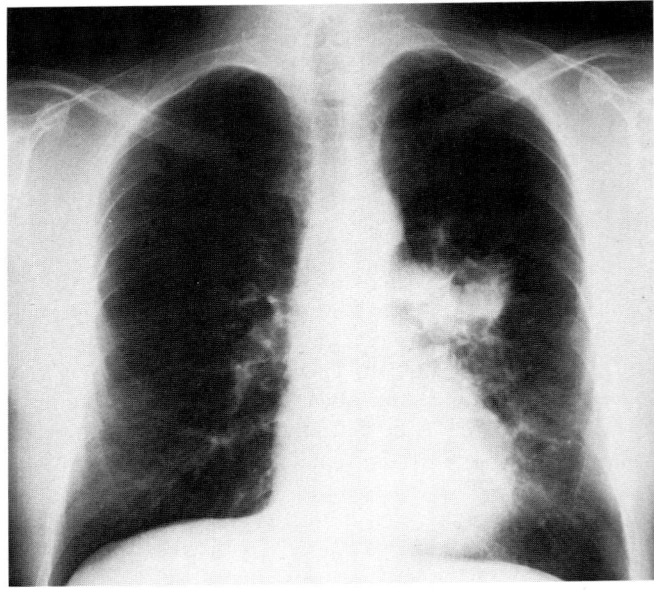

A

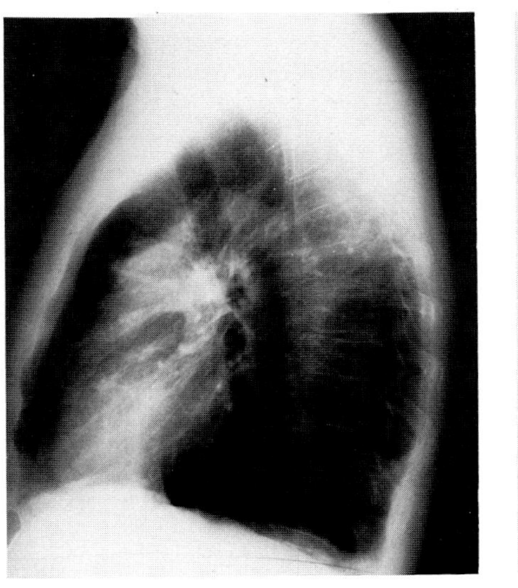

B

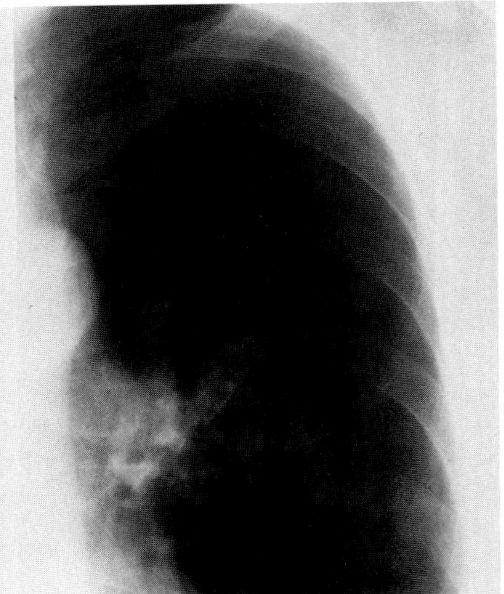

C

Figure 15-2. (*A*) Posteroanterior radiograph of a 52-year-old male with long-standing ABPA. A left hilar lesion is present. (*B*) Lateral view of the same patient. (*C*) The "gloved-finger" shadow in the left upper lobe represents mucus-filled bronchi from the same patient.

therapy.[61,62] In addition, perihilar infiltrates may simulate adenopathy[63] and air–fluid interfaces may be present in dilated, partially obstructed bronchi. Cavitation is rare.[62] Roentgenographic findings other than extensive fibrosis or parenchymal infiltrates do not aid in defining a particular stage, although management is obviously different.[64] Blebs, bullae, and spontaneous pneumothorax have been described.[65]

ASSOCIATED DISEASES

Patients with cystic fibrosis frequently carry *A. fumigatus* in their sputum and are at risk for developing ABPA. In an early study of 46 patients with cystic fibrosis, nearly 40% manifested immediate cutaneous reactivity to *Aspergillus* mix (none had a type III intermediate Arthus-type response), 37% showed positive precipitins to *A. fumigatus*, and 11% (four patients) met criteria for ABPA.[66] The prevalence rate may be lower in Europe.[67] The exact prevalence may be difficult to discern because the underlying lung disease in cystic fibrosis can obscure chest findings considered to be diagnostic criteria for ABPA.[68,69] The bronchiectasis and mucus production characteristic of cystic fibrosis may offer a suitable environment not only for *Aspergillus* species but for other fungi and for some bacteria, and the immunologic reaction against those organisms may play a role in the continued lung destruction seen in the disease.[68,70] Thus, the response of patients with cystic fibrosis to the *Aspergillus* organism in their airways ranges from clinically and serologically apparent ABPA (10%), to a possible variant of ABPA, to serologic manifestation of *Aspergillus* sensitization without clinical manifestation (about 50%).[70–72] It has recently been shown that the activated T- and B-cell response to *Aspergillus* may be important in ABPA complicating cystic fibrosis.

Other variants of ABPA have been reported. One woman developed myalgias, weight loss, fever, and eosinophilia and had skin biopsy–proven leukocytoclastic vasculitis consistent with Churg-Strauss syndrome 17 years after bronchial biopsy and serologically proven ABPA.[74] ABPA secondary to *A. oryzae* has been reported in a young woman exposed to this fermentation starter for soybean products.[6] Allergic *Aspergillus* sinusitis in conjunction with ABPA has been seen in a middle-aged woman with atopic features.[12] A broader spectrum of allergic bronchopulmonary fungoses such as allergic bronchopulmonary candidiasis may exist for which specific serologic tests could become available.[75–77] Some patients have asthma, proximal bronchiectasis, a history of pneumonia of the upper lobes, but inconclusive serologic or culture evidence to confirm a diagnosis of ABPA or other fungosis. Such patients in whom cystic fibrosis has been excluded should be treated as if ABPA is present, and their sera should be saved for future analysis.

TREATMENT

Treatment of ABPA is most dependent upon early recognition. Even in experienced centers, some patients managed for years for asthma may not be identified as having ABPA until pulmonary fibrosis is apparent. Our experience suggests that therapy with

TABLE 15-3. Some Clinical Observations Based on over 20 Years of Experience with ABPA at Northwestern

1. ABPA may occur in childhood and remain undiagnosed for up to 3 decades. ABPA thus should be excluded in childhood asthma.
2. Physicians familiar with the decline in total serum IgE levels after prednisone therapy of the acute phase of ABPA may attempt to treat with prednisone until the IgE level is normal. This is excessive treatment, as the IgE level often remains significantly elevated in the absence of active ABPA. Treatment goals should be a normal chest radiograph and a plateau of the IgE level.
3. Recognition of ABPA at any stage is rarely followed by progression to a more severe stage because exacerbations are treated early with prednisone and progressive lung damage does not occur. Thus, patients may be reassured about the prognosis.
4. Even if Stage V (fibrotic end-stage lung disease) is present at time of diagnosis, careful management with prednisone may permit a comfortable existence for 10 or more years.
5. ABPA may exist in 1% to 2% of all asthmatics, and exclusion at least once is essential.

corticosteroids cannot prevent evolution to Stage IV corticosteroid-dependent asthma but can prevent progression to Stage V (i.e., pulmonary fibrosis).[78]

All patients with chronic asthma should be tested for immediate cutaneous reactivity to *Aspergillus*, especially if there is a history of recurrent pneumonia. All prick (or intradermal) skin test–positive patients need conventional chest roentgenographs. ABPA infiltrates may be associated with little or no symptomatology in about one-third of the cases.[15] If the total serum IgE level is elevated and precipitating antibodies are present to *A. fumigatus*, AP hilar pulmonary tomography should be considered. Serologic studies such as the serum IgE-Af and IgG-Af assays described above should be obtained.[21,28] In addition, atopic family members should be investigated, even though the yield will be low. Once the diagnosis of ABPA is made, prednisone therapy should be initiated, and serial total IgE levels should be obtained (initially monthly) even in asymptomatic patients. The frequency of serum IgE determinations can then be reduced according to clinical status.

Exacerbations should be treated with oral corticosteroids.[54] We recommend initial treatment with prednisone, 35 to 40 mg (0.5 mg/kg/day) given as a single morning dose for 2 weeks, followed by conversion to an alternate-day dosing schedule for 3 months, with eventual tapering and discontinuation. Theophylline, inhaled beta adrenergic agonists, and inhaled corticosteroids are warranted as adjunctive therapy. Comparison total IgE levels and chest roentgenograms should be obtained 1 month after the initiation of therapy. Reduction of the total IgE level to 35% of its pretreatment value along with a clinical response signals the resolution of the exacerbation.[25,26] Close follow-up is required to monitor continued remission. Inflammation and immunologic reactions have been successfully controlled with oral corticosteroids. Recurrent courses of prednisone at lower doses may be required to treat exacerbations of asthma, although these doses are not usually effective in treating exacerbations of ABPA. The distinction is crucial to the prevention of continued lung destruction.

Several antifungal agents have been tested in ABPA patients, including amphotericin B, clotrimazole, natamycin, hystatin, and ketoconazole, with mixed or disappointing results. This is consistent with the presumed immunologic etiology of this disease. Data are not available for the newer antifungal agents, such as itroconazole. Cromolyn may be used to treat the associated asthma but has not been shown to decrease the incidence of roentgenographic infiltrates characteristic of ABPA exacerbations.[17] Inhaled corticosteroids may be useful as adjunctive therapy for the treatment of asthma.

Stage IV and V patients require daily or alternate-day prednisone. The dosage depends on previous tendency to relapse at a given dose, upcoming mold sporulation season in patients with seasonal variation, and other factors. These patients should be examined 1 week before any surgical procedure and should receive 25 mg to 40 mg prednisone every morning for 5 to 7 days prior to the procedure. Surgery should be performed only if absolutely necessary in severely compromised patients (e.g., FEV_1 less than 0.8 L), as in other chronic lung diseases, and only when the patient's respiratory status is optimal.

SUMMARY

Allergic bronchopulmonary aspergillosis is a chronic, relapsing, immunologically mediated disease occurring predominantly in patients with asthma, caused by hypersensitivity to colonized A. *fumigatus*. The immunopathogenesis is not understood fully. The clinical spectrum ranges from a virtual absence of symptoms to end-stage pulmonary fibrosis; ongoing lung damage occurs in both groups. Early detection and management with corticosteroids can prevent end-stage lung disease and fibrosis and are therefore the cornerstones of therapy.

REFERENCES

1. Hinson KFW, Moon AJ, Plummer NS. Bronchopulmonary aspergillosis: A review and a report of eight new cases. Thorax 1952;7:317.
2. Patterson R, Golbert TM. Hypersensitivity disease of the lung. Univ Mich Med Ctr J 1968;34:8.
3. McCarthy DS, Pepys J. Allergic bronchopulmonary aspergillosis. Clinical immunology: (1) Clinical features. Clin Allergy 1971;1:261.
4. Micheli PA. *Nova plantarum genera juxta Tournefortii methodum disposita*. Florence, 1729.
5. Raper KB, Fennell DI. The genus *Aspergillus*. Baltimore: Williams and Wilkins, 1965.
6. Akiyama K, Takizawa H, Suzuki M, Miyachi S, Ichinohe M, Yanagihara Y. Allergic bronchopulmonary aspergillosis due to *Aspergillus oryzae*. Chest 1987;91:285.
7. Savage A, Isa JM. A note on mycotic pneumonia of chickens. Sci Agr 1933;13:341.
8. Witter JF, Chute HL. Aspergillosis in turkeys. J Am Vet Med Assoc 1952;121:387.
9. Solomon WR, Burge HP, Boise JR. Airborne *Aspergillus fumigatus* levels outside and within a large clinical center. J Allergy Clin Immunol 1978;62:56.
10. Radin RC, Greenberger PA, Patterson R, Ghory A. Mold counts and exacerbations of allergic bronchopulmonary aspergillosis. Clin Allergy 1983;13:271.
11. Rosenberg IL, Greenberger PA. Allergic bronchopulmonary aspergillosis and aspergilloma: Long-term follow-up without enlargement of a large multiloculated cavity. Chest 1984;85:123.
12. Sher TH, Schwartz HJ. Allergic *Aspergillus* sinusitis with concurrent allergic bronchopulmonary aspergillosis: Report of a case. J Allergy Clin Immunol 1988;81:844.

13. Imbeau SA, Cohen M, Reed CE. Allergic bronchopulmonary aspergillosis in infants. Am J Dis Child 1977;131:1127.
14. Kiefer TA, Kesarwala HH, Greenberger PA, et al. Allergic bronchopulmonary aspergillosis in a young child: Diagnostic confirmation by serum IgE and IgG indices. Ann Allergy 1986;56:233.
15. Rosenberg M, Patterson R, Mintzer R, Cooper BJ, Roberts M, Harris K. Clinical and immunologic criteria for the diagnosis of allergic bronchopulmonary aspergillosis. Ann Intern Med 1977;86:405.
16. Greenberger PA, Patterson R. Diagnosis and management of allergic bronchopulmonary aspergillosis. Ann Allergy 1986;56:444.
17. Safirstein BH, D'Souza MF, Simon G, Tai E, Pepys J. Five-year follow-up of allergic bronchopulmonary aspergillosis. Am Rev Respir Dis 1973;108:450.
18. Rosenberg M, Mintzer R, Aaronson DW, Patterson R. Allergic bronchopulmonary aspergillosis in three patients with normal chest x-ray films. Chest 1977;72:597.
19. Grammer LC, Greenberger PA, Patterson R. Allergic bronchopulmonary aspergillosis in asthmatic patients presenting with allergic rhinitis. Int Arch Allergy Appl Immunol 1986;79:246.
20. Ricketti AJ, Greenberger PA, Patterson R. Varying presentations of ABPA. Int Arch Allergy Appl Immunol 1984;73:283.
21. Ricketti AJ, Greenberger PA, Patterson R. Immediate-type reactions in patients with allergic bronchopulmonary aspergillosis. J Allergy Clin Immunol 1983;71:541.
22. McCarthy DS, Pepys J. Allergic bronchopulmonary aspergillosis: Clinical immunology: (2) Skin, nasal, and bronchial tests. Clin Allergy 1971;1:415.
23. Henderson AH. Allergic aspergillosis: Review of 32 cases. Thorax 1968;23:501.
24. Patterson R, Fink JN, Pruzansky JJ, et al. Serum immunoglobulin levels in pulmonary allergic aspergillosis and certain other lung diseases, with special reference to immunoglobulin E. Am J Med 1973;54:16.
25. Patterson R, Rosenberg M, Roberts M. Evidence that *Aspergillus fumigatus* growing in the airway of man can be a potent stimulus of specific and nonspecific IgE formation. Am J Med 1977;63:257.
26. Ricketti AJ, Greenberger PA, Patterson R. Serum IgE as an important aid in management of allergic bronchopulmonary aspergillosis. J Allergy Clin Immunol 1984;74:68.
27. Ouchterlony Ö. Diffusion-in-gel methods for immunological analysis. Prog Allergy 1958;5:1.
28. Wang JL, Patterson R, Rosenberg M, Roberts M, Cooper BJ. Serum IgE and IgG antibody activity against *Aspergillus fumigatus* as a diagnostic aid in allergic bronchopulmonary aspergillosis. Am Rev Respir Dis 1978;117:917.
29. Rosenberg M, Patterson R, Roberts M. Immunologic responses to therapy in allergic bronchopulmonary aspergillosis: Serum IgE value as an indicator and predictor of disease activity. J Pediatr 1977;91:914.
30. Rosenberg M, Patterson R, Roberts M, Wang J. The assessment of immunologic and clinical changes occurring during corticosteroid therapy for allergic bronchopulmonary aspergillosis. Am J Med 1978;64:599.
31. Patterson R, Greenberger PA, Ricketti AJ, Roberts M. A radioimmunoassay index for allergic bronchopulmonary aspergillosis. Ann Intern Med 1983;99:18.
32. Gutt L, Greenberger PA, Liotta JL. Serum IgA antibodies to *Aspergillus fumigatus* in various stages of allergic bronchopulmonary aspergillosis. J Allergy Clin Immunol 1986;78:98.
33. Brummund W, Resnick A, Fink JN, Kurup VP. *Aspergillus fumigatus*–specific antibodies in allergic bronchopulmonary aspergillosis and aspergilloma: Evidence for a polyclonal antibody response. J Clin Micro 1987;25:5.
34. Greenberger PA, Patterson R. Allergic bronchopulmonary aspergillosis: Model of bronchopulmonary disease with defined serologic, radiologic, pathologic and clinical findings from asthma to fatal destructive lung disease. Chest 1987;91(suppl):165S.

35. Kauffman HF, Beaumont F, de Monchy JGR, Sluiter HJ, de Vries K. Immunologic studies in bronchoalveolar fluid in a patient with allergic bronchopulmonary aspergillosis. J Allergy Clin Immunol 1984;74:835.

36. Slavin RG, Fischer VW, Levin EA. A primate model of allergic bronchopulmonary aspergillosis. Int Arch Allergy Appl Immunol 1978;56:325.

37. Ricketti AJ, Greenberger PA, Pruzansky JJ, Patterson R. Hyperreactivity of mediator-releasing cells from patients with allergic bronchopulmonary aspergillosis as evidenced by basophil histamine release. J Allergy Clin Immunol 1983;72:386.

38. Cromwell O, Moqbel R, Fitzharris P, et al. Leukotriene C_4 generation from human eosinophils stimulated with IgG–*Aspergillus fumigatus* antigen immune complexes. J Allergy Clin Immunol 1988;82:535.

39. Slavin RG, Hutcheson PS, Knutsen AP. Participation of cell-mediated immunity in allergic bronchopulmonary aspergillosis. Int Arch Allergy Appl Immunol 1987;83:337.

40. Forman SR, Fink JN, Moore VL, Wang J, Patterson R. Humoral and cellular immune responses in *Aspergillus fumigatus* pulmonary disease. J Allergy Clin Immunol 1978:62:131.

41. Geha RS. Circulating immune complexes and activation of the complement sequence in acute allergic bronchopulmonary aspergillosis. J Allergy Clin Immunol 1977;60:357.

42. Marx JJ, Flaherty DK. Activation of the complement sequence by extracts of bacteria and fungi associated with hypersensitivity pneumonitis. J Allergy Clin Immunol 1976;57:328.

43. Kurup VP, Resnik A, Scribner GH, Gunasekaran M, Fink JN. Enzyme profile and immunochemical characterization of *Aspergillus fumigatus* antigens. J Allergy Clin Immunol 1986;78:1166.

44. Longbottom JL. Allergic bronchopulmonary aspergillosis: Reactivity of IgE and IgG antibodies with antigenic components of *Aspergillus fumigatus* (IgE/IgG antigen complexes). J Allergy Clin Immunol 1983;72:668.

45. Longbottom JL. Antigens/allergens of *Aspergillus fumigatus*. Clin Exp Immunol 1983;53;354.

46. Longbottom JL. Antigens and allergens of *Aspergillus fumigatus*. II. Their further identification and partial characterization of a major allergen (Ag 3). J Allergy Clin Immunol 1986;78:18.

47. Harvey C, Longbottom JL. Characterization of a major antigen component of *Aspergillus fumigatus*. Clin Exp Immunol 1986;65:206.

48. Harvey C, Longbottom JL. Characterization of a second major antigen Ag 13 (antigen C) of *Aspergillus fumigatus* and investigation of its immunological reactivity. Clin Exp Immunol 1987;70:247.

49. Taylor ML, Longbottom JL. Partial characterization of a rapidly released antigenic/allergenic component (Ag 5) of *Aspergillus fumigatus*. J Allergy Clin Immunol 1988;81:548.

50. Kurup VP, Greenberger PA, Fink JN. Antibody response to low-molecular-weight antigens of *Aspergillus fumigatus* in allergic bronchopulmonary aspergillosis. J Clin Microbiol 1989;27:1312.

51. Leung PSC, Gershwin ME, Coppel R, Halpern G, Novey H, Castles JJ. Localization, molecular weight, and immunoglobulin subclass response to *Aspergillus fumigatus* allergens in allergic bronchopulmonary aspergillosis. Int Arch Allergy Appl Immunol 1988;85:416.

52. Kurup VP. Production and characterization of a murine monoclonal antibody to *Aspergillus fumigatus* antigen having IgG- and IgE-binding activity. Int Arch Allergy Appl Immunol 1988;86:400.

53. Bosken CH, Myers JL, Greenberger PA, Katzenstein AA. Pathologic features of allergic bronchopulmonary aspergillosis. Am J Surg Pathol 1988;12:216.

54. Patterson R, Greenberger PA, Radin RC, Roberts M. Allergic bronchopulmonary aspergillosis: Staging as an aid to management. Ann Intern Med 1982;96:286.

55. Greenberger PA, Patterson R, Ghory AC, et al. Late sequelae of allergic bronchopulmonary aspergillosis. J Allergy Clin Immunol 1980;66:327.

56. Halwig JM, Greenberger PA, Levine M, Patterson R. Recurrence of allergic bronchopulmonary aspergillosis after seven years of remission. J Allergy Clin Immunol 1984;74:738.

57. Patterson R, Greenberger PA, Halwig MJ, Liotta JL, Roberts M. Allergic bronchopulmonary aspergillosis, natural history, and classification of early disease by serologic and roentgenographic studies. Arch Intern Med 1986;146:916.

58. Lee TM, Greenberger PA, Patterson R, Roberts M, Liotta JL. Stage V (fibrotic) allergic bronchopulmonary aspergillosis. Arch Intern Med 1987;147:319.

59. Nichols D, Dopico GA, Braun S, Imbeau S, Peters M, Rankin J. Acute and chronic pulmonary function changes in allergic bronchopulmonary aspergillosis. Am J Med 1979;67:631.

60. Patterson R, Greenberger PA, Lee T, et al. Prolonged evaluation of patients with corticosteroid-dependent asthma stage of allergic bronchopulmonary aspergillosis. J Allergy Clin Immunol 1987;80:663.

61. Mintzer RA, Rogers LF, Kruglik GD, Rosenberg M, Neiman HL, Patterson R. The spectrum of radiologic findings in allergic bronchopulmonary aspergillosis. Radiology 1978;127:301.

62. Phelan MS, Kerr IH. Allergic bronchopulmonary aspergillosis: The radiological appearance during long-term follow-up. Clin Radiol 1984;35:385.

63. Fisher MR, Mendelson EB, Mintzer RA, Ricketti AJ, Greenberger PA. Use of linear tomography to confirm the diagnosis of allergic bronchopulmonary aspergillosis. Chest 1985;87:499.

64. Mendelson EB, Fisher MR, Mintzer RA, Halwig JM, Greenberger PA. Roentgenographic and clinical staging of allergic bronchopulmonary aspergillosis. Chest 1985;87:334.

65. Ricketti AJ, Greenberger PA, Glassroth J. Spontaneous pneumothorax in allergic bronchopulmonary aspergillosis. Arch Intern Med 1984;144:151.

66. Nelson L, Callerame ML, Schwartz RH. Aspergillosis and atopy in cystic fibrosis. Am Rev Respir Dis 1979;120:86.

67. Schonheyder H, Jensen T, Hoiby N, Koch C. Clinical and serological survey of pulmonary aspergillosis in patients with cystic fibrosis. Int Arch Allergy Appl Immunol 1988;85:472.

68. Feanny S, Forsyth S, Corey M, Levison H, Zimmerman B. Allergic bronchopulmonary aspergillosis in cystic fibrosis: A secretory immune response to a colonizing organism. Ann Allergy 1988;60:64.

69. Laufer P, Fink JN, Bruns WT, et al. Allergic bronchopulmonary aspergillosis in cystic fibrosis. J Allergy Clin Immunol 1984;73:44.

70. Zeaske R, Bruns WT, Fink JN, et al. Immune responses to *Aspergillus* in cystic fibrosis. J Allergy Clin Immunol 1988;82:73.

71. Brueton MJ, Ormerod LP, Shah KJ, Anderson CM. Allergic bronchopulmonary aspergillosis complicating cystic fibrosis in childhood. Arch Dis Child 1980;55:348.

72. Birx DL, Summers R, Berger M. Acute deterioration of pulmonary function in cystic fibrosis illustrating the association of atopy and allergic bronchopulmonary aspergillosis with the underlying disease. Ann Allergy 1984;53:124.

73. Knutsen A, Slavin RG. *In vitro* T cell responses in patients with cystic fibrosis and allergic bronchopulmonary aspergillosis. J Lab Clin Med 1989;113:428.

74. Stephens M, Reynolds S, Gibbs AR, Davies B. Allergic bronchopulmonary aspergillosis progressing to allergic granulomatosis and angiitis (Churg-Strauss syndrome). Am Rev Respir Dis 1988;137:1226.

75. Lee TM, Greenberger PA, Oh S, Patterson R, Roberts M, Liotta JL. Allergic bronchopulmonary candidiasis: Case report and suggested diagnostic criteria. J Allergy Clin Immunol 1987;80:816.

76. Greenberger PA. Allergic bronchopulmonary aspergillosis and fungoses. Clin Chest Med 1988;9:599.

77. Turner ES, Greenberger PA, Sider L. Complexities of establishing an early diagnosis of allergic bronchopulmonary aspergillosis in children. Allergy Proc 1989;10:63.

78. Greenberger PA, Patterson R. Allergic bronchopulmonary aspergillosis and the evaluation of the patient with asthma. J Allergy Clin Immunol 1988;81:646.

16

Hypersensitivity Pneumonitis

Jordan N. Fink

Hypersensitivity pneumonitis, also known as extrinsic allergic alveolitis, is caused by immunologically mediated inflammation in the lung following intermittent exposure and sensitization to any of a wide variety of biologic dusts. Characteristically, the disease affects the peripheral airspaces of the lung and the interstitium and presents as respiratory or systemic symptoms that follow inhalation of the offending agent.[1-3] The disorder presents in acute, insidious or subacute and chronic forms and may ultimately cause permanent damage to the lung parenchyma.[2-4] Both humoral and cellular immune responses to the offending antigen can be identified in the peripheral circulation and in the lung parenchyma.[1-3] The inflammatory response results in symptom patterns associated with restrictive or obstructive defects in pulmonary function; all clinical features of the disorder usually reverse on avoidance of the offending agent or administration of corticosteroids.

CLINICAL FEATURES

Acute Form

Hypersensitivity pneumonitis most commonly manifests as acute, explosive episodes of chills, fever, dyspnea, malaise, and myalgia occurring 4 to 6 hours after a previously sensitized person is exposed to the offending antigen.[1-3] Repeated episodes may be confused with a bacterial or viral illness unless a careful environmental history is obtained. The flu-like episodes are associated with diffuse bibasilar end-inspiratory rales that may persist for days after the episode terminates. No extrapulmonary physical findings have been described. Laboratory abnormalities detected during the episodes include a leukocytosis with a shift to young forms and variable eosinophilia that may reach 20%. Immunoglobulin levels may be elevated as a polyclonal gammopathy,

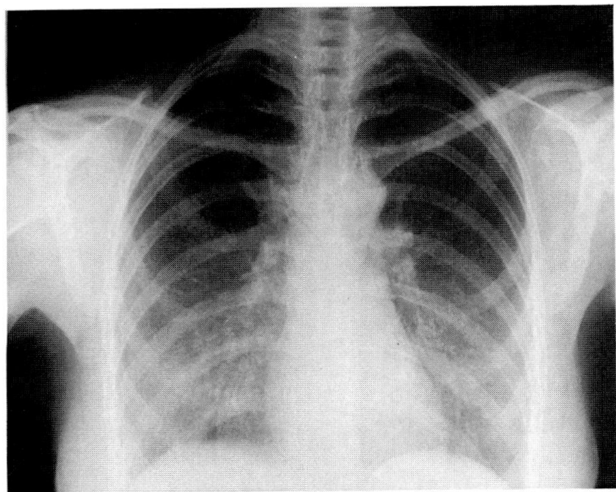

Figure 16-1. Pigeon breeder's disease. Fine nodular bibasilar interstitial infiltrates in the acute form of pigeon breeder's disease.

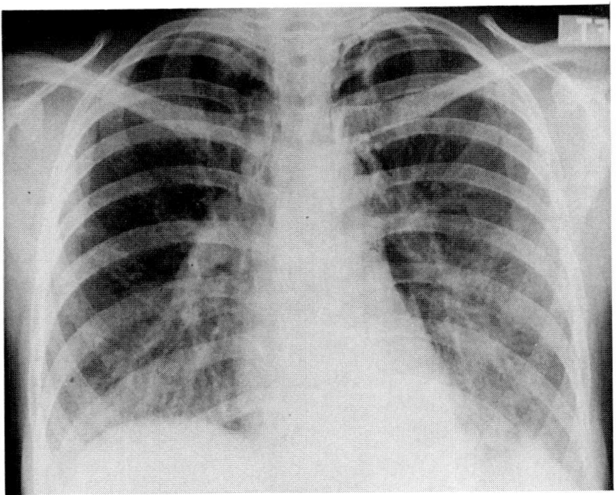

Figure 16-2. Farmer's lung. Diffuse interstitial infiltrates with nodulation in farmer's lung.

especially after repeated episodes; rheumatoid factor can be detected in over 50% of patients. IgE levels are within normal limits except in the 15% of patients with hypersensitivity pneumonitis who are also atopic.[1-3]

Chest radiographic findings are nonspecific and may be normal, especially if the episodes are widely spaced. The acute form of hypersensitivity pneumonitis, however, is usually accompanied by bilateral interstitial nodular changes, predominantly in the lower lobes (Figs. 16-1, 16-2).[4-6] Hazy or fluffy infiltrates may also accompany the nodules, and on occasion hilar adenopathy may be seen. The histopathologic picture accompanying this acute form is characterized by a lymphocytic alveolar and interstitial inflammation with increased numbers of plasma cells, occasional eosinophils, and large numbers of intra-alveolar and intraseptal foamy-appearing macrophages. Giant cells may be seen and early granuloma formation may also be detected (Fig. 16-3).[7,8]

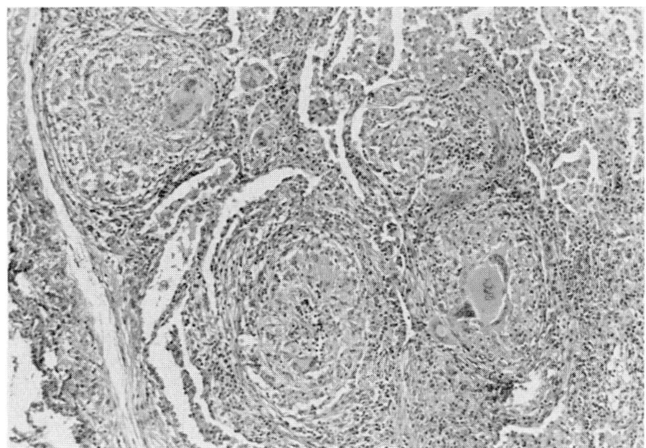

Figure 16-3. Ventilation pneumonitis. Diffuse interstitial pneumonitis with lymphocytic infiltration and granuloma formation in ventilation pneumonitis.

Pulmonary function abnormalities mirror the roentgenographic and histopathologic abnormalities. During an acute episode there is a predominant restrictive impairment peaking at 4 to 6 hours after exposure.[1-3,9] There is a decrease in lung volumes, most pronounced in the forced vital capacity. Diffusion is reduced and oxygen desaturation may be detected; arterial oxygen desaturation following exercise may be an early finding in the disease.[2,3] As the patient recovers from the acute episode, the reduced vital capacity and diffusion may persist for weeks, and in some patients pulmonary function returns to normal but the arterial oxygen desaturation remains. In a few patients an immediate pulmonary response follows inhalation of the offending antigen within minutes and has features of airway obstruction, with a decrease in expiratory flow. This early response has features of airway hyperreactivity with enhanced methacholine reactivity and probably represents bronchial wall inflammation.[9]

Therapy of the acute form of hypersensitivity pneumonitis consisting of avoidance of antigen, a short course of corticosteroids, or both, results in rapid resolution of all clinical abnormalities with normalization of the chest radiographic appearance and pulmonary function. Further episodes are prevented as long as avoidance continues.

Subacute Form

Approximately 15% of patients with hypersensitivity pneumonitis present with a more insidious syndrome. The patient develops symptoms of bronchitis with cough and some sputum production. Anorexia, malaise, and weight loss may be prominent.[2,3] Acute episodes of chills and fever are unusual unless the patient is exposed to and inhales large amounts of antigen, such as by purposeful bronchial challenge. Physical findings in these patients are nonspecific with evidence of weight loss and chronic illness; bibasilar crackling rales may be heard and may disappear after long-term avoidance or therapy.

Laboratory examination of these patients may reveal evidence of long-standing illness, such as polyclonal immunoglobulinemia and low-grade elevation of white blood cell counts. Erythocyte sedimentation rates are usually not elevated in these patients.[2,3] Chest roentgenographic features are similar to those of the acute form, but there may be a further increase in interstitial markings or nodulations, representing more intense inflammation or early fibrosis.[4-6] Histopathologic studies of the lung demonstrate increased numbers of granulomas within the interstitial inflammatory process. Some of the giant cells may contain birefringent material, and bronchiolitis may be detected.[7,8]

Pulmonary function abnormalities are similar to those found in the acute form of hypersensitivity pneumonitis but may take longer to resolve between episodes or after avoidance or even following the use of corticosteroids.[2,3] This suggests that the subacute form of the disease is a more aggressive form associated with lesions that are more difficult to reverse.

Chronic Form

A small number of patients with long-term exposure develop chronic and progressive pulmonary symptoms without systemic features. These patients develop breathlessness, dyspnea with exertion or even at rest, and cough. Late in the disease process there are signs of respiratory failure, and cor pulmonale may occur.[1-3] Physical examination of these patients reveals the findings of chronic interstitial lung disease with tachypnea, cyanosis, and at times nail clubbing. Dry, crackling rales are prominent, and features of right heart strain and failure may be detected.

Chest roentgenographs in these patients demonstrate increased interstitial markings indicative of pulmonary fibrosis. In some patients the peripheral portion of the lungs are more involved, giving a "white-wall" appearance. In others, honeycombing and signs of hyperinflation may develop.[4-6] The prominent histopathologic finding in the lung of these patients is fibrosis with interspersed granulomas and a mild to minimal lymphocytic interstitial infiltrate.[7,8] The fibrosis may be diffuse and associated with areas of alveolar destruction, or it may be localized or focal. In some patients a prominent bronchiolitis obliterans can cause peripheral areas of emphysema.[2,3,7,8]

Pulmonary function tests in these individuals usually demonstrate irreversible restrictive and diffusion defects consistent with interstitial pulmonary fibrosis.[2,9] Some may also have prominent high-grade obstruction, probably related to the chronic obstructive bronchiolitis. All these features are irreversible and may, in fact, progress in spite of avoidance or long-term administration of systemic corticosteroids. Progression of the fibrotic process can lead to end-stage lung disease and death.[2,10,11]

There is some evidence that chronic exposure to antigen may lead to progressive pulmonary fibrosis, as occurred in 30% of farmers who developed pulmonary disability after repeated attacks of farmer's lung due to inhalation of antigen from moldy hay.[11,12] The development of progressive pulmonary disability does not seem to be as prominent in individuals with hypersensitivity pneumonitis due to repeated exposure to avian dusts: their clinical and pulmonary function abnormalities usually reverse after avoidance, even after years of exposure.[13]

ANTIGENS ASSOCIATED WITH THE DISEASE

Several organic dusts have been identified as causative agents of hypersensitivity pneumonitis and many are listed in Table 16-1. In most cases the antigens are inhaled during the course of occupational exposure such as farming, sugar cane harvesting,

TABLE 16-1. Agents Inducing Hypersensitivity Pneumonitis

ANTIGEN	SOURCE	DISEASE
Microorganisms		
THERMOPHILIC ACTINOMYCETES		
Micropolyspora faeni (*Faeni rectivirgula*)	Moldy hay, sugar cane,	Farmer's lung Bagassosis
T. vulgaris, T. viridis	compost,	Mushroom
T. sacharii	contaminated forced-	worker's lung
T. candidus	air systems	Ventilation pneumonitis
Fungi		
Aspergillus clavatus	Moldy malt	Malt worker's lung
Alternaria sp.	Moldy wood chips	Wood worker's lung
Bacillus subtilis	Moldy wood dust	Wood worker's lung
Cephalosporium sp.	Contaminated sewage	Sewage-induced hp
Cryptostroma corticale	Moldy maple bark	Maple bark stripper's lung
Penicillium frequentans	Moldy cork	Suberosis
P. caseii, P. roquefortii	Molding cheese	Cheese worker's lung
Streptomyces albus	Enhanced fertilizer	Fertilizer-induced hp
Mucor stolonifer	Paprika dust	Paprika splitter's lung
Pullularia	Contaminated wood	Sauna taker's lung, sequoiosis
Trichosporium cutaneum	House dust	Summer hp* of Japan
Animal Proteins		
Amoeba	Contaminated humidifiers	Ventilation pneumonitis
Avian proteins	Avian excreta Turkey, pigeon, chicken	Bird breeder's lung
Rodent proteins	Rat urinary proteins	Laboratory worker's lung
Bovine and porcine proteins	Pituitary snuff	Pituitary snuff taker's lung
Insects and Other Organisms		
Sitophilus granarius	Wheat weevils	Grain handler's lung
Naegleria gruberi	Amoeba	Ventilation pneumonitis
Acanthamoeba castellani		
Chemicals		
Toluene diisocyanate	Plasticizers	TDI hp
Phthalic anhydride	Altered respiratory	Phthalate hp
Trimellitic anhydride	proteins	TMA hp
Diphenylmethane diisocyanate		MDI hp
Gold, amiodarone, procarbazine	Drugs	Drug-induced hp

* hp, hypersensitivity pneumonitis

lumber processing, mushroom growing, and cork processing. Some antigens are inhaled during hobby-related activities, such as breeding birds. Other exposures are unrelated to occupation and are caused by contaminants of forced air heating, cooling, or humidification systems. Most antigens are high molecular weight derivatives of bacteria, fungi, amoeba, animals, or plants; others are low molecular weight chemicals or pharmaceuticals, usually encountered in the workplace.

Probably the most important antigens causing hypersensitivity pneumonitis are thermophilic actinomycetes—ubiquitous microorganisms that thrive in decaying vegetable matter or compost. They can also multiply in furnace plenum chambers or in air conditioning or humidification systems, whence they can be dispersed through the environment served by the forced air system.[14-16] It has been estimated that farmers handling moldy hay may be exposed to up to 1.6 billion spores in the air; a significant proportion of those 5 μm spores may be inhaled and retained in the lung.[17] Studies of the antigenic determinants of the actinomycete inducing farmer's lung have revealed over 30 distinct proteins, many with enzymatic activities.[18,19] Perhaps these microorganisms induce pulmonary inflammation by both immunologic and enzymatic mechanisms.

Avian serum proteins may also cause hypersensitivity pneumonitis; several studies have indicated that immunoglobulin A, altered by avian gastrointestinal enzymes and excreted in avian droppings, may be the offending agent.[20] Highly reactive chemicals used largely in the plastic industry may couple to respiratory proteins, become antigenic, and also induce pulmonary hypersensitivity.[21-23] Drugs such as gold, procarbazine, and amiodarone have also been associated with disease resembling hypersensitivity pneumonitis.[24-26]

IMMUNOLOGIC FEATURES

The inhalation of the biologic dusts leads to a number of immune responses in exposed individuals. Individuals with hypersensitivity pneumonitis uniformly demonstrate serum precipitating antibody against the offending agent.[1-3] However, a significant proportion of exposed but asymptomatic individuals develop similar titers of specific serum antibodies to the same antigens. Surveys of farmers and or bird handlers have demonstrated that up to 50% may have detectable precipitating antibodies without clinical features of disease.[27,28] Precipitating antibodies can easily be detected by the double immunodiffusion technique of Ouchterlony; if more sensitive tests such as radioimmunoassays or enzyme-linked immunoassays are used, the prevalence of antibody detection increases. However, since a significant number of exposed but well individuals also have detectable humoral immune responses, the finding of antibody against environmental antigens should be considered as evidence of exposure only; clinical correlation is needed to confirm the diagnosis.

Testing for skin reactivity to the antigens of hypersensitivity pneumonitis is limited by the irritating properties of most of the organic dusts. In pigeon breeders, however, immediate wheal and flare skin reactions followed by a late-onset (4-6 hours) reaction consisting of erythema and edema at the injection site can be demonstrated in most ill individuals, but also in significant numbers of exposed but well subjects.[29]

Studies of peripheral lymphocytes have demonstrated cellular immune responses in patients with hypersensitivity pneumonitis and in variable numbers of well but exposed individuals. Lymphocyte transformation and generation of cytokines such as migration inhibition factor have been detected following stimulation with appropriate antigen,[30,31] and these responses appear to discriminate better between patients and nonpatients than do humoral tests. This suggests that cellular rather than humoral immune mechanisms are important in the pathogenesis of hypersensitivity pneumonitis.

The technique of bronchoalveolar lavage (BAL) has allowed the sampling of the alveolar environment in individuals exposed to organic dusts, which may deposit in the peripheral airways where the inflammation is active. Early studies demonstrated marked increases (often over 60%) in lymphocytes in patients with pigeon breeder's disease. Studies with monoclonal antibodies directed against cell membrane markers indicated that most of the cells were T-cells, which were shown to express surface markers of activation.[32] Evaluation of the T-cell subsets in the lavage fluids demonstrated a preponderance of suppressor over helper cells.[33–35] Subsequent studies demonstrated that the T-cells in the lavage fluid of ill pigeon breeders have a greater response to antigen or mitogen than those of asymptomatic but exposed breeders, and that the T-suppressor cells from ill breeders have demonstrably impaired function.[36] This impairment in immunoregulation may in part explain the unchecked expansion of T-cell populations and active antibody formation in these patients. The preponderance of suppressor T-cells in the pulmonary parenchyma probably mirrors the immunoregulatory imbalance; its significance in the pathogenesis of hypersensitivity pneumonitis has not yet been elucidated.

Other studies have demonstrated activation of lavage macrophages as detected by enhanced cell function and expression of specific membrane markers.[37,38] The activated macrophages appear as large foamy cells with increased cytoplasmic vacuoles and may be present in clumps within and between alveoli.[39] This suggests that these cells have an active and aggressive role in the inflammatory process.

Increases in mast cells and natural killer cells have also been reported in the lavage fluids of patients with hypersensitivity pneumonitis.[40,41] These cells may be involved in the regulation of T-cell responses through the release of cytokines influencing lymphocyte function and also in vascular pulmonary responses through the release of histamine and other mediators of vascular tone. Specific staining of lung biopsy tissues from patients has confirmed the increase in natural killer, cytotoxic, and T cells (specifically, T-suppressor cells) in the lesions.[42,43] This population expansion within the lung is likely related to enhanced local immune responses and to lack of appropriate immunomodulation of that response.

Evaluation of the lavage fluids has revealed marked elevations in total protein and albumin, and antibodies to specific IgG, IgA, and IgM antigens have been detected.[44–46] These features are compatible with the active inflammatory process and are indicative of local pulmonary immune responses to inhalation of the antigen.

Serial lavage studies of ill pigeon breeders before and after purposeful exposure to antigen have elucidated sequential changes in the lung in hypersensitivity pneumonitis.[47] Within 24 hours after challenge, an increase in neutrophils could be detected. By 5 to 8 days, lymphocytes had increased and neutrophils had returned to prechallenge levels. The neutrophilia may have resulted from antigen-antibody complement interaction with release of chemotactic factors and attraction of cells. Subsequent lavage studies revealed that neutrophils were replaced by lymphocytes, probably as a result of the release of cytokines from alveolar macrophages, mast cells, and other T-cells. At each exposure this sequence is repeated, and ultimately the chronic active immunologic inflammatory process leads to granuloma formation and, with cell injury, fibrosis.

Studies of lavage fluids from asymptomatic farmers or pigeon breeders revealed surprising increases in lymphocytes, T-cells, and T-suppressor cells—in some cases, to the degree seen in ill individuals.[32,36,48] Defects in suppressor cell function, however, could not be detected in the lavage fluid of the asymptomatic pigeon breeders.[36] Further, a 2-year follow-up of the farmers with asymptomatic alveolitis demonstrated persistence in the lavage fluid of lymphocytosis without clinical features of disease.[48] Therefore, in asymptomatic but exposed subjects the detection of precipitating antibody and lymphocytic alveolitis is evidence of an immune response but in the absence of the clinical syndrome does not indicate disease.

DIAGNOSIS

The diagnosis of hypersensitivity pneumonitis should be considered in patients with recurrent respiratory or systemic symptoms resembling influenza but temporally associated with a particular environment. Other patients may have features suggestive of chronic bronchitis with anorexia and weight loss or features of progressive pulmonary impairment. Thus, the key to diagnosis is a complete and careful history in which symptoms are related to particular exposures, and in which remission of those symptoms follows avoidance of the environment.

Pulmonary function tests indicating restriction, defects in diffusion capacity, and in some cases obstruction are complementary to the history. Similarly, the chest roentgenographic features of interstitial pneumonitis are not specific unless correlated with the history. The demonstration of serum precipitating antibodies to organic dust antigens indicates exposure and an immune response but not necessarily disease. Bronchoalveolar lavage studies demonstrating a T-suppressor cell alveolitis may be helpful, as may a lung biopsy. These studies point to the diagnosis, but ultimately an association between exposure to the offending or etiologic agent and development of the clinical syndrome must be established.

Inhalation challenge offers a technique for establishing such a relationship.[50] Prior to challenge, the suspected environment may have to be evaluated for potential offending antigens. This can be done by inspecting the workplace or home. Samples from specific areas of the environment, such as water or scrapings from humidifiers or air conditioners, may be cultured for thermophilic actinomycetes or fungi. Other workplace materials that may be inhaled, such as milling coolants, may also need to be cultured. Material safety data sheets must be inspected for potential sensitizing chemicals, especially reactive plasticizers such as anhydrides, phthalates, or isocyanates. Other sources, such as NIOSH documents, may be useful in pinpointing potential offending agents.

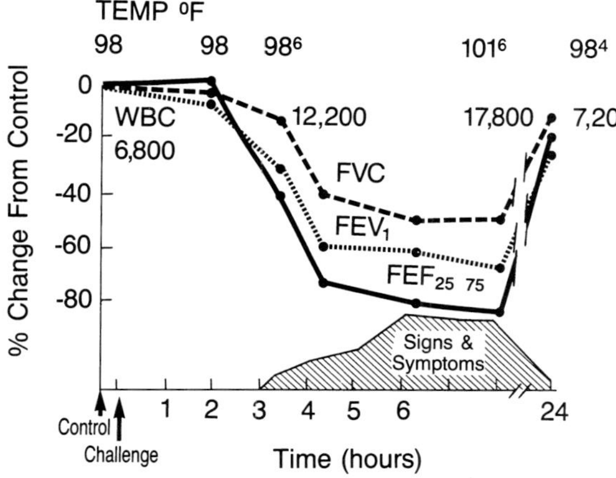

Figure 16-4. Response to challenge in hypersensitivity pneumonitis. Late-onset response to purposeful challenge with pigeon serum in a pigeon breeder with hypersensitivity pneumonitis.

Once potential antigens have been isolated and identified, purposeful challenge can be cautiously undertaken. Baseline pulmonary functions must be assessed initially, and challenge must not be carried out if the impairment is significant. When purposeful challenge is done, suspected agents are used in concentrations as close to natural exposure levels as possible. Usually the agent is placed in a compressed-air–driven nebulizer and is inhaled for 15 minutes. During and after exposure the patient is examined frequently and questioned for signs for illness. Pulmonary function, including measurements of FEV_1, D_LCO, and blood gasses, body temperature, and white blood cell counts are monitored repeatedly for from 12 to 24 hours. Responses are terminated with intravenous corticosteroids when significant clinical symptoms and signs occur. Most patients with hypersensitivity pneumonitis will develop the characteristic chills, fever, dyspnea, malaise, and myalgia 4 to 6 hours after exposure, and these are accompanied by restrictive and gas-transfer changes in pulmonary function, bibasilar rales, and elevations in temperature and white blood cell counts (Fig. 16-4). Some patients will develop a dual response characterized by an immediate asymptomatic drop in flow that is followed by a return to normalcy and then, at 4 to 6 hours, by the development of restrictive and diffusion defects along with a leukocytosis and signs and symptoms characteristic of the episode (Fig. 16-5).

It should be emphasized that purposeful inhalation challenge testing requires caution. The test may exacerbate preexisting inflammation, causing pulmonary damage, and may sensitize normal individuals. Thus, careful clinical, environmental, and immunologic correlation is essential prior to the purposeful challenge.

An alternative to bronchial challenge in the laboratory is challenge in the natural environment, such as the farmer's barn or the breeder's pigeon coop. The duration of such exposure can be judged by the history and, following a baseline evaluation, the patient may be brought back to the laboratory for further testing and observation. This technique is less hazardous than purposeful challenge because the dose of antigen inhaled has essentially been clinically evaluated during prior episodes involving similar exposures.

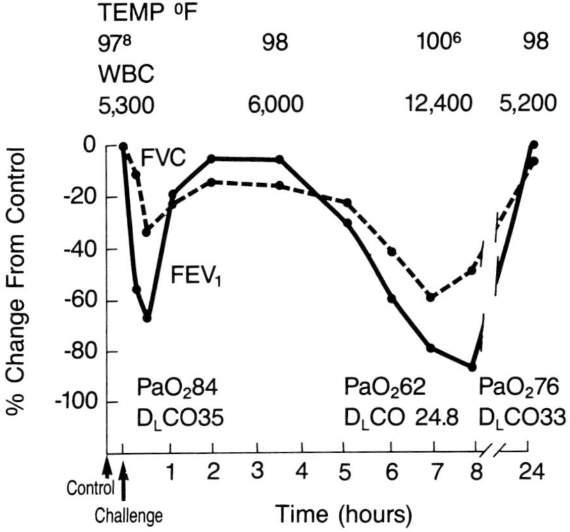

Figure 16-5. Response to challenge in ventilation pneumonitis. Immediate and late systemic and pulmonary response with hypoxia and a diffusion defect in a patient with ventilation pneumonitis after inhalation challenge with humidifier water.

DIFFERENTIAL DIAGNOSIS

The differential diagnosis to be considered in patients with suspected hypersensitivity pneumonitis includes the wide variety of causes of interstitial pneumonitis. The temporal relationship to the environment and the immunologic studies point to the diagnosis of hypersensitivity pneumonitis, which can then be confirmed by additional clinical and laboratory studies and careful observation after environmental challenge. Lymphocytosis on bronchoalveolar lavage is not specific for hypersensitivity pneumonitis but may be found in other interstitial pneumonitides. A predominance of T-suppressor cells in the lavage fluid is characteristic of, but not limited to, hypersensitivity pneumonitis. Lymphocytosis of the lavage fluid is also characteristic of sarcoidosis, but in that case the T-cell population is predominantly of the helper cell rather than the suppressor cell type.[33,37] The physical findings in hypersensitivity pneumonitis are limited to the pulmonary parenchyma; if extrapulmonary features are found, the diagnosis of hypersensitivity pneumonitis is in doubt. Chest roentgenographic and pulmonary function studies are not characteristic but may be helpful if there are significant changes with environmental manipulations.

In the differential diagnosis of hypersensitivity pneumonitis, several other environmentally induced syndromes must be considered. Occupational asthma also has a temporal relationship to the workplace, often beginning 4 to 6 hours after exposure.[50] In contrast to hypersensitivity pneumonitis where the symptoms and signs may be systemic and have features of restrictive lung disease, the clinical features in these patients are those of asthma, with wheezing, obstructive functional changes, and persistent airway hyperreactivity. IgE-mediated mast cell mechanisms may be identified in these patients by in vivo or in vitro tests.

The "sick building syndrome" has recently been described. It has been shown to be related to an increase in volatile substances and particulate matter in energy-efficient buildings, in which air exchanges and intermixing of fresh and recirculated air are significantly reduced. This reduction results in an increase in levels of mold spores, smoke, other volatile fumes, chemicals, and dusts.[51,52] This then leads, in up to 90% of workers, to significant irritant mucosal symptoms: burning sensations in the eyes and nose, cough, and, in some, itching and wheezing. There are few clinical and laboratory findings, and chest roentgenograms and pulmonary function are normal.[52] The symptoms occur mainly at work and are relieved on weekends or on vacation. The high prevalence of affected individuals is in contrast to hypersensitivity environmental disorders, which affect a minority of exposed individuals. IgE-mediated mast cell reactions may be detected in some workers, but immune responses to the workplace environment are not common in the affected population. Once the problem is identified, the treatment rests on improving the ventilation by increasing the air exchanges within the building.

Humidifier fever has been described largely in Europe and is a systemic and respiratory illness with a temporal relationship to the workplace, but with few clinical, laboratory, radiographic, or pulmonary function findings.[53,54] Immune responses to organisms contaminating the humidification system may be demonstrated. The symptoms include chills, fever, shortness of breath, and cough occurring at work. The symptoms persist but do not appear to be disabling or to lead to permanent changes. Contamination of humidification systems with organisms producing endotoxin is thought to be the cause of the disease.[55] Careful maintenance of the humidification system generally controls the symptoms.

TREATMENT

Once the offending agent is identified, the treatment of hypersensitivity pneumonitis consists of avoidance. Maple bark strippers' disease has been eliminated by covering cut maple logs so that they do not get wet: the organisms causing the disease grow under wet bark. The growth of thermoactinomyces in vegetable matter can be prevented by changing farm practices to avoid storage conditions that favor the growth of the organisms. The addition of a 1% solution of propionic acid to compost piles may prevent the growth of organisms as may the use of bottom-loading silos, which reduce conditions favorable to actinomycete growth. Regular maintenance will reduce the growth of microorganisms in forced-air ventilation and humidification systems.

In some cases of work-induced hypersensitivity pneumonitis, changing the patient's job may eliminate exposure to the antigen; if that does not work total avoidance of the workplace may be necessary. Masks that filter out chemicals and particulates may be helpful, but they are often cumbersome and constricting, making prolonged wearing difficult. Workers with hypersensitivity pneumonitis who continue to have even minimal exposure to antigen should be followed regularly with pulmonary function and chest roentgenograms to detect any subtle changes that might indicate continuing damage to the lung parenchyma.

The value of purposeful injection of antigen such as is done in atopic respiratory disorders has not been systematically studied in hypersensitivity pneumonitis. This immunotherapy may in fact be contraindicated because of the possibility of inducing immune complex diseases such as vasculitis when the injected antigen and circulating IgG antibodies interact. In rabbit models of hypersensitivity pneumonitis, long-term inhalation exposure to antigen results in reduction of the pulmonary interstitial or granulomatous response.[56,57] In humans, however, that has not been the result. In fact, in sensitized individuals who continue exposure, clinical features of the disease persist and may progress[11,12].

In those who cannot avoid the offending environment, corticosteroids may reduce the pulmonary inflammation and the episodes of hypersensitivity pneumonitis. Prednisone or its equivalent is administered in doses of up to 60 to 80 mg per day until a clinical response occurs and then is tapered over the next 30 to 60 days. Antihistamines and bronchodilators are not helpful unless bronchospasm accompanies the episodes. Cromolyn sodium may be useful in some patients with mild inflammation. In general, if the offending environment is avoided and drug therapy is instituted quickly, function returns to normal, all signs of the disease resolve, and the patient can return to a normal life.

REFERENCES

1. Pepys J. Hypersensitivity diseases of the lung due to fungi and other organic dusts. Monogr Allergy 1969;4:45.
2. Fink JN: Hypersensitivity pneumonitis. J Allergy Clin Immunol 1984;74:1.
3. Salvaggio JE: Hypersensitivity pneumonitis. J Allergy Clin Immunol 1987;79:558.
4. Rankin J, Kobayashi M, Barbee RA, Dickie HA. Pulmonary granulomatoses due to inhaled organic antigens. Med Clin North Am 1967;51:495.
5. Unger JO, Fink JN, Unger GE. Pigeon breeder's disease: Roentgenographic lung findings in hypersensitivity pneumonitis. Radiology 1968;90:683.
6. Hargreave F, Hinson KF, Reid L, Simon G, McCarthy DS. The radiologic appearance of allergic alveolitis due to bird sensitivity (bird fancier's lung). Clin Radiol 1972;23:1.
7. Hensley GT, Garancis JC, Cherayil GD, Fink JN. Lung biopsies of pigeon breeder's disease. Arch Pathol 1969;87:572.
8. Hammar S. Hypersensitivity pneumonitis. Pathol Annu 1988;23:pt 1:195.
9. Schlueter DP. Response of the lung to inhaled antigen. Am J Med 1974;57:476.
10. Greenberger PA, Pien LC, Patterson R, Robinson P, Roberts M. End-stage lung and ultimately fatal disease in a bird fancier. Am J Med 1989;86:119.
11. Barbee RA, Callies Q, Dickie HA, Rankin J. The long-term prognosis in farmer's lung. Am Rev Respir Dis 1968;97:223.
12. Braun SR, doPico GA, Tsiatis A, Dickie HA, Rankin JA. Farmer's lung disease: Long-term clinical and physiologic outcome. Am Rev Respir Dis 1979;117:185.
13. Schlueter DP, Fink JN. Personal observation.
14. Gregory RP, Lacey ME. Mycological examination of the dust from moldy hay associated with farmer's lung disease. J Gen Microbiol 1963;30:75.
15. Banaszak E, Thiede W, Fink JN. Hypersensitivity pneumonitis due to contamination of an air conditioner. N Engl J Med 1970;283:271.
16. Fink JN, Banaszak EF, Thiede WH, Barboriak JJ. Interstitial pneumonitis due to hypersensitivity to an organism contaminating a heating system. Ann Intern Med 1971;74:80.

17. Lacey J, Lacey M. Spore concentration in the air of farm buildings. Trans Br Mycol Soc 1964;47:547.
18. Roberts R. Studies on micropolyspora faeni antigens. Ann NY Acad Sci 1974;22:202.
19. Roberts R. Fractionation and characterization of thermophilic actinomycete. J Allergy Clin Immunol 1978;61:199.
20. Edwards JH, Barboriak JJ, Fink JN. Antigens in pigeon breeder's disease. Immunology 1970;19:729.
21. Schlueter DP, Banaszak EF, Fink JN, Barboriak JJ. Occupational asthma due to tetrachlorophthalic anhydride. J Occup Med 1978;20:183.
22. Fink JN, Schlueter DP. Bathtub refinisher's lung: An unusual response to toluene diisocyanate. Am Rev Respir Dis 1978;118:955.
23. Malo JL, Zeiss CR. Occupational hypersensitivity pneumonitis after exposure to diphenylmethane diisocyanate. Am Rev Respir Dis 1985;125:113.
24. Franzen P, Patterson T. Alveolitis during chrysotherapy for rheumatoid arthritis. Acta Med Scand 1983;214:249.
25. Lewis LD: Procarbazine associated alveolitis. Thorax 1984;39:206.
26. Venet A, Canbarrere I, Bonan G. Five cases of immune mediated amiodarone pneumonitis. Lancet 1984;i:962.
27. Fink JN, Schleuter DP, Sosman AJ, et al. Clinical survey of pigeon breeders. Chest 1972;62:271.
28. Gruchow HW, Hoffman RG, Marx JJ, Emanuel DA, Rimm AA. Precipitating antibodies to farmer's lung antigens in a Wisconsin farming population. Am Rev Respir Dis 1981;124:411.
29. Fink JN, Sosman AJ, Barboriak JJ, Schlueter DP, Holmes RA. Pigeon breeder's disease: A clinical study of a hypersensitivity pneumonitis. Ann Intern Med 1968;68:1205.
30. Hansen PF, Penny R. Pigeon breeder's disease: Study of the cell-mediated immune response to pigeon antigens by the lymphocyte culture technique. Int Arch Allergy Appl Immunol 1974;47:498.
31. Fink JN, Moore VL, Barboriak JJ. Cell-mediated hypersensitivity in pigeon breeders. Int Arch Allergy Appl Immunol 1974;47:498.
32. Moore VL, Pedersen GM, Hauser WC, Fink JN. A study of lung lavage materials in patients with hypersensitivity pneumonitis: In-vitro response to mitogen and antigen in pigeon breeder's disease. J Allergy Clin Immunol 1980;65:385.
33. Leatherman JW, Michael AF, Schwartz BA, Hoidal R. Lung T-cells in hypersensitivity pneumonitis. Ann Intern Med 1984;100:390.
34. Comier Y, Belanger J, LeBlanc P, Hebert J, Laviolette M. Lymphocyte subpopulations in extrinsic allergic alveolitis. Ann NY Acad Sci 1986;465:370.
35. Haslam PL. Bronchoalveolar lavage in extrinsic allergic alveolitis. Eur J Respir Dis (suppl) 1987;154:120.
36. Keller RH, Schwartz S, Schlueter DP, Bar-Sela S, Fink JN. Immunoregulation in hypersensitivity pneumonitis: Phenotypic and functional studies of bronchoalveolar lavage lymphocytes. Am Rev Respir Dis 1984;130:766.
37. Costabel U, Bross KJ, Ruble KH, Lohr GW, Matthys H. Ia-like antigens on T-cells and their subpopulations in pulmonary sarcoidosis and in hypersensitivity pneumonitis: Analysis of bronchoalveolar and blood lymphocytes. Am Rev Respir Dis 1985;131:227.
38. Mormex JF, Cordier G, Pages J, et al. Activated lung lymphocytes in hypersensitivity pneumonitis. J Allergy Clin Immunol 1984;74:719.
39. Wenzel FJ, EManuel DA, Gary RL. Immunofluorescent studies in patients with farmer's lung. J Allergy Clin Immunol 1971;48:224.
40. Haslam PL, Dewar A, Butchers P, Primett ZS, Newman-Taylor A, Turner-Warwick M. Mast cells, atypical lymphocytes, and neutrophils in bronchoalveolar lavage in extrinsic allergic alveolitis: Comparison with other interstitial lung disease. Am Rev Respir Dis 1987;135:35.

41. Soler P, Nioche S, Valeyre D, et al. Role of mast cells in the pathogenesis of hypersensitivity pneumonitis. Thorax 1987;42:565.

42. Semenzato G, Agostini C, Zambello R, et al. Lung T-cells in hypersensitivity pneumonitis: Phenotypic and functional analyses. J Immunol 1986;137:1164.

43. Semenzato G, Trentin L, Zambello R, et al. Different types of cytotoxic lymphocytes are involved in the cytolitic mechanisms taking place in the lung of patients with hypersensitivity pneumonitis. Am Rev Respir Dis 1988;137:70.

44. Reynolds HY, Fulmer JD, Kazmierowski JA, Roberts W, Frank MM, Crystal RG. Analysis of cellular and protein content of bronchoalveolar lavage fluid from patients with idiopathic pulmonary fibrosis and chronic hypersensitivity pneumonitis. J Clin Invest 1977;59:165.

45. Patterson R, Wang J, Fink JN, Calvanico NJ, Roberts M. IgA and IgG antibody activities of serum and bronchoalveolar fluid from symptomatic and asymptomatic pigeon breeders. Am Rev Respir Dis 1979;120:1113.

46. Calvanico NJ, Ambeganokar SP, Schlueter DP, Fink NJ. Immunoglobulin levels in bronchoalveolar lavage fluid from pigeon breeders. J Lab Clin Med 1980;96:129.

47. Fourmier E, Lahoute C, Wattre P, Tourrel AB, Voisin C. Cellular and humoral characteristics of the local immunological conflict in bird fancier's disease revealed by serial studies of the bronchoalveolar lavage. Eur J Respir Dis 1982;63:268.

48. Cormier Y, Belanger J, Beaudoin J, Laviolette M, Beaudoin R, Hebert J. Abnormal bronchoalveolar lavage in asymptomatic dairy farmers: Study of lymphocytes. Am Rev Respir Dis 1984;130:1046.

49. Cormier Y, Belanger J, Laviolette M. Prognostic significance of bronchoalveolar lymphocytosis in farmer's lung. Am Rev Respir Dis 1987;135:692.

50. Spector SL. Bronchial challenges with antigens. In: Spector SL, ed. Provocative challenge procedures: Bronchial, oral, nasal, and exercise. CRC Press, Boca Raton, FL, 1983, 97.

51. Spengler JD, Sexton K. Indoor air pollution: A public health perspective. Science 1983;221:9.

52. Sterling TD, Sterling E, Dimech-Ward H. Building illness in the white collar workplace. Int J Health Sci 1983;12:277.

53. Edwards JH. Humidifier fever. J R Soc Health 1982;102:7.

54. Pickenny CAC. Humidifier fever. Eur J Respir Dis 1982;123 (suppl):104.

55. Rylander R, Hagland P, Landholm M, Mattshy I, Stengrist I. Humidifier fever and endotoxin exposure. Clin Allergy 1978;8:561.

56. Richerson HB, Richards DW, Swanson PA, Butler JE, Snelzer MT. Antigen specific desensitization in a rabbit model of acute hypersensitivity pneumonitis. J Allergy Clin Immunol 1981;68:226.

57. Wilson B, Mondloch V, Katzenstein A, Moore VL. Hypersensitivity pneumonitis in rabbits: Modulation of pulmonary inflammation by long-term aerosol challenge with antigen. J Allergy Clin Immunol 1984;94:180.

17

Eosinophilic Pneumonias

Manuel Lopez
John E. Salvaggio

The term "pulmonary eosinophilia" was applied by Crofton and co-workers[1] to a group of diseases in which lung shadows were observed radiologically and were accompanied by eosinophilia. They divided the syndromes into five groups: Löffler syndrome; prolonged pulmonary eosinophilia; pulmonary eosinophilia with asthma; tropical pulmonary eosinophilia; and polyarteritis nodosa. Reeder and Goodrich applied the term "pulmonary infiltration with eosinophilia (PIE syndrome)" to the same group of syndromes.[2] Because eosinophilic infiltration of the lung can exist without peripheral blood eosinophilia, Liebow and Carrington suggested the name "eosinophilic pneumonias" as more appropriate.[3]

Throughout the years the classification and terminology of these syndromes have been controversial. Although significant progress has been made in understanding the etiologic factors in some diseases, such as Löffler syndrome, tropical eosinophilia, and allergic bronchopulmonary aspergillosis, in many cases the cause remains unknown and the factors determining the site and nature of the reaction are poorly understood. Any classification of these syndromes remains artificial since there may be significant overlap among the different groups. However, it is useful to classify these syndromes as a framework for evaluating patients with pulmonary infiltrates and eosinophilia. This article will discuss the different eosinophilic pneumonia syndromes classified in Table 17-1. A consideration of the secondary pulmonary eosinophilias (Table 17-2) is also important in differential diagnosis—particularly to rule out infectious etiologies, which necessitate different forms of therapy[4-6] and may be aggravated by the use of steroids.

THE EOSINOPHIL

The eosinophilic granulocyte was so named by Erlich because of the staining of its granules with the acidic dye eosin. Eosinophils are produced in the bone marrow from

TABLE 17-1. Eosinophilic Pneumonias

Acute
1. Associated with helminthic infections (Löffler's syndrome)
2. Drug-induced
3. Idiopathic

Chronic
1. Allergic bronchopulmonary mycosis
2. Associated with asthma
3. Idiopathic

Tropical Eosinophilia

Allergic Granulomatosis and Angiitis

stem cells, different from those of the neutrophil/monocyte stem cell line, under the influence of a variety of eosinophilopoietic factors, including granulocyte-macrophage colony stimulating factor, interleukin 3, and interleukin 5.[7,8] Eosinophils are released into the blood with an emergence time of 60 to 80 hours, a circulatory half-life of 8 to 12 hours, and a tissue half-life of several days. In contrast to other granulocytes, eosinophils are primarily tissue cells with numbers 200 to 400 times greater in tissues than in the blood. The eosinophil has a polymorphic cellular shape, like other granulocytes. Its nucleus is characteristically bilobed and lacks a nucleolus. Its most distinctive microscopic feature is a class of large ellipsoidal cytoplasmic granules termed "secondary" or "specific" granules, which contain an electron-dense crystalloid core enclosed in a less dense matrix. Large spherical primary lysosomal granules proliferate during the early development of eosinophils and many mature into crystalloid granules after the myelocyte stage. A separate class of small and homogeneously dense granules is also present in the cytoplasm.

TABLE 17-2. Secondary Pulmonary
Eosinophilias (Partial List)

Infection
Mycobacterial
Fungal
Brucellosis

Neoplastic
Hodgkin's disease
Sarcoma
Bronchogenic carcinoma

Others
Sarcoidosis
Rheumatoid arthritis
Hypereosinophilic syndrome

TABLE 17-3. Principal Protein Constituents of Human Eosinophils

CONSTITUENT	CELLULAR LOCATION	PUTATIVE FUNCTIONS
Cationic Polypeptides		
Major basic protein	Secondary granules, > 95% of protein in core	Mediates eosinophil adhesion and toxicity for helminths
		Activates mast cells
Eosinophil cationic protein	Secondary granules, matrix	Alters Hageman factor function and enhances plasmin activity
		Helminthicidal
		Neurotoxic
		Activates mast cells
Eosinophil-derived neurotoxin	Secondary granules, matrix	Centrally neurotoxic
Eosinophil protein X	Secondary granules, matrix	Centrally neurotoxic, possibly identical to eosinophil-derived neurotoxin
Enzymes		
Peroxidase	Secondary granules, matrix	Microbicidal and cytotoxic with H_2O_2 and halide
		Activates mast cells
Lysophospholipase (Charcot-Leyden crystal protein)	Plasma membrane	Inactivates lysophospholipids
Phospholipase D	Granules	Inactivates platelet-activating factor
Histaminase	Granules	Inactivates histamine

Eosinophilic Granules

Eosinophilic granules contain many enzymes and cationic polypeptides. Some of these are of special importance in the eosinophilic pneumonias. Their putative functions are listed in Table 17-3. Major basic protein (MBP) is an arginine-rich polypeptide of 9300 daltons that constitutes over 95% of the protein content of the core of the large granules. MBP is toxic to parasites and causes cell damage to a variety of tumor and mammalian cells. Pleural fluid from patients with eosinophilic pneumonia and blood and sputum from patients with asthma have MBP levels similar to those causing cell damage in vitro. This observation suggests that MBP may play an important role in the inflammatory reaction associated with eosinophilic pneumonias. The matrix of the granules contains several enzymes and proteins, including eosinophil cationic protein (ECP), eosinophil-derived neurotoxin (EDN), and eosinophil peroxidase (EPO). It is clear that the eosinophil has all the armamentarium needed to actively participate in inflammation and can produce tissue damage through the release of granular enzymes and cationic proteins.[9–11]

Eosinophil Heterogeneity

As in the case of mast cells, there are distinct subpopulations of eosinophils. When eosinophils are separated by density gradient two populations of cells are obtained: normodense and hypodense. These two subgroups differ in morphology and in biochemical and functional activities. Increased numbers of hypodense eosinophils are found in diseases associated with eosinophilia and their quantity correlates with the degree of eosinophilia. Increased levels of hypodense eosinophils have been reported in chronic helminthic infections,[12] bronchial asthma,[13] idiopathic hypereosinophilic syndrome,[14] and bronchoalveolar lavage (BAL) fluid from patients with PIE syndrome.[15] Hypodense eosinophils are metabolically more active and have increased function. It has been shown that hypodense eosinophils exhibit enhanced antibody-mediated cytotoxicity, such as against *Schistosoma mansoni* larvae, increased ligand-initiated chemotactic activity, enhanced ionophore-induced generation of leukotriene C_4 (LTC$_4$), increased consumption of glucose and O_2, and enhanced expression of low-affinity IgE receptors and other surface receptors. Although the exact mechanism leading to the appearance of hypodense eosinophils is unknown, there is increasing evidence that these cells are the result of hyperstimulation and represent activated cells.[16] T lymphocyte granulocyte-macrophage colony stimulating factor and tumor necrosis factor enhance eosinophil LTC$_4$ production and cytotoxicity against antibody-coated schistosoma and convert the cells to hypodense eosinophils. Chemoattractants, including eosinophilic chemotactic factor of anaphylaxis (ECF-A), histamine, platelet activating factor (PAF), and leukotriene B_4 (LTB$_4$), can induce both nuclear hypersegmentation and hypodense eosinophils. Lung eosinophils are exposed to maximum eosinophil chemotactic activity (ECA), likely resulting in their retention in the lung and further continuous stimulation by ECA and cytokines. This in turn probably induces the appearance of activated hypodense eosinophils.

Eosinophils generate superoxide and hydroxyl radicals at rates equal to or higher than those observed for neutrophils. Other eosinophil enzymatic activities are devoted to the oxidation of arachidonic acid, which in turn generates numerous mediators. In eosinophils the cyclo-oxygenase pathway predominantly produces PGE$_2$. The 5-lipoxygenase pathway in eosinophils generates principally LTC$_4$, with smaller amounts of LTB$_4$, LTD$_4$, and LTE$_4$; 15-lipoxygenation results in the generation of several hydroxy-eicosatetranoic acid (Hete) metabolites. Eosinophils also produce enzymes that down-

TABLE 17-4. Parasites Causing
Acute Eosinophilic Pneumonia

Ascaris species

Ancylostoma duodenale

Necator americanus

Toxocara eanis

Toxocara cetis

Strongyloides stercoralis

Schistosoma species

Trichinella spiralis

regulate hypersensitivity reactions. Components of this downregulatory response include PGE_2-induced suppression of mediator release by mast cells, ingestion of mast cell granules by eosinophils, and binding of heparin by MBP. Another set of specific eosinophil-derived enzymes is also capable of degradating mediators; eosinophil-derived histaminase is capable of inactivating histamine.

It is clear that eosinophils are tissue cells that have the capacity to augment and prolong or inhibit and terminate immediate and late reactions evoked by mast cells and basophils. Eosinophils alone and in concert with mast cells and macrophages also seem to possess the potential to participate in host defense or to promote processes that injure host tissues.

ACUTE EOSINOPHILIC PNEUMONIA

Helminthic Infestation

In 1932, Löffler[17] reported four patients who had developed peripheral blood eosinophilia and transient pulmonary infiltrates associated with minimal or no chest symptoms. In the following 20 years, more than 100 similar cases were reported from Löffler's clinic.[18] The etiology of this syndrome was unknown at the time of the original report but it was subsequently recognized that the syndrome accompanied infestations with *Ascaris lumbricoides*[19,20] and other parasites (Table 17-4). In the migratory larval stage these parasites travel through the lung, where an eosinophilic inflammatory host response ensues. Ingested *Ascaris lumbricoides* eggs hatch in the intestine and the larvae migrate through mesenteric lymphatics and portal-hepatic venules into the pulmonary parenchyma. After several days, larvae penetrate capillary walls, gain access to the alveoli, ascend the major airways to the epiglottis, and are swallowed to complete the life cycle. The parasites ultimately reside in the intestine as mature adults. Parenchymal pulmonary infiltrates are the result of a larval pneumonitis, the intensity of which is proportional to both the size of the inoculum and the degree of protection acquired from previous exposures.[20,21] Symptoms are transient because larvae that fail to emigrate from the lung die within a few weeks.

Clinical Manifestations
Many cases of eosinophilic pneumonia are asymptomatic and are discovered on routine chest radiographs. Symptoms are characterized by mild cough with occasional wheeze, malaise, anorexia, and low-grade fever. Chest radiographs reveal unilateral or bilateral homogenous densities with an alveolar-interstitial pattern classically located in the lung periphery.[22] Physical examination may demonstrate expiratory wheezes and inspiratory crackles[19] (Fig. 17-1). A heavy load of parasites may produce a more severe syndrome characterized by massive pulmonary infiltrates, asthma, pulmonary function abnormalities consistent with airway obstruction, marked eosinophilia, elevated serum IgE levels, and respiratory failure.[21]

Pathology
Typically in acute eosinophilic pneumonia due to helminthic infestation there is infiltration of the alveolar septa and spaces with eosinophils and histiocytes without

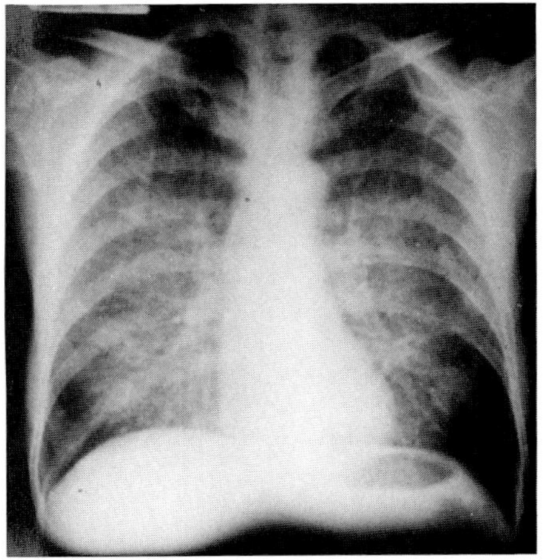

A

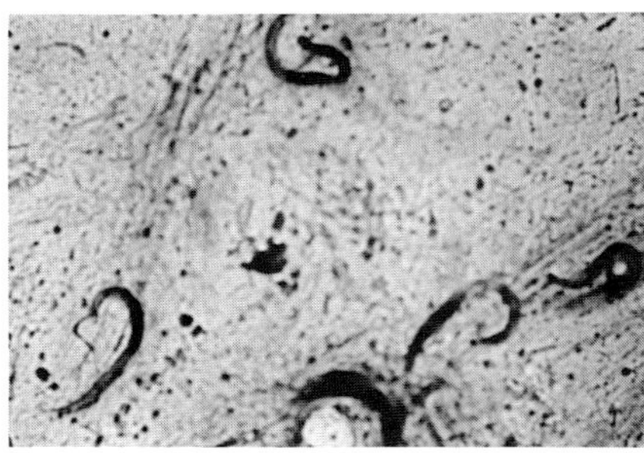

B

Figure 17-1. Acute eosinophilic pneumonia. The patient is a 66-year-old male with a history of cough, dyspnea, chills, and fever. (*A*) The radiograph of the chest revealed diffuse bilateral infiltrates. (*B*) The sputum was positive for *Strongyloides stercoralis.* Treatment with Thiabendazol resulted in gradual improvement of symptoms and clearing of the infiltrates. (Courtesy of G. Alvarez, M.D.)

significant necrosis or vascular lesions.[23] The mast cell–dependent chemotaxis of eosinophils and the helminthicidal properties of MBP and eosinophil cationic protein account for the eosinophilic tissue inflammation at the time of larval migration into the pulmonary parenchyma.

Diagnosis

Diagnosis is difficult and depends on the clinical presentation, the transient nature of the illness, serologic detection of specific anti-parasite antibodies, and a meticulous search for parasites in tissue and body secretions. In rare cases, typical third-stage larvae can be demonstrated in sputum or gastric washings. The appearance of ascaris eggs in the stool several weeks after the illness can also provide retrospective evidence of prior ascaris larvae migration through the lung.

Treatment

Although the pulmonary aspects of parasitic infection are self-limited and typically result in no permanent tissue damage, treatment with an appropriate antihelminthic drug is necessary when eggs are found in the stool in order to prevent other consequences of the infection. For *Ascaris lumbricoides,* mebendazole 100 mg b.i.d. for 3 days is recommended. Because pulmonary symptoms resolve within several weeks but eggs from mature worms are not initially detected until approximately 2 months after ingestion, careful follow-up is essential. Severe cases require a short course of corticosteroids.

Drug-Induced

A variety of drugs have been reported to cause acute eosinophilic pneumonia.[24–45] A partial list of these drugs is given in Table 17-5. Clinically, symptoms vary greatly in

TABLE 17-5. Drugs Capable of Inducing
Acute Eosinophilic Pneumonia (Partial List)

DRUG	REFERENCE
Ampicillin	24
Arsenicals	25
Beclomethasone	26
Bleomycin	27
Carbamazepine	28
Chlorpromazine	29
Chlorpropamide	30
Cromolyn	31
Dilantin	32
Gold salts	25
Imipramine	33
Mephenesin	34
Methotrexate	35
Naproxen	36
Nitrofurantoin	37
Para-amino salicylic acid	38
Penicillin	39
Phenothiazine	25
Propylthiouracil	25
Phenylbutazone	25
Streptomycin	25
Sulfonamide	40
Tetracycline	41

severity and are characterized by low-grade fever, cough, and dyspnea with or without wheezing. Chest radiographs show unilateral or bilateral peripheral lung infiltrates. Peripheral blood eosinophilia is usually but not necessarily present. Some patients may present with cutaneous eruptions, particularly urticaria, as the initial sign of an adverse pulmonary drug reaction. Lung biopsy usually demonstrates alveolar and interstitial eosinophilic, lymphocytic, and histiocytic infiltrates.

In most cases, once the offending agent has been removed, symptoms and infiltrates resolve within a month. Administration of corticosteroids may be indicated in severe cases.

Nitrofurantoin is unique among the drugs causing pulmonary eosinophilia[42,43]; pulmonary reactions to this drug may present as acute or chronic patterns. Acute reactions to nitrofurantoin occur within 1 month of therapy. They comprise approximately 90% of cases and are characterized by nonproductive cough, low-grade fever, dyspnea, and pulmonary crackles. The erythrocyte sedimentation rate is frequently elevated and there is an increase in the total peripheral blood eosinophil count. Chest radiography reveals bibasilar diffuse or patchy infiltrates with frequent pleural effusions. Pathologic changes include interstitial and alveolar infiltrates of mononuclear cells and

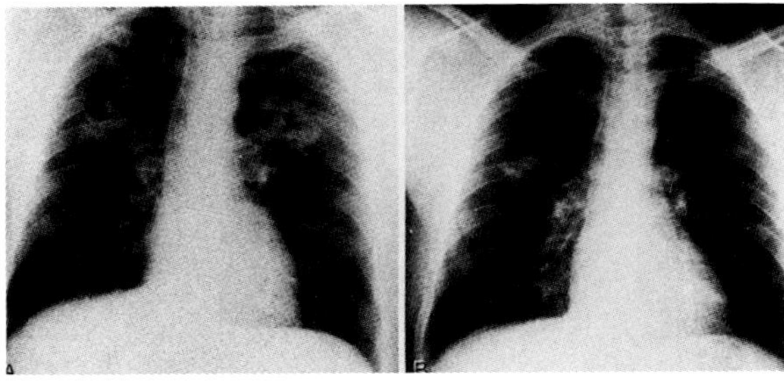

Figure 17-2. Allergic bronchopulmonary aspergillosis. This 34-year-old male had asthma since childhood. During the past year he had been admitted for an episode of "asthmatic bronchitis." More recently, he noted brown flecks and occasional streaks of blood in his sputum. Laboratory data included a leukocyte count of 4500/mm^3 with 14% eosinophils (1330/mm^3), a serum IgE level of 6700 ng/ml, an immediate response to prick testing for *Aspergillus* antigen, presence of precipitating antibodies to *Aspergillus* in the serum, and *Aspergillus* hyphae in the sputum. (*A*) Multiple infiltrates are evident in both upper zones, extending as finger-like projections compatible with peribronchial infiltrates and obstruction of multiple segmental bronchi. (*B*) A follow-up film, taken 3 months after steroid therapy was initiated, shows dramatic resolution of the infiltrates. (Courtesy of H. Buechner, M.D.)

polymorphonuclear leukocytes with variable degrees of tissue eosinophilia. Vascular wall infiltrates consisent with vasculitis may also be noted.

Chronic reactions to nitrofurantoin are less common and occur 2 months to 5 years after initiation of therapy. Symptoms consist of an insidious onset of exertional dyspnea and nonproductive cough. Eosinophilia is less common, and there is an increased incidence of positive antinuclear antibodies and lupus-like symptoms. Chest radiographic findings and pathologic changes resemble those noted in the acute form but interstitial fibrosis is more prominent. Treatment involves simple discontinuation of the drug. In the chronic type of nitrofurantoin reaction, steroids may halt the progression of tissue damage.

Exposure to inorganic chemicals may also result in transient pulmonary infiltrates with eosinophilia. Several cases of nickel-induced Löffler's syndrome have been reported, after either inhalation of nickel carbonyl fumes in an industrial setting or ingestion of a nickel-containing coin.[44,45]

In some patients with acute pulmonary eosinophilia, no etiologic agent can be found. Allen and co-workers[46] reported four cases of eosinophilic pneumonia in which patients presented with symptoms of an acute febrile illness, severe hypoxemia, diffuse pulmonary infiltrates, and an increased number of eosinophils in BAL fluid with no evidence of infection. Two of the patients required mechanical ventilation and all responded to oral prednisone.

Allergic Bronchopulmonary Mycosis

In 1952, Hinson and co-workers[47] reported what is now classified as allergic bronchopulmonary aspergillosis (ABPA) (Fig. 17-2). Their initial report included eight patients with episodes of reversible bronchospasm, recurrent lung infiltrates with fever occurring over months or years, sputum and blood eosinophilia, mucus plugs obstructing airways, sputum, *Aspergillus* hyphae in sputum, and central, saccular bronchiectasis. Currently, the most important diagnostic criteria for ABPA are a history of asthma with peripheral blood eosinophilia, specific serum IgE and precipitating antibodies to *As-*

pergillus species, elevated total serum IgE levels, a history of transient or fixed pulmonary infiltrates, and central bronchiectasis. For a complete review of this syndrome, see Chapter 15. In some patients with a clinical history of ABPA, no *Aspergillus* hyphae are found in the sputum nor are serologic tests positive for anti-aspergillus antibody. Recent reports suggest that hypersensitivity to *Helminthosporium, Curvularia, Dreschlera,* and *Stemphyllium* species can produce a clinical picture identical to that noted in ABPA.[48–50] This suggests the use of the more general term "allergic bronchopulmonary mycosis" to describe this condition. Therefore, in a setting where ABPA is suspected but no evidence of *Aspergillus* hypersensitivity is found, repeated isolation of another fungal species in the sputum should prompt consideration of skin and serologic tests to detect immune reactivity to the particular genus and species isolated.

CHRONIC EOSINOPHILIC PNEUMONIA (CEP)

Chronic eosinophilic pneumonia (CEP) was described by Carrington and co-workers in 1969.[51] Typically, patients present with severe illness characterized by fever, night sweats, weight loss, and progressive dyspnea. Asthma may accompany or precede the onset of symptoms in approximately 50% of cases. Chest radiographic findings are characterized by peripheral lung infiltrates described as the "photographic negative" of the radiologic shadows seen in pulmonary edema.[52] Other radiographic findings are pleural effusion, cavitations, and patchy migratory infiltrates. CEP has been reported in one patient without pulmonary infiltrates who related a history consistent with the syndrome and had increased eosinophils in BAL fluid and positive histologic changes on lung biopsy.[53] When the illness is most severe, lung volumes and diffusion capacity are decreased, hypoxemia is prominent, and mechanical ventilation may be required.[54] Laboratory findings include peripheral blood eosinophilia in two-thirds of the cases,[55] an elevated sedimentation rate, and thrombocytosis[56] (Fig. 17-3). Recently increased total serum IgE levels have been reported in some patients early in the course of the disease.[57,58]

In a recent report[59] that described 19 patients with biopsy-proven chronic eosinophilic pneumonia and reviewed 100 additional cases fulfilling the criteria for CEP, a diagnosis could be made with reasonable certainty in most cases without lung biopsy. Females were affected more than twice as often as males and pre-existing atopic disease was detected in 50% of patients, with asthma being the most common manifestation. The most common symptoms and signs were cough, fever, dyspnea, weight loss, sputum production, wheezing, night sweats, and malaise. In spite of a history of atopy, most patients were asymptomatic in the period immediately before onset of CEP symptoms. Peripheral blood eosinophilia greater than 6% was seen in approximately 90% of the cases, as was a sedimentation rate of more than 20 mm/hour. Weight loss was at times prominent, often exceeding 10 kg. The classic roentgenographic finding of a "photographic negative of pulmonary edema" was seen in less than one-half of the cases, although peripheral infiltrates in the outer two-thirds of the lung fields were the most common radiographic abnormality. The peripheral infiltrates were predominantly located in the upper lung zones in less than one-half of the cases, and they occurred bilaterally. In one-third of the cases, chest films revealed a nonperipheral

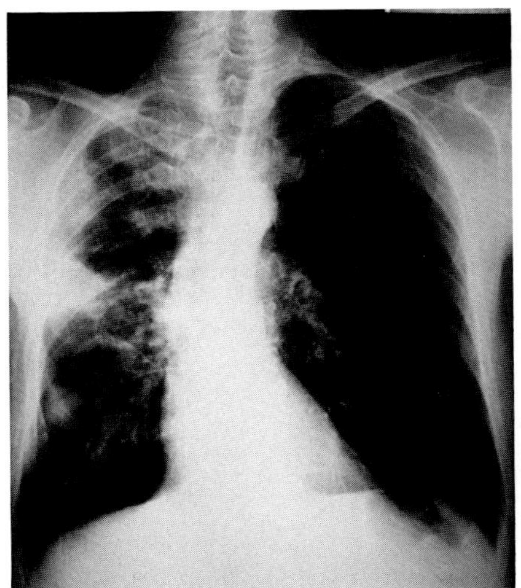 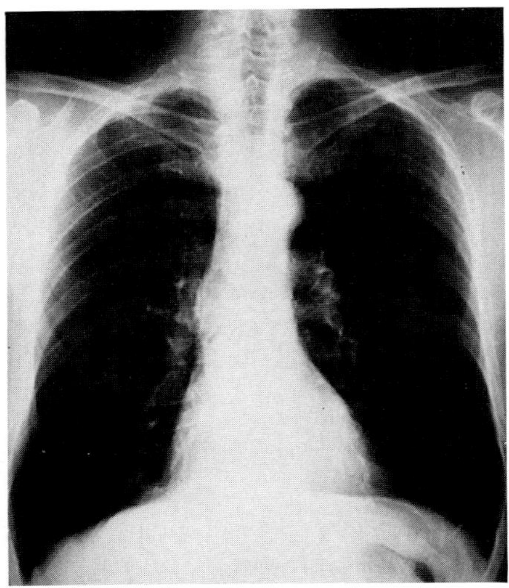

A   **B**

Figure 17-3. Eosinophilic pneumonia. This 57-year-old male had a 40-year history of bronchial asthma and was highly allergic to house dust mites. Two weeks prior to admission, he developed flu-like symptoms, cough, and progressive dyspnea. Laboratory data included a leukocyte count of 14,300/mm^3 with 20% eosinophils, and arterial blood gas analysis revealed a pH of 7.45, a PO_2 of 62 torr, and a PCO_2 of 34 torr. (*A*) In this chest radiograph, dense areas of peripheral consolidation are apparent in the lateral part of the right upper and middle zones, and small areas of consolidation are visible in lower zones. Following evaluation the diagnosis of eosinophilic pneumonia was made, and treatment with prednisone 60 mg/day was initiated. (*B*) A follow-up film taken 1 month later shows a normal appearance.

radiographic distribution—again, usually bilaterally. The asthma was more often of the extrinsic or IgE-mediated variety. It often occurred in association with allergic rhinitis and nasal polyps.

Histologic findings are characterized by interstitial and alveolar infiltrates with activated eosinophils in various stages of degranulation,[52,57] as well as macrophages, lymphocytes, and plasma cells (Fig. 17-4). Multinucleated giant cells with eosinophilic granules and needle-shaped bodies, recognizable as minute Charcot-Leyden crystals, are also present within lesions. In spite of extensive cellular infiltration, the alveolar septa are usually intact and fibrosis is minimal.[60] Electron microscopy has demonstrated the accumulation of eosinophil granules in extracellular areas and in macrophage cytoplasm. Immunofluorescence studies have demonstrated strong staining for MBP in the area of eosinophilic microabscesses.[56,57] BAL fluid characteristically demonstrates increased numbers of eosinophils.[61]

The etiology of CEP is unknown. The clinical presentation, elevated serum IgE levels, eosinophilia, and responsiveness to steroids suggest involvement of IgE-dependent immediate and late-phase hypersensitivity in disease pathogenesis, as would appear to be the case in ABPA. The common characteristic of these patients is marked tissue infiltration by eosinophils, and it is likely that these cells play a key role in disease

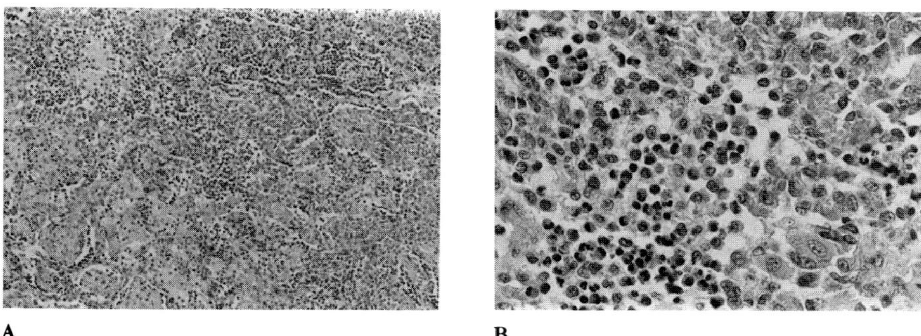

Figure 17-4. Chronic eosinophilic pneumonia. Low-power (*A*) and high-power (*B*) views of lung biopsy tissue from a patient with chronic eosinophilic pneumonia demonstrate extensive interstitial and alveolar infiltrates, mainly of eosinophils. (Courtesy of C. Restrepo, M.D.)

pathogenesis. As more specific etiologic agents are identified, better classification of the pulmonary eosinophilic syndrome will no doubt develop. At present, however, CEP remains a heterogenous group of syndromes with the common feature of lung injury mediated by eosinophils and their products.

Diagnosis

BAL has been alleged to be a useful diagnostic technique in CEP. In one recent study,[46] four patients with an acute form of noninfectious, eosinophilic pneumonia were evaluated using BAL as a diagnostic tool. These individuals presented with severe hypoxemia, pulmonary infiltrates, a marked increase of eosinophils on BAL, and no history of asthma or atopy. The condition resolved completely after administration of corticosteroids and erythromycin and was thought to be distinct from other types of idiopathic eosinophilic lung disease, rather than part of the spectrum of CEP. In these reported cases all subjects had a BAL eosinophil count of over 25% before treatment and a marked reduction after treatment. It remains to be seen whether BAL will be helpful or even necessary in establishing the diagnosis of CEP, but in most studies the correlation between eosinophilia on BAL and evidence of eosinophilic alveolitis has been good. Thus, BAL, with stains and cultures of lavage fluid and cellular analysis, may be a reasonable initial invasive diagnostic procedure to consider in patients presenting with respiratory insufficiency and pulmonary infiltrate of unknown cause.

Computed tomography (CT) has been reported as useful in defining the peripheral distribution of infiltrates in CEP. CT should be considered before lung biopsy in instances where there is a strong clinical suspicion of CEP but conventional radiographs do not reveal a peripheral infiltrate.

Many clinicians feel that lung biopsy is not necessary for the diagnosis of CEP. The diagnosis can be made with careful attention to the characteristic features, roentgenographic and laboratory findings, immunologic evaluation to rule out ABP, BAL with appropriate cultures for infection, and/or therapeutic trial with corticosteroids. In one recent review of 119 cases,[59] the diagnosis was made clinically in one-third of the patients. It was felt that the therapeutic trial of corticosteroids was particularly helpful in confirming the diagnosis. The remaining two-thirds of the patients underwent a lung biopsy, approximately 60% having an open lung biopsy and the remainder transbronchial or needle biopsies.

Treatment

Corticosteroids are the recommended treatment for CEP. Prednisone at doses of 40 to 60 mg daily provides dramatic clinical improvement in most patients, with resolution of radiographic infiltrates in 2 to 4 weeks. In the review by Jederlinic[59] of 78 patients with CEP, there was a complete resolution of the symptoms in 84% of cases within 2 weeks of corticosteroid treatment. In most of the other cases a clinical response was apparent in 2 weeks with complete clinical responses in 1 month. Rapid tapering of steroid dosage frequently resulted in relapse with recurrence of clinical and radiologic changes; the relapse rate after short-term treatment in Jederlinic's study was 80%. For this reason the need for prolonged therapy is clear. It is recommended that corticosteroid treatment be given for at least 6 months, starting with high doses (60 mg/day) and tapering to a low daily or alternate-day dose following the initial clinical response. In patients with repeated episodes, steroids may provide radiologic resolution but permanent pulmonary physiologic impairment and architectural damage may still result.[52]

Prognosis

The duration of therapy must be individualized for each patient. Pearson and Rosenow[55] followed eight cases of CEP for periods ranging from 27 months to 12 years (mean = 6 years) after diagnosis. At the time of follow-up, six of the eight patients had discontinued steroids. Although half continued to have asthma, none had recurrent infiltrates. Steroid therapy appears to shorten the duration of the disease. In those with an aggressive course, it may be lifesaving.

TROPICAL EOSINOPHILIA

There has been considerable confusion over the term "tropical eosinophilia," and clinicians have used the term loosely. Evidence has accumulated indicating that tropical eosinophilia is a syndrome caused by a hypersensitivity reaction to filarial infections.[62] Infection with the filarial species *Wuchereria bancrofti* or *Brugia malayi* typically results in recurrent lymphangitis with fibrosis and lymphatic obstruction. In some patients, a variation of this presentation occurs, characterized by paroxysmal nocturnal cough, wheezing, patchy pulmonary infiltrates, and profound eosinophilia. Disseminated lymphadenopathy, weight loss, and low-grade fever occur with lesser frequency. According to Donohugh[63] the diagnosis of tropical eosinophilia should include history of a dry, irritating, primarily nocturnal cough accompanied by attacks of wheezing and dyspnea; pulmonary infiltrates; eosinophilia above 2000/mm^3, a positive filaria complement fixation test; and a clinical and hemotologic response to diethylcarbamazine (Fig. 17-5).

The clinical manifestations of tropical eosinophilia were initially described in India in the 1940s by Frimodt-Moller and Barton[64] and by Weingarten.[65] Recognition of

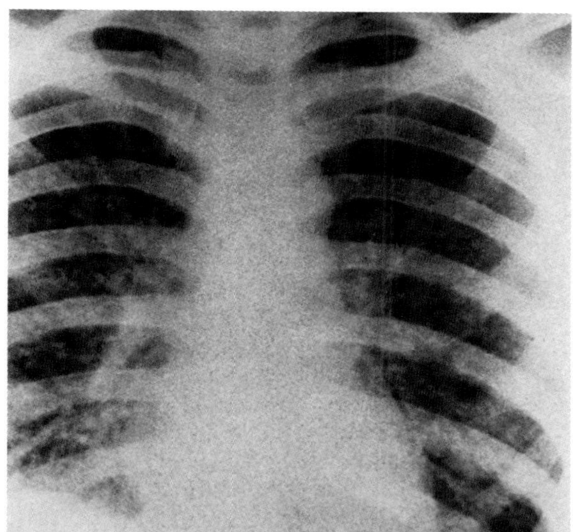

Figure 17-5. Tropical eosinophilia. The patient is a 24-year-old Indian student with worsening asthma and eosinophilia for 3 months. He had lived in India until 3 years prior to hospitalization and had received diethylcarbamazine therapy in the past for similar complaints. On admission his leukocyte count was 54,000/mm³ with 70% eosinophils (37,800/mm³). The sereum IgE level was 4000 ng/ml and a serologic test for filariasis gave markedly positive results. Chest radiograph shows profuse small nodules appearing as mottled infiltrates. Symptoms resolved over several days following initiation of diethylcarbamazide therapy. (Courtesy of P. Weller, M.D.)

the role of filarial infections in tropical eosinophilia has gradually appeared in the literature[66–69] and can be summarized as follows: Patients have very high titers of antifilarial antibodies, and despite the inability to detect filaria in the circulation (typically apparent in blood smears of those with lymphoreticular filariasis), lung and lymph node biopsy specimens contain microfilariae.[70] Patients respond well to diethylcarbamazide, an effective antifilarial agent.

In some patients with filariasis, pulmonary infiltrates can be absent and generalized lymphadenopathy and eosinophilia are the most prominent features. It is not well understood why some patients develop primarily pulmonary-eosinophilic manifestations and others, lymphadenopathy. Apparently, age is important, since pulmonary manifestations increase with advancing age. Ottesen and Neva demonstrated reaginic (IgE) antibodies to antigens from the human filarial parasites *Wuchereria bancrofti* and *Brugia malayi* in seven patients with tropical eosinophilia[71,72]; it is likely that the pathogenesis of this syndrome is similar to that of ABPA, in which immediate IgE-mediated hypersensitivity and late-phase eosinophilic infiltrates play a prominent role.

Laboratory Findings

Tropical eosinophilia is usually characterized by intense eosinophilia (>3000/mm³), elevated total serum IgE levels (typically > 1000 ng/ml),[72] and high titers of antifilarial complement-fixing antibodies in the absence of circulating microfilaria.

Radiographic Findings

A pattern of decreased translucency of the lung fields with an increase in linear markings and hilar prominance is found in 98% of untreated patients with active disease.[73]

Additional findings include diffuse, finely nodular infiltrates and occasional consolidation patterns, usually with ill-defined margins and a subsegmental distribution.

Pathology

Lung biopsies have shown varying degrees of parenchymal changes depending on the duration of illness.[74] The earliest lesions, within 2 weeks of initial symptoms, are patchy and characterized by collections of histiocytes in alveolar, interstitial, peribronchial, and perivascular spaces. Histologic changes in patients who have had symptoms for 1 to 3 months are characterized by eosinophilic infiltrates, eosinophilic abscesses, and bronchopneumonia. Lesions are primarily peribronchial and perivascular in distribution; bronchioles are infiltrated with eosinophils and edematous. Lumens are blocked with mucus and clumps of eosinophils. In patients with disease of long duration (>2 years), marked fibrosis is evident.

Pulmonary Function

Pulmonary function studies show an obstructive defect in patients presenting with symptoms of tropical eosinophilia of less than 1 month duration. In more chronic cases a restrictive defect is superimposed on the obstructive dysfunction.[75] Airway hyperreactivity as demonstrated by histamine challenge has been reported in two patients.[76]

Treatment

Diethylcarbamazine at a dosage of 8 to 12 mg/kg/day for 2 weeks is the drug of choice in tropical eosinophilia.[77] By 2 weeks after initiation of therapy there is marked clinical improvement and a decrease in the total eosinophil count. A gradual decrease in serum IgE levels and antifilarial antibodies is also associated with clinical improvement. Patients who relapse may improve following a second course of therapy. In patients with longstanding illness, restrictive pulmonary dysfunction may persist despite successful treatment.[75]

ALLERGIC GRANULOMATOSIS AND ANGIITIS (CHURG-STRAUSS SYNDROME)

Allergic granulomatosis is an uncommon type of eosinophilic granulomatous inflammation with associated vascular necrosis occurring in an asthmatic patient. In 1951, Churg and Strauss[78] described 14 patients with asthma, fever, vasculitis, and eosinophilia. Throughout the years there has been considerable discussion of this syndrome and its distinction from polyarteritis nodosa.

Although the vascular changes resemble those in polyarteritis nodosa, allergic granulomatosis and angiitis (Churg-Strauss syndrome) has unique features, including the following: (1) frequent involvement of pulmonary vessels; (2) involvement of various types and sizes of vessels; (3) intravascular and extravascular granuloma formation; (4) eosinophilic tissue infiltrates; and (5) association with asthma and peripheral eosinophilia.[79] Lanham[80] has divided the clinical course of the disease into three phases. First, there is a prodromal phase consisting of allergic disease that typically begins with allergic rhinitis and asthma and may persist for years. A second phase follows that is characterized by peripheral blood eosinophilia and eosinophilic tissue infiltrates producing a picture similar to that of chronic eosinophilic pneumonia or eosinophilic gastroenteritis; the third phase is characterized by life-threatening vasculitis that may involve many organs. The severity of the angiitis and granulomatosis varies from patient to patient. Infiltration of abdominal viscera with granulomas and the associated angiitis may result in gastric ulcers, bowel perforation, and colonic obstruction. In some patients, renal and central nervous system symptoms may be the result of granulomas and vasculitis.

Laboratory Findings

An elevated sedimentation rate and leukocytosis are frequently noted. Peripheral blood eosinophilia is prominent in approximately 85% of cases. Serum IgE levels have been elevated in some cases and appear to correlate with the activity of the vasculitis.[81]

Pathology

Histologic hallmarks of Churg-Strauss syndrome are necrotizing vasculitis, tissue infiltration by eosinophils, and extravascular granulomas.[80] The initial step in the formation of these granulomas is a massive invasion by eosinophils, which is followed by necrosis of the involved tissue and the development of the characteristic granulomas. These granulomas may heal and completely resolve or, more typically, scar.[82] The vasculitis affecting small arteries and small veins occurs in association with a predominant eosinophilic infiltration. Typically, lesions progress from an eosinophilic inflammatory vascular and perivascular infiltrate, to necrotizing vasculitis, to a healed, occluded vessel.

The three histologic components, necrotizing vasculitis, tissue infiltration with eosinophils, and extravascular granulomas, often do not coexist, and granulomas may be particularly difficult to find by tissue biopsy.

Polyarteritis nodosa (PAN), a disease characterized by occasional asthma and eosinophilia, is clinically very similar. The primary histologic features of PAN include a neutrophilic cellular infiltrate, the involvement of small and medium arteries, and the absence of necrotizing granulomas outside of the vascular tissue.

Etiology

The cause of Churg-Strauss syndrome is unknown. The clinical presentation of asthma, eosinophilia, and elevated IgE levels suggests an allergic reaction. However, no specific allergen has been identified. The vasculitis may be caused by deposits of immune complexes in blood vessels with complement activation and secondary inflammatory reaction. Circulating immune complexes have been identified in some patients, and renal biopsy specimens are positive for IgM deposits.[83] IgE levels have been elevated in some cases and appear to correlate with activity of the vasculitis.[80,81] It has been suggested that IgE-mediated release of vasoactive amines facilitates the deposition of immune complexes. The factors that cause the progression of the disease from eosinophilic pneumonia to systemic vasculitis with granuloma formation[84,85] are unknown.

Treatment

Untreated Churg-Strauss syndrome can be fatal. High doses of prednisone (60–100 mg/day) are often required. Chumbley and co-workers[86] reported a 5-year survival rate of 62% among patients treated with corticosteroids. In patients deteriorating on high doses of prednisone, pulse therapy with 1.0 g methylprednisone per day for 4 days may be effective.[87] In patients who do not respond to corticosteroids or who have evidence of systemic vasculitis with major organ involvement, therapy with cytotoxic drugs is indicated. Fauci[79,88] recommends a regimen of cyclophosphamide 2 mg/kg/day as a single oral dose or 4 mg/kg intravenously for the first 3 to 4 days in the critically ill patient. When given orally, the cyclophosphamide dosage is adjusted to maintain the leukocyte count between 3000 and 3500 cells/mm^3 and the neutrophil count above 1500/mm^3. Not all patients with Churg-Strauss syndrome have a progressively worsening course,[89] and careful selection of patients for corticosteroid and immunosuppressive therapy is required.

REFERENCES

1. Crofton JW, Livingstone JL, Oswald NC, Roberts ATM. Pulmonary eosinophilia. Thorax 1952;7:1.
2. Reeder WH, Goodrich BE. Pulmonary infiltration with eosinophilia (PIE syndrome). Ann Intern Med 1952;36:1217.
3. Liebow AA, Carrington CB. The eosinophilic pneumonias. Medicine (Baltimore) 1969;48:251.
4. Lombard CM, Tazelaar HD, Krasne DL. Pulmonary eosinophilia in coccidioidal infections. Chest 1987;91:734.
5. Slungaard A, Ascensao J, Zanjani E, Jacobs HS. Pulmonary carcinoma with eosinophilia: Demonstration of a tumor-derived eosinophilopoietic factor. N Engl J Med 1983;309:778.
6. Dawes PT, Smith DH, Scott DL. Massive eosinophilia in rheumatoid arthritis: Report of four cases. Clin Rheumatol 1986;5:62.
7. Gleich GJ, Adolphson CR. The eosinophil leukocyte: Structure and function. Adv Immunol 1986;39:177.
8. Clutterbuck EJE, Hirst EMA, Sanderson CJ. Human interleukin-5 (IL5) regulates the production of eosinophils in human bone marrow cultures: Comparison and interaction with IL1, IL3, IL6, and GM-CSF. Blood 1989;73:1504.
9. Fredens K, Dahl R, Venge P. The Gordon phenomenon induced by eosinophil cationic protein and eosinophil protein X. J Allergy Clin Immunol 1982;70:361.
10. Durack DT, Sumi SM, Klebanoff SJ. Neurotoxicity of eosinophils. Proc Natl Acad Sci USA 1979;76:1443.
11. Young JD, Peterson CGB, Venge P, Cohn ZA. Mechanism of membrane damage mediated by human eosinophil cationic protein. Nature 1986;321:613.
12. DeSimone C, Donneli G, Meli D, et al. Human eosinophils and parasitic diseases. II. Characterization of two cell fractions isolated at different densities. Clin Exp Immunol 1982;48:249.
13. Fukuda T, Dunnette SL, Reed CE, et al. Increased numbers of hypodense eosinophils in the blood of patients with bronchial asthma. Am Rev Respir Dis 1985;132:981.
14. Capron M, Tonnel AB, Bletry O, Capron A. Heterogeneity of human peripheral blood eosinophils: Variability in cell density and cytotoxic ability in relation to the level and the origin of hypereosinophilia. Int Arch Allergy Appl Immunol 1983;72:336.

15. Chihara J, Kino T, Fukuda F, Oshima S. Increases of hypodense eosinophils in bronchoalveolar lavage fluid in patients with PIE syndrome. Jpn J Allergy 1985;34:676.
16. Chihara J, Nakajima S. Induction of hypodense eosinophils and nuclear hypersegmentation of eosinophils by various chemotactic factors and lymphokines in vitro. Allergy Proc 1989;10:27.
17. Löffler W. Zur differential-diagnose der lungeninfiltrierungen: II. Über fluchtige succedan-infiltrate (mit eosinophile). Beitr z Klin d Tuberk 1932;79:368.
18. Maier C. Temporary eosinophilic pulmonary infiltration: Summary of more than one hundred observations, Basel: Helvetica Medica Acta. 1943;10:95. (Abstracted in JAMA 1943;123:868).
19. Gelpi AP, Mustafa A. Ascaris pneumonia. Am J Med 1968;44:377.
20. Beaver PC, Danaraj TJ. Pulmonary ascariasis resembling eosinophilic lung; Autopsy report with description of larvae in the bronchioles. Am J Trop Med Hyg 1958;7:100.
21. Phills JA, Harrold AJ, Whiteman GV, Perelmutter L. Pulmonary infiltrates, asthma and eosinophilia due to *Ascaris suum* infection in man. N Engl J Med 1972;286:965.
22. Citro LA, Gordon ME, Miller WT. Eosinophilic lung disease (or how to slice P.I.E.). Am J Roentgenol Radium Ther Nucl Med 1973;117:787.
23. Bedrossian CW, Greenberg SD, Williams LJ. Ultrastructure of the lung in Löffler's pneumonia. Am J Med 1975;58:438.
24. Poe RH, Condemi JJ, Weinstein SS, Schuster R. Adult respiratory distress syndrome related to ampicillin sensitivity. Chest 1980;77:449.
25. Nutman TB, Ottesen EA, Cohen SG. The eosinophil, eosinophilia, and eosinophil related disorders. III. Clinical assessments. Allergy Proc 1989;10:33.
26. Mollura JL, Bernstein R, Fines SR, et al. Pulmonary eosinophilia in a patient receiving beclomethasone dipropionate aerosol. Ann Allergy 1979;42:326.
27. Yousem SA, Lifson JD, Colby TV. Chemotherapy-induced eosinophilic penumonia: Relation to bleomycin. Chest 1985;88:103.
28. Cullinan SA, Bower GC. Acute pulmonary hypersensitivity to carbamazepine. Chest 1975;68:580.
29. Shear MK. Chlorpromazine-induced PIE syndrome. Am J Psychiatr 1978;135:492.
30. Bell RJM. Pulmonary infiltration with eosinophils caused by chlorpropamide. Lancet 1964;i:1249.
31. Lobel H, Machtey I, Eldror MY. Pulmonary infiltrates with eosinophilia in an asthmatic patient treated with disodium chromoglycate. Lancet 1972;ii:1032.
32. Michael JR, Rudin ML. Acute pulmonary disease caused by phenytoin. Ann Intern Med 1981;95:452.
33. Wilson IC, Gambill JM, Sandifer MG. Löffler's syndrome occurring during imipramine therapy. Am J Psychiatr 1963;119:892.
34. Rodman T, Fraimow W, Meyerson RM. Löffler's syndrome: Report of a case associated with administration of mephenesin carbamate (Tolseram). Ann Intern Med 1958;3:668.
35. Sostman HD, Matthay RA, Putman CE, et al. Methotrexate-induced pneumonitis. Medicine 1976;55:371.
36. Nader DA, Schillaci RF. Pulmonary infiltrates with eosinophilia due to naproxen. Chest 1983;83:280.
37. Israel HL, Diamond P. Recurrent pulmonary infiltration and pleural effusion due to nitrofurantoin sensitivity. N Eng J Med 1962;266:1024.
38. Warring FC, Howlett KS. Allergic reactions to para-amino-salicylic acid: Report of seven cases, including one of Löffler's syndrome. Am Rev Tuberc 1952;65:235.
39. Reichlin S, Loveless MH, Kane EG. Löffler's syndrome following penicillin therapy. Ann Intern Med 1953;38:113.
40. Wang KK, Bowyer BA, Fleming CR, Schroeder K. Pulmonary infiltrates and eosinophilia associated with sulfasalazine. Mayo Clin Proc 1984;59:343.

41. Ho D, Tashkin DP, Bein ME, et al. Pulmonary infiltrates with eosinophilia associated with tetracycline. Chest 1979;76:33.

42. Holmberg L, Boman G. Pulmonary reactions to nitrofurantoin: 447 cases reported to the Swedish Adverse Drug Reaction Committee, 1966–1976. Eur J Respir Dis 1981;62:180.

43. Hailey FJ, Glascock HW, Hewitt WF. Pleuropneumonic reactions to nitrofurantoin. N Engl J Med 1969;281:1087.

44. Sunderman FW, Sunderman FW Jr. Löffler's syndrome associated with nickel sensitivity. Arch Intern Med 1961;107:405.

45. Gray J. Löffler's syndrome following ingestion of a coin. Can Med Assoc J 1982;127:999.

46. Allen JN, Pacht ER, Gadek JE, Davis WB. Acute eosinophilic pneumonia as a reversible cause of noninfectious respiratory failure. N Engl J Med 1989;321:569.

47. Hinson KFW, Moon AJ, Plumner NS. Bronchopulmonary aspergillosis: A review and report of eight cases. Thorax 1952;7:317.

48. Hendrick DJ, Ellithorpe DB, Lyon F, Hattier P, Salvaggio JE. Allergic bronchopulmonary helminthosporiosis. Am Rev Respir Dis 1982;126:935.

49. Benatar SR, Allan B, Hevitson RP, Don PA. Allergic bronchopulmonary stemphyliosis. Thorax 1980;35:515.

50. McAleer R, Kroenert DB, Elder JL, Froudist JH. Allergic bronchopulmonary disease caused by *Curvularia lunata* and *Drechslera hawaiiensis*. Thorax 1981;36:338.

51. Carrington CB, Addington WW, Goff AM, et al. Chronic eosinophilic pneumonia. N Engl J Med 1969;280:787.

52. Gaensler EA, Carrington CB. Peripheral opacities in chronic eosinophilic pneumonia: The photographic negative of pulmonary edema. Am J R 1977;128:1.

53. Dejaegher P, Derueaux L, Dubois P, Demedts M. Eosinophilic pneumonia without radiographic pulmonary infiltrates. Chest 1983;84:637.

54. Libby DM, Murphy TF, Edwards A, Gray G, King KC. Chronic eosinophilic pneumonia: An unusual cause of acute respiratory failure. Am Rev Respir Dis 1980;122:497.

55. Pearson DL, Rosenow EC. Chronic eosinophilic pneumonia (Carrington's): A follow up study. Mayo Clin Proc 1978;53:73.

56. Grantham JG, Meadows JA, Gleich GJ. Chronic eosinophilic pneumonia: Evidence of eosinophil degranulation and release of major basic protein. Am J Med 1986;80:89.

57. Gonzalez EB, Swedo JL, Rajaraman S, et al. Ultrastructural and immunohistochemical evidence for the release of eosinophilic granules in vivo: Cytoxic potential in chronic eosinophilic pneumonia. J Allergy Clin Immunol 1986;79:755.

58. McEvoy JD, Donald KJ, Edwards RL. Immunoglobulin levels and electron microscopy in eosinophilic pneumonia. Am J Med 1978;64:529.

59. Jederlinic PJ, Siciliau L, Gaensler EA. Chronic eosinophilic pneumonia: A report of 19 cases and a review of the literature. Medicine 1988;67:154.

60. Quinonez GE, Simon GT, Kay JM. Electron microscopy of chronic eosinophilic pneumonia. Clin Invest Med 1986;9:238.

61. Dejaegher P, Demedts M. Bronchoalveolar lavage in eosinophilic pneumonia before and during corticosteroid therapy. Am Rev Respir Dis 1984;129:631.

62. Ottesen EA, Neva FA, Paranjape RS, et al. Specific allergic sensitization to filarial antigens in tropical eosinophilia syndrome. Lancet 1979;i:1158.

63. Donohugh DL. Tropical eosinophilia: An etiologic inquiry. N Engl J Med 1963;269:1357.

64. Frimodt-Moller C, Barton RM. A pseudo-tuberculosis condition associated with eosinophilia. Indian Med Gaz 1940;75:607.

65. Weingarten RJ. Tropical eosinophilia. Lancet 1943;i:103.

66. Danaraj TJ. Treatment of eosinophilic lung (tropical eosinophilia) with diethyl-carbamazide. Proc Alum Assoc Malaya 1956;9:172.

67. Webb JK, Cob CK, Gault EW. Tropical eosinophilia: Demonstration of microfilariae in lung, liver and lymph nodes. Lancet 1960;i:835.
68. Lie Kian Joe. Occult filariasis: Its relationship with tropical pulmonary eosinophilia. Am J Trop Med 1962;11:646.
69. Joshi VV, Udwadia FE, Gadgil RK. Etiology of tropical eosinophilia: A study of lung biopsies and review of published reports. Am J Trop Med 1969;18:231.
70. Beaver PC. Filariasis without microfilaremia. Am J Trop Med 1970;19:181.
71. Neva FA, Ottesen EA. Tropical (filarial) eosinophilia. N Engl J Med 1978;298:1129.
72. Neva FA, Kaplan AP, Pacheco G, Gray L, Danaraj TJ. Tropical eosinophilia: A human model of parasitic immunopathology, with observations on serum IgE levels before and after treatment. J Allergy Clin Immunol 1975;55:422.
73. Herlinger H. Pulmonary changes in tropical eosinophilia. Br J Radiol 1963;36:889.
74. Udwadia FE. Tropical eosinophilia: A correlation of clinical, histopathologic, and lung function studies. Dis Chest 1967;52:531.
75. Nesarajah MS. Pulmonary function in tropical eosinophilia. Thorax 1972;27:185.
76. Chhabra SK, Gaur SN. Airway hyper-reactivity in tropical pulmonary eosinophilia. Chest 1988;93:1105.
77. Spry CJF, Kumaraswami V. Tropical eosinophilia. Semin Hematol 1982;19:107.
78. Churg J, Strauss L. Allergic granulomatosis, allergic angiitis and periarteritis nodosa. Am J Pathol 1951;27:277.
79. Fauci AS. Vasculitis. J Allergy Clin Immunol 1983;72:211.
80. Lanham JG, Elkon KB, Pusey CD, Hughes GR. Systemic vasculitis with asthma and eosinophilia: A clinical approach to the Churg-Strauss syndrome. Medicine 1984;63:65.
81. Sale S, Patterson R. Recurrent Churg-Strauss vasculitis, with exophthalmos, hearing loss, nasal obstruction, amyloid deposits, hyperimmunoglobulinemia E, and circulating immune complexes. Arch Intern Med 1981;141:1363.
82. Churg J. Allergic granulomatosis and granulomatous-vascular syndromes. Ann Allergy 1963;21:619.
83. Koss MN, Antonovych T, Hochholzer L. Allergic granulomatosis (Churg-Strauss syndrome): Pulmonary and renal morphologic findings. Am J Surg Pathol 1981;5:21.
84. Cogen FC, Mayock RL, Sweiman B. Chronic eosinophilic pneumonia followed by polyarteritis nodosa complicating the course of bronchial asthma: Report of a case. J Allergy Clin Immunol 1977;60:377.
85. Stephens M, Reynolds S, Gibbs AR, Davies B. Allergic bronchopulmonary aspergillosis progressing to allergic granulomatosis and angiitis (Churg-Strauss syndrome). Am Rev Respir Dis 1988;137:1226.
86. Chumbley LC, Harrison EG, DeRemee RA. Allergic granulomatosis and angiitis (Churg-Strauss syndrome): Report and analysis of 30 cases. Mayo Clin Proc 1977;52:477.
87. Mac Fadyen R, Tron V, Keshmiri M, Road JD. Allergic angiitis of Churg and Strauss syndrome: Response to pulse methylprednisolone. Chest 1987;91:629.
88. Leavitt RY, Fauci AS. Pulmonary vasculitis. Am Rev Respir Dis 1986;134:149.
89. Ford RM. Transient pulmonary eosinophilia and asthma: A review of 20 cases occurring in 5,702 asthma sufferers. Am Rev Respir Dis 1966;93:797.

18

Pulmonary Eosinophilic Granuloma

Udaya B. S. Prakash

Pulmonary eosinophilic granuloma, or primary pulmonary histiocytosis-X, is a granulomatous disease of unknown etiology characterized by abnormal proliferation of histiocytes and an unpredictable natural history, although the disease generally tends to be slowly progessive. Pulmonary eosinophilic granuloma belongs to the group of diseases collectively known as histiocytic reticulocytosis or histiocytic reticuloendotheliosis. This category of diseases encompasses Letterer-Siwe disease (acute disseminated histiocytosis-X), Hand-Schüller-Christian disease (chronic disseminated histiocytosis-X), and localized histiocytosis-X, or eosinophilic granuloma. The term histiocytosis-X was proposed in 1953 by Lichtenstein[1] to describe these three related disease complexes. Lieberman and associates[2] challenged this unitary concept, and on the basis of their experience with 113 cases concluded that the Hand-Schüller-Christian triad is nonspecific and the term "multifocal eosinophilic granuloma" should be used to describe the abnormalities observed in various organs. More recently, the Writing Group of the Histiocyte Society[3] has suggested that the syndromes belonging to the histiocytosis-X family of diseases be called Langerhans-cell histiocytosis. Further, the group has recommended that this new classification based on histogenetic criteria should replace the terms histiocytosis-X, pulmonary eosinophilic granuloma, Letterer-Siwe syndrome, Hand-Schüller syndrome, Hashimoto-Pritzker syndrome, self-healing histiocytosis-X, pure cutaneous histiocytosis, Langerhans-cell granulomatosis, type II histiocytosis, and the generic term non-lipid reticuloendotheliosis. Even though the term "eosinophilic granuloma" has been applied to involvement of an isolated organ such as lung or bone, the term pulmonary eosinophilic granuloma or histiocytosis-X will be used in this chapter.

ETIOLOGY

The etiology of pulmonary eosinophilic granuloma remains unknown. Although electron microscopy has shown intramitochondrial crystalline inclusion bodies, which suggests a viral etiology, there have been no studies to document that pulmonary eosinophilic granuloma is caused by an infectious agent.[4] Auld[5] in 1957 proposed that pulmonary histiocytosis-X was a hypersensitivity disease because of the presence of granulomas and eosinophils, but this concept has not been proven. The presence of circulating immune complexes and granular IgG and complement components in alveolar walls and capillaries of patients with pulmonary eosinophilic granuloma has suggested an immune mechanism as the basis for the pathology.[6] Immune deficiency has been shown in a small group of patients with histiocytosis-X.[7] The most striking association, however, is between pulmonary eosinophilic granuloma and tobacco smoking. This relationship strongly indicates that an external irritant, namely inhaled tobacco smoke, may be one of the major culprits in the causation of this disorder. A history of tobacco smoking has been observed in the majority of patients with this disease.[8] In a review by Friedman and colleagues[9] of 100 cases of eosinophilic granuloma diagnosed by open lung biopsy, a history of tobacco smoking was noted in 97% of patients, in contrast to a smoking prevalence of 35% in the general population. A similar prevalence of tobacco smoking was reported by Hance and associates,[10] who theorized, on the basis of results of bronchoalveolar lavage (BAL) in patients with pulmonary eosinophilic granuloma, that smoking-induced macrophage alveolitis may somehow initiate the pathologic process. Exposure to chemicals was mentioned in one publication, but most reports do not mention this association.[11] Accumulation of Langerhans cells on the epithelial surface of the lower respiratory tract in normal subjects in association with cigarette smoking indicates that the initial stimulus to the causation of pulmonary eosinophilic granuloma may start here.[12] Results of special staining techniques, discussed below, in the diagnosis of this disorder strongly suggest an immune-mediated mechanism or mechanisms, the details of which remain unclear.[13]

PATHOLOGY

Early in the disease, gross examination of the lung discloses prominent small subpleural nodules measuring 2 mm to over 10 mm, and varying number of small irregular cystic lesions. The effector cell accountable for producing eosinophilic granuloma is derived from the mononuclear phagocyte system, and although the monocytes are usually referred to as "histiocytes," they are actually a combination of pigment-laden alveolar macrophages and "histiocytosis-X cells," commonly referred to as H-X cells (Figs. 18-1, 18-2), which are closely related to Langerhans cells in normal skin.[14,15] Langerhans cells are seldom if ever seen in normal lungs.[16-18] H-X cells are therefore considered to be reactive or activated Langerhans cells, and therefore, pulmonary eosinophilic granuloma is considered to represent a pathologic proliferation of Langerhans cells.[12,16,19,20] Barbey and co-workers[21] studied the expression of HLA-DR 1 i blood group antigen and T6 antigen in H-X cells and pulmonary alveolar macrophages and

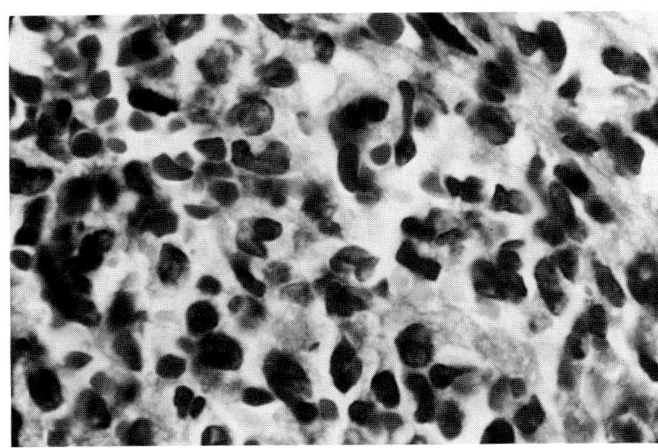

Figure 18-1. Transbronchoscopic lung biopsy showing Langerhans cells with folded and lobulated nuclei; H&E. (Photomicrograph courtesy of T. V. Colby, M.D.).

confirmed the hypothesis that H-X cells constitute a specialized subpopulation of the mononuclear phagocyte system. Although these mononuclear cells are distinct from macrophages, they are identical in antigen transport mechanisms. Electron microscopy confirms the unity of the disorders under the generic term "histiocytosis-X" by identifying a common marker organelle,[22] known as X-body or Birbeck granule (Fig. 18-3), in the H-X cell in all three forms of the disease (acute disseminated histiocytosis-X or Letterer-Siwe disease; chronic disseminated histiocytosis-X or Hand-Schüller-Christian disease; localized histiocytosis-X or eosinophilic granuloma). These inclusion bodies, however, are not specific for eosinophilic granuloma since they have been found in pulmonary fibrosis and other diffuse diseases.[16,23–25] This marker organelle of H-X cell is also found in normal Langerhans cells. The definition of the H-X cell includes the following criteria: lack of pigment bodies, presence of a convoluted nucleus, and X-bodies (pentalaminar cytoplasmic inclusions) that measure 40 to 45 nm in width.[20] BAL studies have demonstrated that Langerhans cells constitute 2% to 20% of the effector cells in pulmonary eosinophilic granuloma.[16] H-X cells are not normally present in the

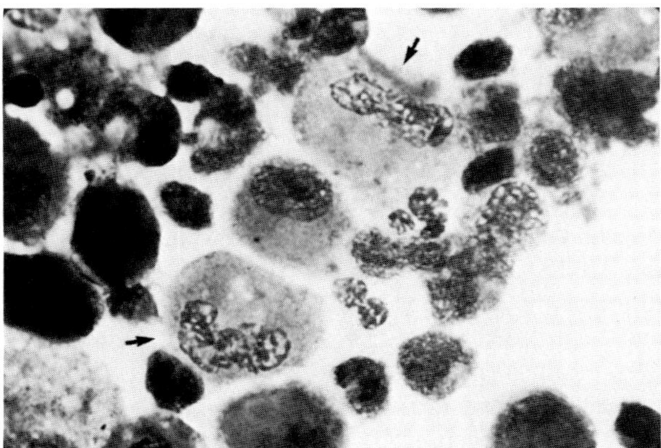

Figure 18-2. Diff-Quick stain of bronchoalveolar lavage effluent showing three histiocytes, two of which (*arrows*) are consistent with Langerhans cells (Photomicrograph courtesy of T. V. Colby, M.D.).

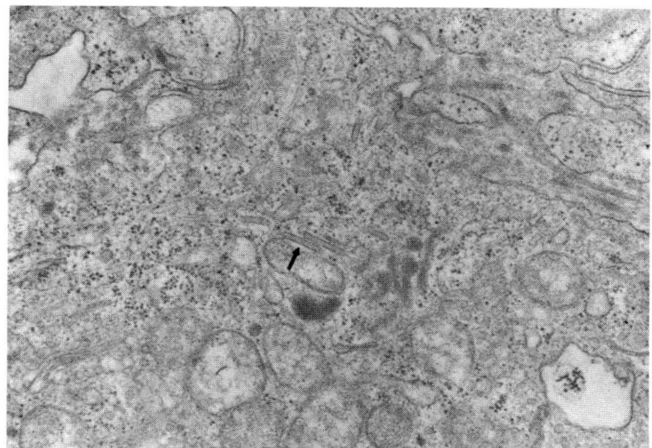

Figure 18-3. High-magnification electron micrograph showing characteristic Birbeck granules (*arrow*). The Birbeck granules (X-bodies) have a rod-shaped configuration and a pentalaminar composition when cut in cross section. Magnification × 38,000. (Electron micrograph courtesy of J. Meyers, M.D.).

alveolar wall and rarely seen in the bronchiolar wall.[16] Crystal and colleagues[26] theorized that the alveolitis in pulmonary eosinophilic granuloma develops because normal mononuclear phagocytes differentiate into H-X cells or the latter are formed elsewhere and accumulate in the lower respiratory tract. Studies have shown that H-X cells replicate in the alveolar structures, indicating that alveolar proliferation of these cells probably has a role in maintaining active alveolitis.[26] The essential histology of lesions in the histiocytosis-X group of disorders is uniform and consists of a proliferation of H-X cells in nodular or sheet-like masses with interspersion of numerous eosinophils, either singly or in clumps. During the early stages of the disease, histologic examination reveals widespread nodules measuring up to a few millimeters in diameter. These foci contain a wide variety of cells, including cells with large vesicular nuclei, cells with vacuolated cytoplasm, giant cells, eosinophils, lymphocytes, polymorphonuclear leukocytes, and histiocytes.[3] The degree of lymphocytic and plasma cell infiltration, eosinophilia, the number of foam cells, and the amount of necrosis or fibrosis vary considerably from lesion to lesion.[27] The histiocytes seldom exhibit mitotic figures but fuse to form multinucleated giant cells, and accumulation of so-called foam cells—vacuolated histiocytes with sudanophilic material in the cytoplasm—may also be found. Further, three types of histiocytes have been observed in electron-microscopic studies: typical pulmonary macrophages, "foamy macrophages," and the type containing Langerhans bodies and fibrils in cytoplasm. The latter histiocytes may have a part in increasing the fibrogenesis.[28] The H-X cells are seen in large numbers in acute and active forms of pulmonary eosinophilic granuloma, diminishing in number as the disease becomes chronic. In pulmonary eosinophilic granuloma, H-X cells are found in granulomas, alveolar interstitium, and between epithelial cells of the lower respiratory system.[18] The H-X cells freely migrate into airspaces, as shown by their presence in BAL fluid. In fibrotic lung disorders, on the contrary, the mobility of Langerhans cells is apparently restricted and these cells are limited to the epithelial layer of bronchioles and alveoli containing proliferating epithelial cells.[16] The granulomatous lesions tend to be vascular and are predominantly located in the peribronchial and perivascular interstitial tissues and in the septa beneath the pleura.[29,30] Microscopically, differentiation

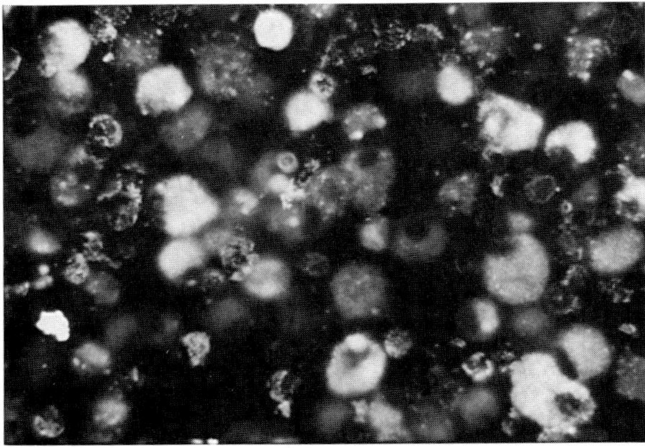

Figure 18-4. Immunofluorescent staining (*bright-appearing cells*) of the Langerhans cells, obtained from bronchoalveolar lavage effluent, with OKT6 antibody. Under the microscope, these cells reveal a positive yellow-orange immunofluorescence. (Photomicrograph courtesy of W. J. Martin II, M.D.).

from desquamative interstitial pneumonia and chronic eosinophilic pneumonia may occasionally be difficult. The latter can be caused by a number of drugs, parasites, and fungi and can also be idiopathic.[31] As the disease progresses, fibrosis replaces the granulomatous process, and formation of characteristic honeycomb cysts results. In the later stages microscopy reveals nonspecific fibrosis.

IMMUNOLOGY

The general assumption that the histiocytosis-X group of disorders is an immune-mediated disease is based on the finding of immune reactivity in H-X cells. Shelley and Juhlin[32] demonstrated that Langerhans cells in skin form a reticuloepithelial trap for external contact antigens and interact with them. It has been surmised that inhaled tobacco smoke may play a similar role in the pathogenesis of pulmonary eosinophilic granuloma.[9,33] Fithian and colleagues[33] showed that Langerhans cells express surface antigen that can be identified by the monoclonal antibody OKT6. Another technique used to identify H-X cells is immunoperoxidase staining of the cytoplasm, but positive staining for S-100 is not specific for H-X cells.[34] Soler and associates[35] performed detailed immunologic studies in patients with pulmonary eosinophilic granuloma and reported that the major cellular components of H-X cells from patients with pulmonary eosinophilic granuloma showed labeling of the plasma membranes by OKT6 antibody (Fig. 18-4) and of the cytoplasm by the anti–S-100 protein antibody, and immunoelectron microscopy showed that the reactive cells had all the structural characteristics of Langerhans cells, including Langerhans cell granules. Chollet and co-workers[36] utilized the monoclonal OKT6 antibody to label H-X cells obtained from BAL fluid in patients with pulmonary eosinophilic granuloma, pulmonary sarcoidosis, and other pulmonary disorders. All patients with pulmonary eosinophilic granuloma exhibited OKT6-reactive cells in their bronchoalveolar effluent. Although H-X cells are present in nearly one-fourth of patients with idiopathic pulmonary fibrosis and hypersensitivity pneumonitis, they are absent in inorganic pneumoconioses, pulmonary lymphangioleiomyomatosis, or sarcoidosis.

Other studies have suggested immune deficiency in some patients with histiocytosis-X. Osband and colleagues[7] found immunologic abnormalities in 12 of 17 patients with histiocytosis-X. Notable were the lack of histamine H_2 surface receptors in T lymphocytes and a deficiency of suppressor cells. Serologic studies in patients with pulmonary eosinophilic granuloma have shown the presence of circulating immune complexes as well as granular deposits of IgG and complement (C3) in the walls of alveoli and pulmonary blood vessels. Using these criteria, King and associates[6] reported that circulating immune-complex–like activity is present in patients with the cellular form of the disease, and deposition of such substances may contribute to the pathogenesis of pulmonary eosinophilic granuloma. These tests, however, are nonspecific and do not aid in the diagnosis of histiocytosis-X. Prostaglandin synthesis by H-X cells has been reported but its implications are unclear.[37]

CLINICAL CONSIDERATIONS

The three major clinical forms of histiocytosis-X are acute disseminated histiocytosis-X, or Letterer-Siwe disease; chronic disseminated histiocytosis-X, or Hand-Schüller-Christian disease; and eosinophilic granuloma, or localized histiocytosis-X. In clinical practice, however, it may be difficult to classify all cases of histiocytosis-X into these neat categories because many patients present with combinations of features of two or all three entities. Even in the same patient clinical features may change during the course of the disease and make it difficult to classify the illness into one of the three distinct categories. Because of the extensive overlap among the three types, staging according to the number and extent of organs involved is more important than classification.[12,38,39]

Letterer-Siwe Disease

Letterer-Siwe disease almost always occurs in infants and children and becomes evident before the age of 2 years and is characterized by extensive dissemination and a fulminating, fatal course. Appearance of symptoms after the age of 2 years is reported to be associated with an 85% 10-year survival, whereas among patients who present prior to this age, the 10-year survival is 40%.[40,41] Adult forms of Letterer-Siwe disease have been reported. Novice and co-workers,[42] in their review of the literature, found 17 cases of Letterer-Siwe disease in adults. Another review of the literature by Crowe and associates[43] revealed 26 cases of patients with Letterer-Siwe disease over the age of 30 years; only 6 of these were over the age of 70 years. Pulmonary involvement was noted in 12 of the 26 cases. The term "progressive differentiated histiocytosis" has been suggested to describe this entity.

Hand-Schüller-Christian Disease

Hand-Schüller-Christian disease usually becomes evident during later childhood or adolescence and progresses rather slowly, so most patients reach adulthood. One or all of the classic triad of signs (exophthalmos, diabetes insipidus, and osteolytic lesions of the skull) may be present. The characteristic triad, however, is observed in only 10% of children with multifocal eosinophilic granuloma.[44] Lieberman and associates,[2] on the basis of their experience with 113 cases, suggested that Hand-Schüller-Christian triad is nonspecific and that the term "multifocal eosinophilic granuloma" should be used to describe the abnormalities observed in various organs. Histiocytosis-X limited to the hypothalamus and complicated by endocrine dysfunction has also been described.[45]

Pulmonary Eosinophilic Granuloma

Eosinophilic granuloma limited to the lung was first reported by Farinacci and colleagues,[46] who suggested that it was pathologically related to the histiocytic proliferation seen in Letterer-Siwe disease and Hand-Schüller-Christian disease. Eosinophilic granuloma is generally a disease of adults and is more commonly limited to the lungs or the bones or both. Pulmonary eosinophilic granuloma is a relatively rare condition, although more than 1000 cases have been reported.[26] More than 300 cases of pulmonary eosinophilic granuloma reported in the literature[9,26,28,46–48] have exhibited diffuse abnormalities on chest roentgenography and an interstitial pulmonary process on pathologic examination. The precise incidence of pulmonary eosinophilic granuloma is not known. In a review of 100 cases of pulmonary eosinophilic granuloma diagnosed by open lung biopsy, the male to female ratio was 2 to 3,[9] even though most series have shown male predominance.[8] Most patients are 20 to 40 years of age.[26] The disorder occurs most frequently in Caucasians, is rare in blacks, and has never been reported in Asians.[4,47,49,50] One instance of familial occurrence has been reported.[8]

Clinical presentations of pulmonary eosinophilic granuloma vary widely. Approximately one-fourth of patients with pulmonary eosinophilic granuloma remain asymptomatic, the disease being uncovered by a routine chest roentgenograph. Up to 30% of patients have nonspecific symptoms, such as fatigue, fever, and weight loss. Symptoms vary depending on the stage of the disease. A nonproductive cough is the most common symptom and is observed in nearly 65% of patients. Dyspnea is observed in 40%. Chest pain is reported by about 25% of patients; it may result from a spontaneous pneumothorax or an osteolytic rib lesion.[51] Unusual pulmonary symptoms include hemoptysis and wheezing.[8,52] Spontaneous pneumothorax occurs in about 10% to 20% of patients,[9] and recurrent pneumothorax is observed in some.[50] Pneumothorax is the result of rupture of subpleural cystic lesions. Pleural effusion, a rare complication, has been noted as a complication of solitary eosinophilic granuloma of the rib.[53] Eosinophilic granuloma of bone is reported in 20% of patients, although the incidence of solitary bone lesions is probably higher. Most patients do not have symptoms referable to the bone lesion and in patients with pulmonary eosinophilic granuloma, skeletal roentgenograms are not routinely performed to assess eosinophilic granuloma of bone. McCullough[54] noted that among 43 patients with histologically proven histiocytosis-X localized to bone who were followed for 10 years, 36 (84%) presented with solitary bone lesions and 31 of these resolved without complication. Another nonpulmonary manifestation of pulmonary eosinophilic granuloma is the occurrence of diabetes insipidus, seen in about 20% of patients.[55] Isolated pulmonary eosinophilic granuloma is rare in chidren, although several cases have been described.[56,57] An unusual case of endobronchial eosinophilic granuloma in the absence of pulmonary parenchymal disease or other manifestations of eosinophilic granuloma was described in a 12-year-old male who presented with atelectasis of the left lung.[58]

Among the unusual manifestations of histiocytosis-X are the examples of this disease affecting extrapulmonary organs. Artzi and colleagues[59] discovered 28 cases of histiocytosis-X involving the head and neck region during a 20-year period; 15 cases were confined to this anatomic area, and periodontal disease was observed in 22 cases (79%). Otologic manifestations of histiocytosis-X are also reported in the literature.[60] Approximately two dozen cases of histiocytosis-X involving the gynecologic system have been reported.[61] Renal involvement has been reported in one patient.[62] Marked elevation of serum alkaline phosphatase associated with rapid destructive changes in the lung has been observed in a patient with pulmonary eosinophilic granuloma.[63] Multiple intrahepatic nodules and hepatic cirrhosis have been described in histiocytosis-X.[64,65]

PHYSIOLOGY

It is usual for relatively good pulmonary function to be maintained when roentgenography reveals extensive abnormalities. Nearly 15% of patients in the series reported by Bassett and colleagues[66] had normal lung function. The slow and gradual loss of lung function suggests more advanced disease or the beginning of fibrosis. A restrictive type of pulmonary dysfunction with decreased lung volumes, normal flow rates, and diminished carbon monoxide diffusion capacity is the most common pattern of abnormality.[9,67] The reduction of gas transfer probably cannot be accounted for by the slight thickening of alveolar capillary membranes demonstrated in ultrastructural studies but rather is due primarily to ventilation-perfusion inequalities.[68] Severe obstructive airway disease, however, is not uncommon in advanced cases.[69,70] In the series of 100 patients reported by Friedman and associates,[9] 20% demonstrated major obstructive defects on routine spirometry. Peribronchial fibrosis and the compression of airways by cystic lesions are very likely the cause of this phenomenon. Obliterative bronchiolitis due to infiltration of bronchial walls by cells and granulomas is another cause of obstructive pulmonary disease.[4,5,66] An additional mechanism of obstructive pulmonary disease is related to tobacco smoking. Severe airway obstruction may be the presenting symptom in some patients.[69]

ROENTGENOLOGY

The chest roentgenologic findings vary with the stage of the disease. Characteristically, the involvement is diffuse, bilateral, and most pronounced in the upper two-thirds of the lung fields.[33,51] In the earlier stages, the chest roentgenograms demonstrate a nodular pattern with lesions ranging from 1 mm to 12 mm in diameter. Alveolar consolidation and cavitation of nodules have been described but are rare.[71,72] In the later stages of the disease, chest roentgenograms may exhibit a reticulonodular pattern (Fig. 18-5) and honeycomb appearance, with the cysts varying from 5 mm to 30 mm, with an average size of less than 1 cm. This honeycomb pattern (Fig 18-6), when located in upper lung zones, is highly suggestive of eosinophilic granuloma. Spontaneous pneumothorax is reported in 6% to 20% of patients with eosinophilic granuloma and may

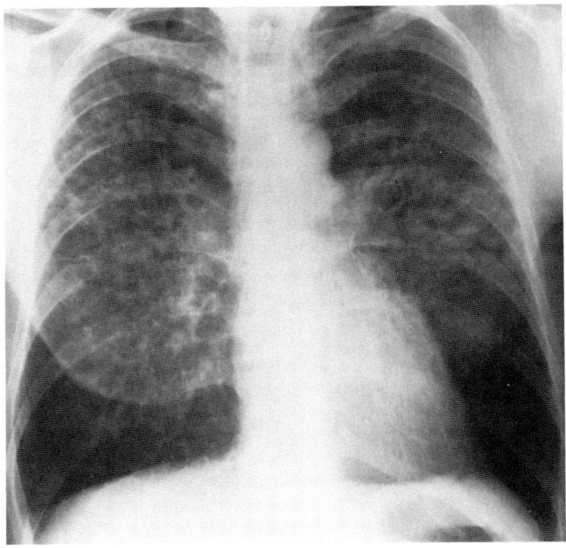

Figure 18-5. Chest roentgeno-graph of a patient with early stage of pulmonary eosino-philic granuloma. Diffuse bilat-eral reticulonodular infiltrates with predominant distribution in upper and middle lung fields are evident. Sparing of the costophrenic angles is noteworthy.

be the first indicator of the condition.[8,30,51,73,74] Involvement of the upper two-thirds of the lungs by diffuse reticulonodular or cystic processes is also seen in sarcoidosis, cystic fibrosis, silicosis, fungal infections, ankylosing spondylitis, and tuberculosis.

The costophrenic angles are usually spared; sparing of both costophrenic angles has been associated with a good prognosis.[75] Pleural reaction or thickening is uncommon, even in patients with recurrent pneumothoraces.[9] Hilar prominence, seen in less than 25% of patients with pulmonary eosinophilic granuloma, is more likely a result of enlarged pulmonary arteries (Fig. 18-7) than of hilar lymphadenopathy, although the latter has been described.[9,76] Lacronique and co-workers[75] studied the chest roentgenograms of 50 adult patients with histologically confirmed pulmonary eosinophilic granuloma and noted that the lesions predominated in the mid-lung fields, usually sparing the costophrenic angles, and that the infiltrates were typically micronodular, reticular, or cystic. These features should suggest pulmonary eosinophilic granuloma if the following clinical features are present: lung volume is normal or increased, there is an associated pneumothorax, disease occurs in a young male, and there are no other intrathoracic (pleural or mediastinal) changes. Nevertheless, solid mediastinal masses with development of cavitation within the mass have been observed in children with pulmonary histiocytosis-X.[77,78] There also have been isolated reports of mass lesions of the anterior chest wall,[79] mass in the neck with tracheal involvement,[80] and hilar lymphadenopathy.[76]

High-resolution computed tomography of the chest (Fig. 18-8) has been used to further define the pulmonary parenchymal abnormalities. Brauner and colleagues[81] studied 18 patients by this method and observed the following abnormalities: thin-walled cysts (94%), nodules (78%), cavitated nodules (17%), thick-walled cysts (39%), reticulation (22%), ground-glass opacities (22%), and irregular interfaces (22%). The lesions were most often diffuse (89%), with a predominant distribution in the upper or

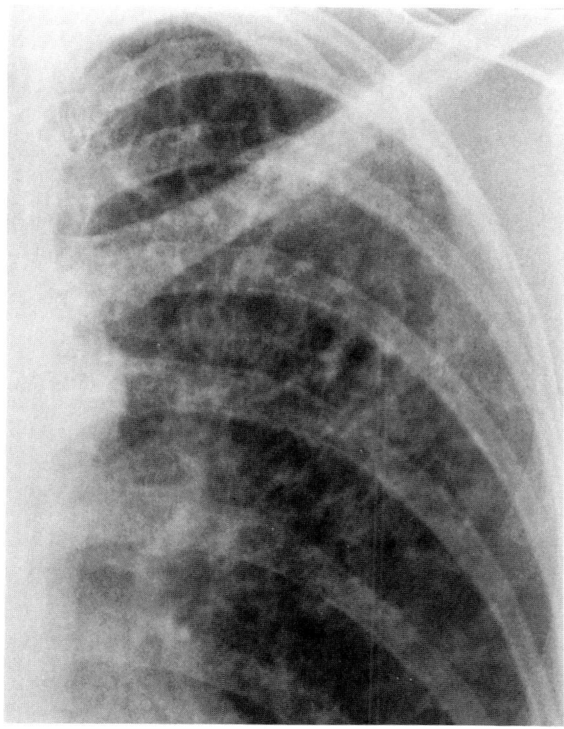

Figure 18-6. Localized view of the chest roentgenograph in a patient with slightly advanced pulmonary eosinophilic granuloma. Diffuse honeycombing and cyst formation are evident.

middle lung zones in nine (50%) patients. Comparison of computed tomography and chest roentgenograms showed that small and large cysts and micronodules were better detected with computed tomography. Longitudinal studies in some patients suggested that computed tomographic patterns progressed from nodules to cavitated nodules, thick-walled cysts to cysts, and distinct cysts to confluent cysts. Moore and associates,[82] in their retrospective study of 11 patients with biopsy-proven pulmonary eosinophilic granuloma in whom high-resolution computed tomography was used, reported that many lesions that appeared reticular on chest roentgenograms were actually cystic. This study also showed that many small nodules were distributed in the centers of secondary lobules around small airways and that computed tomographic findings correlated better with the diffusing capacity than did the chest roentgenologic findings. Magnetic resonance imaging has been used in staging and in monitoring response to therapy.[14]

DIAGNOSIS

Previously, virtually all cases of pulmonary eosinophilic granuloma were diagnosed by open lung biopsy. Subsequently, transbronchoscopic lung biopsy has been applied. It should be noted, however, that in the proper clinical setting, the diagnosis can

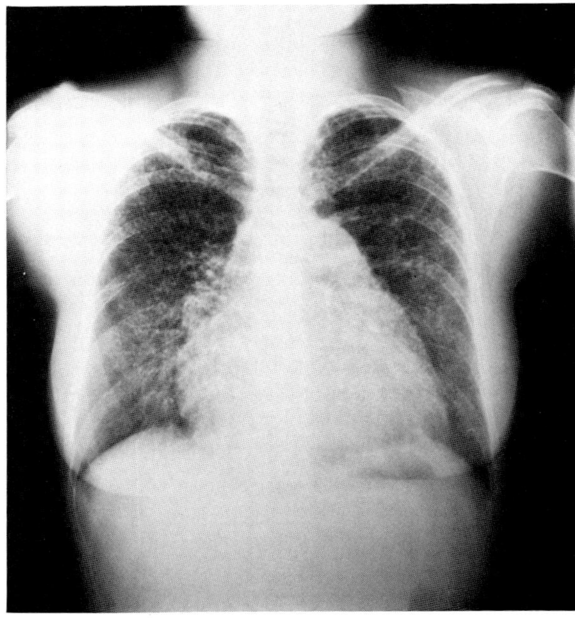

Figure 18-7. Chest roentgenograph of a patient with progressive fibrosis and cor pulmonale secondary to pulmonary eosinophilic granuloma. A bilateral diffuse interstitial process, prominence of hilar vasculature, and cardiomegaly are evident.

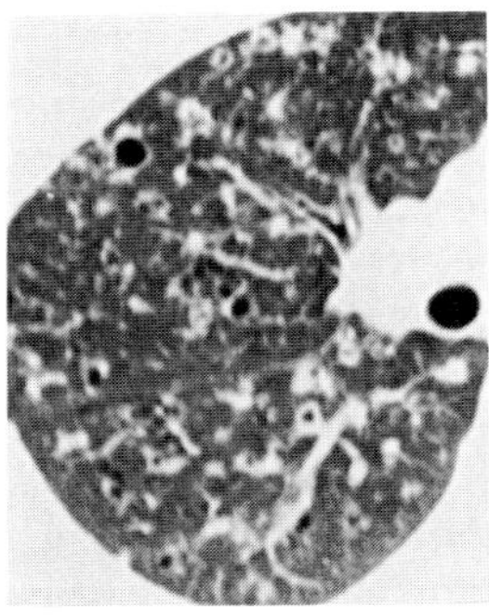

Figure 18-8. High-resolution computed tomography of right lung in a patient with pulmonary eosinophilic granuloma. Multiple nodules with some showing cavitation, cystic spaces, thick-walled cysts, and institial process are common findings.

be made on clinical grounds alone. The most important aspects of establishing the diagnosis are the awareness of this unusual entity and correlation of clinical, roentgenologic, and physiologic data. For instance, if one encounters a young adult male who presents with a spontaneous pneumothorax and the chest roentgenogram reveals diffuse honeycombing or reticulonodular process, one can be almost certain of the diagnosis. The physical examination in patients with pulmonary eosinophilic granuloma may be normal, and therefore of little help. In advanced cases, decreased lung sounds and crackles are occasionally detectable. In the minority of patients who develop obstructive lung disease, expiratory slowing of lung sounds may be present. Clubbing is observed in a minority of patients, particularly in those with advanced disease. Hepatosplenomegaly and lymphadenopathy are conspicuously absent in pulmonary eosinophilic granuloma, although disseminated histiocytosis-X may exhibit these features. Routine hematologic and serologic data are generally normal. The sedimentation rate is either normal or only minimally elevated. Peripheral eosinophilia is not a feature of eosinophilic granuloma.

Roentgenologic abnormalities in pulmonary eosinophilic granuloma mimic other diseases and one should consider these in the differential diagnosis when faced with a diffuse infiltrative process that is predominantly upper and middle lobe in distribution. The following diseases produce diffuse upper-lobe abnormalities: cystic fibrosis, sarcoidosis, allergic bronchopulmonary aspergillosis, lymphangioleiomyomatosis, silicosis, mycoses, and tuberculosis. One important roentgenologic feature is that although involvement of the upper and lower lung fields is common, it is the middle lung fields that are consistently involved.

A variety of special techniques can be used to discover or confirm the presence of Langerhans cells. Electron microscopy is useful since the cytoplasmic Langerhans cell inclusion bodies (Birbeck granules or X-bodies) can be seen. Electron microscopy can be performed on biopsy material as well as lavage material, although few centers are equipped to use this technique on a routine basis. Bronchoalveolar lavage is a safe and useful technique for the diagnosis of pulmonary eosinophilic granuloma.[17,83] The cells harvested from lavage can be studied for their immune properties and functions, tested with specific antigens, and examined for the presence of unique surface antigens using OKT6 monoclonal antibodies, antibodies to S-100 protein, or antibodies to the HLA-DR protein. Although these immunologic methods have been used in clinical practice to detect the Langerhans cells, none is specific. The most specific of these for diagnostic purposes is the OKT6 monoclonal antibody.[36] Transbronchoscopic lung biopsy is an excellent method of establishing the diagnosis of pulmonary eosinophilic granuloma. It is essential, however, that the clinician communicate with the pathologist regarding the possibility of the diagnosis, since not infrequently the biopsies are interpreted as showing idiopathic pulmonary fibrosis or nonspecific changes, and only a repeated examination, particularly with the clinician's input, will authenticate the diagnosis. Initially incorrect diagnoses such as desquamative interstitial pneumonitis, lymphoma, and eosinophilic pneumonitis have caused confusion in several cases.[80]

THERAPY AND PROGNOSIS

Because of the fluctuating course and frequent propensity toward spontaneous resolution, it is clinically difficult to objectively assess any form of treatment. Therefore, use of toxic drugs should be undertaken with caution.[84] Treatment with corticosteroid and vinca alkaloid derivatives is of varying efficacy. Asymptomatic patients and those with stable chest roentgenologic abnormalities should be observed without specific therapy. Smoking cessation should be stressed even though there are no data to show that this will result in resolution of the disease. In progressive disease, high-dose corticosteroid therapy has been the treatment of choice. Prednisone 0.75 to 1.0 mg/kg/day for as long as 6 to 12 months may be necessary. In refractory and widely disseminated cases, trial of therapy using vinca alkaloids (vinblastine or vincristine) is recommended.[85] In children with histiocytosis-X, use of vinca alkaloids has proved to be equally efficacious with or without corticosteroids.[86] Enlarging or symptomatic bone lesions are treated by steroids, excision-curettage, or radiation. Radiation is not indicated in pulmonary eosinophilic granuloma. Crude extract of thymus gland has induced complete remission in patients who had certain immunologic deficiencies (suppressor-cell deficiency, lack of histamine H_2 surface receptors) associated with histiocytosis-X.[7] The prognosis is poor in patients with large bullous lesions, progressive obstructive airways disease, severe hypoxemia, secondary pulmonary hypertension, and involvement of costophrenic angles on chest roentgenography. In the pediatric population, patients younger than 2 years are more responsive to therapy than older children, and maintenance therapy prolongs the duration of remission.[87,88] The natural history in pulmonary eosinophilic granuloma of adults is one of fluctuating illness and, not uncommonly, spontaneous resolution.[89] Therefore, the clinical course of pulmonary eosinophilic granuloma is usually benign, despite the persistence of severe roentgenographic abnormality. Friedman and co-workers[9] reviewed 100 cases of eosinophilic granuloma diagnosed by open lung biopsy and reported that nearly one-quarter of patients were asymptomatic and the outcome was generally benign; persistent symptoms were noted in 22%, progressive disease in 4%, and death in 1%. The clinical manifestations were more severe in younger men, who had a higher incidence of pneumothorax, fibrosis, honeycombing, and diabetes insipidus.[9] The overall prognosis is good in adults with pulmonary eosinophilic granuloma; mortality rates are below 5%.

The mortality and morbidity rates in pediatric patients with pulmonary involvement is higher, even though a Mayo Clinic study[90] of 12 children noted that lung involvement rarely caused symptoms and almost invariably cleared. Sims[91] observed that among 43 children under the age of 12 years with histiocytosis-X, evaluated over a 29-year period, 67% survived; of these, 52% had a detectable disability. The majority of deaths were associated with pulmonary involvement. Komp and colleagues[92,93] also noted late deaths from respiratory failure associated with opportunistic infections. Nezelof and colleagues,[38] in their retrospective review of 50 cases of disseminated histiocytosis-X in children, collected over a period of 27 years, observed that 24 children died. The prognosis was dependent neither on age nor on histologic findings but on the extent of the lesions. Patients with a favorable prognosis were characterized by skin lesions, diabetes insipidus, roentgenologic evidence of pulmonary involvement, and multiple bone lesions. Lewis[51] reported that 5 of his 12 proven cases were fatal. Acute fulminating cases in children have been reported.[94,95] Unfavorable prognostic factors include extremes of age, multiple pneumothoraces, extensive multisystem disease, prolonged constitutional disturbance, extensive cysts or honeycombing on chest roentgenograms, and markedly decreased diffusing capacity for carbon monoxide.[26]

Greenberger and colleagues[40] reported that radiation and chemotherapy used to treat histiocytosis-X may be associated with at least a 50% chance of inducing malignancy. Histiocytosis-X can mimic recurrent malignant disease,[96] and hence the term "malignant histiocytosis-X" (unrelated to malignant histiocytosis) has been used to describe rapidly progressive histiocytosis-X.[97] This appears to be an inappropriate terminology. The disease itself is known to be nonmalignant,[98] even though Lombard and colleagues[99] described four patients who developed both pulmonary histiocytosis-X and carcinoma of the lung. Additional factors, such as cigarette smoking, may better explain this association.

REFERENCES

1. Lichtenstein L. Histiocytosis-X: Integration of eosinophilic granuloma of the bone, "Letterer-Siwe disease," and "Schüller-Christian disease" as related manifestations of a single nosologic entity. Arch Pathol 1953;56:84.
2. Lieberman PH, Jones CR, Dargeon HWK, Begg CF. A reappraisal of eosinophilic granuloma of bone, Hand-Schüller-Christian syndrome, and Letterer-Siwe syndrome. Medicine 1969;48:375.
3. The Writing Group of the Histiocyte Society. Histiocytosis syndromes in children. Lancet 1987;i:208.
4. Prophet D. Primary pulmonary histiocytosis-X. Clin Chest Med 1982;3:643.
5. Auld D. Pathology of eosinophilic granuloma of the lung. Arch Pathol 1957;63:113.
6. King TE Jr, Schwarz MI, Dreisin RE, Pratt DS, Theofilopoulos AN. Circulating immune complexes in pulmonary eosinophilic granuloma. Ann Intern Med 1979;91:397.
7. Osband ME, Lipton JM, Lavin P, Levey R, Vawter G, Greenberger JS, McCaffrey RP, Parkman R. Histiocytosis-X: Demonstration of abnormal immunity, T-cell histamine H_2-receptor deficiency, and successful treatment with thymic extract. N Eng J Med 1981;304:146.
8. Colby TV, Lombard C. Histiocytosis X in the lung. Hum Pathol 1983;14:847.
9. Friedman PJ, Liebow AA, Sokoloff J. Eosinophilic granuloma of lung: Clinical aspects of primary histiocytosis in the adult. Medicine (Baltimore) 1981;60:385.
10. Hance AJ, Basset F, Saumon G, Danel C, Valeyre D, Battesti JP, Chretien J, Georges R. Smoking and interstitial lung disease: The effect of cigarette smoking on the incidence of pulmonary histiocytosis X and sarcoidosis. Ann NY Acad Sci 1986;465:643.
11. Huhn D, Konig G, Weig J, Schneller W. Pulmonary histiocytosis X in adult patients. Klin-Wochenschr 1981;59:377.
12. Lahey ME. Prognostic factors in histiocytosis-X. Am J Pediatr Hematol Oncol 1981;3:57.
13. Favara BE, McCarthy RC, Mierau GW. Histiocytosis-X. Hum Pathol 1983;14:663.
14. Moore JB, Kulkarni R, Crutcher DC, Bhimani S. MRI in multifocal eosinophilic granuloma: Staging disease and monitoring response to therapy. Am J Pediatr Hematol Oncol 1989;11:174.
15. McLelland J, Newton J, Malone M, Camplejohn RS, Chu AC. A flow cytometric study of Langerhans cell histiocytosis. Br J Dermatol 1989;120:485.
16. Kawanami O, Basset F, Ferrans VJ, Soler P, Crystal RG. Pulmonary Langerhans' cells in patients with fibrotic lung disorders. Lab Invest 1981;44:227.
17. Basset F, Soler P, Jaurand MC, Bignon J. Ultrastructural examination of broncho-alveolar lavage for diagnosis of pulmonary histiocytosis X: Preliminary report on 4 cases. Thorax 1977;32:303.
18. Basset F, Soler P, Wyllie L, Mazin F, Turiaf J. Langerhans cells and lung interstitium. Ann NY Acad Sci 1976;278:599.
19. Nezelof C, Basset F, Rousseau MF. Histiocytosis-X: Histogenetic arguments for a Langerhans cell origin. Biomedicine 1973;18:366.
20. Corrin B, Basset F. A review of histiocytosis X with particular reference to eosinophilic granuloma of the lung. Invest Cell Pathol 1979;2:137.
21. Barbey S, Monnet JP, Nezelof C, Gane P, Nogues C. Failure of histiocytosis X cells to express i blood group antigen. Pathol Res Pract 1985;180:584.
22. Birbeck MS, Breathnach AS, Everall JD. An electron microscope study of basal melanocytes and high level clear cells (Langerhans cells) in vitiligo. J Invest Dermatol 1961;37:51.

23. Mercy TW, Reynolds HY. Pulmonary histiocytosis-X. Lung 1985;163:129.
24. Kullberg FC, Funahashi A, Siegesmund KA. Pulmonary eosinophilic granuloma: Electron microscopic detection of X-bodies on lung lavage cells and transbronchoscopic lung biopsy in one patient. Ann Intern Med 1982;96:188.
25. Hammar S. Langerhans cells. Pathol Annu 1988;23(pt 2):293.
26. Crystal RG, Bitterman PB, Rennard SI, Hance AJ, Keogh BA. Interstitial lung diseases of unknown causes: Disorders characterized by chronic inflammation of the lower respiratory tract. (Second of two parts) N Engl J Med 1984;310:235.
27. Oberman HA. Idiopathic histiocytosis: A clinicopathologic study of 40 cases and review of the literature on eosinophilic granuloma of bone, Hand-Schüller-Christian disease and Letterer-Siwe disease. Pediatrics 1961;28:307.
28. Brody AR, Kanich RE, Graham WG, Craighead. Cyst wall formation in pulmonary eosinophilic granuloma. Chest 1974;66:576.
29. Knudson RJ, Badger TL, Gaensler EA. Eosinophilic granuloma of the lung. Med Thoracales 1966;23:248.
30. Nadeau PJ, Ellis FH, Harrison EG, et al. Primary pulmonary histiocytosis X. Dis Chest 1960;37:325.
31. Fox B, Seed W. Chronic eosinophilic pneumonia. Thorax 1980;35:578.
32. Shelley WB, Juhlin L. Langerhans cells form a reticuloepithelial trap for external contact antigens. Nature 1976;261:46.
33. Fithian E, Kung P, Goldstein G, Rubenfeld M, Fenoglio C, Edelson R. Reactivity of Langerhans cells with hybridoma antibody. Proc Natl Acad Sci 1981;78:2541.
34. Flint A, Lloyd RV, Colby TV, Wilson BW. Pulmonary histiocytosis X: Immunoperoxidase staining for HLA-DR antigen and S-100 protein. Arch Pathol Lab Med 1986;110:930.
35. Soler P, Chollet S, Jacque C, Fukuda Y, Ferrans VJ, Basset F. Immunocytochemical characterization of pulmonary histiocytosis X cells in lung biopsies. Am J Pathol 1985;118:439.
36. Chollet S, Soler P, Dournova P, Richard MS, Ferrans VJ, Basset F. Diagnosis of pulmonary histiocytosis X by immunodetection of Langerhans cells in bronchoalveolar lavage fluid. Am J Pathol 1984;115:225.
37. Gonzalez-Crussi F, Hsueh W, Wiederhold MD. Prostaglandins in histiocytosis-X: PG synthesis by histiocytosis-X cells. Am J Clin Pathol 1981;75:243.
38. Nezelof C, Frileux-Herbet F, Cronier-Sachot J. Disseminated histiocytosis X: Analysis of prognostic factors based on a retrospective study of 50 cases. Cancer 1979;44:1824.
39. Pritchard J. Histiocytosis X: Natural history and management in childhood. Clin Exp Dermatol 1979;4:421.
40. Greenberger JS, Crocker AC, Vawter G. Results of treatment of 127 patients with systemic histiocytosis (Letterer-Siwe syndrome, Schüller-Christian syndrome, and multifocal eosinophil granuloma). Medicine 1981;60:311.
41. Tsunematsu Y, Koide R, Watanabe S, Takahashi H, Morikawa Y, Shimizu K. A clinicopathological study of histiocytosis X. Jpn J Clin Oncol 1984;14:633.
42. Novice FM, Collison DW, Kleinsmith DM, Osband ME, Burdakin JH, Coskey RJ. Letterer-Siwe disease in adults. Cancer 1989;63:166.
43. Crowe MJ, O'Loughlin S, Noel J, Dervan P. Histiocytosis X with pulmonary and cutaneous manifestations (Letterer-Siwe disease) in an elderly woman. Ir J Med Sci 1981;150:278.
44. Avery ME, McAfee JG, Guild HG. The course and prognosis of reticuloendotheliosis (eosinophilic granuloma, Schüller-Christian disease, and Letterer-Siwe disease): A study of forty cases. Am J Med 1957;22:636.
45. Ober KP, Alexander E Jr, Challa VR, Ferree C, Elster A. Histiocytosis X of the hypothalamus. Neurosurgery 1989;24:93.
46. Farinacci C, Jeffrey H, Lackey R. Eosinophilic granuloma of the lung: Report of two cases. U.S. Armed Forces Med J 1951;2:1085.

47. Dunmore LA Jr, El-Khoury SA. Eosinophilic granuloma of the lungs: A report of three cases in Negro patients. Am Rev Respir Dis 1964;90:789.
48. Hirsch MS, Hong CK. Familial pulmonary histiocytosis-X. Am Rev Respir Dis 1973;107:831.
49. Morley TF, Silverstein SD, Giudice JC, Csere RS. Multifocal eosinophilic granuloma. Respiration 1988;54:89.
50. Adam A, Berson D, Levine C, Marchand P. Recurrent spontaneous pneumothoraces associated with pulmonary histiocytosis X: A case report. S Afr Med J 1977;51:594.
51. Lewis JG. Eosinophilic granuloma and its variants with special reference to lung involvement: A report of 12 patients. Q J Med 1964;33:337.
52. Knight RK. Haemoptysis in eosinophilic granuloma. Br J Dis Chest 1979;73:181.
53. Pappas CA, Rheinlander HF, Stadecker MJ. Pleural effusion as a complication of solitary eosinophilic granuloma of the rib. Hum Pathol 1980;11:765.
54. McCullough CJ. Eosinophilic granuloma of bone. Acta Orthop Scand 1980;51:389.
55. Case records of the Massachusetts General Hospital (case 5-1978). N Engl J Med 1978;298:327.
56. McDowell HP, Macfarlane PI, Martin J. Isolated pulmonary histiocytosis. Arch Dis Child 1988;63:423.
57. Nondahl SR, Finlay JL, Farrell PM, Warner TF, Hong R. A case report and literature review of "primary" pulmonary histiocytosis X of childhood. Med Pediatr Oncol 1986;14:57.
58. O'Donnell AE, Tsou E, Awh C, Fallat ME, Patterson K. Endobronchial eosinophilic granuloma: A rare cause of total lung atelectasis. Am Rev Respir Dis 1987;136:1478.
59. Artzi Z, Grosky M, Raviv M. Periodontal manifestations of adult onset of histiocystosis X. J Periodontal 1989;60:57.
60. Cunningham MJ, Curtin HD, Jaffe R, Stool SE. Otologic manifestations of Langerhans cell histiocytosis. Arch Otolaryngol Head Neck Surg 1989;115:807.
61. Thomas R, Barnhill D, Bibro M, Hoskins W, Hambidge W. Histiocytosis-X in gynecology: A case presentation and review of the literature. Obstet Gynecol 1986;67(3 suppl):46S.
62. Volmer J. Histiocytosis X of lungs and kidneys. Virchows Arch (Pathol-Anat) 1975;369:81.
63. Hansen PB. Histiocytosis X characterized by marked elevation of serum alkaline phosphatase and rapid destructive changes in the lung parenchyma. Eur Respir J 1989;2:188.
64. Hara T, Mizuno Y, Ishii E, Ueda K, Hirata T, Daimaru Y, Nakagawara A. Histiocytosis X presenting as multiple intrahepatic nodules. Nippon Ketsueki Gakkai Zasshi 1988;51:1059.
65. Pirovino M, Jeanneret C, Lang RH, Luisier J, Bianchi L, Spichtin H. Liver cirrhosis in histiocytosis X. Liver 1988;8:293.
66. Basset F, Corrin B, Spencer H, Lacronique J, Roth C, Soler P, Battesti JP, Georges R, Chretien J. Pulmonary histiocytosis-X. Am Rev Respir Dis 1978;118:811.
67. Hoffman L, Cohn JE, Gaensler EA. Respiratory abnormalities in eosinophilic granuloma of the lung: Long-term study of five cases. N Engl J Med 1962;267:577.
68. Divertie MB, Cassan SM, Brown AL Jr. Application of ultrastructural morphometry to lung specimens in pulmonary histiocytosis X. Thorax 1975;30:326.
69. Elliott JA. Severe airways obstruction as a presenting feature of pulmonary histiocytosis-X: A case report. Br J Dis Chest 1983;77:299.
70. Sopko JA, Bedell J. A severe, stable obstructive defect in the airways in primary pulmonary histiocytosis X. Chest 1979;75:205.
71. Clark RL, Margulies SI, Mulholland JH. Histiocytosis X: A fatal case with unusual pulmonary manifestations. Radiology 1970;95:631.
72. Weber WN, Margolin FR, Nielsen SL. Pulmonary histiocytosis X. AJR 1969;107:280.
73. Gelfand ET, Sheiner NM. Pneumothorax in pulmonary eosinophilic granuloma. Can Med Assoc J 1974;110:937.
74. Roland AS, Merdinger WF, Froeb HF. Recurrent spontaneous pneumothorax: A clue to the diagnosis of histiocytosis X. N Engl J Med 1964;270:73.

75. Lacronique J, Roth C, Battesti JP, Basset F, Chretien J. Chest radiological features of pulmonary histiocytosis X: A report based on 50 adult cases. Thorax 1982;37:104.
76. Masson R, Tedeschi L. Pulmonary eosinophilic granuloma with hilar adenopathy simulating sarcoidosis. Chest 1978;73:682.
77. Abramson SJ, Berdon WE, Reilly BJ, Kuhn JP. Cavitation of anterior mediastinal masses in children with histiocytosis-X: Report of four cases with radiographic and pathologic findings and clinical follow up. Pediatr Radiol 1987;17:10.
78. Nakata H, Suzuki H, Sato Y, Kawahara H, Horie A. Histiocytosis-X with anterior mediastinal mass as its initial manifestation. Pediatr Radiol 1982;12:84.
79. Konno K, Hayashi I, Oka S. Eosinophilic granuloma (histiocytosis-X) involving anterior chest wall and lung. Am Rev Respir Dis 1969;100:391.
80. Pomeranz S, Proto A. Histiocytosis-X: Unusual confusing features of eosinophilic granuloma. Chest 1986;89:88.
81. Brauner MW, Grenier P, Mouelhi MM, Mompoint D, Lenoir S. Pulmonary histiocytosis X: Evaluation with high-resolution CT. Radiology 1989;172:255.
82. Moore AD, Godwin JD, Muller NL, Naidich DP, Hammar SP, Buschman DL, Takasugi JE, de Carvalho CR. Pulmonary histiocytosis X: Comparison of radiographic and CT findings. Radiology 1989;172:249.
83. Daniele RP, Elias JA, Epstein PE, Rossman MD. Bronchoalveolar lavage: Role in the pathogenesis, diagnosis, and management of interstitial lung disease. Ann Intern Med 1985;102:93.
84. McLelland J, Broadbent V. Histiocytosis X: Response to chemotherapy [letter]. J R Soc Med 1989;82:122.
85. Komp DM. Langerhans cell histiocytosis. N Engl J Med 1987;316:747.
86. Lahey ME. Histiocytosis X: Comparison of three treatment regimens. J Pediatr 1975;87:179.
87. Lahey M. Prognosis in reticuloendotheliosis in children. J Pediatr 1962;60:664.
88. Zinkham WH. Multifocal eosinophilic granuloma: Natural history, etiology, and management. Am J Med 1976;60:457.
89. Corbeel L, Eggermont E, Desmyter J, Surmont I, De Vos R, De Wolf Peeters C, Cobbaert C, Eykens A. Spontaneous healing of Langerhans cell histiocytosis (histiocytosis X). Eur J Pediatr 1988;148:32.
90. Carlson RA, Hattery RR, OConnell EJ, Fontana RS. Pulmonary involvement by histiocytosis X in the pediatric age group. Mayo Clin Proc 1976;51:542.
91. Sims DG. Histiocytosis X: Follow-up of 43 cases. Arch Dis Child 1977;52:433.
92. Komp DM. Long-term sequelae of histiocytosis X. Am J Pediatr Hematol Oncol 1981;3:163.
93. Komp DM, El-Mahdi A, Starling KA, Easley J, Vietti TJ, Berry DH, George SL. Quality of survival in histiocytosis X: A Southwest Oncology Group study. Med Pediatr Oncol 1980;8:35.
94. Melhem RE, Hajjar JJ, Balassanian N. Histiocytosis X: A report of 15 cases in the paediatric age group. Br J Radiol 1964;37:898.
95. Recant L, Hartroft WS (eds). Rapidly progressive pulmonary infiltration, fever and coma (clinicopathologic conference). Am J Med 1958;24:437.
96. Murray PA, Hall PA. Histiocytosis X mimicking recurrent malignant disease: A report of two cases. Clin Radiol 1988;39:310.
97. Wood C, Wood GS, Deneau DG, Oseroff A, Beckstead JH, Malin J. Malignant histiocytosis X: Report of a rapidly fatal case in an elderly man. Cancer 1984;54:347.
98. Rabkin MS, Wittwer CT, Kjeldsberg CR, Piepkorn MW. Flow-cytometric DNA content of histiocytosis X (Langerhans cell histiocytosis). Am J Pathol 1988;131:283.
99. Lombard CM, Medeiros LJ, Colby TV. Pulmonary histiocytosis X and carcinoma. Arch Pathol Lab Med 1987;111:339.

19
Pulmonary Alveolar Proteinosis

Robert M. Hoffman
Robert M. Rogers

Initially described in 1958 by Rosen and co-workers,[1] pulmonary alveolar proteinosis (PAP) remains an enigmatic disease. This chapter will discuss the epidemiology, clinical presentation, diagnosis, and treatment of PAP in detail. We will also focus on some of the unanswered questions regarding PAP, particularly those dealing with its pathogenesis. First, however, a brief history of PAP will be presented, beginning with Rosen's landmark article.

HISTORICAL PERSPECTIVE

The initial description of PAP was a retrospective pathologic review, consisting of pathologic material from 27 patients from 19 states, Canada, Italy, and the United Kingdom referred to Samuel Rosen at the Armed Forces Institute of Pathology, Benjamin Castleman at the Massachusetts General Hospital, and Averill Liebow at Yale University School of Medicine. The authors were somewhat reluctant to publish their findings since they had not yet found a causative agent, but the histologic and radiographic appearance of the disease was so striking that they felt a report was warranted. It is fortunate they opted to submit their report at that time rather than wait for the discovery of an etiology for PAP, or else the disease might still be undescribed. Their biopsy material (20 open lung biopsies and 7 autopsies) showed the presence of "granular and floccular acidophilic material, which filled large groups of alveoli, with minimal or no changes in the interalveolar septa." In addition, this intra-alveolar material, which they called "proteinaceous," was strongly positive for the periodic acid-Schiff (PAS) reagent and remained so after digestion with diastase. The authors also described exfoliating "septal cells," large mononuclear cells in the alveolar walls that contained strongly PAS-positive granules. It was their supposition that these cells eventually sloughed into the lumen with subsequent disintegration of the cytoplasm into floccular

449

masses and granules that remained PAS-positive. The results of subsequent studies using electron microscopy suggested that these degenerating cells were most likely alveolar macrophages.[2,3] The authors also noted that the pathologic process bore a close resemblance to *Pneumocystis* pneumonia.

The patients in the series ranged from 2 years old to 57 years of age. There was a male to female ratio of 2.5:1. The authors noted an interesting assortment of occupational exposures, including four lumberyard workers, two electricians, a fruit sprayer, a rat-cage cleaner, a printing plant employee, and a machinist in a plastics factory. The clinical presentation was variable but in most patients was characterized by the insidious onset of dyspnea and cough, which was usually productive. The number of patients who smoked cigarettes was not noted. The chest radiographs of the patients showed "fine, diffuse, perihilar, radiating, feathery or vaguely nodular" infiltrates in a butterfly pattern resembling pulmonary edema. The patients were treated with a variety of therapeutic regimens, including steroids and antibiotics, none of which was particularly successful. Eight patients in the series eventually died, three with superimposed infection (two cases of nocardiosis and one case of cryptococcosis).

Rosen's report has withstood the test of time to a remarkable degree. The reader will note that within this chapter repeated references will be made to this seminal work since so many of the initial observations are still valid today. The major advance since 1958 has been the introduction of lung lavage as an effective treatment for PAP. Our knowledge of the nature of the intra-alveolar material in PAP has also grown over the past 30 years, and this has prompted several suggestions for a more appropriate name for the disease, including pulmonary alveolar phospholipidosis,[4] lipoproteinosis,[5] and even phospholipoproteinosis.[6]

CLINICAL FEATURES

Epidemiology

The true incidence of PAP is unknown. It is thought to be an extremely rare disease. By 1980, 260 cases had been described in the world's literature,[7] but since case reports are more difficult to publish today unless there is a new insight into the disease process or a new complication, these reports probably grossly underestimate the true occurrence of the disease. In our local geographic area, we have seen four new cases in the past 5 years. Assuming that we see all of the new cases in this area, one can estimate the incidence of PAP to be approximately one case per million adults per 5-year period. There has been little change in terms of patient characteristics since Rosen's report. There is still probably a male preponderance of 2–3:1. Patients with PAP have been described from infancy[8] to age 87,[9] but most cases occur in the 3rd and 4th decades.[10]

Symptoms

Rosen's report was a retrospective study based on pathologic material; many of the clinical data pertaining to the original 27 patients were unknown. However, his emphasis on a clinical presentation characterized by an "unheralded onset" with "creepingly progressive dyspnea" still holds true. There were also complaints of fatigability, chest pain, slight weight loss, and cough, which was usually productive. The sputum was sometimes described as thick and yellow and in one case as composed of "chunks." This description of chunky, yellow sputum continues to be associated with PAP, but in our experience is extremely unusual. In fact, we have rarely observed productive cough to be a predominant symptom in patients with PAP, except in those patients who smoke cigarettes. Hemoptysis is extremely rare in our experience, although streaky hemoptysis associated with hard coughing was reported in almost a fourth of patients in one series.[6] Fever has been noted in patients with PAP, but when this occurs, it usually signals the presence of infection. As mentioned previously, in Rosen's article there were two patients with nocardia and one with cryptococcal infection. The association of PAP with these infections as well as tuberculosis, atypical mycobacterial infection, other fungal infections, and bacterial and viral infections has been confirmed in subsequent reports.[11-15] The number of cases of PAP associated with infection is heavily weighted by the early literature. Bedrossian and co-workers estimated that 40 out of 260 of the cases of PAP described prior to 1975 were accompanied by infections with opportunistic pathogens.[7] However, the frequency of these infections has markedly decreased in the recent literature, perhaps due to earlier and more effective therapeutic intervention for the disease. We have not seen a patient with active infection in our series of approximately 80 patients, although one or two of them have been treated at their local hospital for pneumonia.

Physical Examination and Laboratory Data

The results of physical examination in PAP are nonspecific. Rales, clubbing, and cyanosis occur in varying percentages, as shown in Table 19-1. Pulmonary function tests usually show a mild restrictive pattern with a low diffusing capacity. Arterial hypoxemia with an elevated shunt fraction is also seen in almost all patients.[16] In addition, several studies have documented that arterial oxygen desaturation with exercise is a universal finding in patients with untreated PAP[6,16,17] and in our experience with this disease dyspnea on exertion seems to correlate with exercise desaturation before and after whole lung lavage.

Laboratory test data are generally normal, except for the serum lactate dehydrogenese (LDH) concentration, which was first noted by Ramirez-R. to be elevated in 1963.[18] This observation was extended by Martin, Rogers, and Myers, who noted that 14 out of 18 patients with PAP had elevated serum LDH levels prior to treatment.[19,20]

The classic chest radiographic appearance of PAP described by Rosen still applies today. However, atypical radiographic presentations are not uncommon.[4,21,22] The infiltrate is usually symmetric and alveolar and predominates in the lower lung fields (Fig. 19-1). However, nodular and interstitial patterns can occur, and the distribution of the infiltrate may have a unilateral or upper lobe predominance. Occasionally, the chest radiograph shows pneumatoceles and atelectasis secondary to occlusion of small airways. Cavitary lesions, which are extremely rare, should suggest the presence of infection. Hilar or mediastinal adenopathy is also extremely rare and should suggest an alternative diagnosis. Roentgenographically, the differential diagnosis in PAP includes a host of other lung diseases characterized by alveolar filling, including cardiogenic pulmonary edema (except that the heart size and pulmonary vasculature are normal in

TABLE 19-1. Reported Clinical Characteristics of Pulmonary Alveolar Proteinosis

CHARACTERISTIC	SERIES			
	*Rogers et al** (14 pts)	*Prakash et al*[†] (34 pts)	*Kariman et al*[‡] (23 pts)	*DuBois et al*[§] (10 pts)
Symptoms				
Dyspnea	100%	79%		
Cough	100% (86% non-productive)	59% (100% non-productive)		
Chest Pain		32%		
Fatigue	64%			
Weight loss	29%	18%		
Hemoptysis		24%		
Signs				
Diffuse rales	86%	18%		30%
Cyanosis		24%		
Clubbing		29%		40%
Pulmonary Function				
TLC	71% predicted	76% predicted	66% predicted	66% predicted
FVC	69% predicted	79% predicted	67% predicted	63% predicted
FEV_1	70% predicted	86% predicted	67% predicted	
D_LCO	49% predicted	52% predicted	46% predicted	44% predicted
PaO_2	57 mm Hg	63 mm Hg	56 mm Hg	68 mm Hg
$PaCO_2$	33 mm Hg	33 mm Hg	34 mm Hg	
$P(A - a)O_2$	47 mm Hg		51 mm Hg	
PaO_2, (100% O_2)	284 mm Hg		367 mm Hg	

* (Data from Rogers RM, Levin DC, Gray BA, Moseley LW Jr. Physiologic effects of bronchopulmonary lavage in alveolar proteinosis. Am Rev Respir Dis 1978;118:255.).

[†] (Data from Prakash UBS, Barham SS, Carpenter HA, Dines DE, Marsh HM. Pulmonary alveolar phospholipoproteinosis: Experience with 34 cases and a review. Mayo Clin Proc 1987;62:499.).

[‡] (Data from Kariman K, Kylstra JA, Spock A. Pulmonary alveolar proteinosis: Prospective clinical experience in 23 patients for 15 years. Lung 1984;162:223.).

[§] (Data from DuBois RM, McAllister WAC, Branthwaite MA. Alveolar proteinosis: Diagnosis and treatment over a 10-year period. Thorax 1983;38:360.).

PAP and pleural effusions are absent). The differential diagnosis should also include desquamative interstitial pneumonitis; alveolar hemorrhage syndromes, such as idiopathic pulmonary hemosiderosis and Goodpasture's syndrome; pulmonary lymphoma; pulmonary alveolar microlithiasis; alveolar sarcoidosis; bronchiolo-alveolar cell carcinoma; uremic pneumonitis; and *Pneumocystis* pneumonia.

Thus far, the CT scan of the chest does not add a great deal to the plain chest radiograph in terms of diagnostic utility, but we find it useful in planning treatment with lung lavage.[23] A CT scan certainly shows more clearly the surprisingly patchy nature of parenchymal involvement in PAP, which may not be evident on the plain film. It

TREATMENT

Rationale

Prior to initiating treatment for PAP, the clinician must carefully consider the indications for therapy in light of the natural history of the disease. In Rosen's article, 6 out of 27 patients had spontaneous improvement in either radiographic appearance or symptoms. Every subsequent series has included some patients who went on to spontaneous remission (usually 20–30%).[6,9,10] This remission can be prolonged.[27] In light of this possibility, if the patient is not too disabled, the option of observation should be offered. However, if pulmonary function tests continue to decline and symptoms worsen, then treatment is indicated.

There is another theoretical reason for early intervention with whole lung lavage. It is our impression, both from our own experience and the literature, that the incidence of serious superinfection in PAP has declined in recent years. As will be described subsequently, alveolar macrophage function is decreased in PAP and the intra-alveolar material in PAP is an excellent culture medium for certain microorganisms.[28] Removing this material by lavage substantially decreases the amount of this culture medium and also seems to restore macrophage function.[29] Consequently, early intervention with whole lung lavage may decrease the infection rate in these patients. As stated previously, the infection rate in our series of patients is very low.

History

The treatment of PAP has evolved considerably since Rosen's report, in which details concerning therapy were available on only 14 patients. Most of them had received antibiotics or steroids, or both. Three patients had received isoproterenol nebulizer treatments and postural drainage, and one of these improved. In 1959, the first report of a PAP patient to be treated with the inhalation of trypsin was published.[30] Other agents, including heparin and acetylcysteine, have been administered by the inhalational route, and although there are reports of clinical improvement associated with this form of therapy,[31,32] the high incidence of side effects, including bronchospasm (which can be life-threatening), fever, and bronchitis and the long period of treatment required have resulted in a justified decline in its use.

There are two recent case reports in which ambroxol has been used to successfully treat PAP, either by inhalation or orally.[33,34] Of course, these reports may represent spontaneous remissions. Since ambroxol causes phospholipidosis and increased phospholipid secretion in experimental animals,[35] it is difficult to conceive of a mechanism by which this drug would cause clinical improvement.

The first use of lung lavage in the treatment of PAP was by Ramirez-R. in 1963.[18,36,37] The technique was called "segmental endobronchial flooding," and involved the blind transtracheal insertion of a polyethylene catheter into the lower respiratory tract, after which 50-ml to 100-ml aliquots of saline were infused into various lung segments through the catheter. The success of this method depended greatly on patient expectoration of thick, lipoproteinaceous material mobilized by the saline infusion. Interestingly, one of the first patients to receive this therapy has remained in remission for 25 years.[38]

In 1965, the technique of whole lung lavage was first used by Ramirez-R.[39] to treat PAP. Additional descriptive terms in the literature include massive bronchial pulmonary lavage, total bronchial pulmonary lavage, and volume controlled bronchial pulmonary lavage. Many series have shown whole lung lavage to be a safe and effective treatment for PAP when performed by an experienced team of pulmonologists, anesthesiologists, respiratory therapists, and nursing personnel.[6,9,16,17,40]

Technique of Whole Lung Lavage

The lavage is usually performed in the operating room under general anesthesia. At least 50 liters of sterile saline solution must be on hand. The saline should be warmed to 37°C prior to the procedure to avoid hypothermia. There is probably no advantage to adding heparin or any other additive to the saline. The patient is placed on a rotating Stryker frame table so that he/she can be axially rotated during the procedure and lavaged in both the prone and supine positions to augment clearance of intra-alveolar material. Routine monitoring of the patient includes an indwelling arterial catheter, pulse oximeter, and an esophageal stethoscope and temperature probe. Monitoring of central venous pressure or pulmonary artery pressure has never been used in any of our patients. It makes little sense to use such monitoring unless the patient has a compromised cardiovascular status, and under these circumstances we would hesitate to do the procedure. After several minutes of preoxygenation with 100% oxygen, general anesthesia is induced with thiopental and either isofluorane or halothane in 100% oxygen. Neuromuscular blockade with a nondepolarizing muscle relaxant is induced after bronchospirometry (if this is to be performed) and monitored with a peripheral nerve stimulator. When a suitable level of anesthesia is reached, the trachea is intubated with the largest left-sided, double-lumen endotracheal tube that can be passed through the glottis atraumatically. A clear polyvinyl chloride disposable tube is used because it molds to the contour of the airway and causes less trauma to the bronchial musosa and cartilage than the stiffer red rubber tubes used in the past. Also, a clear tube is preferable since during the procedure one can observe the side leading to the ventilated lung for leaking lavage fluid and the side leading to the lavaged lung for leaking air bubbles. The largest tube is recommended because the left endobronchial cuff will make contact over a greater area of the bronchial mucosa with less air in the cuff than if a smaller tube is used. In addition, a large tube facilitates better suctioning and more rapid instillation and drainage of fluid.

One cannot overemphasize the importance of precise placement of the double-lumen tube prior to initiating the lavage. Placement should be checked anatomically with a pediatric flexible fiberoptic bronchoscope and physiologically by checking for leaks with a water seal technique: that is, one lung is ventilated and held at a plateau ventilatory pressure of 40 cm of water while the tube to the non-ventilated lung is held underwater. The patient must be paralyzed for the water seal test, since the patient will aspirate water with a spontaneous breath. Any bubbling implies inadequate separation of the airway to each lung. Water seal is checked in this fashion on both sides. Since the newer polyvinyl chloride tubes are so flexible, the tip of the endobronchial tube has a tendency to migrate past the left upper lobe orifice into the left lower lobe, thereby occluding the left upper lobe. If this occurs while the left lung is being venti-

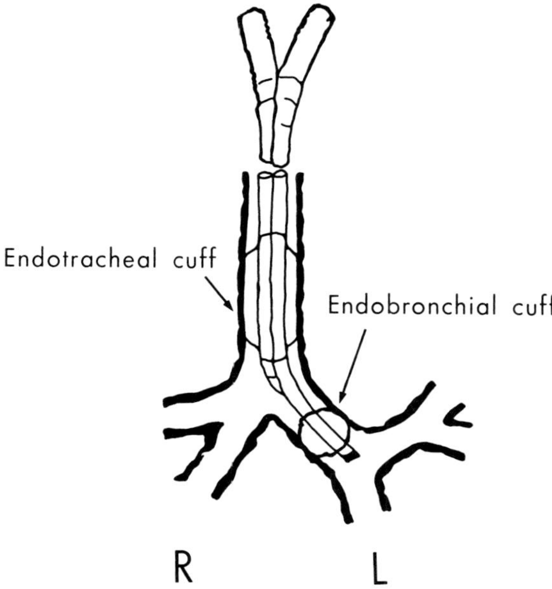

Figure 19-3. Correct positioning of double-lumen tube for whole lung lavage. Note that the left upper lobe is easily occluded if the endobronchial tube is advanced too far distally. Proximal displacement of the tube will result in an inadequate seal of the left mainstem bronchus. (From Hoffman RM, Rogers RM. Pulmonary alveolar proteinosis. In: George RB, ed. Pulmonary and critical care update. Vol. 3, lesson 13. Princeton: CPEC, 1987:1.).

lated and the right lung is being lavaged, a sudden increase in airway pressure may result. Similarly, if the left lung is being lavaged, occlusion of the left upper lobe will result in a sudden decrease in the amount of saline that can be infused into the lung. On the other hand, the endobronchial tube must not be moved too far proximally or else it will slip out of the left mainstem bronchus. Repeat visualization with the fiberoptic bronchoscope may be necessary several times during the lavage procedure in order to verify proper positioning of the tube. Utilizing the bronchoscope to position the double-lumen endotracheal tube has taken all of the guesswork out of tube placement and is an absolute necessity in order to perform an uneventful lavage. Correct tube placement is illustrated in Figure 19-3.

It is our practice to lavage the most severely affected lung first, since one would like to ventilate the "good" lung during the patient's initial lavage in order to facilitate the best possible gas exchange. Determining which lung is worse in a functional sense can be done preoperatively on the basis of a CT scan of the chest. It can also be done intraoperatively, with the patient under general anesthesia but spontaneously breathing, by comparing the oxygen uptake in each lung as determined by differential bronchospirometry using 100% oxygen.[41,42] If lung function appears to be the same bilaterally, then the left lung is lavaged first while the right lung is ventilated because the right lung has a larger volume.

The pros and cons of performing whole lung lavage in the decubitus versus the supine position have been reviewed in detail by Benumof[43] and it is his conclusion that the supine position offers the best compromise between the risk of spillage and blood flow distribution problems. The saline reservoir is suspended approximately 100 cm above the carina and connected to the tube leading to the lung to be lavaged. This inflow line and drainage line are arranged as in Kylstra's initial description.[42] Before proceeding with the lavage, however, the inflow tube is clamped and the lung to be lavaged is not ventilated for 5 minutes in order to allow intra-alveolar gas (which has been preoxygenated with 100% oxygen) to be absorbed into the bloodstream. After this period of "degassing," the clamp is released and saline is allowed to flow into the lung in small amounts (50–100 ml) at a time. If there are no obvious leaks as determined by auscultation, fluid can be infused in increasing amounts. Usually, the largest volume that the lung can accept is roughly equal to the inspiratory capacity (IC) (total lung capacity minus functional residual capacity) of the lung being lavaged. For the left lung, this is estimated as being 45% of the IC for both lungs, while the IC of the right lung is 55% of the IC for both lungs. When the infusion of saline is complete, the fluid is immediately allowed to drain. Initially, one should see the return of turbid, yellowish-brown effluent. Not all of the fluid instilled will drain out, since one can usually anticipate that a volume of saline roughly equivalent to the functional residual capacity of the lung being lavaged will remain in that lung during the course of the lavage. After the first 10 liters of saline have been infused and returned the effluent usually begins to clear. When this occurs, a team of respiratory therapists is called upon to administer chest physiotherapy over the lavaged lung during the emptying phase of the lavage. This results in a prompt increase in the turbidity of the lavage fluid and increases the yield of particulate matter removed.[44] The lavage is continued in this fashion until the lavage effluent is almost totally clear. At this point the patient is rotated to the prone position and the lavage is continued until there is a final clearing of the turbidity of the fluid. The exact endpoint of the lavage is difficult to determine. Usually one reaches a point where no further clearing of the fluid is observed. Small bronchial casts usually persist in the lavage material and never completely disappear. We usually find that it takes about 50 liters of saline (range of 40–70 liters) to bring about maximal clearing of the lavage fluid, but there is significant variability among patients.

There are certain physiologic alterations that occur during lavage that the lavage team should be aware of.[45] Characteristically, arterial blood oxygenation varies during the phases of the lavage cycle, with the highest arterial saturation occurring near completion of the infusion phase when the airway pressure in the lavaged lung is at its peak, thereby causing shunting of pulmonary blood flow to the contralateral lung being ventilated. On the other hand, the PaO_2 will customarily drop as the lavaged lung is being emptied, because as the airway pressure decreases, perfusion returns to the totally unventilated lavaged lung, thereby creating a large shunt effect. The other problem that the operating team must be aware of is the potential for leakage and hydrothorax. It is necessary to keep a continuous record of the total volume of saline infused and recovered. If the cumulative retention of lavage fluid (amount infused minus amount emptied) exceeds 1500 ml or if the negative balance per filling and emptying cycle exceeds 200 ml, then either of these possibilities must be considered. Leakage of fluid into the contralateral lung should be fairly obvious to both the anesthesiologist and the pulmonologist and usually the following may be observed sequentially if this is the case: (1) the appearance of bubbles in the lavage fluid draining from the lavaged lung; (2) rales and rhonchi over the ventilated lung; and (3) a fall in arterial oxygen saturation.

Any of these findings should warrant a repeat check of endotracheal tube positioning with the fiberoptic bronchoscope. Repositioning of the tube or adjustment of bronchial balloon cuff pressure may be necessary in order to correct the leak. The occurrence of hydrothorax is much more subtle and may only be assumed in the presence of a large negative fluid balance without an obvious leak of fluid to the contralateral side.

After the lavage is terminated, the lavaged lung is drained for the final time, thoroughly suctioned, and then ventilated. Our anesthesiologist often inflates the lavaged lung with positive end-expiratory pressure while occluding the airway to the other lung in order to bring about uniform reinflation of the lavaged lung. Most patients can be extubated while still in the operating room, but if a patient is not a candidate for this, the double-lumen tube is changed to a single-lumen endotracheal tube and the patient is mechanically ventilated in the recovery room until extubation is possible. A chest film is taken in the recovery room, primarily to check for hydrothorax. The lung that has just been lavaged frequently is totally opacified in the immediate postoperative chest film, but this opacification clears fairly rapidly.[46] On the day following the lavage procedure, the patient is encouraged to deep breathe with incentive spirometry. Chest percussion and postural drainage may be continued in order to remove the remaining fluid and to enable the patient to bring up secretions.

Special Cases

The vast majority of patients can be lavaged using the aforementioned technique. It has even been used safely on a pregnant patient.[47] However, there are extremely rare patients who cannot tolerate unilateral lung lavage either because (1) they cannot achieve adequate oxygenation (PaO_2 >100 mm Hg) by ventilating one lung with 100% O_2; (2) they do not have another lung due to prior surgical excision[48]; or (3) it is anatomically impossible due to the small size of the airway (as in children). In these patients there are a number of alternative treatments that can be tried. Extracorporeal membrane oxygenation (ECMO) has been used to provide adequate gas exchange during standard unilateral lung lavage or bilateral lung lavage, either with partial venoarterial cardiopulmonary bypass[49–51] or with venovenous bypass.[52,53] Another technique that has been employed, especially in patients in whom there is excessive oxygen desaturation during the drainage phase of the lavage (when shunt increases due to the return of blood flow to the unventilated lung), is the use of a flow-directed balloon-tipped pulmonary artery catheter.[54,55] In these reports the pulmonary artery catheter balloon was inflated in the main pulmonary artery of the lung being lavaged during the period of lung drainage until the phasic pulmonary artery trace just began to dampen; in every patient an increase in PaO_2 occurred. However, because of the potential hazard of pulmonary artery rupture,[56] this method must be used with extreme caution and as a last resort. It should be emphasized that in our experience the vast majority of PAP patients can be lavaged with the conventional method without having to resort to the aforementioned techniques. The only time we have had to use ECMO was in a patient who had undergone a right middle and lower lobectomy prior to developing PAP.

A novel approach to the problem of hypoxemia during lavage was used by Jansen and co-workers,[57] who performed whole lung lavage under hyperbaric oxygen conditions. Another alternative to whole lung lavage is the use of the fiberoptic bronchoscope to lavage the lungs one lobe at a time.[58] With this technique, a cuffed bronchoscope is inserted into a lobar bronchus and saline irrigation is carried out. The procedure is carried out under topical anesthesia with the patient breathing high flow O_2 by face mask. For maximum control of the airway, the procedure should probably be done through an endotracheal tube. Continuous monitoring of O_2 saturation is advised because of the risk of hypoxemia associated with any bronchoscopic procedure.[59] One or two lobes may be done at a time and the lavage may be repeated as needed. Although the recovery of material is clearly not as great as with whole lung lavage and no series has been reported outlining the potential hazards of this procedure in severely hypoxic patients, the relative ease with which it can be performed would seem to make it a reasonable technique to try before using a system as complicated as ECMO. Furthermore, this technique could conceivably improve the patients' gas exchange enough to make them suitable candidates for whole lung lavage.

Finally, the lavage of children poses a particularly vexing problem, since the smallest double-lumen tube is 28 French, with each lumen being slightly less than 4.5 mm in diameter. In such patients a single-lumen tube has been used to perform bilateral lavage using partial cardiopulmonary bypass to provide adequate oxygenation.[49,60,61] In very small infants, in whom cardiopulmonary bypass may be hazardous, an ingenious technique has been used to perform unilateral whole lung lavage using a balloon-tipped pulmonary artery catheter, which is introduced into the lung that is to be lavaged through the side-arm of a rigid bronchoscope. The infant can be ventilated through the bronchoscope while the lavage is performed through the pulmonary artery port of the catheter.[62]

Outcome

The response of patients to whole lung lavage is variable. In 1978, Rogers and co-workers[16] reported on 14 patients who underwent lavage with follow-up from 2 to 96 months. In addition to subjective improvement, there was significant improvement in the following parameters 5 days after lavage: vital capacity, total lung capacity, resting room air PaO_2, exercise PaO_2, shunt, and diffusing capacity. However, the long-term effects varied. Some patients required annual or semi-annual lavages (5/12) whereas others remained in remission for 36 to 96 months of follow-up (6/12). Repeat lavage was successful in reversing clinical and physiological abnormalities in those patients who experienced a recurrence except in one patient who failed to show a response to treatment after 21 lavages and in whom a repeat open lung biopsy showed significant pulmonary fibrosis.

In Selecky's series, all patients had radiographic, physiological, and symptomatic improvement with lavage.[17] Seven out of twelve patients did not need a second lavage, but the follow-up period in this report was only 5 to 21 months. Five patients needed a repeat lavage within 18 months of the initial lavage. In Dubois' series, all 10 patients improved and eventually returned to work after lung lavage.[40] Kariman reported that 76% (11/14) of his patients who were lavaged had a good response with most requiring one to four lavages performed over 1 to 3 years, but one patient needed twelve lavages over 5 years before a remission was achieved. Three out of fourteen patients either had no response to lavage or a gradually diminishing effect with repeated lavage. No tissue was obtained in these patients.[9] In Prakash's series, 13 of 21 (62%) patients who were lavaged had no recurrence after a single lavage. Five patients (24%) had a recurrence after a single lavage. Five patients (14%) showed no response to lavage (no details were given).[6]

There are a few well-described cases of interstitial pulmonary fibrosis in association with PAP in the literature. Hudson and co-workers described a patient with PAP who spontaneously resolved. He then developed pulmonary fibrosis 13 years later.[63] Kaplan and Sabin reported the development of pulmonary fibrosis in a PAP patient after three whole lung lavages.[64] In Clague's report the development of fibrosis occurred early in the course of the patient's PAP.[65]

PATHOPHYSIOLOGY

Rosen's speculation on the cause of PAP was intriguing. He thought that the genesis of the PAS-positive material was from transformed attached and exfoliated "septal" cells— large mononuclear cells observed within the alveolar walls. Since immunocytochemistry or electron microscopy was not performed in his report, it is difficult to say whether or not these septal cells represented type II pneumocytes or alveolar macrophages. What caused these cells to transform was conjectured to be an environmental toxin (chemical inhalants, detergents, or new antibiotics were entertained as possibilities) and therefore the disease was thought to be possibly a "penalty for the convenience of modern living." This hypothesis, although attractive, has yet to be proved and the etiology of PAP is still a mystery.

Animal Models: Inhalational

Most studies on the etiology of PAP have focused on animal models or on studies of the material obtained from whole lung lavage. The animal models are of two types: inhalational and drug-induced. A wide variety of fine dust particles, including silica,[5,66–73] aluminum,[66,74] nickel,[75,76] pyrite,[77] lignite coal,[78] antimony trioxide,[79] bismuth orthovanadate,[80] crushed fiberglass,[81] and volcanic ash,[82,83] have induced a pathologic process similar to PAP in experimental animals. In most of these models the disease process is initiated when the inhaled or directly instilled particulate matter causes an influx of macrophages into the alveolar space.[66,69,73,76,77,79–83] There is a subsequent proliferation of type II pneumocytes associated with an accumulation of phospholipid in the surfactant pool.[70–72,75] The alveolar macrophages ingest the phospholipid, become markedly overloaded with this material, and then the alveolar spaces become filled with lipoproteinaceous material derived from hyperplastic type II pneumocytes and disintegrating phospholipid-laden alveolar macrophages. The description is reminiscent of the disintegrating septal cells described by Rosen.[1] However, Corrin and King found that the type II cells in their model were intact.[66] In the silica model, the development of classic silicotic nodules as opposed to proteinosis was a function of the animal strain and particle type, size, and concentration.[84]

What evidence is there that inhalation of dust is a causative agent in human PAP? As stated previously, Rosen suspected that inhalation of toxic solvents had something to do with the etiology. Davidson and MacLeod found that in 50% of the 139 cases they reviewed patients had been exposed to a variety of dusts and fumes. They concluded, however, that the information in most of the published reports to that time was too scanty to permit an adequate assessment for environmental causes.[10] Heppleston and Young[85] demonstrated remarkable ultrastructural similarity between the animal and human forms of PAP. However, the fact remains that there are very few reports in the literature that convincingly show a link between environmental exposure and PAP. Buechner and Ansari described four cases of acute silicosis in sandblasters in which there was intra-alveolar filling with PAS-positive material.[86] However, in contrast to Rosen's initial description of the histopathology of PAP, the sandblasters also had marked interstitial pneumonitis and fibrosis. Rosen felt that these patients had two independent pulmonary diseases: PAP and diffuse interstitial pneumonitis. Interstitial fibrosis and silicotic nodules were also observed in subsequent reports of acute "silicoproteinosis."[87–89] A temporal correlation between high-intensity exposure to aluminum dust,[90] cement dust,[91] and kaolin[92] at the workplace and the development of PAP has also been reported. Based on our own experience and the few reports cited above, we think that dust-induced PAP in humans is rare, occurs only with very intense and massive exposures, and is associated with more interstitial abnormalities than one finds in a typical case of PAP.

In a review of 37 cases of PAP,[93] McEwen and Abraham found that 13 patients had been exposed to various dusts and fumes. Using light microscopy, the authors found markedly increased numbers of small, inorganic birefringent particles in the lung tissue of 20 of the PAP patients when compared with control patients with other lung diseases characterized by alveolar filling. A follow-up study utilizing scanning electron microscopy and energy-dispersive X-ray analysis confirmed that the concentration of particulates was much higher in the tissue of the patients with PAP.[94] However, on average the distribution of particles among silica, silicates, and other particles was the same as in the controls. Individual patients occasionally did show markedly increased percentages of certain particulates (increased silica in a sandblaster; increased iron, chromium, and tin particles in a welder; and increased silicates in a cement finisher). In three out of five infants examined there were increased silicates containing both silicon and magnesium in a ratio consistent with talc. Of course, these analyses do not clearly establish a cause and effect relationship between dust exposure and PAP, merely an association. Patients with underlying PAP probably have impaired alveolar clearance mechanisms and are therefore more susceptible to the accumulation of intra-alveolar particles.

Animal Models: Drug-induced

Other models of PAP in experimental animals are based on drug ingestion. The most commonly used drug in this model is the anorectic agent chlorphentermine,[95] although over 20 compounds, including amiodarone[96] and iprindole,[97] have induced similar pathologic changes. These drugs are all cationic amphiphilic compounds. The effect of these agents is to cause the accumulation of lamellar inclusions consisting primarily of phospholipids within a variety of cell types throughout the organism. In the lung, alveolar macrophages become engorged with these inclusions and accumulate in the alveolar space.[98] If the drug is administered for a long enough period, PAP may appear after these cells disintegrate.[97] The mechanism is thought to be decreased phospholipid degradation both in alveolar macrophages and in alveolar lavage fluid.[99] Chlorphentermine may bind to phospholipids and render this complex resistant to the action of phospholipase.[100,101] There are no reported cases of drug ingestion being implicated in a case of PAP in humans, but the animal model of drug-induced phospholipidosis has been very valuable in elucidating possible mechanisms for PAP.

Biochemical Constituents of Lavage Fluid

Many investigators have focused on the lavage fluid itself as a way of determining the pathophysiology of PAP. Larson and Gordinier[102] first speculated that the intra-alveolar material in PAP may represent an excessive accumulation of pulmonary surfactant, and this hypothesis was subsequently confirmed by several investigators. The composition of the fluid obtained from whole lung lavage was shown by Ramirez-R. and Harlan[103] to consist of 73% protein, 27% lipid, and less than 1.5% carbohydrate, similar proportions to those Rosen measured in whole lung.[1] They also noted that there was an excessive accumulation of lipid in PAP washings compared with those from patients with asthma and chronic bronchitis (10–40 times greater) but the lipid composition was very similar in both sets of washings. The predominant lipid component was phospholipid (60% of total lipid) and the main phospholipid constituent was phosphatidylcholine (60% of total phospholipid). The high proportion of phosphatidylcholine was very suggestive of the composition of pulmonary surfactant. McClenahan and Mussenden[104] also found that the lipid profile of PAP washings was the same as washings from normal patients without lung disease, adding more support to the concept that there was an inordinate accumulation of qualitatively normal pulmonary surfactant in PAP. Finally, Sahu and co-workers[105] showed that the fatty acid composition of the phosphatidylcholine isolated from PAP lavage was primarily palmitic acid, again the same as in normal pulmonary surfactant.

The proteinaceous component of PAP lavage has also been studied in considerable detail. In 1966, Hawkins and co-workers[106] found that the soluble proteins in alveolar washings from three cases of PAP could be identified in the patients' plasma by immunoelectrophoresis and thus were derived from serum. Rupp[107] was the first to describe a selective increase in IgG and a lesser increase in IgA in lavage fluid. These findings were later confirmed by Bell and Hook,[108] who also found two soluble proteins of molecular weight 47 kDa and 52 kDa in PAP lavage that were not found in serum or in lung washings from normals. They hypothesized that the accumulation of soluble proteins in the lavage material of PAP patients was best explained by the diffusion of proteins from capillary to alveolus through channels of normal size and selectivity. However, this mechanism could not account for the increased immunoglobulin levels in lavage, which would imply enhanced local synthesis or enhanced transport of immunoglobulins to the alveolar surface.

The presence of phospholipases,[109] prostaglandins, and leukotrienes[110] has also been noted in PAP lavage fluid. In addition to these soluble components, a great deal of attention has been focused on several proteins that are insoluble in aqueous solution, beginning with the work of Passero and co-workers.[111] The principal protein identified in this study had a molecular weight of 36 kDa. Although the relative proportion of this protein in PAP lavage varies depending on the methods used for its isolation,[112] it is likely that this protein is the major surfactant apoprotein SP-A,[113] and that other higher molecular weight proteins found in PAP lavage are oligomers of SP-A. Ross and co-workers[114] demonstrated immunologic reactivity, detailed tryptic fragment analysis, amino acid composition, and collagenase and endoglycosidase digests all supporting the close identity of SP-A and alveolar proteinosis protein. Partial amino acid sequencing of the 32 kDa alveolar proteinosis protein was also identical to human SP-A.[115] Alveolar proteinosis protein did have an increased propensity to form dimers and oligomers even after treatment with sulfhydryl-reducing agents when compared to normal human SP-A.[114] Whether this propensity has anything to do with the pathogenesis of PAP requires further study. Antibody against SP-A stains the intra-alveolar material in PAP intensely, as shown by Singh and co-workers.[116,117] SP-A is also heavily glycosylated, which may account for the carbohydrate content and the positive PAS staining of the intra-alveolar material seen in PAP.[111] It should also be noted that PAP lavage is a plentiful source of SP-A and the other known surfactant proteins SP-B and SP-C[113] and has been utilized in many recent studies on the structure and function of these important proteins.[118–121] Lynn[122] has described a glycoprotein of molecular weight 250 kDa in PAP lavage fluid and several proteolytic fragments of this protein of molecular weights 130 kDa, 80 kDa, 62 kDa, 36 kDa, and 26 kDa. It is not clear whether these proteins are also related to any of the pulmonary surfactant proteins.

Ultrastructure of Lavage Fluid Constituents

Electron microscope studies of PAP lavage material have shown that it is not the bland, amorphous, finely granular acellular material one sees under light microscopy. Costello and co-workers described many foamy macrophages when PAP material was viewed under the electron microscope.[2] The cells contained many complex inclusions that were thought to represent lipid contained within phagolysosomes. The acellular fraction contained numerous lamellated structures, later called multilamellated structures by Hook[123] and subclassified into four types by subsequent investigators.[124,125] These structures consisted of alternating layers of light and dark lamellae. The darker lamellae consisted of trilaminar membranes 80–100 angstroms thick, probably representing a phospholipid bilayer, and the lighter lamellae were 150–300 angstroms thick and amorphous in appearance, probably representing protein. The shapes and sizes of the multilamellated structures were quite variable. They accounted for about 50% of the volume of the insoluble material in lavage fluid.[112,126] The authors concluded that multilamellated structures were an abnormal form of tubular myelin, and that even though some regions of multilamellated structures contained the quadratic lattice of normal tubular myelin, deviations from this pattern predominated. The multilamellated structures could be formed in vitro by mixing extracted proteins from the lungs of patients with PAP with liposomes prepared from normal human lung surfactant.[127] Whether these structures form because of an abnormal protein or simply because of excessive amounts of SP-A is not clear.

Alveolar Macrophage Function in PAP

The function of alveolar macrophages has been scrutinized in PAP since the work of Golde and co-workers.[128] They showed that alveolar macrophages obtained from PAP lavage survived poorly in culture, showed impaired chemotaxis, and had decreased adhesiveness to glass. The macrophages phagocytosed normally but had decreased ability to kill yeast. The authors thought that this abnormal alveolar macrophage function represented an acquired defect since normal peripheral blood monocytes incubated in PAP lavage effluent assumed morphologic abnormalities similar to alveolar macrophages recovered from patients with PAP. Harris[129] reported that alveolar macrophages from PAP patients showed decreased phagocytosis of *Staphylococcus aureus* compared with normal alveolar macrophages. Nugent and Pesanti made similar observations.[130] They also studied the effect of PAP lavage on the phagocytic and degradative activities of mouse peritoneal macrophage monolayers. Exposure to PAP lavage resulted in a decrease in phagocytic capacity for both *Staphylococcus aureus* and *Candida*. Intracellular bacterial killing was normal. Finally, Gonzalez-Rothi and Harris[131] demonstrated decreased ingestion of yeast and decreased phagolysosome fusion by PAP alveolar macrophages. Cultured normal human and rat alveolar macrophages exposed to PAP lavage became abnormal in appearance and displayed decreased phagocytic indices. We have shown that the abnormal function of alveolar macrophages recovered from PAP patients may be reversible after whole lung lavage, although the mechanism for this is as yet undescribed.[29] Recently, a protein was found in the lavage and the serum of a patient with PAP that inhibited the respiratory burst of normal blood monocytes.[132] Abnormal alveolar macrophage function has also been described in some of the inhalational animal models for PAP, particularly the nickel-induced model.[133]

Speculations on Pathogenesis

How do these studies impact on our understanding of the pathogenesis of PAP? The development of PAP is probably a complex chain of events involving dysfunction of both type II pneumocytes and alveolar macrophages. Ramirez and Harlan[103] reported that the incorporation of radiolabeled palmitate and glycerol into phospholipid by lung tissue homogenates was the same in biopsy material from PAP patients and normal lung tissue. However, radiolabeled palmitate that had been injected intravenously into PAP patients persisted for a much longer time in the washings of these patients than in washings from patients with asthma or chronic bronchitis. The authors concluded that the problem in PAP was defective clearance of intra-alveolar material and not overproduction. In the inhalation model of PAP, as in the human disease, there is also an increase in surfactant phospholipid, but whether this increase in surfactant represents increased production or decreased metabolism is controversial. In some animal models it appears to be a combination of both.[67] This discrepancy between the animal and human data may be due to the fact that in the animal model surfactant turnover was determined in an early phase of the disease marked by a degree of type II cell proliferation not seen in humans.[85]

Only recently has the clearance of normal surfactant been recognized as primarily involving reuptake by type II pneumocytes.[134–136] The ingestion of pulmonary surfactant by alveolar macrophages is probably not a significant clearance mechanism in the normal lung.[137] Therefore, the defect in the clearance and degradation of intra-alveolar phospholipoproteinaceous material in PAP likely represents dysfunction of type II cells. The reason for this defect remains to be determined in the inhalational animal model and in human PAP; in the drug-induced animal model it is probably due to inhibition of phospholipase.[101]

In the inhalational model, one of the initial events in PAP is the accumulation of alveolar macrophages in the alveolar space. The macrophages then ingest the accumulating intra-alveolar lipoproteinaceous material and become morphologically and functionally abnormal, disintegrate, and release their intracellular contents. This may further contribute to the accumulation of intra-alveolar material and perhaps further suppress type II cell–mediated alveolar clearance mechanisms, thereby creating a vicious cycle. Whether alveolar macrophages are functionally abnormal to begin with in PAP or merely "innocent phagocytes" engulfed in a sea of lipoprotein is unclear, although most reports favor the latter.[29,128]

This entire process has been called an atypical reaction to tissue injury.[138] The initiating factors, however, are poorly understood. Inhalation may play a role in some cases but other factors, especially genetic predisposition,[49,139–141] infection, drug ingestion, and immune status, may be important. Perhaps the individual who develops PAP has acquired or inherited a subtle abnormality in SP-A structure (an increased tendency to oligomerize, for example) leading to dysfunctional reuptake of pulmonary surfactant by type II pneumocytes. This would seem to be a promising area for future research.

SECONDARY PROTEINOSIS

Since the initial description of PAP, there has been an increase in the recognition of lesions identical to PAP in the lung tissue of patients with other diseases, usually hematologic malignancies,[7] but also described in association with AIDS,[142] solid tumors,[143] tuberculosis,[144] and interstitial pneumonitis.[89,145] This entity, known as secondary PAP, shows a strong PAS positivity in the involved areas, but the involvement is much more focal and patchy than in primary PAP. Immunoperoxidase staining using a specific antibody to SP-A has shown that the intra-alveolar material stains intensely and diffusely in primary PAP, but there is only faint staining in secondary proteinosis.[116] It is thought that the areas of PAS positivity in secondary PAP represent the accumulation of necrotic debris and exudate secondary to the primary disease process or therapy thereof and not the surfactant material that one sees in primary PAP. Patients with leukemia and secondary PAP have undergone whole lung lavage,[53] but the outcome has generally been disappointing owing to the patient's underlying disease.

REFERENCES

1. Rosen SH, Castleman B, Liebow AA. Pulmonary alveolar proteinosis. N Engl J Med 1958;258:1123.
2. Costello JF, Moriarty DC, Branthwaite MA, Turner-Warwick M, Corrin B. Diagnosis and treatment of alveolar proteinosis: The role of electron microscopy. Thorax 1975;30:121.
3. Kuhn C, Gyorkey F, Levine BE, Ramirez-R J. Pulmonary alveolar proteinosis: A study using enzyme histochemistry, electron microscopy, and surface tension measurement. Lab Invest 1966;15:492.

4. Claypool WD, Rogers RM, Matuschak GM. Update on the clinical diagnosis, management, and pathogenesis of pulmonary alveolar proteinosis (phospholipidosis). Chest 1984;85:550.
5. Heppleston AG, Wright NA, Stewart JA. Experimental alveolar lipo-proteinosis following the inhalation of silica. J Pathol 1970;101:293.
6. Prakash UBS, Barham SS, Carpenter HA, Dines DE, Marsh HM. Pulmonary alveolar phospholipoproteinosis: Experience with 34 cases and a review. Mayo Clin Proc 1987;62:499.
7. Bedrossian CWM, Luna MA, Conklin RH, Miller WC. Alveolar proteinosis as a consequence of immunosuppression: A hypothesis based on clinical and pathological observations. Hum Pathol 1980;11(suppl):527.
8. Coleman M, Dehner LP, Sibley RK, Burke BA, L'Heureux PR, Thompson TR. Pulmonary alveolar proteinosis: An uncommon cause of chronic neonatal respiratory distress. Am Rev Respir Dis 1980;121:583.
9. Kariman K, Kylstra JA, Spock A. Pulmonary alveolar proteinosis: Prospective clinical experience in 23 patients for 15 years. Lung 1984;162:223.
10. Davidson JM, MacLeod WM. Pulmonary alveolar proteinosis. Br J Dis Chest 1969;63:13.
11. Andriole VT, Balla M, Wilson GL. The association of nocardiosis and pulmonary alveolar proteinosis: A case study. Ann Intern Med 1964;60:266.
12. Carlsen TT, Hill RB Jr, Rowlands DT Jr. Nocardiosis and pulmonary alveolar proteinosis. Ann Intern Med 1964;60:275.
13. Ranchod M, Bissell M. Pulmonary alveolar proteinosis and cytomegalovirus infection. Arch Pathol Lab Med 1979;103:139.
14. Reyes JM, Putong PB. Association of pulmonary alveolar lipoproteinosis with mycobacterial infection. Am J Clin Pathol 1980;74:478.
15. Hartung M, Salfeder K. Pulmonary alveolar proteinosis and histoplasmosis: Report of three cases. Virchows Arch (Pathol Anat) 1975;368:281.
16. Rogers RM, Levin DC, Gray BA, Moseley LW Jr. Physiologic effects of bronchopulmonary lavage in alveolar proteinosis. Am Rev Respir Dis 1978;118:255.
17. Selecky PA, Wasserman K, Benfield JR, Lippmann M. The clinical and physiological effect of whole-lung lavage in pulmonary alveolar proteinosis: A ten-year experience. Ann Thor Surg 1977;24:451.
18. Ramierez-R. J, Nyka W, McLaughlin J. Pulmonary alveolar proteinosis: Diagnostic technics and observations. N Engl J Med 1963;268:165.
19. Martin RJ, Rogers RM, Myers NM. Pulmonary alveolar proteinosis: Shunt fraction and lactic acid dehydrogenase concentrations as aids to diagnosis. Am Rev Respir Dis 1978;117:1059.
20. Martin RJ, Coalson JJ, Rogers RM, Horton FO, Manous LE. Pulmonary alveolar proteinosis: The diagnosis by segmental lavage. Am Rev Respir Dis 1980;121:819.
21. Preger L. Pulmonary alveolar proteinosis. Radiology 1969;92:1291.
22. Ramirez-R. J. Pulmonary alveolar proteinosis: A roentgenographic analysis. Am J Roentgenol 1964;92:571.
23. Godwin JD, Muller NL, Takasugi JE. Pulmonary alveolar proteinosis: CT findings. Radiology 1988;169:609.
24. Yeh SDJ, White DA, Stover-Pepe DE, Caravelli JF, Van Uitert C, Benua RS. Abnormal gallium scintigraphy in pulmonary alveolar proteinosis (PAP). Clin Nucl Med 1986;12:294.
25. Vidone RA, Hoffman L, Hukill PB, Nesbitt KA, McMahon FJ. The diagnosis of pulmonary alveolar proteinosis by sputum examination. Dis Chest 1966;49:326.
26. Rubinstein I, Mullen BM, Hoffstein V. Morphologic diagnosis of idiopathic pulmonary alveolar lipoproteinosis—revisited. Arch Intern Med 1988;148:813.
27. Wilson DO, Rogers RM. Prolonged spontaneous remission in a patient with untreated pulmonary alveolar proteinosis. Am J Med 1987;82:1014.
28. Ramirez-R. J, Savard EV, Hawkins JE. Biologic effect of pulmonary washings from cases of alveolar proteinosis. Am Rev Respir Dis 1966;94:244.

29. Hoffman RM, Dauber JH, Rogers RM. Improvement in alveolar macrophage migration after therapeutic whole lung lavage in pulmonary alveolar proteinosis. Am Rev Respir Dis 1989;139:1030.

30. Sieracki JC, Horn RC Jr, Kay S. Pulmonary alveolar proteinosis: Report of 3 cases. An Intern Med 1959;51:728.

31. Brodsky I, Mayock RL. Pulmonary alveolar proteinosis: Remission after therapy with trypsin and chymotrypsin. N Engl J Med 1961;265:935.

32. Jay SJ. Pulmonary alveolar proteinosis: Successful treatment with aerosolized trypsin. Am J Med 1979;66:348.

33. Diaz JP, Manresa Presas F, Benasco C, Guardiola J, Munoz L, Clariana A. Response to surfactant activator (ambroxol) in alveolar proteinosis (letter). Lancet 1984;i:1023.

34. Naito M, Kunieda T, Yoshioka T, Okubo S, Yutani C. A case of pulmonary alveolar proteinosis treated with oral administration of ambroxol. Nippon Kyobu Shikkan Gakkai Zasshi 1985;23:912.

35. Cerutti P, Kapanci Y. Effects of metabolite VIII of bromhexine (NA 872) on type II epithelium of the lung. Respiration 1979;37:241.

36. Ramirez-R. J, Schultz RB, Dutton RE. Pulmonary alveolar proteinosis: A new technique and rationale for treatment. Arch Intern Med 1963;112:419.

37. Ramirez-R. J, Campbell GD. Pulmonary alveolar proteinosis: Endobronchial treatment. Ann Intern Med 1965;63:429.

38. Green D, Criner GJ. Twenty-five year follow-up of a patient treated with lung lavage for pulmonary alveolar proteinosis (letter). N Engl J Med 1987;317:839.

39. Ramirez-R. J, Kieffer RJ Jr, Ball WC Jr. Bronchopulmonary lavage in man. Ann Intern Med 1965;63:819.

40. DuBois RM, McAllister WAC, Branthwaite MA. Alveolar proteinosis: Diagnosis and treatment over a 10-year period. Thorax 1983;38:360.

41. Rogers RM, Kuhl DE, Hyde RW, Mayock RL. Measurement of the vital capacity and perfusion of each lung by fluoroscopy and macroaggregated albumin lung scanning: An alternative to bronchospirometry for evaluating individual lung function. Ann Intern Med 1967;67:947.

42. Kylstra JA, Rausch DC, Hall KD, Spock A. Volume-controlled lung lavage in the treatment of asthma, bronchiectasis, and mucoviscidosis. Am Rev Respir Dis 1971;103:651.

43. Benumof J. Anesthesia for thoracic surgery. Philadelphia: WB Saunders, 1987:358.

44. Kao D, Wasserman K, Costley D, Benfield JR. Advances in the treatment of pulmonary alveolar proteinosis. Am Rev Respir Dis 1975;111:361.

45. Rogers RM, Szidon JP, Shelburne J, Neigh JL, Shuman JF, Tantum KR. Hemodynamic response of the circulation to bronchopulmonary lavage in man. N Engl J Med 1972;296:1230.

46. Gale ME, Karlinsky, Robins AG. Bronchopulmonary lavage in pulmonary alveolar proteinosis: Chest radiograph observations. Am J Roentgenol 1986;146:981.

47. Matuschak GM, Owens GR, Rogers RM, Tibbals SC. Progressive intrapartum respiratory insufficiency due to pulmonary alveolar proteinosis. Chest 1984;86:496.

48. Heymach GJ, Shaw RC, McDonald JA, Vest JV. Fiberoptic bronchopulmonary lavage for alveolar proteinosis in a patient with only one lung. Chest 1982;81:508.

49. Seard C, Wasserman K, Benfield JR, Cleveland RJ, Costley DO, Heimlich EM. Simultaneous bilateral lung lavage (alveolar washing) using partial cardiopulmonary bypass. Am Rev Respir Dis 1970;101:877.

50. Freedman AP, Pelias A, Johnston RF, et al. Alveolar proteinosis lung lavage using partial cardiopulmonary bypass. Thorax 1981;36:543.

51. Altose MD, Hicks RE, Edwards MW. Extracorporeal membrane oxygenation during bronchopulmonary lavage. Arch Surg 1976;111:1148.

52. Zapol WM, Wilson R, Hales C, et al. Venovenous bypass with a membrane lung to support bilateral lung lavage. JAMA 1984;251:3269.

53. Cooper JD, Duffin J, Glynn MFX, Nelems JM, Teasdale S, Scott AA. Combination of membrane oxygenator support and pulmonary lavage for acute respiratory failure. J Thorac Cardiovasc Surg 1976;71:304.

54. Alfrey DD, Zamost BG, Benumof JL. Unilateral lung lavage: Blood flow manipulation by ipsilateral pulmonary artery balloon inflation. Anesthesiology 1981;55:376.

55. Spragg RG, Benumof JL, Alfery DD. New methods for performance of unilateral lung lavage. Anesthesiology 1982;57:535.

56. Matthay MA, Chatterjee K. Bedside catheterization of the pulmonary artery: Risks compared with benefits. Ann Intern Med 1988;109:826.

57. Jansen HM, Zuurmond WWA, Roos CM, Schreuder JJ, Bakker DJ. Whole-lung lavage under hyperbaric oxygen conditions for alveolar proteinosis with respiratory failure. Chest 1987;91:829.

58. Brach BB, Harrell JH, Moser KM. Alveolar proteinosis: Lobar lavage by fiberoptic bronchoscopic technique. Chest 1976;69:224.

59. Albertini RE, Harrell JH II, Kurihara N, Moser KM. Arterial hypoxemia induced by fiberoptic bronchoscopy. JAMA 1974;230:1666.

60. Lippmann K, Mok MS, Wasserman K. Anaesthetic management for children with alveolar proteinosis using extracorporeal circulation. Br J Anaesth 1977;49:173.

61. Hiratzka LF, Swan DM, Rose EF, Ahrens RC. Bilateral simultaneous lung lavage utilizing membrane oxygenator for pulmonary alveolar proteinosis in an 8-month-old infant. Ann Thorac Surg 1983;35:313.

62. Moazam F, Schmidt JH, Chesrown SE, et al. Total lung lavage for pulmonary alveolar proteinosis in an infant without the use of cardiopulmonary bypass. J Pediatr Surg 1985;20:398.

63. Hudson AR, Halprin GM, Miller JA, Kilburn KH. Pulmonary interstitial fibrosis following alveolar proteinosis. Chest 1974;65:700.

64. Kaplan AI, Sabin S. Case report: Interstitial fibrosis after uncomplicated pulmonary alveolar proteinosis. Postgrad Med 1977;61(5):263.

65. Clague HW, Wallace AC, Morgan WKC. Pulmonary interstitial fibrosis associated with alveolar proteinosis. Thorax 1983;38:865.

66. Corrin B, King E. Pathogenesis of experimental pulmonary alveolar proteinosis. Thorax 1970;25:230.

67. Heppleston AG, Fletcher K, Wyatt I. Changes in the composition of lung lipids and the "turnover" of dipalmitoyl lecithin in experimental alveolar lipo-proteinosis induced by inhaled quartz. Br J Exp Pathol 1974;55:384.

68. Heppleston AG. Atypical reaction to inhaled silica. Nature 1967;213:199.

69. Heppleston AG. Animal model of human disease: Pulmonary alveolar lipo-proteinosis. Am J Pathol 1975;78:171.

70. Dethloff LA, Gilmore LB, Brody AR, Hook GER. Induction of intra- and extra-cellular phospholipids in the lungs of rats exposed to silica. Biochem J 1986;233:111.

71. Gabor S, Zugravu E, Kovats A, Bohm B, Andrasoni D. Effects of quartz on lung surfactant. Environ Res 1978;16:443.

72. Richards RJ, Curtis CG. Biochemical and cellular mechanisms of dust-induced lung fibrosis. Environ Health 1984;55:393.

73. Gross P, de Treville RTP. Alveolar proteinosis. Arch Pathol 1968;86:255.

74. Gross P, Harley RA, deTreville RTP. Pulmonary reaction to metallic aluminum powders. Arch Environ Health 1973;26:227.

75. Casarett-Bruce M, Camner P, Curstedt T. Changes in pulmonary lipid composition of rabbits exposed to nickel dust. Environ Res 1981;26:353.

76. Johansson A, Camner P, Robertson B. Effects of long-term nickel dust exposure on rabbit alveolar epithelium. Environ Res 1981;25:391.

77. Governa M, Valentino M, Tosi P, et al. Pulmonary alveolar lipoproteinosis in rats following intratracheal injection of pyrite particles. J Toxicol Environ Health 1986;19:403.

78. Gross P, Nau CA. Lignite and the derived steam-activated carbon: The pulmonary response to their dust. Arch Environ Health 1967;14:450.

79. Gross P, Brown JHU, Hatch TF. Experimental endogenous lipid pneumonia. Am J Pathol 1952;28:211.

80. Lee KP, Gillies PJ. Pulmonary response and intrapulmonary lipids in rats exposed to bismuth orthovanadate dust by inhalation. Environ Res 1986;40:115.

81. Lee KP, Barras CE, Griffith FD, Waritz RS. Pulmonary response to glass fiber by inhalation exposure. Lab Invest 1979;40:123.

82. Sanders CL, Conklin AW, Gelman RA, Adee RR, Rhoads K. Pulmonary toxicity of Mount St. Helen's volcanic ash. Environ Res 1982;27:118.

83. Wehner AP, Dagle GE, Clark ML. Lung changes in rats inhaling volcanic ash for one year. Am Rev Respir Dis 1983;128:926.

84. Heppleston AG. Determinants of pulmonary fibrosis and lipidosis in the silica model. J Exp Pathol 1986;67:879.

85. Heppleston AG, Young AE. Alveolar lipo-proteinosis: An ultrastructural comparison of the experimental and human forms. J Pathol 1972;107:107.

86. Buechner HA, Ansari A. Acute silicoproteinosis: A new pathologic variant of acute silicosis in sandblasters characterized by histologic features resembling alveolar proteinosis. Dis Chest 1969;55:274.

87. Xipell JM, Ham KN, Price CG, Thomas DP. Acute silicoproteinosis. Thorax 1977;32:104.

88. Suratt PM, Winn WC Jr, Brody AR, Bolton WK, Giles RD. Acute silicosis in tombstone sandblasters. Am Rev Respir Dis 1977;115:521.

89. Rubin E, Weisbrod GL, Sanders DE. Pulmonary alveolar proteinosis: Relationship to silicosis and pulmonary infection. Radiology 1980;135:35.

90. Miller RR, Churg AM, Hutcheon M, Lam S. Pulmonary alveolar proteinosis and aluminum dust exposure. Am Rev Respir Dis 1984;130:312.

91. McCunney RJ, Godefroi R. Pulmonary alveolar proteinosis and cement dust: A case report. J Occup Med 1989;31:233.

92. Abraham JL, Auchincloss JH. Pulmonary alveolar proteinosis associated with kaolin exposure (abstract). Am Rev Respir Dis 1985;131:A208.

93. McEuen DD, Abraham JL. Particulate concentrations in pulmonary alveolar proteinosis. Environ Res 1978;17:334.

94. Abraham JL, McEuen DD. Inorganic particulates associated with pulmonary alveolar proteinosis: SEM and X-ray microanalysis results. Appl Pathol 1986;4:138.

95. Lullmann-Rauch R. Drug-induced lysosomal storage disorders. In: Dingle JT, Jacques PJ, Shaw IH, eds. Lysosomes in applied biology and therapeutics, vol. 6. Amsterdam: North-Holland, 1979:49.

96. Reasor MJ, Ogle CL, Walker ER, Kacew S. Amiodarone-induced phospholipidosis in rat alveolar macrophages. Am Rev Respir Dis 1988;137:510.

97. Vijeyaratnam GS, Corrin B. Pulmonary alveolar proteinosis developing from desquamative interstitial pneumonitis in long term toxicity studies of iprindole in the rat. Virchows Arch (Anat Pathol) 1973;358:1.

98. Reasor MJ. Phospholipidosis in the alveolar macrophage induced by cationic amphiphilic drugs. Federation Proc 1984;43:2578.

99. Miles PR, Bowman L, Tucker J, Reasor MJ, Wright JR. Alterations in rat alveolar surfactant phospholipids and proteins induced by administration of chlorphentermine. Biochim Biophys Acta 1986;877:167.

100. Ma JYC, Ma JKH, Weber KC. Fluorescence studies of the binding of amphiphilic amines with phospholipids. J Lipid Res 1985;26:735.

101. Hostetler KY, Matsuzawa Y. Studies on the mechanism of drug-induced lipidosis: Cationic amphiphilic drug inhibition of lysosomal phospholipases A and C. Biochem Pharmacol 1981;30:1121.
102. Larson RK, Gordinier R. Pulmonary alveolar proteinosis: Report of six cases and a review of the literature. Ann Intern Med 1965;62:292.
103. Ramirez-R. J, Harlan WR Jr. Pulmonary alveolar proteinosis: Nature and origin of alveolar lipid. Am J Med 1968;45:502.
104. McClenahan JB, Mussenden R. Pulmonary alveolar proteinosis. Arch Intern Med 1974;133:284.
105. Sahu S, DiAugustine RP, Lynn WS. Lipids found in pulmonary lavage of patients with alveolar proteinosis and in rabbit lung lamellar organelles. Am Rev Respir Dis 1976;114:177.
106. Hawkins JE, Savard EV, Ramirez-R. J. Pulmonary alveolar proteinosis: Origins of proteins in pulmonary washings. Am J Clin Pathol 1967;48:14.
107. Rupp GH, Wasserman K, Ogawa M, Heiner DC. Bronchopulmonary fluids in pulmonary alveolar proteinosis. J Allergy Clin Immunol 1973;51:227.
108. Bell DY, Hook GER. Pulmonary alveolar proteinosis: Analysis of airway and alveolar proteins. Am Rev Respir Dis 1979;119:979.
109. Sahu S, Lynn WS. Phospholipase A in pulmonary secretions of patients with alveolar proteinosis. Biochim Biophys Acta 1977;487:354.
110. Zijlstra FJ, Vincent JE, van den Berg B, Hoogsteden HC, Neyens HJ, van Dongen JJM. Pulmonary alveolar proteinosis: Determination of prostaglandins and leukotrienes in lavage fluid. Lung 1987;165:79.
111. Passero MA, Tye RW, Kilburn KH, Lynn WS. Isolation and characterization of two glycoproteins from patients with alveolar proteinosis. Proc Natl Acad Sci USA 1973;70:973.
112. Hook GER, Gilmore LB, Talley FA. Multilamellated structures from the lungs of patients with pulmonary alveolar proteinosis. Lab Invest 1984;50:711.
113. Possmayer F. Pulmonary perspective: A proposed nomenclature for pulmonary surfactant-associated proteins. Am Rev Respir Dis 1988;138:990.
114. Ross GF, Ohning BL, Tannenbaum D, Whitsett JA. Structural relationships of the major glycoproteins from human alveolar proteinosis surfactant. Biochim Biophys Acta 1987;911:294.
115. White RT, Damm D, Miller J, et al. Isolation and characterization of the human pulmonary surfactant apoprotein gene. Nature 1985;317:361.
116. Singh G, Katyal SL, Bedrossian CWM, Rogers RM. Pulmonary alveolar proteinosis: Staining for surfactant apoprotein in alveolar proteinosis and in conditions simulating it. Chest 1983;83:82.
117. Singh G, Katyal SL. Surfactant apoprotein in nonmalignant pulmonary disorders. Am J Pathol 1980;101:51.
118. Wright JR, Wager RE, Hawgood S, Dobbs L, Clements JA. Surfactant apoprotein M_r = 26,000–36,000 enhances uptake of liposomes by type II cells. J Biol Chem 1987;262:2888.
119. Young SL, Wright JR, Clements JA. Cellular uptake and processing of surfactant lipids and apoprotein SP-A by rat lung. J Appl Physiol 1989;66:1336.
120. Jacobs KA, Phelps DS, Steinbrink R, et al. Isolation of a cDNA clone encoding a high molecular weight precursor to a 6-kDa pulmonary surfactant-associated protein. J Biol Chem 1987;262:9808.
121. Weaver TE, Sarin VK, Sawtell N, Hull WM, Whitsett JA. Identification of surfactant proteolipid SP-B in human surfactant and fetal lung. J Appl Physiol 1988;65:982.
122. Lynn WS. Alveolyn-structure and source: A review. Exp Lung Res 1984;6:191.
123. Hook GER, Bell DY, Gilmore LB, Nadeau D, Reasor MJ, Talley FA. Composition of bronchoalveolar lavage effluents from patients with pulmonary alveolar proteinosis. Lab Invest 1978;39:342.
124. Sato S, Takishima T. A new myelin-like laminated body found in two cases of pulmonary alveolar proteinosis. Tohoku J Exp Med 1978;126:257.

125. Takemura T, Fukuda Y, Harrison M, Ferrans VJ. Ultrastructural, histochemical, and freeze-fracture evaluation of multilamellated structures in human pulmonary alveolar proteinosis. Am J Anat 1987;179:258.

126. Gilmore LB, Talley FA, Hook GER. Classification and morphometric quantitation of insoluble material from the lungs of patients with alveolar proteinosis. Am J Pathol 1988;133:252.

127. Hook GER, Gilmore LB, Talley FA. Dissolution and reassembly of tubular myelin-like multilamellated structures from the lungs of patients with pulmonary alveolar proteinosis. Lab Invest 1986;55:194.

128. Golde DW, Territo M, Finley TN, Cline MJ. Defective lung macrophages in pulmonary alveolar proteinosis. Ann Intern Med 1976;85:304.

129. Harris JO. Pulmonary alveolar proteinosis: Abnormal in vitro function of alveolar macrophages. Chest 1979;76:156.

130. Nugent KM, Pesanti EL. Macrophage function in pulmonary alveolar proteinosis. Am Rev Respir Dis 1983;127:780.

131. Gonzalez-Rothi RJ, Harris JO. Pulmonary alveolar proteinosis: Further evaluation of abnormal alveolar macrophages. Chest 1986;90:656.

132. Muller-Quernheim J, Schopf RE, Benes P, Schulz V, Ferlinz R. A macrophage-suppressing 40-kD protein in a case of pulmonary alveolar proteinosis. Klin Wochenschr 1987;65:893.

133. Johansson A, Camner P, Jarstrand C, Wiernik A. Morphology and function of alveolar macrophages after long-term nickel exposure. Environ Res 1980;23:170.

134. Wright JR, Clements JA. State of the art: Metabolism and turnover of lung surfactant. Am Rev Respir Dis 1987;135:426.

135. Hallman M, Epstein BL, Gluck L. Analysis of labeling and clearance of lung surfactant phospholipids in rabbit: Evidence of bi-directional surfactant flux between lamellar bodies and alveolar lavage. J Clin Invest 1981;68:742.

136. Jacobs H, Jobe A, Igekami M, Conaway D. The significance of reutilization of surfactant phosphatidylcholine. J Biol Chem 1983;258:4156.

137. Desai R, Tetley TD, Curtis CG, Powell GM, Richards RJ. Studies on the fate of pulmonary surfactant in the lung. Biochem J 1978;176:455.

138. Smith FB. Alveolar proteinosis: Atypical response to injury. NY State J Med 1980;80:1372.

139. Wilkinson RH, Blanc WA, Hagstrom JWC. Pulmonary alveolar proteinosis in three infants. Pediatrics 1968;41:510.

140. Webster JR, Battifora H, Furey C, Harrison RA, Shapiro B. Pulmonary alveolar proteinosis in two siblings with decreased immunoglobulin A. Am J Med 1980;69:786.

141. Teja K, Cooper PH, Squires JE, Schnatterly PT. Pulmonary alveolar proteinosis in four siblings. N Engl J Med 1981;305:1390.

142. Ruben FL, Talamo TS. Secondary pulmonary alveolar proteinosis occurring in two patients with acquired immune deficiency syndrome. Am J Med 1986;80:1187.

143. Schiller V, Aberle DR, Aberle AM. Pulmonary alveolar proteinosis: Occurrence with metastatic melanoma to lung. Chest 1989;95:466.

144. Steer A. Focal pulmonary alveolar proteinosis in pulmonary tuberculosis. Arch Pathol 1969;87:347.

145. Bhagwat AG, Wentworth P, Conen PE. Observations on the relationship of desquamative interstitial pneumonitis and pulmonary alveolar proteinosis in childhood: A pathologic and experimental study. Chest 1970;58:326.

20

Diffuse Alveolar Hemorrhage in Immune and Idiopathic Disorders

James W. Leatherman

Diffuse alveolar hemorrhage occurs in a number of immunologic disorders, including antibasement membrane antibody (ABMA) disease, systemic vasculitides, and the collagen vascular disorders.[1-6] Diffuse alveolar hemorrhage also occurs in certain conditions for which an immune etiology is suspected but is less well established, such as idiopathic pulmonary hemosiderosis,[1] idiopathic glomerulonephritis,[5] and responses to certain drugs or chemicals.[7-11] For the most part the clinicopathologic features of immune/idiopathic alveolar hemorrhage (IAH) are similar regardless of the specific underlying disorder. Differential diagnosis of IAH is therefore usually based on the clinical pattern of extrapulmonary disease, special serologic studies, and renal biopsy. This chapter will address the subject of IAH primarily from a clinical perspective. First, a scheme for classifying the many different disorders that may cause IAH will be presented. Next, the most common causes of IAH will be briefly reviewed. Finally, an approach to the diagnosis and management of the patient who presents with features that are suggestive of IAH will be outlined.

CLASSIFICATION OF IAH SYNDROMES

The various conditions that have been associated with IAH can be divided into five major categories: ABMA disease; systemic vasculitides and collagen vascular diseases; glomerulonephritis unrelated to ABMA or vasculitis; drugs or chemicals; and idiopathic pulmonary hemosiderosis (Table 20-1). Sometimes the etiology of IAH is easily defined. For example, there are established serologic and immunopathologic criteria for diagnosing ABMA disease. Similarly, the cause of IAH that is accompanied by typical clinicopathologic features of systemic lupus erythematosus (SLE) or Wegener's granulomatosis (WG) may be readily apparent. In other cases the etiology of IAH is not so easily defined. Not infrequently, IAH occurs in association with features of a systemic

TABLE 20-1. Causes of Immune/Idiopathic Diffuse Alveolar Hemorrhage (IAH)

CAUSES	REFERENCES
Antibasement membrane antibody disease	3,23,24,37
Systemic vasculitides/collagen vascular diseases	
Wegener's granulomatosis	41,52,54–56
Nonspecific systemic necrotizing vasculitis, "overlap vasculitis" (includes "microscopic polyarteritis")	2,4,5,52
Systemic lupus erythematosus	6,72
Henoch-Schönlein syndrome	45,46
Behçet's disease	47
Essential mixed cryoglobulinemia	48
Rheumatoid arthritis	14,18,51
Progressive systemic sclerosis	50
Mixed connective tissue disease	49
Alveolar hemorrhage and glomerulonephritis unrelated to ABMA, vasculitis, or collagen vascular disease*	
Thrombotic thrombocytopenic purpura	103, present
Membranoproliferative glomerulonephritis	5,104
IgA nephropathy	105
Diffuse endocapillary proliferative glomerulonephritis	5
Focal proliferative glomerulonephritis	5
Alveolar hemorrhage due to drugs or chemicals	
D-penicillamine	7,8
Trimellitic anhydride	9
Isocyanates	10
Nitrofurantoin	11
Idiopathic pulmonary hemosiderosis	1

* IAH with pauci-immune necrotizing and/or crescentic glomerulonephritis is classified as nonspecific systemic vasculitis (presumptive)

small vessel vasculitis, but without sufficient clinicopathologic criteria to permit a diagnosis of WG, SLE, or another of the more distinctive vasculitic syndromes.[4] We have used the term nonspecific systemic necrotizing vasculitis in reference to these cases[2] whereas others classify such cases as microscopic polyarteritis[4] or polyangiitis overlap syndrome.[12] Another diagnostic problem is posed by the patient who presents with IAH and crescentic glomerulonephritis unrelated to ABMA and without other features of multisystem vasculitis. We and others have previously classified cases of IAH with idiopathic crescentic glomerulonephritis separately from the vasculitides.[2,5] However, the renal lesion in these cases (i.e., necrotizing and crescentic glomerulonephritis with a paucity of immune deposits by immunofluorescence and electron microscopy) is identical to that found in WG and systemic necrotizing vasculitis. Furthermore, Falk and Jennette[13] have detected anti-neutrophil cytoplasmic antibody (ANCA) in a similar percentage of cases classified as systemic vasculitis or kidney-limited necrotizing glomerulonephritis (see below). Currently, we would classify cases of IAH associated with pauci-immune necrotizing and crescentic glomerulonephritis under the category of systemic vasculitis. Finally, diagnostic criteria for idiopathic pulmonary hemosiderosis (i.e., isolated IAH not due to drugs or chemicals, vasculitis, SLE, or ABMA) lack precision, because this diagnosis is fundamentally one of exclusion.[2] As the clinicopathologic features in a particular case of IAH may evolve over time, a change in diagnosis may be required.[14-17] Thus, the clinician should not expect to precisely define every case of IAH at the outset. Rather, one should assign the most appropriate diagnosis given the information available at presentation and be prepared to modify this diagnosis as new clinicopathologic features develop.

Standard medical texts usually emphasize ABMA disease and idiopathic pulmonary hemosiderosis when dealing with the subject of pulmonary hemorrhage, leaving the impression that these two disorders are the most common causes of IAH. This, however, is not the case. Local experience at four affiliated teaching hospitals with 41 cases of adult IAH (38 with concomitant glomerulonephritis) included the following distribution of cases: ABMA disease, 13 (32%); vasculitides/collagen vascular disease, 27 (66%), including 5 (12%) cases of idiopathic crescentic glomerulonephritis (presumptive vasculitis); thrombotic thrombocytopenic purpura (TTP), 1 (2%). Thus, the vasculitides have accounted for two-thirds of cases, whereas ABMA has been responsible for only one-third of cases. During the 12 years that these cases have been encountered we have not seen a single instance of idiopathic pulmonary hemosiderosis. A somewhat similar distribution of cases was found by Holdsworth and associates, who reported on their experience with 45 cases of IAH and glomerulonephritis.[5] Of the 45 cases, 7 (18%) had ABMA disease, 25 (55%) had systemic vasculitis, and 12 (27%) were classified as idiopathic glomerulonephritis with IAH. As noted previously, it may be difficult to define with precision the specific underlying disorder in many cases of IAH. Given these limitations, the 27 cases of vasculitis-related IAH encountered locally were classified as follows: WG, 6; SLE or overlap connective tissue disease, 5; nonspecific systemic vasculitis, 16. Patients given the latter diagnosis did not meet established histopathologic or clinical criteria for WG or SLE. A diagnosis of nonspecific systemic necrotizing vasculitis was made when IAH occurred in conjunction with pauci-immune necrotizing or crescentic glomerulonephritis (14 cases), with or without extrarenal disease, or when there was evidence for leukocytoclastic vasculitis in the skin when there was only pulmonary and cutaneous disease (2 cases). In keeping with a "lumper's" rather than a "splitter's" approach to systemic vasculitis, no attempt was made to further subdivide these 16 cases. However, 2 of the 16 patients had widespread vasculitis affecting multiple organs in the setting of seropositive rheumatoid arthritis and thus might be considered to have an atypical presentation of rheumatoid vasculitis.[14-18]

ANTIBASEMENT MEMBRANE ANTIBODY DISEASE

In 1919 Ernst Goodpasture described the association of fatal lung hemorrhage and necrotizing glomerulonephritis that followed apparent recovery from a bout of influenza.[19] Four decades later Stanton and Tange coined the eponym Goodpasture's syndrome in reference to the coexistence of lung hemorrhage and glomerulonephritis.[20] The pathogenesis of this syndrome was unknown. With the development of immunofluorescent

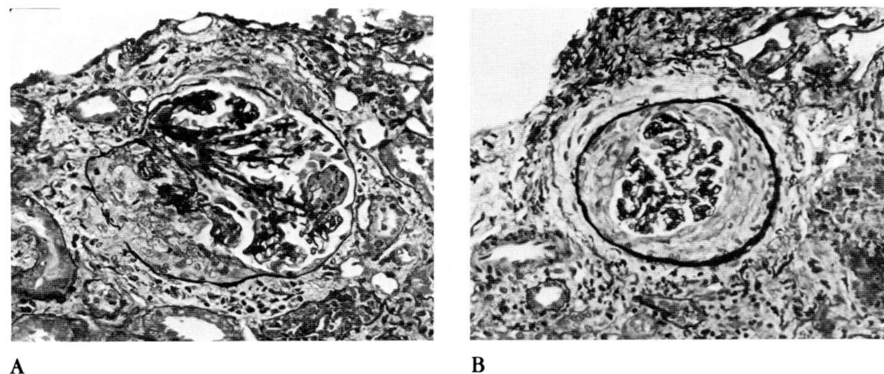

Figure 20-1. Segmental necrotizing and crescentic glomerulonephritis. (*A*) Glomerulus shows crescent at 6–9 o'clock. (*B*) Another glomerulus in same biopsy specimen shows circumferential crescent. Immunofluorescence and electron microscopy were negative. Diagnosis: systemic necrotizing vasculitis (microscopic polyarteritis). (Masson trichrome, ×320)

techniques it later became apparent that in certain instances Goodpasture's syndrome was associated with deposition of IgG antibody along the glomerular basement membrane, suggesting a possible immunologic mechanism.[21] In 1967 Lerner, Glassock, and Dixon produced glomerulonephritis in animals injected with this anti-glomerular basement membrane antibody, thereby demonstrating its pathogenicity.[22] Subsequently, the term Goodpasture's syndrome has been widely used in specific reference to IAH and glomerulonephritis caused by ABMA, although some prefer the original clinical definition of lung hemorrhage and glomerulonephritis regardless of pathogenesis. Goodpasture noted the presence of splenic arteritis in his original report.[19] Since arteritis is an uncommon feature of ABMA disease, it is likely that ABMA-mediated injury was not the mechanism of the disease that now bears his name.

Antibasement membrane antibody demonstrates a high degree of specificity, reacting only with the basement membranes of the alveolus, glomerulus, renal tubule, and choroid plexus.[23] The antigenic components to which ABMA binds have been localized to the $\alpha3(IV)$ chain of type IV collagen.[24,25] This molecule has structural heterogeneity that is tissue-specific and this may help explain the limitation of clinical disease to the lungs and kidneys despite the presence of type IV collagen in other organs.[24] There is considerable evidence that ABMA causes glomerulonephritis, although the precise mechanisms of tissue injury are not fully understood. Early studies showed that both heterologous antisera to renal tissue[26] and ABMA eluted off involved human kidneys[22] were nephrotoxic when injected into experimental animals. Furthermore, recurrence of ABMA-mediated glomerulonephritis in kidneys transplanted into recipients who still have circulating ABMA in serum provides additional evidence for the nephritogenic importance of ABMA.[22,27] The mechanisms through which tissue-bound ABMA injures glomeruli are not fully understood. It is believed that complement components and attraction of neutrophils and monocytes are important aspects of renal injury.[24] Lymphocytes are also important in the pathogenesis of ABMA disease, because B lymphocytes make the antibody and recognition of antigen within the context of HLA molecules is a function of the T lymphocyte.[24,28] The nature of the stimulus causing antibody to be produced in the first place is not known. Since an upper respiratory infection precedes the onset of clinical findings in roughly 50% of cases,[23] it has been proposed that a virus-induced injury to alveolar basement membrane could serve as the initial stimulus for production of ABMA. A similar role for hydrocarbons has been suggested,[29] but a history of an appropriate exposure is lacking in most cases of ABMA disease.[23]

The role of ABMA in the pathogenesis of IAH is not well defined. Animals injected with ABMA eluted off glomeruli develop glomerulonephritis, but the lungs are unaffected.[22] Even when heterologous antibody has been developed in response to injections of alveolar basement membrane, recipients of this antibody again develop glomerulonephritis without IAH.[30] Humans who have ABMA-mediated glomerulonephritis without IAH have similar titers of ABMA in serum as those who have both lung and kidney involvement.[31] These and other data have suggested the need for a cofactor or cofactors whose presence may be required for circulating ABMA to gain access to alveolar basement membrane, bind, and cause lung injury. Animals given ABMA together with a sublethal exposure to 100% oxygen that alters capillary permeability develop fatal lung injury, but the lungs of animals given ABMA alone are unaffected.[32] In humans, bouts of IAH have been correlated with concurrent infection in some patients.[33] Finally, Donaghy and Rees have reported that cigarette smoking could be an important determinant of IAH in patients who have ABMA in serum.[31] Among 47 patients with ABMA disease in whom a smoking history was obtained, pulmonary hemorrhage was detected in all 37 smokers but in only 2 of 10 nonsmokers. This relationship between smoking and ABMA-mediated IAH has not been found by all investigators,[34] however, and at present the pathogenesis of IAH in ABMA disease remains poorly understood.

As would be predicted by the binding specificity of ABMA, the salient features of ABMA disease are restricted to IAH and glomerulonephritis. Organs other than the lungs and kidneys are rarely affected. Patients often present with hemoptysis, but renal involvement is generally evident at the time of initial evaluation.[23,35–37] The majority of patients have renal dysfunction and those who have a normal serum creatinine level will usually have microscopic hematuria.[37] Rarely, ABMA-mediated IAH will occur with no clinical evidence of glomerulonephritis.[38] A diagnosis of ABMA disease must therefore be considered in all cases of IAH, with or without obvious glomerulonephritis, in which clinical examination fails to disclose objective evidence of a vasculitis or SLE.

Diagnosis of ABMA disease is established relatively easily by the combination of serum assay for ABMA and immunofluorescent examination of a renal biopsy specimen. Serum ABMA can be detected by radioimmunoassay, enzyme-linked immunosorbent assay (ELISA), and indirect immunofluorescence. The reported sensitivity and specificity of radioimmunoassay for detecting ABMA are each in excess of 95%.[23] ELISA is similarly accurate in detecting or excluding the presence of circulating ABMA.[39] Indirect immunofluorescence is highly specific for ABMA provided that the result is strongly positive and controls are negative,[40] but a negative result does not preclude the presence of ABMA in serum, as some investigators have found indirect immunofluorescence to be negative in a significant number of cases in which radioimmunoassay, ELISA, or both, were positive (A Fish, M.D., personal communication). The major

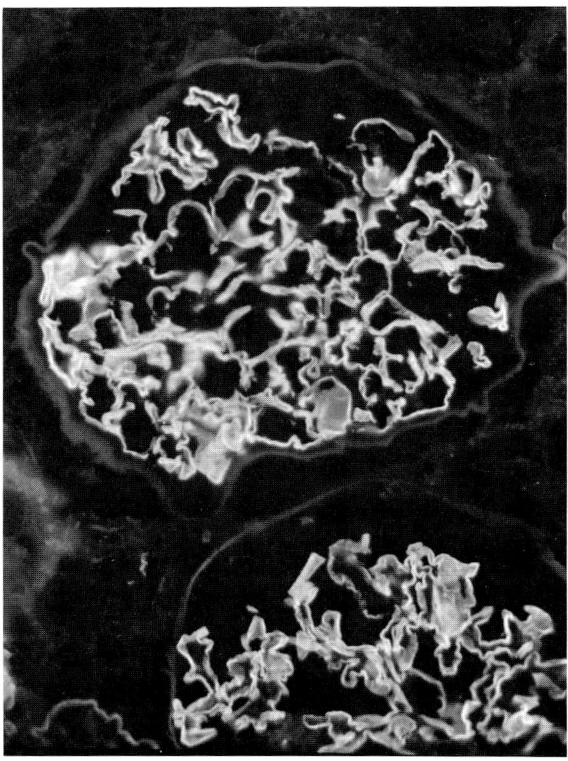

Figure 20-2. Antibasement membrane antibody disease. Two glomeruli show linear, ribbon-like staining for IgG along capillary walls by immunofluorescence. ($\times$320)

advantage of indirect immunofluorescence is that it is more widely available than are radioimmunoassay or ELISA.

Unless prohibitively risky, renal biopsy should be performed in patients with possible ABMA disease. Histopathology often shows crescent formation and segmental necrosis, but glomeruli may appear only minimally altered or even normal.[40] The segmental, necrotizing, and crescentic glomerulonephritis of ABMA disease is identical to that seen in vasculitis by light microscopic criteria. The hallmark of ABMA-mediated glomerulonephritis is strongly positive linear staining for IgG along glomerular capillaries (Fig. 20-2).[23,40] Less intense linear staining can be observed in other conditions,[40] emphasizing the complementary diagnostic roles of renal biopsy and serum ABMA assay. It could be argued that a positive assay for serum ABMA would obviate the need for diagnostic renal biopsy. Nonetheless, no serologic test has 100% accuracy and when dealing with a potentially lethal disease that requires treatment with intensive immunosuppression, it seems prudent to gather diagnostic information from both serology and renal biopsy whenever possible.

Unlike renal biopsy, lung biopsy is seldom indicated for establishing a diagnosis of ABMA disease. Although some patients with ABMA-related IAH have demonstrable linear deposits of IgG along alveolar septa, others do not. In fact, one study found negative immunofluorescent staining of transbronchial lung biopsies in 7 of 10 patients with ABMA disease and IAH.[36] Furthermore, the ease and reliability with which a diagnosis of ABMA disease can be established by serology and renal biopsy render lung biopsy unnecessary. If a lung biopsy is obtained in the setting of isolated IAH, it is important that tissue be frozen for examination by immunofluorescence. Pulmonary capillaritis has been found in some cases of ABMA disease, so that this finding will not reliably differentiate ABMA disease and vasculitis.[41]

The most common cause of death in untreated ABMA disease is renal failure, with fewer patients succumbing to respiratory failure. Currently recommended treatment of ABMA disease consists of plasma exchange in combination with immunosuppression (prednisone, cyclophosphamide, with or without the addition of azathioprine).[42] The rationale for this approach is that ABMA will be rapidly removed from serum by plasma exchange and the immunosuppression will prevent a rebound rise in antibody and have an anti-inflammatory effect. Unfortunately, neither this form of combination therapy nor other regimens have been evaluated in large prospective studies. A small randomized study compared immunosuppression alone versus immunosuppression plus plasma exchange in patients with ABMA disease.[36] Although there was no statistically significant difference in outcome between the two groups, there was a trend in favor of combined therapy with respect to ultimate renal function. However, the degree of renal insufficiency and number of glomerular crescents at the time therapy was begun appeared to be more important determinants of outcome than the type of therapy received.[36] The importance of baseline renal function in determining the ultimate response to therapy has been clearly demonstrated by Peters and colleagues.[42] They treated 41 patients with ABMA-mediated glomerulonephritis with combined plasma exchange and immunosuppression. Renal function was preserved or improved in 15 of 17 patients who were nonoliguric and had a serum creatinine below 6 mg/dl at the start of treatment. In contrast, 23 of 24 patients who had either a serum creatinine level greater than 6 mg/dl or oliguria required dialysis for end-stage renal disease.[42] This experience, together with the risks of therapy, has led these investigators to recommend foregoing treatment of ABMA-mediated glomerulonephritis if renal failure is far advanced at presentation and there is no active IAH that would require treatment.[43] According to this approach, patients would simply be supported with dialysis until circulating ABMA is no longer detectable, at which time renal transplantation could be offered.

Although IAH may be somewhat less of a threat to patients with ABMA disease than is glomerulonephritis, it may nonetheless become severe enough to cause acute respiratory failure (Fig. 20-3). Thus, prompt diagnosis and treatment of ABMA-related IAH are imperative. There have been reports of ABMA-related IAH that responded well to pulse methylprednisolone.[36,44] However, some clinicians feel that the addition of plasma exchange to immunosuppression yields better control of IAH.[42] In the largest reported series, 29 of 33 cases of ABMA-related IAH responded to combination therapy.[42] The effect of treatment on IAH is difficult to evaluate because spontaneous remissions can occur. Nonetheless, based on the available evidence it would seem prudent to employ combined immunosuppression and plasma exchange for ABMA-related IAH when IAH is moderate to severe, and especially if empiric corticosteroids have

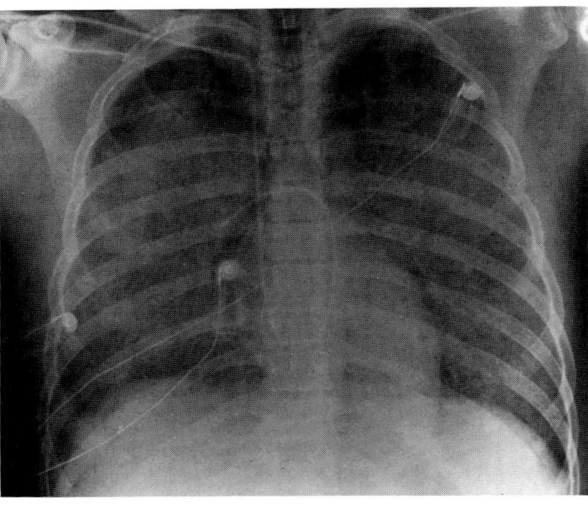

Figure 20-3. Massive IAH in ABMA disease. Chest roentgenogram of a young man who had presented 3 days earlier with isolated glomerulonephritis. After receiving daily plasma exchange and immunosuppression for 3 days he had developed hemoptysis and rapidly progressive respiratory failure. Plasma exchange and immunosuppression were continued. Despite initially severe hypoxemia (PaO_2 < 50 mm Hg on FI_{O_2} 1.0 and PEEP 15 cm H_2O), the patient recovered and was extubated after 7 days. Patient had not smoked cigarettes for several days prior to the onset of hemoptysis, but during the 16 hours prior to onset of respiratory failure he had smoked approximately 20 cigarettes.

failed to control IAH within 24 to 48 hours. Pulse corticosteroids might be considered as initial therapy when IAH is relatively mild and there is virtually no hope for recovery of renal function. Previously reported data indicate that cigarette smoking should be strongly discouraged.[31]

SYSTEMIC VASCULITIDES AND COLLAGEN VASCULAR DISEASES

The systemic vasculitides and collagen vascular diseases are responsible for the majority of cases of IAH.[2,5] By far the most common causes of vasculitis-related IAH are WG, SLE, and nonspecific systemic necrotizing vasculitis (microscopic polyarteritis, polyangiitis overlap syndrome). In addition, IAH has been described in Henoch-Schönlein syndrome,[45,46] Behçet's disease,[47] cryoglobulinemia,[48] endocarditis-related vasculitis,[5] tumor-related vasculitis,[5] mixed connective tissue disease,[49] progressive systemic sclerosis,[50] and rheumatoid arthritis.[14,18,51] In rheumatoid arthritis IAH may occur with[14,18] or without[51] evidence of systemic rheumatoid vasculitis.

Until recently there were few data regarding the underlying pathology of IAH in systemic vasculitis and SLE. This may have been due in part to the difficulty of recognizing small vessel vasculitis in the setting of severe lung hemorrhage and in part to the relative infrequency with which lung biopsies have been performed to evaluate presumed vasculitis-related IAH. In 1985, Mark and Ramirez described the histopathologic features of 13 cases of vasculitis-related IAH, including cases of presumed WG, nonspecific systemic vasculitis, and SLE.[52] Capillaritis was observed in all 13 cases and venulitis or arteriolitis in 4 cases, but larger vessels were uniformly spared. Myers and Katzenstein have also detected small vessel vasculitis in SLE-related IAH and have referred to this lesion as "acute microangiitis,"[53] a term coined by Liebow to emphasize both the neutrophilic nature of the inflammatory infiltrate and the small size of involved vessels. Pulmonary capillaritis has also been detected by others in cases of WG[41,52,54–56] and the Henoch-Schönlein syndrome.[45] It should be noted, however, that capillaritis has been detected in cases of IAH related to ABMA disease and idiopathic pulmonary hemosiderosis,[41] so that pulmonary capillaritis does not necessarily indicate the presence of a systemic vasculitis.

Recognition of acute microangiitis in the lung may be easy if small arteries and arterioles are involved because the pathologist can readily appreciate the neutrophils, many of which appear necrotic with abundant nuclear dust, within vessel walls.[52,53] Recognition of capillaritis, however, may be more challenging. Capillaries themselves are usually obscured by neutrophils so that the presence of capillaritis is inferred by the location of inflammatory cells within alveolar septa.[53] Entire portions of alveolar septa may appear necrotic and this may account for the associated intra-alveolar hemorrhage.[53] Due to the potential difficulty in recognizing capillaritis in the background of severe alveolar hemorrhage, referral of slides to experts in the field of lung pathology would seem advisable.

The immunopathogenesis of IAH in SLE and the systemic vasculitides has been examined by use of immunofluorescent staining of lung tissue. Granular immune deposits of IgG, sometimes with C3, have been found along alveolar septa in some,[6] but not all,[53,57] cases of SLE-related IAH. Pulmonary immune complexes containing IgA have also been detected in the Henoch-Schönlein syndrome.[45] There is however, no convincing evidence that immune complexes mediate IAH in vasculitides other than SLE and Henoch-Schönlein syndrome. When immune complexes have been sought by immunofluorescent examination of the lungs in vasculitis-related IAH they have generally not been found.[52] Similarly, glomeruli seldom contain immune deposits in renal vasculitis.[58,59] Furthermore, hypocomplementemia, a common feature of immune complex disease, is usually absent in WG and systemic necrotizing vasculitis. In sum, the available evidence does not support a major role for immune complexes in the pathogenesis of IAH and glomerulonephritis related to nonspecific systemic vasculitis or WG. Preliminary data suggest that ANCA could play a role in the pathogenesis of necrotizing vasculitis.[58]

Wegener's Granulomatosis

Two patterns of vasculitis occur in WG: (1) necrotizing granulomatous vasculitis involving primarily the upper airway and lung, and (2) a nonspecific small vessel vasculitis that usually affects the kidneys and may involve almost any organ system. It is the granulomatous vasculitis that confers distinction upon WG and sets it apart from the other vasculitides. Pathologic diagnosis of WG requires demonstration within tissue of necrotizing granulomatous inflammation and vasculitis and exclusion of infection by special stains and cultures. The histopathologic features of the small vessel nongranulomatous vasculitis of WG are not specific for this disorder.

The spectrum of disease that may be seen in WG is broad, ranging from indolent and isolated involvement of the upper airway to fulminant multisystem vasculitis. The pattern of disease that one is likely to encounter will depend in part on one's area of specialization, on local referral patterns, and on the type of hospital in which one practices. For instance, the type of WG seen at the National Institutes of Health (NIH) is characterized by nearly universal involvement of the upper airway and lungs and a high incidence (85%) of renal involvement.[60] Patients referred to this tertiary center had generally had symptoms for many months and very few had renal failure. The reported experience with WG at the Mayo Clinic includes almost 30% of patients who had isolated upper airway disease, and renal involvement was seen in only 42% of cases.[61] A smaller series of 13 patients from a community-based hospital reported a much more fulminant pattern of disease, with an incidence of renal failure and early death far in excess of that which would likely be encountered at a tertiary referral center.[62] Finally, in a series of 18 cases of WG reported from a renal unit there was a 100% incidence of renal involvement, frequent need for early dialysis, and early death in 7 of 18 cases.[63] The crucial point is that WG is a disease that has an extremely varied presentation, and physicians involved in the care of patients with this disease should be familiar with literature emanating from a variety of sources in order to have a more complete appreciation of the potential spectrum of disease.

In this regard, IAH as an early manifestation of WG has been underemphasized in the literature, in part because of the rarity with which it was observed in large, widely quoted series from tertiary centers. In a paper published in 1982 we described two cases of WG presenting as IAH, reviewed three additional cases, and commented that IAH was a rare manifestation of WG.[14] Subsequent personal experience and the reported experience of others[4,41] have altered this view considerably. The assertion that IAH is not an uncommon manifestation of WG is most convincingly supported by the fact that Haworth and associates found evidence for "definite" alveolar hemorrhage in 13 of 53 (25%) patients with WG seen at a single renal unit.[4]

Unlike other, more "typical," patterns of lung involvement in WG, IAH is due not to a granulomatous vasculitis, but rather to pulmonary capillaritis.[41,52,54–56] Thus, IAH, like segmental necrotizing glomerulonephritis and palpable purpura, is a manifestation of nongranulomatous small-vessel vasculitis that occurs in this disorder. As the histopathology of WG-related IAH may show only capillaritis without granulomatous inflammation,[52,54–56] definitive diagnosis of WG by open lung biopsy, generally the procedure of choice for diagnosing WG, may not be possible when IAH occurs without coexistent nodules. Travis and associates did find evidence for subtle granulomatous inflammation in three of five cases of WG-related IAH,[41] sometimes only after obtaining deeper sections, emphasizing the need for a meticulous inspection of slides that show capillaritis-related hemorrhage.

In most of the reported cases IAH has occurred early in the course of WG. Not infrequently, severe IAH coexisted with other evidence of a widespread, fulminant vasculitis. In some cases a diagnosis of WG could not be established at presentation but only became apparent some months to years later when more typical manifestations related to necrotizing granulomatous vasculitis (cavitary lung nodules, sinus or other upper airway disease) appeared.[14–17,41] Thus, a diagnosis of WG must be considered in all cases of vasculitis-related IAH, even when a thorough evaluation fails to delineate upper airway pathology or pulmonary nodules.

In 1985 VanderWoude described the presence of an autoantibody (ANCA) against neutrophils and monocytes in patients with active WG.[64] Control sera from individuals with granulomatous infection were uniformly negative, as were sera obtained from patients who had other types of vasculitis.[64] Additional work from several centers has indicated that serum ANCA is present in 84% to 96% of cases of active generalized WG and is generally absent in patients with infection or healthy controls.[65,66] There is some disagreement, however, as to whether the ANCA assay differentiates WG from other systemic vasculitides. One large study found that ANCA was frequently present in serum obtained from patients who had systemic necrotizing vasculitis and idiopathic crescentic glomerulonephritis.[13] Others have found the ANCA assay to be negative in most vasculitides other than WG.[64-66] This disparity in results may be due in part to the way in which the test is interpreted. As originally described, a positive ANCA assay was based on the presence of cytoplasmic staining of neutrophils (and monocytes) that had been fixed in ethanol. Falk and Jennette have reported that in addition to this cytoplasmic (c-ANCA) staining pattern, another perinuclear (p-ANCA) staining pattern is seen in patients with systemic vasculitis. They consider the p-ANCA pattern to be positive and have determined that it is due to antibody against myeloperoxidase.[58] (The c-ANCA pattern appears to be due to a different antibody that recognizes a 30 kDa component of the primary granule.)[58] Centers that have reported negative serum ANCAs in patients with vasculitides other than WG reported only the c-ANCA as positive.[65,66] Although titers may fluctuate, the pattern observed (c-ANCA or p-ANCA) does not change in individual patients assessed repeatedly over time.[58] There does seem to be some correlation between the staining pattern for ANCA and the clinico-pathologic features of pulmonary vasculitis. Pulmonary capillaritis with IAH occurs in association with either c-ANCA or p-ANCA.[58] In contrast, necrotizing granulomatous inflammation is observed in c-ANCA positive patients but not in p-ANCA positive patients.[58] Much remains to be clarified about the role of ANCA in the diagnosis and management of patients with systemic vasculitis and its possible role in the pathogenesis of the disease. The evidence to date suggests that a positive serum ANCA (c-ANCA or p-ANCA) is found in the great majority (80–96%) of patients who have active generalized WG[64-66] or systemic necrotizing vasculitis,[58,67] in fewer than 10% of control sera obtained from patients with glomerulonephritis unrelated to vasculitis,[13] and rarely in healthy controls. Differentiation of WG from nonspecific systemic vasculitis on the basis of the ANCA pattern would seem unwarranted at this time. Diagnosis of WG should therefore be based on traditional histopathologic criteria or the combination of features of a small vessel vasculitis (IAH, segmental necrotizing glomerulonephritis) together with highly suggestive clinical or radiologic evidence of WG (e.g., cavitary lung nodules, extensive sinus and other upper airway disease).

Treatment of IAH in WG should include corticosteroids, initially as pulse methylprednisolone, and cyclophosphamide. In our experience the response of IAH to therapy has generally occurred too quickly to ascribe the benefit to cyclophosphamide. Also, in some cases IAH was treated successfully with empiric corticosteroids before cyclophosphamide was begun.[2] However, cyclophosphamide is the more important agent for controlling other aspects of the disease and has changed the long-term outlook from almost certain death or end-stage renal disease in the pre-cyclophosphamide era to an overall "cure" rate of 90% in the large series from the NIH.[60] It should be appreciated that few patients in the NIH series had fulminant disease at the time therapy was begun and that the outlook for patients with fulminant WG and renal failure at

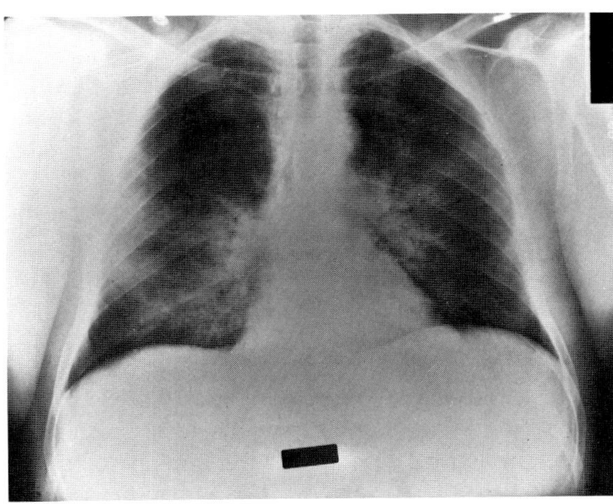

Figure 20-4. Vasculitis-related IAH. Chest roentgenogram shows bilateral infiltrates. This middle-aged man developed isolated IAH that progressed over 24 to 48 hours, leading to acute respiratory failure 1 day after this film was obtained. Open lung biopsy was reviewed by consulting pathologist and was interpreted as showing pulmonary capillaritis with hemorrhage. Serum ANCA strongly positive. Diagnosis: systemic necrotizing vasculitis presenting as isolated IAH. (Courtesy of Ralph Nietrzebe, M.D.)

presentation may be considerably less favorable.[62,63] Nonetheless, cyclophosphamide offers the best chance for control of disease and even combined respiratory and renal failure at presentation may completely reverse after management with corticosteroids, cyclophosphamide, and supportive measures such as dialysis and ventilatory support.

Systemic Necrotizing Vasculitis

In certain instances IAH occurs in the setting of a systemic necrotizing vasculitis whose clinicopathologic features are not sufficiently unique as to permit classification into one of the distinctive vasculitic syndromes such as WG, SLE, Henoch-Shönlein syndrome, or Behçet's disease. In such cases IAH nearly always coexists with glomerulonephritis. Additional manifestations of small vessel vasculitis (e.g., palpable purpura, mononeuritis multiplex, synovitis, serositis) may or may not be present. In our experience, this nonspecific systemic necrotizing vasculitis has been the single most common cause of IAH, accounting for 39% of all cases. Haworth and associates have found evidence for "definite" IAH in 20% of their patients with microscopic polyarteritis.[4] It should be appreciated that although this is predominantly a disease of small vessels (arterioles, capillaries, venules), its course and prognosis differ markedly from classic hypersensitivity vasculitis. Hypersensitivity vasculitis typically has a good prognosis, often has prominent skin manifestations, and is caused by immune complexes.[12] In contrast, small vessel systemic necrotizing vasculitis (microscopic polyarteritis) typically causes organ failure or death if left untreated and there is seldom evidence of immune complex deposits in glomeruli or other tissues.

A pathologic diagnosis of systemic necrotizing vasculitis is often most easily obtained by kidney biopsy. The typical renal lesion is a segmental, necrotizing, crescentic pauci-immune glomerulonephritis (see Fig. 20-1).[58,59,68] An identical lesion is found in WG. Unequivocal arteriolitis or arteritis in the kidney biopsy specimen is seen in less than 20% of cases.[68] Although unusual, vasculitis-related IAH can occur without any evidence of glomerulonephritis or other extrapulmonary disease (Fig. 20-4). In this circumstance, lung biopsy is required for diagnosis and will show alveolar hemorrhage, capillaritis, and occasionally arteriolitis or venulitis.[52] Lung immunofluorescence, as in the kidney, is usually negative.[52] As noted previously, systemic necrotizing vasculitis has been associated with a high frequency of serum ANCA positivity when both the cytoplasmic and perinuclear staining pattern are considered to be positive.[58]

The optimal treatment of systemic necrotizing vasculitis is not certain. Many clinicians, perhaps the majority, favor use of combined corticosteroids with cyclophosphamide, whereas others feel that corticosteroids alone are equally effective. In a study of renal vasculitis, Jennette and Falk found a 75% 1-year survival without end-stage renal disease (ESRD) in patients who received corticosteroids and cyclophosphamide.[69] The outcome with respect to mortality and ESRD was the same for patients with renal-limited disease and for those with systemic vasculitis. Several patients in this study died of massive IAH. In contrast, our experience has been that life-threatening IAH usually abates after a few days of high-dose corticosteroid therapy and patients generally require no more than 7 to 10 days of mechanical ventilatory support.

Systemic Lupus Erythematosus

Systemic lupus erythematosus is associated with many different patterns of pleuropulmonary disease, including IAH. The clinicopathologic features of IAH in SLE are similar to those seen in WG and nonspecific systemic vasculitis, with the previously mentioned exception that immune complexes are sometimes found along alveolar septa.[4,53] In most reported cases, IAH has occurred in patients who already have an established diagnosis of SLE. Usually, there is other evidence for activation of the underlying disease (e.g., glomerulonephritis). Affected individuals are usually acutely ill with fever and other signs of systemic toxicity that may suggest an infectious etiology for the respiratory illness. Additional factors that may contribute to difficulty in differentiating IAH from infection are that hemoptysis may be absent or trivial in some cases (Fig. 20-5), SLE-related immune hemolysis may render a sudden unexplained drop in hemoglobin less useful as a diagnostic criterion for IAH, and the presence of SLE-related thrombocytopenia can increase the amount of bleeding from nonimmune insults. Furthermore, the patient who is receiving immunosuppressive therapy is at risk for developing opportunistic angioinvasive infections (e.g., invasive aspergillosis) that may lead to considerable bleeding.[70] Suffice it to say that confident clinical diagnosis of IAH in SLE may be difficult and that careful and thorough evaluation to exclude infection is mandatory. Despite these considerations, differentiation of IAH from other conditions can often be accomplished without recourse to open lung biopsy.[71]

For reasons that are unclear, the reported mortality of SLE-related IAH seems to be very high. Published reports suggest a mortality rate in excess of 50%. In one series, six of seven patients died.[72] Our experience with five cases of IAH related to SLE or overlap connective tissue disease does not support this grim prognosis in that only one of five patients died, although all five required mechanical ventilatory support for respiratory failure. It is possible that there has been a greater tendency to report cases of IAH in which autopsy has excluded infection than cases diagnosed clinically.

The clinical syndrome of acute lupus pneumonitis, like IAH, is associated with marked systemic toxicity and a high likelihood of respiratory failure.[73] Whether IAH

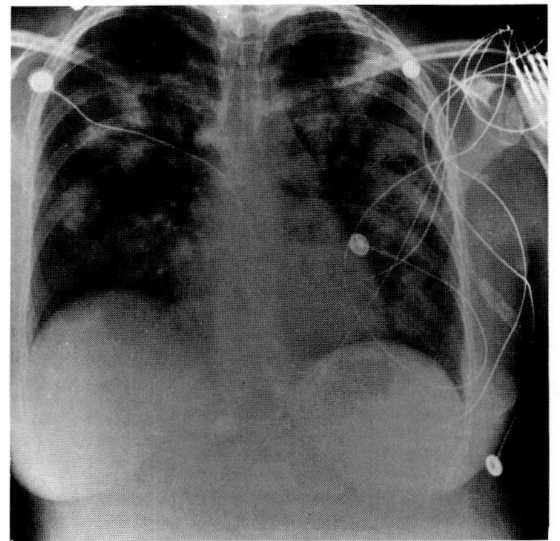

A

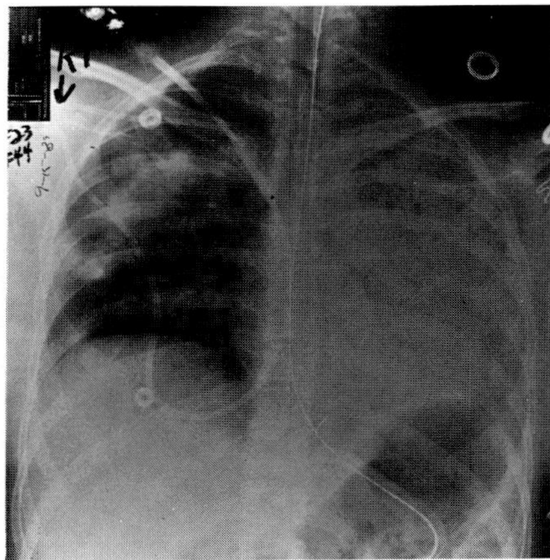

B

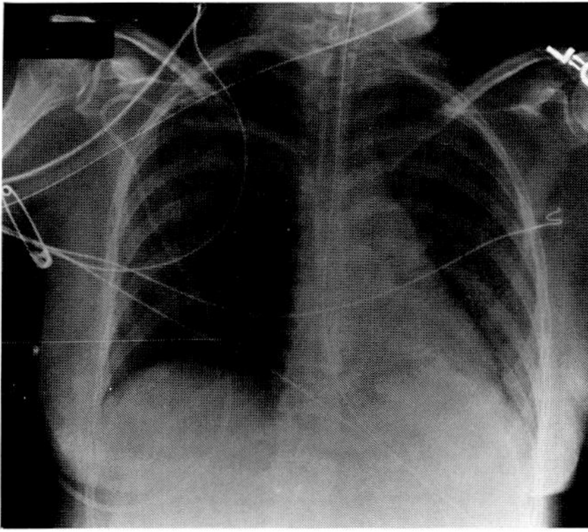

C

Figure 20-5. Alveolar hemorrhage in SLE. (*A*) Initial chest roentgenogram of young woman with known SLE who presented with cough, one episode of trivial hemoptysis, high fever, and dyspnea. Bilateral infiltrates are apparent. Broad-spectrum antibiotics were begun and amphotericin B was started because of pathologist's interpretation of sputum smear as indicating blastomycosis. Intital hemoglobin 11 g/dl. (*B*) Chest roentgenogram several days later at time of transfer showing progression with asymmetry. There was no further hemoptysis, but hemoglobin remained in the 9–10 g/dl range despite four units packed RBC's. Bronchoscopy revealed blood welling up from numerous subsegmental bronchi and a grossly bloody lavage effluent, but surprisingly little hemosiderin in macrophages. Empiric methylprednisolone was begun for presumed IAH. (*C*) Chest roentgenogram 4 days later after receiving daily methylprednisolone. The rate of resolution is consistent with IAH but not with an infectious cause of respiratory failure. Antimicrobials were discontinued. The patient was extubated next day and recovered fully. Patient never showed evidence of extrapulmonary features of SLE. No blastomycosis was apparent on culture; the initial KOH stain was misinterpreted because of the presence of RBC "ghosts."

and acute lupus pneumonitis are truly distinct entities or basically belong to the same spectrum of lung disease is uncertain.[74] There does seem to be overlap in the clinicopathologic features of these two entities, but there certainly are cases of lethal acute pulmonary disease related to SLE in which alveolar hemorrhage is not a prominent pathologic feature.[74] Diagnosis of acute lupus pneumonitis is based on compatible clinicopathologic features and, as with IAH, careful exclusion of infectious etiologies.

Optimal treatment of SLE-related IAH is not apparent from the available literature. Based on anecdotal reports and a favorable local experience, treatment with pulse methylprednisolone followed by oral prednisone is recommended. Cyclophosphamide is recommended when major extrapulmonary organs (e.g., CNS, kidney)[58,75] appear to be in jeopardy or when pulmonary disease fails to respond to corticosteroids. Thus, the therapeutic approach is basically the same as that used in WG and nonspecific systemic necrotizing vasculitis.

IDIOPATHIC PULMONARY HEMOSIDEROSIS

The term idiopathic pulmonary hemosiderosis refers to isolated IAH that is unrelated to drugs or chemicals, ABMA, SLE, or vasculitis.[1,2] Since the diagnosis is one of exclusion, a confident diagnosis of idiopathic pulmonary hemosiderosis requires that a clinical, serologic, and histopathologic assessment has excluded other disorders known to produce diffuse alveolar hemorrhage. As patients given this diagnosis may later develop evidence of a systemic disorder,[17,76] idiopathic pulmonary hemosiderosis must remain a tentative diagnosis until prolonged follow-up over several years has failed to demonstrate disease evolution.

Idiopathic pulmonary hemosiderosis occurs most often in children and young adults, but may be seen at almost any age.[1] Most of the literature regarding this disorder preceded the discovery of techniques for detecting ABMA, ANCA, and ANA in serum.[77] It is likely that many of the previously diagnosed cases of idiopathic pulmonary hemosiderosis would be reclassified with the currently available serologic tools. Furthermore, some cases classified as idiopathic pulmonary hemosiderosis have had pathologic evidence for acute capillaritis.[41] There is no consensus as to whether such cases should be classified as idiopathic pulmonary hemosiderosis or vasculitis. Certainly, cases of isolated IAH with a positive serum ANCA would be more reasonably classified as vasculitis (see Fig. 20-4).

Treatment of idiopathic pulmonary hemosiderosis is of uncertain benefit. Apparent responses to corticosteroids,[77] other immunosuppressive agents,[78] and plasmapheresis[79] have been reported. Assessment of therapeutic efficacy is difficult, because spontaneous exacerbations and remissions of IAH occur and there are no extrapulmonary features to follow. Given these limitations, it would seem that initial management with corticosteroids, followed by a tapering dosage schedule over the ensuing weeks to months if a good response is apparent, would be reasonable. Other agents might be considered if corticosteroids fail to show benefit.

DIAGNOSIS OF IAH

There are several essential steps involved in the approach to patients with suspected IAH. First, it must be determined that the alveoli-filling process is indeed IAH rather than another more common pulmonary disorder. Second, the underlying disorder responsible for IAH must be defined. Third, empiric therapy aimed at arresting life-threatening IAH must be instituted. Finally, definitive therapy appropriate for the specific underlying disorder must be given in order to treat both the pulmonary and the extrapulmonary manifestations of disease.

The essential features of IAH per se are basically the same regardless of the responsible disorder. The fundamental process is bleeding from the pulmonary microvasculature, usually due to capillaritis, that leads to alveolar shadows on chest roentgenogram, hemoptysis, anemia, and dyspnea. Most often bleeding is diffuse, or at least multifocal, giving rise to bilateral infiltrates (see Figs. 20-3 to 20-5). A pulmonary edema–like pattern is common, but other distributions also occur.[80,81] Sparing of the apices and costophrenic angles is common (see Fig. 20-3).[80] Sometimes, there is marked asymmetry in the distribution of infiltrates (see Fig. 20-5*B*) and on occasion an entirely unilateral process is seen.[2] In general, the chest roentgenographic pattern does not allow differentiation of IAH from other alveoli-filling disorders but it will affect the differential diagnosis. Hemoptysis typically accompanies active IAH. Some authors have reported that hemoptysis is absent in many cases of IAH,[82] but this has not been our experience. Some degree of hemoptysis, albeit often trivial, has occurred in almost all cases of IAH that we have recognized. As the origin of bleeding is from parenchymal microvessels rather than airways, extensive IAH may give rise only to minor hemoptysis. Perhaps a better indicator of the extent of IAH is the change in the hemoglobin concentration that occurs during active bleeding. Anemia is a nearly constant feature of IAH and during major episodes of intra-alveolar bleeding the hemoglobin concentration may fall by 2–4 g/dl, or sometimes more, over a period of 24 to 48 hours (see Fig. 20-5). A stable hemoglobin concentration in the face of progressive alveolar shadowing on the chest roentgenogram argues strongly against a diagnosis of IAH. Additional causes for anemia in patients with IAH include iron deficiency and concomitant renal failure. Iron deficiency results from loss of hemoglobin-bound iron into alveoli, where macrophages convert it into hemosiderin. This sequence results in hemosiderin-laden macrophages and failure of iron to be re-utilized by the reticuloendothelial system for erythropoiesis.[83]

The characteristic triad of IAH (i.e., hemoptysis, anemia, and alveolar infiltrates on chest roentgenogram) should alert the clinician to the possibility of IAH. However, other more common pulmonary disorders also present with hemoptysis and pulmonary infiltrates and may be accompanied by anemia that is due to another disease process. Although many pulmonary processes might be considered in the differential diagnosis, the disorders with which IAH is most often confused are pulmonary edema due to high pulmonary venous pressure, pneumonia, and the adult respiratory distress syndrome (ARDS). In approaching this differential diagnosis, it is useful for the clinician to ask two questions: Do the alveolar shadows seen on chest roentgenogram represent frank alveolar hemorrhage? Is there evidence of glomerulonephritis or other extrapulmonary disease consistent with a systemic immunologic disorder? Determining that alveoli are blood-filled is helpful, because although the conditions considered in the differential diagnosis of IAH may give rise to hemoptysis, they seldom result in frank, confluent alveolar hemorrhage. As noted earlier, correlation of serial hemoglobin values with chest roentgenograms is very helpful in assessing the likelihood of alveolar hemorrhage. More direct evidence for alveolar hemorrhage can be obtained by measurement of the carbon monoxide diffusing capacity (D_LCO)[84–86] or by bronchoscopy. The D_LCO increases during acute alveolar hemorrhage because extravascular as well as intravascular erythrocytes will bind the inhaled CO.[84] Although precise data are not available, it has been suggested that a D_LCO that is 30% above a baseline value, or greater than 130% of the predicted value if no previous value is available, would indicate active alveolar hemorrhage.[84,86] A markedly elevated DLCO (e.g., $\geq$200% of predicted), as can occasionally be seen with IAH, would represent almost unequivocal evidence of alveolar hemorrhage.

Bronchoalveolar lavage during acute IAH typically reveals a grossly bloody lavage effluent and abundant hemosiderin-laden macrophages. However, we have seen two cases of unequivocal IAH of several days duration in which the lavage effluent was grossly bloody, yet for some unexplained reason the macrophages contained very little hemosiderin. Hemosiderin-laden macrophages can be seen in congestive heart failure and in other conditions associated with entry of red blood cells into alveoli,[70,87–97] so their presence in no way provides a specific diagnosis. This is especially true in the immunocompromised host, in whom marked alveolar hemorrhage can occur as a result of certain angioinvasive infections (e.g., aspergillosis) or thrombocytopenia or both.[70] A recent study has called into question the reliability of hemosiderin-laden macrophages as a marker for diffuse alveolar hemorrhage, noting that positive iron stains were often related to cigarette smoking and dust-laden macrophages.[98] However, Travis and associates have commented that the Prussian blue staining in smokers is generally fainter and less granular than the staining seen in hemosiderosis.[41] We believe that a grossly bloody lavage with abundant hemosiderin-laden macrophages supports the presence of frank alveolar hemorrhage and, in the appropriate clinical setting, is of value in differentiating IAH from other disorders, especially when combined with the information provided by culture and stains for microorganisms. Also, bronchoscopy of patients with severe IAH reveals evidence of major diffuse hemorrhage prior to lavage, in that fresh blood may be seen welling up from numerous subsegmental bronchi.

It is crucial to appreciate that documenting frank alveolar hemorrhage by whatever means does not establish the presence of IAH. Diffuse intrapulmonary bleeding can result from other disease processes.[87–97] Thus, it is always imperative that infection, increased pulmonary venous pressure, ARDS, and other conditions be excluded with reasonable certainty before a clinical diagnosis of IAH is made. In particular, high pulmonary venous pressure must be excluded, particularly in patients with oliguric renal failure.[96] In some instances, this may require only clinical evaluation of central venous pressure, perhaps supplemented by echocardiography to exclude mitral stenosis or left ventricular dysfunction. If there is any doubt, however, direct measurement of the wedge pressure is recommended. Although unusual, we have seen patients who had extensive pulmonary hemorrhage due solely to high pulmonary venous pressure in the absence of mitral stenosis.

Careful evaluation of the patient's physical examination and the urinalysis are of great importance in the differential diagnosis of suspected IAH. Although isolated IAH does occur in idiopathic pulmonary hemosiderosis and occasionally in other disorders, the vast majority of patients with IAH have concomitant glomerulonephritis and they may also have involvement of other organs if the underlying disorder is one of the systemic vasculitides. Thus, failure to find any abnormalities in the urine sediment, serum creatinine, or extrapulmonary physical examination should always lead to a reconsideration of a clinical diagnosis of IAH.

A "pulmonary-renal" syndrome may be due to a variety of conditions other than IAH with glomerulonephritis. Acute renal failure with hypervolemia and acute tubular necrosis with concomitant adult respiratory distress syndrome (ARDS) or bilateral pneumonia

TABLE 20-2. Differential Diagnosis of the Major Causes of Immune/Idiopathic Alveolar Hemorrhage

DISORDER	EXTRAPULMONARY FEATURES	SEROLOGY	GLOMERULAR PATHOLOGY		ESSENTIAL DIAGNOSTIC CRITERIA
			Histopathology	*IF/EM*	
ABMA disease	GN > 90% Extrarenal disease rare	+ ABMA	Variable-segmental necrosis, crescents common	Linear IgG by IF	+ Serum ABMA Linear IgG in glomeruli
SLE	GN > 90% Extrarenal disease common (arthritis, serositis, purpura, photosensitivity, etc.)	+ ANA	Variable-segmental necrosis, crescents in minority	Granular IgG by IF, electron dense deposits by EM	Clinical features, + ANA, immune complexes in glomeruli by IF, EM
WG	GN > 90% Extrarenal disease a. Distinctive: upper airway disease, pulmonary nodules b. Nonspecific (arthritis, purpura, mononeuropathy, etc.)	+ ANCA	Segmental necrosis, cresents	Negative (granular IF in minority)	1. Necrotizing granulomatous vasculitis in upper airway or lung biopsy *or* 2. Pauci-immune necrotizing GN with extensive upper airway disease or cavity lung nodules
Nonspecific systemic necrotizing vasculitis (microscopic polyarteritis, polyangiitis, overlap syndrome)	GN > 90% Extrarenal disease variably present (arthritis, purpura, mononeuropathy, etc.)	± ANCA (usually + if include p-ANCA)	Segmental necrosis, crescents	Negative (granular IF in minority)	Necrotizing, crescentic GN (or pathologic evidence of vasculitis elsewhere) and exclude WG to extent possible
Idiopathic pulmonary hemosiderosis	None	None	Normal		Exclusion of all other causes

ABMA = Antibasement membrane antibody; ANA = antinuclear antibody; ANCA = antineutrophil cytoplasmic antibody; p-ANCA = perinuclear ANCA; EM = elecron microscopy; GN = glomerulonephritis; IF = immunofluorescence; SLE = systemic lupus erythematosus; WG = Wegener's granulomatosis may on occasion be difficult to differentiate from IAH with glomerulonephritis. As noted earlier, determining whether or not the pulmonary process likely represents frank hemorrhage by DLCO or bronchoscopy and measurement of the wedge pressure are of obvious diagnostic value. In addition, it is crucial to quickly determine the etiology of the elevated serum creatinine level because IAH is strongly associated with glomerulonephritis, but not with acute tubular necrosis. Careful inspection of the urine sediment is mandatory. Red blood cell casts indicate the presence of glomerular disease. Recent data suggest that a glomerular origin for hematuria may be predicted by the presence of abnormalities in the red cell membrane.[99] Early renal biopsy is recommended if glomerulonephritis is not readily excluded through noninvasive evaluation.

In especially confusing cases, open lung biopsy might be considered to help differentiate pulmonary capillaritis with IAH from pneumonia, ARDS, or other processes. However, generally the information available from the clinical setting, physical examination, simple laboratory studies, serologic studies, bronchoscopy with lavage, pulmonary artery catheterization, and early renal biopsy provides sufficient data to establish a diagnosis. The use of open lung biopsy to evaluate suspected IAH would have greatest utility when there is evidence of isolated alveolar hemorrhage and a negative serum ABMA assay or where there is concern about the presence of an opportunistic infection in a patient who is receiving immunosuppressive therapy for an established immunologic disorder.[70]

The etiology of IAH is generally established by clinical evaluation, serologic studies, and renal biopsy (Table 5-2). Antibasement membrane antibody disease is readily diagnosed by detecting ABMA in serum and by the presence of linear deposits of IgG along glomerular capillaries. Systemic lupus erythematosus is diagnosed by a positive ANA, an appropriate clinical syndrome, and detection of a renal biopsy pattern consistent with lupus nephritis. The latter may take many forms on light microscopy, but immune deposits are a regular feature by immunofluorescence and electron microscopy. Wegener's granulomatosis can be diagnosed most confidently by a biopsy of lung or upper airway that reveals necrotizing granulomatous inflammation with vasculitis. Importantly, lung biopsy in WG may not provide a specific diagnosis when IAH occurs as the sole pulmonary manifestation of disease: that is, no focal nodules or cavitary lesions are seen on chest roentgenogram. A presumptive diagnosis of WG is reasonable if IAH is associated with segmental necrotizing glomerulonephritis and there are highly suggestive clinical features of upper airway involvement, such as a combination of several of the following: sinus involvement, nasopharyngeal ulceration, otitis media, conjunctivitis, and episcleritis. A diagnosis of nonspecific systemic necrotizing vasculitis, or microscopic polyarteritis, is made when IAH coexists with segmental necrotizing glomerulonephritis, with or without extrarenal features of vasculitis, and there is neither evidence for ABMA in serum or glomeruli nor clinicopathologic features that allow a confident diagnosis of WG. A serum ANCA assay will typically be positive in WG and may also be positive in nonspecific systemic vasculitis. However, this assay alone should probably not be relied upon to make a diagnosis of vasculitis without a corroborative biopsy specimen from the kidney or another involved organ.

In many cases it may not be possible to determine whether IAH and glomerulonephritis is due to WG or to nonspecific systemic vasculitis, even with clinical and pathologic examination of the upper airway and measurement of a serum ANCA. Indeed, some patients diagnosed as having nonspecific systemic vasculitis may later demonstrate classic features of WG. Recent data suggest that in some cases of IAH in WG, open lung biopsy may reveal not only the relatively nonspecific finding of hemorrhage and capillaritis but also subtle evidence of granulomatous inflammation.[41] However, differentiation between WG and nonspecific vasculitis as the cause of IAH is often not possible. Similarly, biopsy of the paranasal sinuses in an attempt to establish a precise diagnosis of WG is often unproductive.[60] It may be reasonable to simply recognize the potential for overlap with regard to clinical and pathologic features of these disorders and not proceed to invasive and often unproductive diagnostic procedures in order to differentiate the two, especially since therapy may not differ substantially.[59,60,69,100]

Lung biopsy has little role in defining the cause of IAH. If one considers the causes of IAH, it is difficult to think of many circumstances in which lung biopsy is likely to provide diagnostic information unavailable through other, less invasive approaches. The major role for open lung biopsy in defining the etiology of IAH is when there is no evidence for extrapulmonary disease. In the few instances of ABMA disease in which there is no apparent renal involvement, the serology would still be expected to be positive. If tissue confirmation of a serologically based diagnosis of ABMA-mediated IAH is desired, then it may still be appropriate to begin with percutaneous renal biopsy even though the serum creatinine level and urine sediment may be normal. In the few reported cases of apparently isolated ABMA-mediated IAH in which renal biopsy was performed, the diagnostic linear immunofluorescent pattern was seen in glomeruli despite a normal histopathologic picture.[38] Indeed, there are problems with both false positive[101] and false negative[36] immunofluorescent studies of the lung as regards diagnosis of ABMA disease. If the serum ABMA assay is negative, then lung biopsy, together with measurement of serum ANCA level, would be helpful in determining whether isolated IAH should be classified as idiopathic pulmonary hemosiderosis or pulmonary vasculitis. Even this distinction may be rather murky, because, as noted previously, cases classified as idiopathic pulmonary hemosiderosis have shown evidence of pulmonary capillaritis.[41] Nonetheless, a lung biopsy and serum ANCA assay are recommended when IAH occurs without extrapulmonary features and in the absence of circulating ABMA.

TREATMENT OF IAH

There have been no prospective randomized studies that have evaluated treatment of IAH. Treatment recommendations are therefore based on a combination of personal experience, similarly anecdotal observations reported by others, and data obtained regarding treatment of the extrapulmonary manifestations of the systemic diseases that cause IAH.

Treatment of the patient with acute IAH involves two aspects—rapid control of active IAH in order to prevent or reverse respiratory failure and prevention or reversal of extrapulmonary organ failure, especially renal failure. A large body of anecdotal experience has been accumulated in support of the concept that treatment with pulse methylprednisolone is frequently followed by cessation of active IAH within 24 to 48 hours, as evidenced by a reduction in hemoptysis, stabilization of hemoglobin concentration, and a stable or improving course with regard to gas exchange and the chest roentgenogram.[2] Once active IAH ceases, resolution usually occurs over a period of a few days to 1 or 2 weeks, depending in large part upon the initial severity of the process. Indeed, respiratory failure caused by massive IAH can be reversed in many instances whereas a similar degree of physiological impairment caused by ARDS would predict a high likelihood of death. Because of the potential reversibility of respiratory failure, it is advocated that when there is strong clinical evidence of IAH, pulse methylprednisolone (1–2 g/day in divided doses for 2 to 3 days) be given empirically while efforts are undertaken to define the underlying immune disorder. Indeed, in some cases suspected IAH should be treated empirically before the clinician has conclusively differentiated IAH from other conditions, as long as the clinical evidence for IAH is reasonably convincing. For instance, a patient who presents with combined acute respiratory failure and acute renal failure with hemoptysis, bilateral infiltrates, and anemia would be reasonably treated with corticosteroid therapy while efforts are undertaken to differentiate IAH from hypervolemia due to renal failure by pulmonary artery catheterization and observation of the acute response to volume contraction by dialysis. Even if the pulmonary process proved to be volume overload rather than IAH, there would likely be little harm in having given a short course of empiric corticosteroids. Although acute IAH usually abates soon after administration of high-dose corticosteroids, it is possible that in some cases spontaneous resolution would have occurred. However, given the potentially dire consequences of withholding treatment for moderate to severe IAH and the apparent efficacy and relative lack of toxicity of pulse methylprednisolone, it is unlikely that a placebo-controlled trial of treatment for active IAH will ever be conducted.

Corticosteroid therapy of acute IAH has been reported to be beneficial in almost all conditions, including ABMA disease[36] and WG.[2] However, it is the impression of Peters and associates that ABMA-related IAH responds better if plasmapheresis is given in addition to immunosuppression.[42] An issue that often arises when a patient initially presents with evidence for acute IAH and glomerulonephritis is whether to use plasmapheresis as part of the empiric regimen until ABMA disease has been excluded. There are no good data upon which to base such a decision. Our approach is to use pulse methylprednisolone alone and try to define the underlying disorder quickly by renal biopsy and serology. If IAH is progressive despite corticosteroids, use of empiric plasmapheresis would be reasonable, even if the underlying disorder proved to be a condition other than ABMA disease.

The absence of prospective randomized studies also renders firm recommendations regarding definitive treatment of the disorders underlying IAH difficult. A combination of plasmapheresis with immunosuppression is recommended for ABMA disease. Definitive treatment of the systemic vasculitides is controversial. Cyclophosphamide plus prednisone has been used with success in treating WG and is considered the treatment of choice for this disorder. Cyclophosphamide has also been recommended as therapy for nonspecific systemic necrotizing vasculitis[59,100] and SLE.[75] Balow has suggested that cyclophosphamide be used in addition to corticosteroids whenever systemic vasculitis jeopardizes vital organs that have a low threshold for vascular insufficiency (i.e., brain, heart, kidney, intestine).[59] This recommendation would certainly apply to most patients with IAH. Although vasculitis-related IAH typically responds to corticosteroids, in the great majority of cases there will be concomitant renal vasculitis, and many clinicians, including the author, feel that for this reason both cyclophosphamide and corticosteroids should be used. Unlike ABMA disease, acute renal failure due to vasculitis may completely reverse with therapy so that a policy of intensive therapy for 4 to 6 weeks with dialysis support is reasonable.[102]

REFERENCES

1. Morgan PGN, Turner-Warwick M. Pulmonary hemosiderosis and pulmonary hemorrhage. Br J Dis Chest 1981;75:225–42.
2. Leatherman JW, Davies SF, Hoidal JR. Alveolar hemorrhage syndromes: Diffuse microvascular lung hemorrhage in immune and idiopathic disorders. Medicine 1984;63:343–61.
3. Rees AJ. Pulmonary injury caused by anti-basement membrane antibody. Semin Respir Med 1984;5:264–72.
4. Haworth SJ, Savage COS, Carr D, Hughes JMB, Rees AJ. Pulmonary hemorrhage complicating Wegener's granulomatosis and microscopic polyarteritis. Br Med J 1985;290:1775.
5. Holdsworth S, Boyce N, Thomson NM, Atkins RC. The clinical spectrum of acute glomerulonephritis and lung hemorrhage (Goodpasture's syndrome). Q J Med 1985;216:75–86.
6. Eagen JW, Memoli VA, Roberts JL, Matthew GR, Schwartz MM, Lewis EJ. Pulmonary hemorrhage in systemic lupus erythematosus. Medicine 1978;57:545–60.
7. Sternlieb I, Bennet B, Scheinberg IW. D-penicillamine-induced Goodpasture's syndrome in Wilson's disease. Ann Intern Med 1975;82:673–76.
8. Matloff DS, Kaplan MM. D-penicillamine-induced Goodpasture's syndrome in primary biliary cirrhosis: Successful treatment with plasmapheresis and immunosuppressives. Gastroenterol 1980;78:1046–49.
9. Herbert FA, Orford R. Pulmonary hemorrhage and edema due to inhalation of resins containing trimellitic anhydride. Chest 1979;76:546–57.
10. Patterson R, Nugent KM, Harris KE, Eberle ME. Immunologic hemorrhagic pneumonia caused by isocyanates. Am Rev Respir Dis 1990;141:226–230.
11. Bucknall CE, Adamson MR, Bauham SW. Nonfatal pulmonary hemorrhage associated with nitrofurantoin. Thorax 1987;42:475–476.
12. Leavitt RJ, Fauci AS. Pulmonary vasculitis. Am Rev Respir Dis 1986;134:149–66.
13. Falk FJ, Jennette JC. Anti-neutrophil cytoplasmic autoantibodies with specificity for myeloperoxidase in patients with systemic vasculitis and idiopathic necrotizing and crescentic glomerulonephritis. N Engl J Med 1988;318:1651–1657.
14. Leatherman JW, Sibley RK, Davies SF. Diffuse intrapulmonary hemorrhage and glomerulonephritis unrelated to antiglomerular basement membrane antibody. Am J Med 1982;72:401–10.
15. Hensley MJ, Feldman NT, Lazarus JM, Galvanek EG. Diffuse pulmonary hemorrhage and rapidly progressive renal failure: An uncommon presentation of Wegener's granulomatosis. Am J Med 1979;66:894–898.
16. Schachter EN, Finkelstein FO, Bastl C, Smith GJW. Diagnostic problems in pulmonary-renal syndromes. Am Rev Respir Dis 1977;115:155–59.
17. O'Donohue WJ. Idiopathic pulmonary hemosiderosis with manifestations of multiple connective tissue and immune disorders. Am Rev Respir Dis 1974;109:473–79.
18. Naschitz JE, Yeshurun D, Scharf Y, et al. Recurrent massive alveolar hemorrhage, crescentic glomerulonephritis, and necrotizing vasculitis in a patient with rheumatoid arthritis. Arch Intern Med 1989;149:406–408.
19. Goodpasture EW. The significance of certain pulmonary lesions in relation to the etiology of influenza. Am J Med Sci 1919;158:863–870.

20. Stanton MC, Tange JD. Goodpasture's syndrome (pulmonary hemorrhage associated with glomerulonephritis). Aust Ann Med 1958;7:132–44.
21. Duncan DA, Drummond KN, Michael AF, Vernier FL. Pulmonary hemorrhage and glomerulonephritis: Report of six cases and study of the renal lesion by the fluorescent antibody technique and electron microscopy. Ann Intern Med 1965; 62:920–938.
22. Lerner RA, Glassock RJ, Dixon FJ. The role of antiglomerular basement membrane antibody in the pathogenesis of human glomerulonephritis. J Exp Med 1967;126:989–1004.
23. Wilson CB, Dixon FJ. Renal injury from immune reactions involving antigens in or of the kidney. In: Brenner BM, Stein J, eds. Contemporary issues in nephrology. Vol 3. New York: Churchill-Livingstone, 1979:46.
24. Young KR. Pulmonary-renal syndromes. In: Matthay R, ed. Pulmonary manifestations of systemic disease. Clin Chest Med, 1989;10:655–675.
25. Saus J, Wieslander J, Lageveld JPM, et al. Identification of the Goodpasture antigen as the $\alpha3(IV)$ chain of collagen IV. J Biol Chem 1988;263:1374–1380.
26. Steblay RW. Glomerulonephritis induced in sheep by injections of heterologous glomerular basement membrane and Freund's complete adjuvant. J Exp Med 1962;116:253–264.
27. Case Records of the Massachusetts General Hospital. N Engl J Med 1976;294:944–951.
28. Oliveira DBG, Peters DK. Autoimmunity and the kidney. Kidney Int 1989;35:923–928.
29. Bierne GJ, Brennan JT. Glomerulonephritis associated with hydrocarbon solvents. Mediated by antiglomerular basement membrane antibody. Arch Environ Health 1972;25:365–369.
30. Steblay RW, Rudofsky VH. Experimental autoimmune anti-glomerular basement membrane antibody-induced glomerulonephritis. I. The effects of injecting sheep with human, homologous and autologous lung basement membranes and complete Freund's adjuvant. Clin Immunol Immunopathol 1983;27:65–80.
31. Donaghy M, Rees AJ. Cigarette smoking and lung hemorrhage in glomerulonephritis caused by autoantibodies to glomerular basement membrane. Lancet 1983;ii:1390–92.
32. Jennings I, Rohold JA, Pressman D, et al. Experimental antialveolar basement membrane antibody mediated pneumonitis. J Immunol 1981;127:129–134.
33. Rees AJ, Lockwood CM, Peters DK. Enhanced allergic tissue in Goodpasture's syndrome by intercurrent bacterial infections. Br Med J 1977;2:723–26.
34. Leaker B, Walker RG, Becker GJ, Kincaid-Smith P. Cigarette smoking and lung hemorrhage in anti-glomerular basement membrane nephritis (letter). Lancet 1984;ii:1039.
35. Wilson CB. Nephritogenic immune responses involving basement membrane and other antigens in or of the glomerulus. In: Cummings N, Michael AF, Wilson CB, eds. Immune mechanisms in renal disease. New York: Plenum Press, 1983, 233.
36. Johnson JP, Moore J, Austin HA, Balow JE, Antonovych TT, Wilson CB. Therapy of anti-glomerular basement membrane antibody disease: Analysis of prognostic significance of clinical, pathology, and treatment factors. Medicine 1985;64:219–27.
37. Teague CA, Doak PB, Simpson IJ, Rainer SP, Herdson PB. Goodpasture's syndrome: Analysis of 29 cases. Kidney Int 1978:13:492–504.
38. Zimmerman SW, Varanasi VR, Hoff B. Goodpasture's syndrome with normal renal function. Am J Med 1979;66:163–71.
39. Fish AJ, Kleppel M, Jeraj K, Michael AF. Enzyme immunoassay of antiglomerular basement membrane antibodies. J Lab Clin Med 1985;105:700–05.
40. Glassock RJ. Goodpasture's syndrome. In: Massry SG, Glassock RJ, eds. Textbook of nephrology. Baltimore: Williams & Wilkins, 1983;6.108–6.113.
41. Travis WD, Colby TV, Lombard C, Carpenter HA. A clinicopathologic study of 33 cases of diffuse pulmonary hemorrhage with lung biopsy confirmation. Am J Surg Path 1990 (in press).
42. Peters DK, Rees AJ, Lockwood CM, Pusey CD. Treatment and prognosis of antibasement membrane antibody mediated nephritis. Transplant Proc 1982;14:513–21.

43. Flores JC, Savage COS, Lockwood CM, Taube D, Cameron JS, Williams DG, et al. Clinical and immunological evolution of oligoanuric anti-GMB nephritis treated by hemodialysis. Lancet 1986;i:5–8.
44. deTorrente A, Popovtzer MM, Guggenheim SJ, Schier RW. Serious pulmonary hemorrhage, glomerulonephritis, and massive steroid therapy. Ann Intern Med 1975;83:281.
45. Kathuria S, Cheifac G. Fatal pulmonary Henoch-Schönlein syndrome. Chest 1982;82:654–56.
46. Weiss VF, Naidu S. Fatal pulmonary hemorrhage in Henoch-Schönlein purpura. Cutis 1979;23:687.
47. Cadman EC, Lundberg WB, Mitchell MS. Pulmonary manifestations in Behçet's syndrome. Arch Intern Med 1976;136:944.
48. Martinez JS, Kohler PF. Variant "Goodpasture's syndrome"? Ann Intern Med 1971;67–75.
49. Germain MJ, Davidman M. Pulmonary hemorrhage and acute renal failure in a patient with mixed connective tissue disease. Am J Kidney Dis 1984;3:420–24.
50. Kallenbach J, Prinsloo I, Zinc S. Progressive systemic sclerosis complicated by diffuse pulmonary hemorrhage. Thorax 1977;32:767–70.
51. Smith BS. Idiopathic pulmonary hemosiderosis and rheumatoid arthritis. Br Med J 1966;1:1403.
52. Mark EJ, Ramirez JF. Pulmonary capillaritis and hemorrhage in patients with systemic vasculitis. Arch Pathol Lab Med 1985;109:413–18.
53. Myers JL, Katzenstein A-LA. Microangiitis in lupus-induced pulmonary hemorrhage. Am J Clin Pathol 1986;85:552–556.
54. Stokes TC, McCann BG, Rees RT, Sims EH, Harrison DEW. Acute fulminating intrapulmonary hemorrhage in Wegener's granulomatosis. Thorax 1982;37:315–16.
55. Travis WD, Carpenter HA, Lie JT. Diffuse pulmonary hemorrhage: An uncommon manifestation of Wegener's granulomatosis. Am J Surg Pathol 1987;11:702–708.
56. Myers JL, Katzenstein A-LA. Wegener's granulomatosis presenting with massive pulmonary hemorrhage and capillaritis. Am J Surg Pathol 1987;11:895–898.
57. Marino CT, Pertschuk LP. Pulmonary hemorrhage in systemic lupus erythematosus. Arch Intern Med 1981;141:201.
58. Jennette JC, Wilkman AS, Falk RJ. Anti-neutrophil cytoplasmic antibody-associated glomerulonephritis and vasculitis. Am J Pathol 1989;135:921–930.
59. Balow JE. Renal vasculitis. Kidney Int 1985;27:954–64.
60. Fauci AS, Haynes BF, Katz P, Wolff SM. Wegener's granulomatosis: Prospective clinical and therapeutic experience with 85 patients over 21 years. Ann Intern Med 1983;98:76–85.
61. McDonald TJ, DeRemee RA. Wegener's granulomatosis. Laryngoscope 1983;93:220–231.
62. Brandwein S, Esdaile J, Danoff D, et al. Wegener's granulomatosis: Clinical features and outcome in 13 patients. Arch Intern Med 1983;143:476–479.
63. Pinching AJ, Lockwood CU, Russell BA, et al. Wegener's granulomatosis: Observations on 18 patients with severe renal disease. Q J Med 1983;208:435–460.
64. VanderWoude FJ, Rasmussen N, Lobatto S, et al. Autoantibodies against neutrophils and monocytes: Tool for diagnosis and marker of disease activity in Wegener's granulomatosis. Lancet 1985;i:425–429.
65. Specks V, Wheatly CL, McDonald TJ, Rorhbach MS, DeRemee RA. Anticytoplasmic autoantibodies in the diagnosis and follow-up of Wegener's granulomatosis. Am J Surg Pathol 1987;11:702–708.
66. Nölle B, Specks U, Lüdemann G, et al. Anticytoplasmic autoantibodies: Their immunodiagnostic value in Wegener's granulomatosis. Ann Intern Med 1989;111:28–40.
67. Savage COS, Jones S, Winearls CG, et al. Prospective study of radioimmunoassay for antibodies against neutrophil cytoplasm in diagnosis of systemic vasculitis. Lancet 1987;i:1389–1393.
68. Savage COS, Winearls CG, Evans DJ, Rees AJ, Lockwood CM. Microscopic polyarteritis: Presentation, pathology, and prognosis. Q J Med 1985;56:467–83.

69. Jennette JC, Falk RJ. Anti-neutrophil cytoplasmic autoantibodies: New insights into crescentic glomerulonephritis, pulmonary-renal syndrome, and systemic vasculitis. AKF Nephrology Letter 1989;6:11–18.

70. Kahn FW, Jones JM, England DN. Diagnosis of pulmonary hemorrhage in the immunocompromised host. Am Rev Respir Dis 1987;136:155–160.

71. Carette S. Macher AM, Nussbaum A, Plotz P. Severe, acute pulmonary disease in patients with systemic lupus erythematosus: Ten years of experience at the National Institutes of Health. Semin Arthritis Rheum 1984;14:52–9.

72. Mintz G, Galindo LF, Fernandez-Diez J, Jimenez FJ, Robles Saavedra E, Enriquez-Casilas RD. Acute massive pulmonary hemorrhage in systemic lupus erythematosus. J Rheumatol 1978;5:39–50.

73. Matthay RA, Schwartz MT, Petty TL, et al. Pulmonary manifestations of systemic lupus erythematosus: Review of twelve cases of acute lupus pneumonitis. Medicine (Baltimore) 1975;54:397–409.

74. Wiedemann HP, Matthay RA. Pulmonary manifestations of the collagen vascular diseases. In: Matthay R, ed: Pulmonary manifestations of systemic disease. Clin Chest Med 1989;10:677–722.

75. Balow JE, Austin HA, Tsokos GC, et al. Lupus nephritis. Ann Intern Med 1987;106:79–94.

76. Kuhn C. Systemic lupus erythematosus in a patient with ultrastructural lesions of the pulmonary capillaries previously reported in the *Review* as due to idiopathic pulmonary hemosiderosis. Am Rev Respir Dis 1972;106:931–32.

77. Soergel KH, Sommers SC. Idiopathic pulmonary hemosiderosis and related syndromes. Am J Med 1962;32:499–511.

78. Byrd RB, Gracey DR. Immunosuppressive treatment of idiopathic pulmonary hemosiderosis. JAMA 1973;226:458–59.

79. Pozo-Rodriquez F, Friene-Campo JM, Guitierrez-Millet V, Barbosa-Ayucar C, Diazde Atauri J, Martin-Escribano P. Idiopathic pulmonary hemosiderosis treated by plasmapheresis. Thorax 1980;35:399.

80. Bowley NB, Steiner RE, Chin WS. The chest x-ray in antiglomerular basement membrane antibody disease (Goodpasture's syndrome). Clin Radiol 1979;30:419–29.

81. Abelda SM, Gefter WB, Epstein DM, Miller WT. Diffuse pulmonary hemorrhage: A review and classification. Radiology 1985;154:289–97.

82. Abud-Mendoya C, Diaz-Jovaneu E, Alarcon-Segovia D. Fatal pulmonary hemorrhage in systemic lupus erythematosus: Occurrence without hemoptysis. J Rheum 1985;12:558–61.

83. Apt L, Pollycone M, Ross JF. Idiopathic pulmonary hemosiderosis: A study of the anemia and iron distribution using radioiron and radiochromium. J Clin Invest 1957;36:1150–59.

84. Ewan PW, Jones HA, Rhodes CG, Hughes JMB. Detection of intrapulmonary hemorrhage with carbon monoxide uptake. N Engl J Med 1976;295:1391–96.

85. Addleman M, Logan AS, Grossman RF. Monitoring intrapulmonary hemorrhage in Goodpasture's syndrome. Chest 1985;87:119–20.

86. Bowley NB, Hughes JMB, Steiner RE. The chest x-ray in pulmonary capillary hemorrhage: Correlation with carbon monoxide uptake. Clin Radiol 1979;30:413–17.

87. Drew WL, Finley TN, Golde DW. Diagnostic lavage and occult pulmonary hemorrhage in thrombocytopenic immunocompromised patients. Am Rev Respir Dis 1977;116:215.

88. Godwin JE, Harley RA, Miller KS, Hefner JE. Cocaine, pulmonary hemorrhage, and hemoptysis. Ann Intern Med 1989;110:843.

89. Wierty LM, Gagnon JH, Anthonisen NR. Intrapulmonary hemorrhage with anemia after lymphography. N Engl J Med 1971;288:1264–65.

90. Finley TN, Aronow A, Cosentino AM, Golde DW. Occult pulmonary hemorrhage in anticoagulated patients. Am Rev Respir Dis 1975;142:23–9.

91. Robboy SJ, Minna JD, Colman RW, Birudorf NI, Lopas H. Pulmonary hemorrhage syndrome as a manifestation of disseminated intravascular coagulation: Analysis of ten cases. Chest 1973;63:718–21.
92. Smith LT, Katzenstein A-LA. Pathogenesis of massive pulmonary hemorrhage in acute leukemia. Arch Intern Med 1982;142:2149–52.
93. Schwartz R, Myerson RM, Lawrence LT, Nichols WT. Mitral stenosis, massive pulmonary hemorrhage, and emergency valve replacement. N Engl J Med 1966;275:755–58.
94. Clinicopathologic conference. N Engl J Med 1978;298:1014–21.
95. Berrigan TJ, Carsky EW, Heitzman ER. Fat embolism: Roentgenographic pathologic correlation in three cases. Am J Roentgenol 1967;96:967–71.
96. Schwartz EE, Teplick JG, Onesti G, Schwartz AB. Pulmonary hemorrhage in renal disease: Goodpasture's syndrome and other causes. Radiology 1977;122:39–46.
97. Spragg RG, Wolf P, Haghiglin P, Abraham JL, Astarita RW. Angiosarcoma of the lung with fatal pulmonary hemorrhage. Am J Med 1983;74:1072–1076.
98. Kim CC, Saleba K, Baughman RP, Wesseler TA. Iron staining on bronchoalveolar lavage smears for detecting occult pulmonary hemorrhage: Is it reliable? Acta Cytol 1989;33:716 (Abstract).
99. Fasset RG, Hogan BA, Matthew TH. Detection of glomerular bleeding by phase contrast microscopy. Lancet 1982;i:1432.
100. Fauci AS, Katz P, Haynes BF, Wolff SM. Cyclophosphamide therapy of severe systemic necrotizing vasculitis. N Engl J Med 1979;301:235–238.
101. Herzog CA, Miller RR, Hoidal JR. Bronchiolitis and rheumatoid arthritis. Am Rev Respir Dis 1984;124:636–639.
102. Hind CRK, Lockwood CM, Peters DK, Paraskevakou H, Evans DJ, Rees AJ. Prognosis after immunosuppression of patients with crescentic nephritis requiring dialysis. Lancet 1983;i:263–65.
103. Green J, Brenner B, Gery R, et al. Case report: Adult hemolytic uremic syndrome associated with nonimmune deposit crescentic glomerulonephritis and alveolar hemorrhage. Am J Med Sci 1988;296:121–125.
104. Zell SC, Duxbury G, Shankel SW. Alveolar hemorrhage associated with a membranoproliferative glomerulonephritis and smooth muscle antibody. Am J Med 1987;82:1073–1076.
105. Yurn MN, Lampton LM, Bloom PM, Edwards JL. Asymptomatic IgA nephropathy associated with pulmonary hemosiderosis. Am J Med 1978;64:1056–1060.

21

Laboratory Techniques for the Study of Immunologically Mediated Pulmonary Diseases

Mark R. Wick
Paul E. Swanson

In the past 10 years, technical advances have enhanced the immunopathologic evaluation of pulmonary disorders a great deal. Some of these developments fall into the realm of clinical serology and will be considered only perfunctorily in the following discussion. Others, however, enable the pathologist to visualize immune complexes, complement deposits, and cellular infiltrates directly in excised tissues and to relate these disease components to morphologic abnormalities at a light microscopic level.

This chapter will present the elements of current immunohistopathologic practice as applied to the lung. Nonneoplastic diseases, because they comprise the majority of diseases necessitating studies of this type, provide the major focus for discussion. Nonetheless, a significant group of disorders appears to bridge the gap between inflammatory and neoplastic aberrations, necessitating a consideration of neoplastic disorders as well. Differential diagnostic approaches to immunologic pulmonary diseases will also be presented. The information contained in this chapter represents a distillation of the published literature supplemented by our own observations.

METHODOLOGY

At present, several techniques exist for the utilization of antibodies as diagnostic tissue probes. The most widely used of these techniques are direct and indirect immunofluorescence, the peroxidase-antiperoxidase (PAP) method, the avidin-biotin-peroxidase complex (ABC) procedure, the alkaline phosphatase–anti-alkaline phosphatase (APAAP) technique, the immunogold procedure, and combinations thereof. In addition, it is sometimes desirable to validate immunohistochemical results with alternative techniques that enable the visualization of deoxyribonucleic acid (DNA) or ribonucleic acid (RNA) sequences that encode the protein targets of antibody reagents. This goal can be accomplished through the use of in situ hybridization analyses.

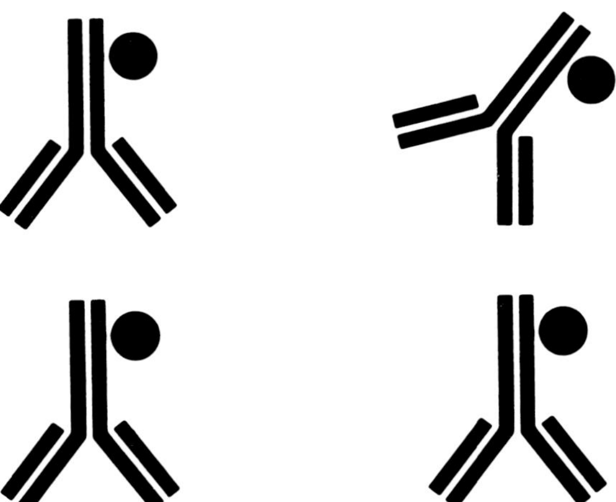

Figure 21-1. "Direct" immuno-fluorescence methods employ a fluoresceinated label that is attached chemically to the Fc fragment of a reagent antibody.

Immunofluorescence Methods

The first immunohistochemical technique devised for clinical use was the direct immunofluorescence (IF) procedure.[1] This method makes use of the knowledge that fluorescent dyes such as fluorescein or rhodamine can be conjugated to intact immunoglobulin or the Fab fragments thereof. If the immunoglobulin has specificity for a given tissue antigen, one obtains a means of directly visualizing the determinant subsequent to antibody binding (Fig. 21-1). Indirect fluorescence procedures are similar, but use a two-step antibody complex in which the second (labeled) antiserum bears the fluorescent tag and has immunologic specificity for the species from which the primary antibody is procured.

Both of these immunofluorescent techniques are widely employed but are usually applied in well-defined, restricted settings. This is because IF methods typically necessitate the use of frozen tissue as a substrate to attain an acceptable signal-to-noise ratio. Even with frozen tissue, immunofluorescent microscopy is plagued by a relatively high level of nonspecific antibody binding. In addition, it is nearly impossible to correlate the targets of antibody binding with morphologic aspects of the specimen, because of the need for specialized illumination.

Such drawbacks notwithstanding, IF procedures are the most effective means of labeling immune complexes in tissue. These complexes do not usually remain intact after fixation of the specimen in routine mordants; furthermore, they are seen only indistinctly in stained tissues visualized by conventional light microscopy.

The Peroxidase-Antiperoxidase Procedure

The introduction of the peroxidase-antiperoxidase (PAP) method by Sternberger and associates in 1970[2] set the stage for a veritable explosion in applied tissue immunology.

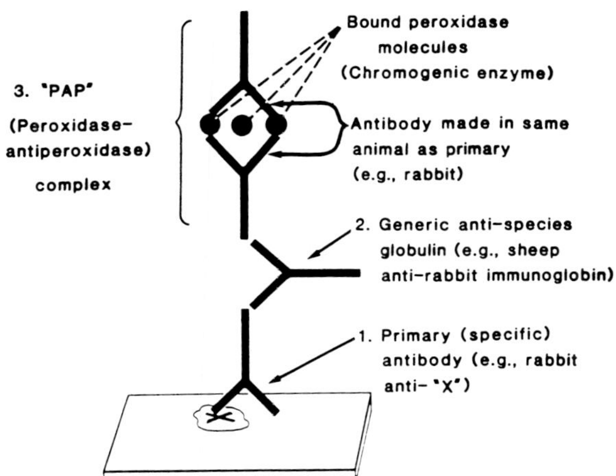

Figure 21-2. The peroxidase-antiperoxidase (PAP) method of immunohistochemistry employs a chromogenic complex (#3) composed of two antibodies from the same source as that of primary reagent (#1). These constituents are bound together by a generic anti-species antibody (#2).

This procedure involves the use of a four-antibody "sandwich," in which the first element is the reagent directed at the specific determinant of interest. The second "link" antibody has generic anti-species specificity against the primary and also recognizes a two-antibody couplet joined to three peroxidase molecules that represents the tertiary chromogenic moiety (Fig. 21-2). Because a free Fc fragment is available for further binding to additional secondary antibody after completion of this sequence, the PAP technique can be extended in a reiterative fashion (Fig. 21-3).[3] Reiteration increases the sensitivity of the method because of amplified peroxidase coupling.

The Avidin-Biotin-Peroxidase Complex Technique

Within a few short years after general implementation of the PAP procedure, it was recognized that Fc fragments of antibodies could easily be joined to biotin, and that avidin could similarly be coupled to several peroxidase molecules. This advance resulted in the avidin-biotin-peroxidase complex (ABC) procedure.[4] In contrast to the PAP method, therefore, ABC technology uses only two antibodies: a primary reagent and a secondary biotinylated antiserum. The tertiary component is a complex preformed matrix of biotin, avidin, and peroxidase, which binds to the secondary antibody with a much higher avidity than that seen between two immunoglobulin molecules (Fig. 21-4). Consequently, the ABC procedure is a powerful, sensitive detection system for localizing tissue antigens. Recent stoichiometric alterations in the structure of the tertiary complex have further increased the efficiency of this technique.[5]

Other Antibody Enzyme Methods

Building on the concepts underlying the PAP procedure, several other antibody-enzyme techniques have been developed in the past few years. These are basically identical in principle to the PAP and ABC systems, but differ from the latter in substituting catalysts other than peroxidase in the chromogenic tertiary complex. Examples

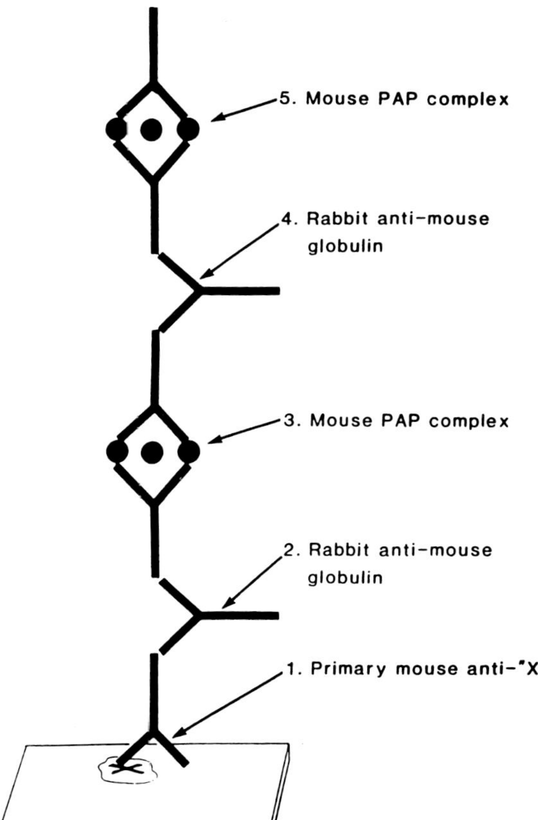

Figure 21-3. The "reiterative" PAP procedure is performed by repeating the second and third steps of the peroxidase-antiperoxidase technique. This amplifies the number of bound peroxidase molecules in the final antibody assembly.

are the alkaline phosphatase–anti-alkaline phosphatase (APAAP),[6] glucose oxidase–anti-glucose oxidase (GAG),[7] avidin-biotin-glucose oxidase (ABGO),[8] and avidin-biotin-beta glucuronidase (ABBG) methods. This diversification of enzymatic coupling allows the immunohistochemist to eliminate from the final staining product background (non-specific) signals that are due to unquenched endogenous tissue peroxidase. The intestinal isozyme of alkaline phosphatase is employed in the APAAP method, making it especially suitable for the analysis of pulmonary tissues. Moreover, glucose oxidase and beta-glucuronidase are not found in human lungs, providing strong support for the use of GAG, ABGO, or ABBG procedures in this context. In our experience and that of others,[8] all of the techniques just cited have sensitivities that are similar to those of more traditional antibody detection methods.

Combined Antibody-Enzyme Procedures

Occasionally, one is faced with the need to label a low-density cellular antigen in tissue, mandating the use of an extremely high-efficiency detection system. Although the

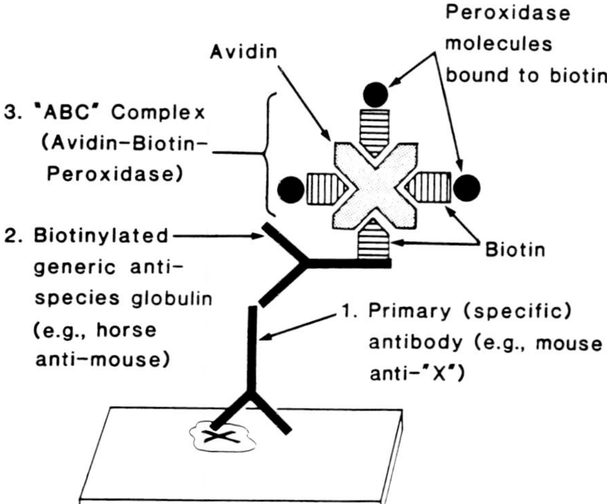

Figure 21-4. The avidin-biotin-peroxidase complex (ABC) procedure utilizes a performed assembly of avidin and biotin, bound to peroxidase. This complex attaches to a biotinylated secondary antibody.

systems presented thus far do have excellent capabilities in this regard, it may be desirable to combine them to multiply their individual avidities. An example of this approach is the avidin-biotin-peroxidase-antiperoxidase (ABPAP) method, as applied with murine monoclonal primary antibodies.[9] In this system, the mouse-PAP procedure is performed first, followed by the ABC technique using a biotinylated secondary anti-mouse antiserum. Following a final reaction step with avidin-biotin-peroxidase complex, a five-layer immunochemical assembly is obtained that contains numerous chromogenic enzyme molecules (Fig. 21-5). We have shown that this procedure is extremely sensitive to minute quantities of antigen, particularly in formalin-fixed and parafffin-embedded specimens.[9]

Immunogold Microscopy; Ultrastructural Immunohistochemistry

Gold particles may be coupled to intact immunoglobulins, to provide a visible marker of antibody binding by means of direct (one-step) or multiple-reagent (indirect) procedures. These differ principally in which antibody bears the gold conjugate.[10] Staphyloccal protein A may be linked to gold as well, serving as another tool for the detection of primary antibodies of the IgG class. The gold signal can be amplified by subsequent exposure to a silver emulsion, which acts much like the developing solutions used in photography.

Immunogold methods are applicable in routine light microscopy, but are much more expensive than antibody-enzyme procedures. They have their greatest use in immunoelectron microscopy, because gold particles are electron-dense.[11] Ultrastructural immunohistochemistry is more complicated than light microscopic methods, because of the need for special fixation and processing of specimens. Tissue preservation in cold paraformaldehyde has yielded good results in most cases, as opposed to fixation

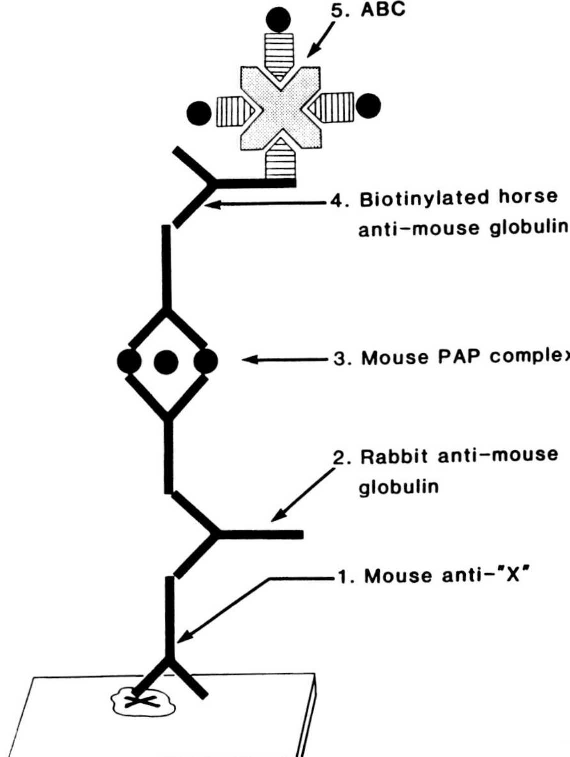

Figure 21-5. Sequential performance of the PAP and ABC procedures yields the "ABPAP" complex, with amplified peroxidase labeling.

with glutaraldehyde, formalin, or other mordants. Fresh tissue also can be used if one has access to a freezing ultramicrotome.

Incubation of the specimen with primary antibody may be done either before or after embedding in polymeric resin (Lowacryl) and preparation of thin tissue sections for electron microscopy. These variations are known as "pre-embedding" and "post-embedding" procedures,[11] and are left to the individual preferences of the investigator.

The value of immunoelectron microscopy lies in its ability to delineate antibody reactivity on a subcellular level. It is possible by such means to determine whether the plasmalemma, nuclear membrane, basal lamina, tissue matrix, or specific intracytoplasmic organelles are the sites of antigen localization.

In Situ Nucleic Acid Hybridization

Although it is not an immunologic technique, in situ nucleic acid hybridization (ISH) utilizes some of the same methodology as antibody-mediated procedures, and it provides information that is adjunctive to immunostaining results.[12]

ISH methods rely on the fact that DNA denatured in tissue specimens in vitro will reanneal to complementary nucleic acids. Nucleic acid sequences (either DNA or RNA) that correspond to known protein-antigen amino acid chains may be synthesized ex vivo and labeled with either radionuclides or biotin. These labeled reagents are referred to as "probes."

Fixed and paraffin-embedded or fresh tissues may be used for ISH assays. The tissue samples are heated to denature endogenous nucleic acids, and then hybridized to the probe under stringent ionic and acid-base conditions. The resulting signal is "developed" by autoradiography of the specimen if radionuclide labels are used or by avidin-biotin-peroxidase methodology if biotinylated probes are employed.

Sequential immunohistochemical and ISH procedures have been developed to enable covisualization of nucleic acid sequences and their protein products in the same cells. For these procedures, it is best to immunostain first and then hybridize, because ISH techniques will denature most cellular proteins, interfering with antibody binding.

Special Processing Requirements

As already mentioned, fresh tissue is needed for immunologic assessment of immune complex deposition in the lung, and it is preferred for ISH procedures on pulmonary tissue. In fact, snap-frozen tissue is desirable in *every* case that may need immunologic evaluation, because fixation procedures adversely affect several antigen systems. For example, formalin is capable of cross-linking many proteinaceous determinants, rendering them unavailable to corresponding antibody reagents.[13]

Other alternatives to freezing specimens have been devised, with inconstant success. For example, cold acetone fixation, preservation in paraformaldehyde, and freeze-drying have been reported by some investigators to preserve antigenic integrity.[14,15] In addition, protease digestion (with trypsin, pepsin, pronase, ficin, or bromelain) of fixed tissues before immunostaining procedures sometimes enhances final results.[16] Nevertheless, given the wide range of markers that are of interest in immunologic lung disease (see below), all of these techniques must be judged inferior to the use of fresh specimens.

ANALYSES OF INTEREST IN IMMUNOLOGIC DISEASES OF THE LUNG

The study of immunologic pulmonary disorders has gone far beyond the simple desire to locate immune complexes in the lung. Most investigators are currently interested in evaluating the interactions among pulmonary tissue compartments in these processes, necessitating the application of a broad variety of antibody reagents. These reagents (Table 21-1) are discussed in the following section.

Immunoglobulins

Many commercial antibodies are available for the localization of immunoglobulins in tissue sections. These include reagents directed at intact IgG, IgA, IgM, IgD, and IgE, as well as specific isotypes of these molecules. In addition, other antibodies are directed at heavy chains only, or against kappa and lambda light chain immunoglobulins. Monoclonal (hybridoma) reagents are preferable in this realm of immunohistochemistry

TABLE 21-1. Immunohistologic Reagents Applicable to Nonneoplastic Diseases of the Lung

REAGENT	DOMINANT REACTIVITY	SOURCE
Fluoresceinated anti-immunoglobulins	Human immunoglobulins	Sternberger Laboratories
PAP complexes	Non-human immunoglobulins	Sternberger Laboratories
ABC, APAAP, GAG, ABGO, and ABBG Universal Kits	Non-human immunoglobulins	Vector Laboratories
Gold-labeled secondary antibodies	Non-human immunoglobulins	Sigma Laboratories
Anti-kappa and lambda light chain immunoglobulins	Human kappa and lambda light chain immunoglobulins	DakoPatts Co., Inc.
Anti-IgG, -IgA, -IgM, -IgD, -IgE	Human immunoglobulins	DakoPatts Co., Inc.
Anti-C3/C4	Human complement fractions 3 & 4	Calbiochem Co.
Anti-cytokeratin CAM 5.2 Mak-6 AE1/AE3	Epithelial cells	Becton-Dickinson Co. Triton BioSciences Hybritech, Inc.
Anti-epithelial membrane antigen	Epithelial cells	DakoPatts Co., Inc.
Anti-Ber-EP4	Epithelial cells	DakoPatts Co., Inc.
Anti-Clara cell antigen	Bronchiolar Clara cells	Dr. G. Singh University of Pittsburgh
Anti-surfactant apoprotein	Type II pneumocytes	Dr. G. Singh University of Pittsburgh
Anti-vimentin	Mesenchymal cells	BioGenex Co.
Anti-desmin	Myogenous cells	BioGenex Co.
Anti-factor VIII related antigen	Endothelial cells	DakoPatts Co., Inc.
BMA-120	Endothelial cells	Behringwerke Co. (Marburg, Germany)
EN-4	Endothelial cells	Dr. E. Wilson-Jones Guy's Hospital, London, UK
Ulex europaeus I lectin	Endothelial and epithelial cells	Vector Laboratories
Anti-collagen type I	Collagen type I	Dr. Edmond Crouch Washington University
Anti-collagen type III	Collagen type III	Dr. Edmond Crouch Washington University
Anti-collagen type IV	Collagen type IV	DakoPatts Co., Inc.
Anti-laminin	Laminin	Dr. Leo Furcht University of Minnesota
Anti-leukocyte common antigen	Human leukocytes	DakoPatts Co., Inc.

(continued)

TABLE 21-1. *(continued)*

REAGENT	DOMINANT REACTIVITY	SOURCE
LN-1 through LN-3	B-lymphocytes; Monocytes/histiocytes	BioGenex Co.
MB-2	B-lymphocytes	BioGenex Co.
L-26	B-lymphocytes	DakoPatts Co., Inc.
MT-1	T-lymphocytes	BioGenex Co.
UCHL-1	T-lymphocytes	DakoPatts Co., Inc.
MAC-387; KP-1	Monocytes/histiocytes	DakoPatts Co., Inc.
Anti-cathepsin B	Monocytes/histiocytes	ICN Laboratories
Anti-HLA-DR	Class II HLA antigens	DakoPatts Co., Inc.
Anti-interleukin 1–6	Human cytokines	Calbiochem, Inc.
Anti-cytomegalovirus	Cytomegalovirus	DakoPatts Co., Inc.
Anti-Herpes virus	Herpes I and II	DakoPatts Co., Inc.
Anti-*Pneumocystis carinii*	*Pneumocystis carinii*	DakoPatts Co., Inc.
Anti-*Toxoplasma*	*Toxoplasma gondii*	BioGenex Co., Inc.
Anti-human immunodeficiency virus	HTLV-III	Abbott Laboratories
Anti-*Mycobacterium tuberculosis;—avium*	Tubercle bacilli	Chemicon, Inc.
Anti-adenovirus	Adenovirus	Chemicon, Inc.
Anti-respiratory syncitial virus	Respiratory syncitial virus	Chemicon, Inc.
CD group antibodies	Human leukocytes	DakoPatts Co. Becton-Dickinson Co. (*See Table 2*)

Abbreviations: PAP = Peroxidase-antiperoxidase
ABC = Avidin-biotin-peroxidase complex
APAAP = Alkaline phosphatase-anti-alkaline phosphatase
GAG = Glucose oxidase-anti-glucose oxidase
ABGO = Avidin-biotin-glucose oxidase
ABBG = Avidin-biotin-beta-glucuronidase
HLA = Human leukocyte antigen

because of their superior specificity over heteroantisera. If immunoglobulin analysis is desired, one must ensure that a portion of diagnostic biopsy specimens is snap-frozen because of the gross inferiority of fixed tissues for this purpose. Indeed, light chains are totally stripped from lymphocytes in conventionally processed specimens, rendering them useless for assessment of cell surface immunoglobulin expression.[17] We have already alluded to the problems encountered in evaluating immune complex deposition in fixed lung tissues.

Complement Proteins

Because the complement cascade commonly participates in humorally mediated immunologic diseases, most pulmonary pathologists assess the presence of bound complement components (e.g., C3, C5, properdin) when such disorders are suspected. Although many commercial antibodies are available, they again require frozen tissue for reliable results.

Epithelial Determinants

The participation by, or alteration of, pulmonary epithelial cells in immunologic diseases has only recently been addressed. Fortunately, several antigen systems that are most commonly analyzed in neoplastic conditions also provide useful information in inflammatory disorders. These include the cytokeratins, epithelial membrane antigen (EMA), the Ber-EP4 antigens, Clara cell antigens, surfactant apoprotein, and various glycoproteinaceous components of epithelial mucins.

Cytokeratins

The cytokeratins are a family of intracellular intermediate filament proteins[18] currently thought to function in the restriction of RNA binding domains at the level of the ribosome.[19] They range in molecular weight from 40 kDa to 69 kDa, and may be detected with many specific monoclonal antibodies. Lung tissue expresses predominantly lower molecular weight proteins in this family of antigens, although metaplastic squamoid cells may shift their synthesis of cytokeratins to the 67 to 69 kDa range.[18] Type I and II alveolar pneumocytes express such proteins, as do all lining cells of the bronchi, bronchioles, and alveolar ducts.

Epithelial Membrane Antigen

"Epithelial membrane antigen" is actually a cluster of glycoproteins that are displayed within the plasmalemma of most epithelial cells, including those of the lung.[20] They were first isolated from human milk fat globule proteins, and have a distribution like that of cytokeratin in pulmonary tissues. Unlike cytokeratins, however, epithelial membrane antigen moieties have molecular weights ranging from 265 kDa to over 440 kDa.

The Ber-EP4 Antigens

The Ber-EP4 antigens are represented by a couplet of 34 kDa and 49 kDa glycoproteins, which are present on the surfaces and within the cytoplasm of nearly all epithelia.[21] Exceptions include squamous cells, hepatocyte parenchyma, and serosal lining (mesothelial) cells. Nearly identical determinants are recognized by the monoclonal antibody HEA-125.

Clara Cell Antigens

A restricted set of glycoproteins has been isolated from the cytoplasm and plasmalemmae of Clara cells within the terminal airways. The most well-characterized of these markers has a molecular weight of 10 kDa, and is labeled by a heteroantiserum raised in rabbits.[22] Immunoreactivity in other lining epithelia of the airway is not observed with this reagent.

Surfactant Apoproteins

Apoproteinaceous components of the surfactant lipoprotein family of molecules may also be detected immunohistochemically with rabbit antisera or monoclonal antibodies.[23] Type II pneumocytes (and to a lesser extent, Clara cells) are recognized by this reagent group.

Glycoproteinaceous Mucin Antigens

Finkbeiner and Basbaum have generated a series of monoclonal antibodies directed against glycoproteinaceous constituents of airway mucins.[24] These hybridoma products label serous, goblet, and mucinous cells of the tracheobronchial tree. Immunoblotting studies indicate that their biochemical targets vary in molecular weight from 14 kDa to 435 kDa.

Generic Mesenchymal Antigens

It is occasionally difficult to distinguish between fibroblastic and myogenic proliferations in routinely stained tissues. However, antibodies to muscle-related proteins enable the immunohistochemist to do so easily.

Desmin is a 53-kDa intermediate filament protein that is universally expressed by nonneoplastic striated and smooth muscle cells.[25] Accordingly, it provides an effective marker for such populations. Vimentin, another intermediate filament moiety with a molecular weight of 57 kDa, is present in all fibroblasts, as well as in many other more differentiated mesenchymal cells.[26]

Endothelial Determinants

A number of monoclonal antibodies are now commercially available to selectively identify endothelial cells, including anti-factor VIII–related antigen, PAL-E, EN4, and BMA-120.[27,28] The molecular structures of the corresponding antigens for these reagents are dissimilar in biochemical constituency and molecular weight, but all of them are restricted to vascular lining cells.

In addition, a plant lectin derived from *Ulex europaeus* I has been used extensively as an endothelial marker.[28] This agglutinin has the disadvantage that it can label epithelial cells of the airway and erythrocytes as well as endothelia.[28] Hence, because of the intricate microanatomy of the alveolar vasculature, it may be extremely difficult to separate reactive endothelial cells from pneumocytes that also bind *Ulex*. Although similarly nonspecific, antisera to angiotensin-converting enzyme also have been employed to label pulmonary blood vessels.

Antibodies to Collagen Types

The morphologic entity known to all pathologists and anatomists as "collagen" represents, in reality, a group of immunologically dissimilar biochemical moieties; these have been designated numerically (I through X).[29] Collagen types I, III, IV, and V are of interest for the pulmonologist and pulmonary pathologist because their synthesis differs in various interstitial pneumonitides that may have an immunopathologic basis.[30] Types I, III, and V are "stromal" or "interstitial" collagens, being synthesized primarily by fibroblasts. Type IV collagen, on the other hand, is an integral part of basement membranes and may be produced by epithelia or diverse mesenchymal cells (e.g., smooth muscle, Schwann cells, and endothelia).[31]

Monoclonal antibodies to the collagen subtypes may be procured commercially, and they provide useful tools to evaluate the elaboration of excess matrix tissue in diseases of the lung. Several of these reagents are active in routinely processed specimens, whereas others require fresh tissue.

Other Basement Membrane Antigens

As well as type IV collagen, basement membranes also contain fibronectin, laminin, and the Goodpasture antigen (GPA),[31,32] all of which have been localized with monoclonal antibodies. Goodpasture antigen has been detected in renal glomeruli, pulmonary alveoli, choroid plexus, thyroid, pituitary, adrenal gland, breast, cornea, and intrahepatic blood vessels.[33] It is still uncertain whether GPA is merely a distinctive antigenic domain of collagen type IV or an independent but related molecule.

Hematopoietic Determinants

The past 10 years have witnessed an outpouring of antibody reagents that may be applied to the characterization of hematopoietic cells. These have been categorized functionally into "cluster designations" (CD), referring to their recognition of related groups of antigenic determinants,[34] and are listed in Table 21-2. In addition, as-yet-unclassified

TABLE 21-2. Cluster Designations (CD) of Anti-Leukocyte Antibodies of Interest in Pulmonary Pathology

CLUSTER DESIGNATION	MAJOR REACTIVITY WITH NORMAL CELLS
1	Thymocytes; Langerhans cells
2	T-cells; natural killer cells
3	Mature T-cells
4	T-helper cells
5	T-cells; some B-cell subsets
6	Mature T-cells
7	T-cells
8	Cytotoxic/suppressor T-cells
9	B-cell progenitors
10	B-cell progenitors
11	Macrophages; monocytes
12	Macrophages; granulocytes
13	Macrophages; granulocytes
14	Macrophages; granulocytes
15	Macrophages; monocytes; granulocytes
16	Granulocytes; natural killer cells
17	Macrophages; granulocytes
18	T-cells
19	B-cells
20	Peripheral B-cells
21	Subset of B-cells
22	Peripheral B-cells
23	Follicular B-cells
24	B-cells; granulocytes
25	Activated T-cells (IL2 receptor)

(continued)

TABLE 21-2. *(continued)*

CLUSTER DESIGNATION	MAJOR REACTIVITY WITH NORMAL CELLS
26	Activated T-cells
27	T-cells; plasma cells
28	T-cell subset
29	T-cell subset
30	Activated lymphoid cells (T- and B-)
31	Monocytes; granulocytes; T-cells
32	Endothelial cells
33	Myeloid cell progenitors
34	Granulocytes; endothelial cells
35	Granulocytes; monocytes
36	Monocytes
37	B-cells
38	Activated T-cells
39	B-cell subsets
40	B-cells
43*	T-cells; granulocytes
44	T-cells; granulocytes
45	All leukocytes (equivalent to anti-leukocyte common antigen)
46	Leukocytes
48	Leukocytes
49	Monocytes; T-cells; B-cells
50	Leukocytes
52	Leukocytes
53	Leukocytes
56	Natural killer cells; activated lymphocytes
57	Natural killer cells; T- and B-cell subsets
58	Leukocytes
60	T-cell subset
64	Monocytes
65	Granulocytes; monocytes
66	Granulocytes
67	Granulocytes
68	Macrophages
69	Activated T- and B-cells
70	Activated T- and B-cells
71	Proliferating lymphocytes
72	B-cells
73	B-cell subset
74	B-cells; monocytes
75	Mature B-cells; T-cell subset
76	Mature B-cells; T-cell subset
77	B-cell subset
78	B-cells

* CD groups 41, 42, 47, 51, 54, 55, 59, and 61–63 label non-lymphoid cells

reagents are available that may well add to our understanding of differentiation and function in this cellular grouping.

Once again, most of these antibodies are best applied to frozen sections. Nevertheless, new hybridoma products and polyclonal heteroantisera allow fixed specimens to be studied for their content of lymphocytes, granulocytes, Langerhans cells, and histiocytes. Because all these cell types can participate in immunologic pulmonary diseases, such reagents are extremely useful in the analysis of routinely processed lung biopsy specimens. LN-1, LN-2, MB-2, and L-26 are reagents that label B-cells, irrespective of their stage of differentiation.[35,36] Likewise, UCHL-1 and MT-1 recognize most T-cells; MAC-387, KP-1, anti-cathepsin B, and anti-Leu M1 are directed at monocytes, histiocytes, and neutrophils[35,37,38]; anti–S-100 protein recognizes Langerhans cells[39–41]; and anti-eosinophil basic protein selectively binds to eosinophilic granulocytes.[42]

In addition, Akiyama and associates have described a series of four monoclonal antibodies (AMH-1 through AMH-4) that recognize differing subsets of mono-histiocytic cells in the lung.[43] These were reported to distinguish between alveolar and pulmonary interstitial macrophages; moreover, AMH2–4 appeared to label epithelioid histiocytes selectively in sarcoidosis and hypersensitivity pneumonitis. More widespread reactivity was seen in alveolar macrophages using anti–PAM-1, a monoclonal reagent developed by Kobzik and colleagues.[44] All five of the antibodies just cited were applied to frozen sections exclusively, and it is not currently known if they are active in fixed specimens.

Histocompatibility Antigens

It is now well known that certain histocompatibility locus antigen (HLA) haplotypes predispose certain individuals to autoimmune or alloimmune diseases. In addition, a growing body of literature supports the contention that epithelial, endothelial, and hematopoietic cells may alter their expression of HLA determinants in immunologic tissue reactions.[45]

Therefore, specific antibodies recognizing class I HLA (A,B,C,) and class II HLA (HLA-DR; HLA-DP; HLA-DQ) are being widely used in immunopathology. These are, again, most active in frozen sections or cytologic preparations; nonetheless, some reagents in this category (LN-3; LK8D3) can also label fixed tissues.[45]

Cytokines

The family of cytokines has occasioned intense interest over the past several years, inasmuch as these substances are intercellular "messengers" that effect changes in function or proliferation of lymphoreticular and stromal elements in inflammatory processes.[46] They include such moieties as gamma-interferon; macrophage migration inhibitory factor (MIF); interleukins (IL) 1 through 6; tumor necrosis factor-alpha; fibroblast growth factor (FGF); prostaglandin E_2; and leukotrienes.

Infectious Agents

The detection of infectious agents in lung biopsy specimens admittedly has only an indirect relationship to the diagnosis of immunologic pulmonopathies. However, many viruses and protozoan organisms can produce tissue alterations that perfectly simulate those seen in immunopathergic states.[47] Fungal infections also sometimes serve as the stimulus for an ongoing hyperimmune pulmonary response.

Hence, it is necessary to analyze some biopsy tissues with antibodies to cytomegalovirus, herpesvirus, adenovirus, respiratory syncytial virus, human immunodeficiency virus, tubercle bacilli, *Pneumocystis carinii,* or *Toxoplasma gondii,* before a definitive diagnostic interpretation can be made. Furthermore, given that the sensitivity of such reagents is less than absolute, ISH often is desirable as well in this context. Most of the agents just cited may be detected with commercially available nucleic acid probes, complementing the efficacy of antibodies directed at microorganisms.[48] Infection with the Epstein-Barr virus (EBV) is usually demonstrable *only* with ISH methods, inasmuch as antibodies to intact virions of this agent typically yield negative results in tissue sections. Lastly, antibodies to fungal or mycobacterial antigens may be used to document the presence of degenerating organisms that would be missed by conventional histochemical studies.[49]

IMMUNOHISTOLOGIC FINDINGS IN SELECTED PULMONOPATHIES

To date, studies are incomplete on pulmonary diseases thought to have at least a partial immunologic pathogenesis. The following section summarizes cumulative knowledge in this area as related to specific microscopic disease groupings. Because of overlaps in cellular injury patterns, the classification system used is not mutually exclusive or incontrovertible. Although the system is based on *predominant* histologic changes seen in each disease entity, some disorders appear in more than one category. Because an all-inclusive discussion of pulmonary disorders is clearly beyond the scope of this presentation, only diseases in which meaningful immunopathologic data have been obtained will be considered.

Diseases Characterized by Cytotoxic Antibody Formation or Deposition of Immune Complexes

A confined set of pulmonary diseases features the presence of specific antibodies that are bound to constituents of the lung or the deposition of immune complexes in the pulmonary vasculature. Among these diseases are usual interstitial pneumonitis ([UIP]—also known as idiopathic pulmonary fibrosis or chronic interstitial pneumonia); interstitial pneumonitis accompanying collagen vascular diseases, such as lupus erythematosus, rheumatoid arthritis, or systemic sclerosis; Goodpasture's syndrome; hypersensitivity pneumonitis; allergic bronchopulmonary aspergillosis (ABPA); and pulmonary polyarteritis nodosa (PAN).

Usual Interstitial Pneumonitis
UIP is a patchy interstitial process manifesting chronic inflammation and progressive fibrosis of the lung, with reactive hyperplasia of type II pneumocytes and the accumulation of macrophages within remaining alveoli. Because immune complex deposition

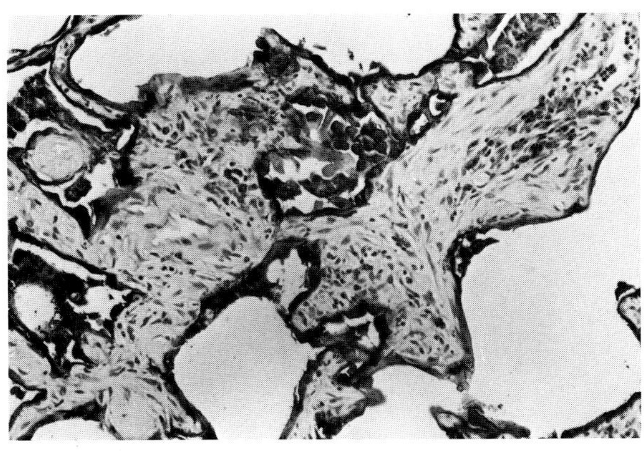

Figure 21-6. Epithelial membrane antigen expression by remaining alveolar pneumocytes, in usual interstitial pneumonitis.

may be observed in alveolar septa, a number of studies have suggested that UIP is a serologically mediated disorder.[50,51] For example, Eisenberg and colleagues demonstrated tissue-bound IgG, IgM, and IgA in this disorder, as well as C3.[50] Moreover, such autoantibodies as rheumatoid factor are overrepresented in patients with UIP. However, it should be noted that these relationships do not prove causation, inasmuch as immunoglobulins may also be detected in pneumocystosis and other "nonimmune" interstitial pneumonitides.[50] No antigenic target molecule has been well characterized in UIP, and entrapment of circulating immunoglobulin by damaged endothelium may therefore be considered as an alternative explanation for the immunofluorescence. Similarly, the enhanced expression of class II HLA determinants by macrophages and alveolar lining cells in the latter condition has been cited as evidence in favor of an immune etiology[52]; nevertheless, it may likewise be an epiphenomenon occasioned by inflammation, since it is also seen in other pneumonitides.

Hammar and colleagues have found that immunostains for cytokeratins may be used to separate alveolar epithelium from macrophages or endothelial cells, which may be morphologically similar in the late stages of UIP.[53] We have observed comparable results with antibodies to EMA, Ber-EP4, Clara cell antigen, and pulmonary surfactant (Fig. 21-6). MAC-387 and KP1 have sufficient specificity to distinguish alveolar macrophages from other cell types in UIP, as do antibodies in the CD11, CDw12, CD14, CD15, and CD17 groups. Vimentin is expressed by proliferating interstitial fibroblasts in UIP, whereas desmin is not. Similarly, these cellular elements are associated with positive immunostaining for collagens type I and III; labeling for collagen type IV is amplified in the basement membranes of damaged blood vessels (Fig. 21-7).[54–56]

Parenthetically, desquamative interstitial pneumonitis (DIP) has been linked closely with UIP by some investigators, because of certain clinicopathologic similarities. However, we are not aware of any studies showing immunoglobulin binding in DIP. The nature of intra-alveolar cells in DIP may be demonstrated by the monocyte-macrophage markers described above, and contrasted with negative results for pulmonary surfactant. This set of observations further disproves early contentions that the latter disease was caused by "desquamation" of alveolar lining cells.

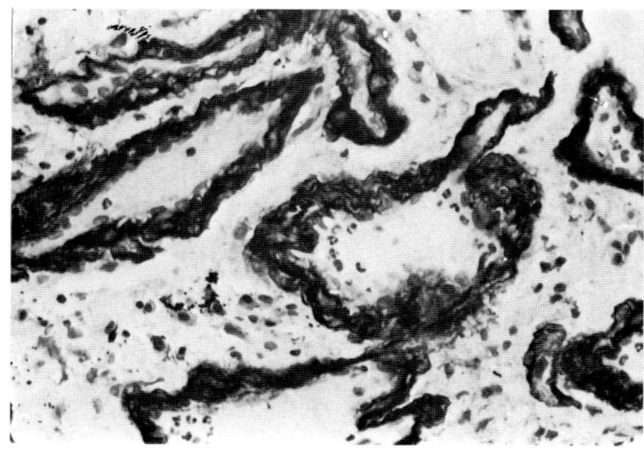

Figure 21-7. Redundant perivascular collagen type IV is apparent in this example of usual interstitial pneumonitis.

Interstitial Pneumonitis of Collagen Vascular Diseases

It is well known that patients with lupus erythematosus, systemic sclerosis, or rheumatoid arthritis may develop pulmonary interstitial disease that closely simulates that observed in idiopathic UIP.[57–61] However, these conditions are almost universally associated with granular immunoglobulin deposition in alveolar capillary walls, unlike UIP. In addition, elution studies demonstrate that native DNA, other nuclear antigens, or IgG partially compose the immune complexes of collagen vascular diseases, together with IgM or IgA and C3.[57,58] Otherwise, the immunohistologic features of these disorders are identical to those of idiopathic UIP.

Hypersensitivity Pneumonitis

Hypersensitivity pneumonitis is an interstitial inflammatory condition caused by a hyperimmune reaction to inhaled thermophile fungal antigens, molds, or animal products such as bird droppings. Precipitins to these allergens are regularly seen in the sera of affected individuals[62,63]; hence, it should not be surprising that immune complexes may be found by immunofluorescent microscopy within alveolar walls or pulmonary blood vessels in hypersensitivity pneumonitis, and that they are composed of the offending antigens along with IgG, IgM, or IgA.[64] Interestingly, Smets and associates have shown that the active allergen of bird feces may be ornithic IgA.[65]

In contrast to UIP and pneumonitis of collagen vascular disease, hypersensitivity pneumonitides feature a prominent lymphoid infiltrate, with focal formation of microgranulomas. These constituents will be discussed below.

Allergic Bronchopulmonary Aspergillosis: Bronchocentric Granulomatosis

Another group of hypersensitivity diseases of the lung is represented by allergic bronchopulmonary aspergillosis (ABPA) and bronchocentric granulomatosis (BG). These differ from the conditions considered in the previous section in that they are mediated by IgE bound to antigenic components of *Aspergillus* or other inhaled allergens and occur predominantly in asthmatic patients. To date, immunohistochemical studies localizing the offending antigens have not been performed, but fungal hyphae of *Aspergillus* are regularly visible on conventional microscopy of ABPA and in approximately 50% of BG cases. Likewise, tissue analyses showing IgE in bronchial walls are lacking. However, in view of the clinical data available on these disorders,[66] it would be expected that IgE-fungal antigenic complexes should indeed be demonstrable in the bronchial mucosa by specialized microscopic techniques. The leukocytic infiltrate in ABPA and BG is mainly eosinophilic, and therefore deposits of eosinophil basic protein are evident immunohistologically in and around diseased airways.

Polyarteritis Nodosa

Polyarteritis nodosa (PAN) rather uncommonly affects the pulmonary arterial vasculature. Nevertheless, it may do so, and therefore enters into differential diagnosis with other vasculitides such as Wegener's granulomatosis and allergic (Churg-Strauss) angiitis (see below). PAN is unique among this group of disorders in that it is the only condition that regularly is associated with circulating immune complexes; these are also demonstrable within the walls of inflamed medium-sized arteries in the lung. Roughly 30% of PAN cases show deposition of IgG and C3 together with hepatitis B surface antigen in such complexes[59,67]; the antigenic moieties in remaining cases are less well defined but may include biochemical constituents of other infectious agents. Healing vascular lesions exhibit reduplication of basement membranes, as detected with immunostains for collagen type IV; in contrast, evolving foci of vasculitis manifest interrupted collagen type IV reactivity because of damage to the endothelial basal lamina. The number of endothelial cells, and their location in PAN lesions, can be elucidated with the use of such antibodies as anti-factor VIII–related antigen; EN4; or BMA-120. *Ulex europaeus* I lectin also may be utilized for the same purpose.

Goodpasture's Syndrome

Goodpasture's syndrome (anti-glomerular basement membrane [GBM] disease) is the prototype of cytopathic antibody-mediated lung disease. In this condition, autoantibody formation occurs against a restricted basement membrane antigen shared by glomerular and pulmonary alveolar capillaries (as well as other vessels), and usually is represented by IgG subclasses 1 and/or 3.[68] Historically, it has been thought that conjugation of these antibodies with basement membranes was sufficient in and of itself to effect tissue damage, by activation of the complement cascade. However, recent investigations have questioned this premise, at least in regard to the pulmonary capillary vasculature. It is now thought that other factors, such as cigarette smoking, may be necessary for autoantibody to produce fully developed lesions in the lung in Goodpasture's syndrome.

Although this issue is of pathobiological interest, it has little bearing on the use of immunohistology for the diagnosis of pulmonary anti-glomerular basement membrane disease. Transbronchial or open biopsy specimens in this disorder demonstrate *linear* staining for IgG along alveolar capillary walls, usually along with C3 (Fig. 21-8).[69] The pattern of reactivity has been emphasized here to distinguish Goodpasture's syndrome from the pneumonitides of collagen vascular disease, which exhibit *granular* deposits of immunoglobulin.[70] As described above, damage to vascular basement membranes

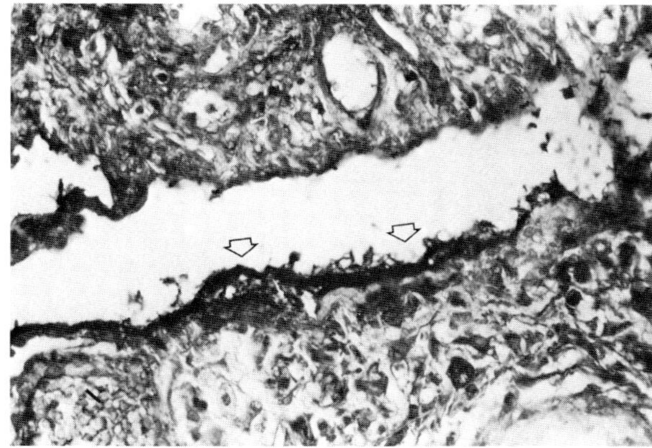

Figure 21-8. Linear staining for IgG in an alveolar ductal wall (arrows) in a case of Good-pasture's (anti-glomerular basement membrane) syndrome.

and lining cells may be assessed with antibodies to collagen type IV, laminin, and endothelial determinants.

Diseases Typified by Prominent Interstitial Fibrosis

Despite the fact that a multitude of pneumonitides may eventuate in end-stage interstitial fibrosis ("honeycomb lung"), the number of lung diseases dominated by amplified collagen deposition is relatively low. These are represented by diffuse alveolar damage, idiopathic pulmonary fibrosis (UIP, see above), the pneumoconioses, and bronchiolitis obliterans-organizing pneumonia.

Diffuse Alveolar Damage

Diffuse alveolar damage may be caused by diverse insults to the lung, including, among others, infection with viruses, mycoplasma, or protozoans; inhaled toxins; various medications; irradiation; and shock.[71] Regardless of its etiology, this disorder progresses through two reproducible tissue phases: first, exudation of serum proteins into alveolar spaces, inflammation, and denudation of alveolar epithelium; and second, fibroblast proliferation with organization.

In the initial stages of diffuse alveolar damage, one may therefore detect loss of types I and II alveolar pneumocytes with immunostains for cytokeratin, EMA, Ber-EP4, and pulmonary surfactant (Fig. 21-9). Loss of vascular integrity and damage to basement membranes are demonstrable with appropriate endothelial and basal laminar determinants. Inflammatory cells are heterogeneous in phase I of the disease and are labeled by myeloid, lymphoid, and monocyte/macrophage antibodies. Suppressor-cytotoxic lymphocytes, recognized by UCHL-1, MT-1, and by CD3, CD5, and CD6–8, predominate among mononuclear cells.

One of the most intriguing facets of diffuse alveolar damage concerns which cases will progress to severe interstitial fibrosis, as opposed to those that show remodeling with recovery of normal tissue structure. In recent years, cytokines derived from infiltrating lymphocytes and monocytes in phase I have come under scrutiny in this regard.

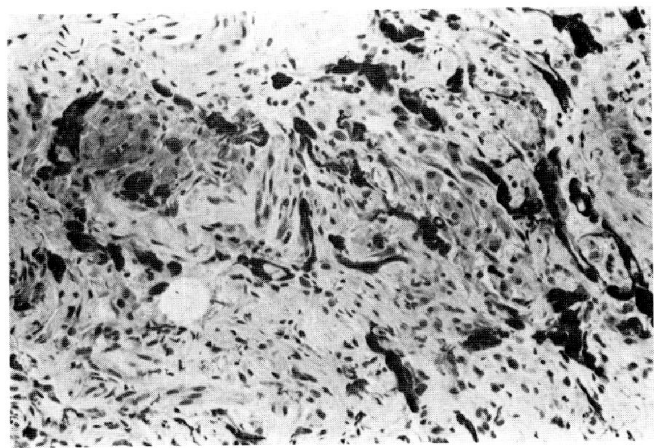

Figure 21-9. Focal loss of alveolar pneumocytes in diffuse alveolar damage, as shown by immunostaining for low molecular weight cytokeratin.

One possible explanation for adverse clinical outcomes in diffuse alveolar damage is that in some cases, monocytes/macrophages may secrete various fibrogenic moieties that stimulate ongoing collagen synthesis (e.g., IL1 or FGF), under the "direction" of T-lymphocytes producing macrophage migration-inhibitory factor, IL2, and angiogenic factors. Angiogenic factors are thought to act as an integral part of collagenesis by stimulating granulation tissue ingrowth, and they have been detected in bronchoalveolar lavage fluids and cell-culture models of diffuse alveolar damage (P. Bitterman, personal communication). In the intermediate stages of the disease, we have demonstrated an excess of small-caliber, intra-alveolar blood vessels using antibodies to endothelial markers (Fig. 21-10). The number of type II pneumocytes seen at the end of stage I also may have a bearing on the ability of the lung to re-epithelialize alveolar spaces, and may be evaluated with anti-surfactant immunostains.

The late stages of unresolved, fibrosing diffuse alveolar damage are characterized by an increase in types I and III matrix collagen.[54,72] As in other conditions featuring vascular damage and repair, the quantity of type IV collagen is also increased (Fig. 21-11).

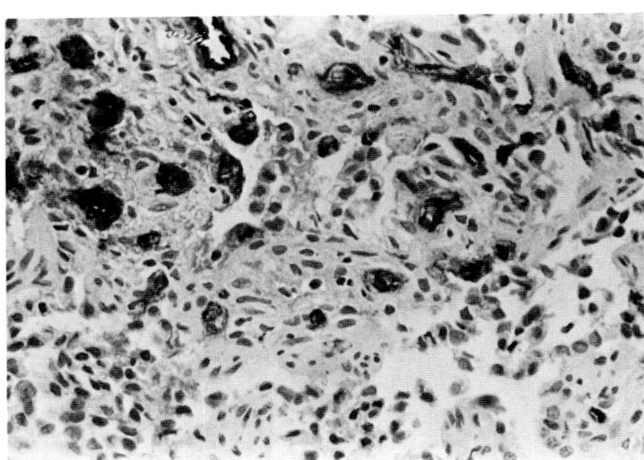

Figure 21-10. Numerous small blood vessels are evident within proliferating granulation tissue in this example of intermediate-phase diffuse alveolar damage, as shown with an immunostain for factor VIII-related antigen.

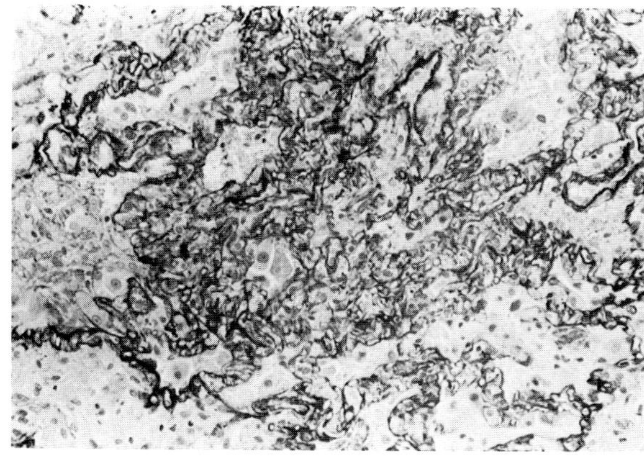

Figure 21-11. Increased deposition of collagen type IV is seen in late-stage diffuse alveolar damage, as shown by an immunostain for this collagen type.

Idiopathic Pulmonary Fibrosis and the Pneumoconioses

The end stage of UIP (idiopathic pulmonary fibrosis) and fibrosing pneumoconioses such as silicosis and asbestosis are similarly typified by progressive augmentation of pulmonary interstitial collagen and loss of normal epithelia/endothelia, as discussed above. However, little has been done to date to assess the impact of cytokines on the evolution of these disorders, at least immunohistologically. This topic should be of considerable interest in light of the fact that several occupational lung diseases are now thought to be partly immunologic in origin, in that lymphoreticular cell products are released by macrophages that have ingested foreign materials.[73] Hence, studies of interleukin localization, as well as the presence of other inflammatory cell products, are warranted in this group of pneumonopathies.

Bronchiolitis Obliterans-Organizing Pneumonitis

The constellation of bronchiolitis obliterans-organizing pneumonitis (BOOP) is now recognized as a distinctive pathologic entity, characterized by effacement of bronchiolar lumina by proliferating fibrous tissue.[74] This reaction pattern shows certain similarities to that of lung allograft rejection, but demonstrates a greater degree of organizing inflammation in the parenchyma surrounding affected bronchioles.

The dynamics of epithelial cell loss, granulation tissue ingrowth, and progressive intraluminal fibrosis have not been well studied immunohistochemically in BOOP. One may employ stains for epithelial markers to enumerate remaining bronchial lining cells; the predominant luminal collagen subclass in the early stages of this disorder is type III.[54,75] Detailed assessments of inflammatory cells in BOOP have not yet been undertaken.

Diseases Characterized by Cellular Infiltrates

Predominant cellular infiltrates are observed in several interstitial pneumonitides. Histiocytosis-X, sarcoidosis, hypersensitivity pneumonitis, allograft rejection, lymphocytic

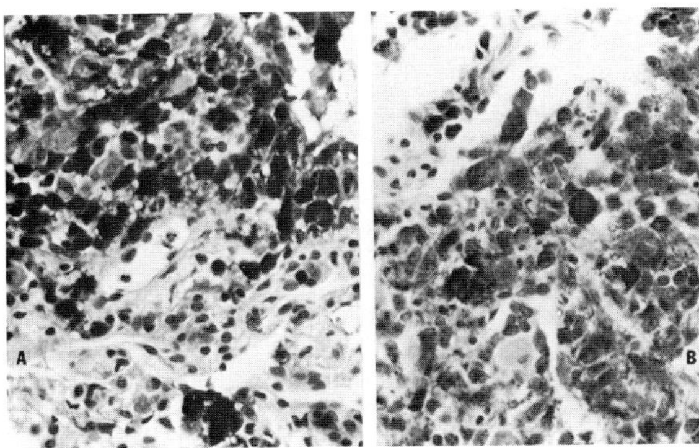

Figure 21-12. Immunoreactivity for S-100 protein (*A*) and HLA-DR antigen (*B*) in an example of pulmonary histiocytosis-X.

interstitial pneumonitis, and angiocentric immunoproliferative lesions ("lymphomatoid granulomatosis") must be included in this category.

Histiocytosis-X

Histiocytosis-X ("eosinophilic granuloma;" Langerhans cell granulomatosis) is a potentially systemic disease that can, in selected instances, affect the lung alone. In such instances the disorder may be confused with other interstitial pneumonitides.

As its name suggests, histiocytosis-X is characterized by the proliferation of a unique cell type; namely, the Langerhans cell. In viscera or lymph nodes, the Langerhans cell shows morphological identity with intraepidermal dendritic cells of the skin and has an analogous immunophenotype. Langerhans cells exhibit conjoint reactivity with CD1 antibodies (T6; Leu 6) and anti–S-100 protein, and express class II HLA determinants as well (Fig. 21-12).[39–41,76] They are often accompanied by eosinophilic infiltrates of variable intensity, which may be highlighted with reagents against eosinophil basic protein. Immunoreactivity for monocyte/macrophage antigens is heterogeneous, but we have observed positivity with anti-cathepsin B and MAC-387 in some cases of histiocytosis-X. Pan-T, pan-B, and lymphocyte subset markers are absent in the histiocytoid cells of eosinophilic granuloma, with the exception of MT-1.

The mere identification of Langerhans cells in a pulmonary infiltrate is not sufficient to establish the diagnosis of histiocytosis-X, because several other conditions may demonstrate variable numbers of these elements. However, Webber and co-workers found that immunoreactivity for S-100 protein was invariably associated with histiocytosis-X when more than 75 positive cells were found per ten high-power (× 400) microscopic fields. Clustering of cells marking for S-100 protein also was an important criterion in their study.[39]

Sarcoidosis and Hypersensitivity Pneumonitis

Although they are quite different clinically in most cases, sarcoidosis and hypersensitivity pneumonitis share significant similarities under the microscope. Both may feature a lymphoid cellular infiltrate in the pulmonary interstitium, punctuated by epithelioid granulomas.[77,78]

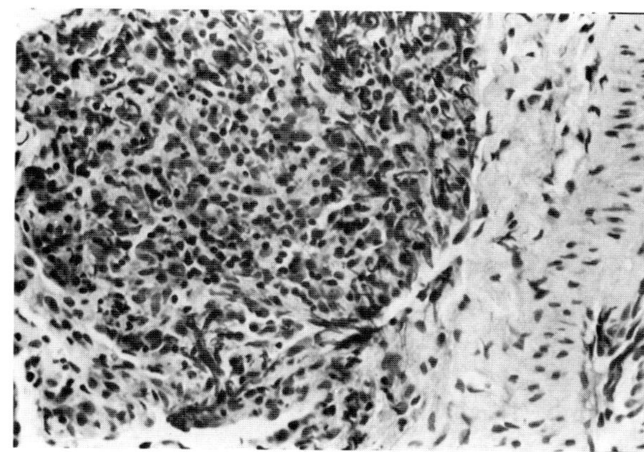

Figure 21-13. Expression of CD8 antigen on the surfaces of infiltrating lymphocytes, in an immunostained biopsy specimen from a case of allograft rejection.

In cases where a definitive separation of these pathologic entities cannot be obtained by other means, immunohistologic evaluation is helpful. Participating lymphocytes in sarcoidosis are primarily T-helper (CD4+) cells,[79–81] whereas those in hypersensitivity pneumonitis belong to the T-suppressor/cytotoxic (CD8+) group.[81] Akiyama and co-workers demonstrated a similar antigenic profile for the epithelioid histiocytes in both diseases,[43] and Costabel and associates showed that lymphoid cells in both conditions expressed class II HLA determinants.[82] Using in situ hybridization for class II HLA mRNA, Spurzem and colleagues claimed that alveolar epithelium was negative for HLA-DR, HLA-DP, and HLA-DQ in sarcoidosis,[83] but this contention was not upheld by immunohistologic results reported by Kallenberg and associates.[52] As mentioned earlier in this discussion, some cases of hypersensitivity pneumonitis exhibit immunoreactivity for interstitial immune complexes, whereas sarcoidosis has not been reported to do so.

Allograft Rejection

Inasmuch as advances in immunomodulatory therapy have now made lung transplantation a practical reality, pulmonologists are faced with the need to evaluate lung allograft rejection. Although data on this topic are still preliminary, it would appear that most examples of lung transplant rejection are cellular in nature. Lymphocytes are seen in and around alveolar ducts, small pulmonary arteries, and bronchioles in this condition, and they typically express T-suppressor/cytotoxic or natural killer (positive for pan-T, CD2, CD8, and CD16) phenotypes (Fig. 21-13). Bronchial and alveolar duct epithelium also demonstrates class II HLA determinants in rejection, as do the infiltrating lymphoid cells.

Another prominent tissue change in failing allografts is the presence of bronchiolitis obliterans. Indeed, this may be so prominent that airway lumina are completely effaced, necessitating the use of special stains for epithelial cells and smooth muscle (cytokeratin, EMA, Ber-EP4, desmin) in order to outline bronchiolar structures. To date, immunohistochemistry has not been employed to determine whether or not bronchiolitis obliterans–rejection reactions differ in any way from BOOP. For example,

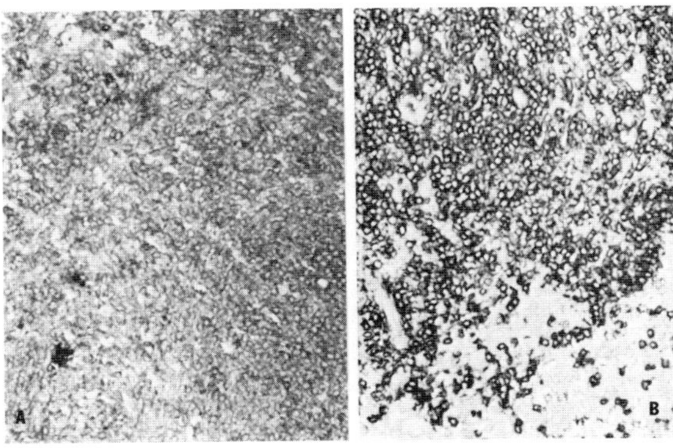

Figure 21-14. Lack of immunoreactivity for kappa light chain immunoglobulin (*A*) contrasts with positivity for lambda light chain (*B*), in a monotypic example of "lymphocytic interstitial pneumonitis."

it may be possible that lymphocytes in allograft rejection will express CD26 and CD30 antigens, whereas such a profile would not be expected in other inflammatory pneumonopathies.

Lymphocytic Interstitial Pneumonitis

Lymphocytic interstitial pneumonitis (LIP) now appears to represent a nonuniform group of disorders, most of which are probably neoplastic rather than inflammatory in nature.[84–87] With this premise in mind, the immunohistologic features of three tentatively identified subsets will be discussed. These are idiopathic polytypic LIP; idiopathic monotypic LIP; and LIP associated with infection by human immunodeficiency virus (HIV) or Epstein-Barr virus (EBV).

Idiopathic polytypic LIP reflects the original conception of this disease as a benign lymphoproliferative interstitial pulmonary disorder.[85] Morphologically, it is composed of aggregates of small lymphocytes, which expand alveolar septa and focally form nodules within the lung parenchyma. Germinal centers are often apparent as well. Immunohistologically, this form of LIP demonstrates polymorphism of the constituent lymphocytes; they are predominantly B-cells, showing a mixture of lambda and kappa light chain surface immunoglobulin (polyclonality); a lesser number of T-cells are evident.

It was formerly thought that germinal center formation was an inviolate indicator of benignancy in LIP; nevertheless, the monotypic idiopathic variant of this disease proves otherwise. The monotypic subtype is identical to polytypic LIP in nearly all morphologic respects, but it differs importantly in exhibiting monoclonality for either lambda or kappa surface immunoglobulin (defined by a ratio of at least 10:1) (Fig. 21-14).[86] This observation is crucial to prognosis, because long-term follow-up studies indicate that monotypic LIP is, in fact, a low-grade malignant lymphoma.[86,87]

The recent availability of ISH procedures is responsible for the delineation of the third category of LIP cases—those associated with HIV or EBV.[88–90] Viral genomic segments are detectable in proliferating lymphocytes in these examples of the disease, which usually occur in clinically immunocompromised individuals. Relatively few studies have been published on the immunophenotype of virus-related LIP, but it would appear that CD8 cells are overrepresented therein.[88,89] Clonality analyses of participating B cells have not been undertaken; however, the clinical course of the disorder has been indolent in most instances.

Angiocentric Immunoproliferative Lesions (AIL)

Pulmonary lymphoid lesions originally classified as "lymphomatoid granulomatosis"[91] are currently known as AIL.[92] These peculiar proliferations feature the presence of variably mature lymphocytes in pulmonary perivascular arrays, often with foci of geographic necrosis and arterial mural necrosis. A minority exhibit overt cytologic anaplasia and are microscopically identical to large cell lymphomas in extrapulmonary sites.

The NIH group has proposed that AIL be considered as a unified group of clonal T-lymphoid malignancies, regardless of their histologic characteristics.[92] These lesions show a predominance of T lymphocytes having abnormal phenotypes, such as the expression of subset markers (CD4, CD8) in the absence of pan-T determinants (CD3, CD5, CD7) or the presence of "activation" markers (e.g., CD30). Variable numbers of B lymphocytes are detectable in AIL, but they occasionally may be so numerous as to obscure the underlying T-cell clone.

Diseases Featuring the Presence of Vasculitis

Relatively few pulmonary diseases are characterized by the presence of large-vessel vasculitis; they include polyarteritis nodosa, Wegener's granulomatosis, allergic angiitis (Churg-Strauss syndrome), and infectious vasculitides. PAN has already been discussed and will be considered only in contrast to the other entities in this category. In addition, it is now generally accepted that Wegener's disease and Churg-Strauss lesions probably represent points in a continuum, and they will be presented accordingly.

Wegener's Granulomatosis/Churg-Strauss Syndrome

Both Wegener's granulomatosis and the Churg-Strauss syndrome are characterized by prominent intramural vascular inflammation affecting both pulmonary arteries and veins. Both also feature the presence of regional parenchymal necrosis and the formation of extravascular granulomas. However, they differ clinically in that classic Churg-Strauss syndrome occurs in patients with a history of atopic tendencies and tends to affect the heart and splenic artery, whereas Wegener's granulomatosis does not. Lastly, lesions of Churg-Strauss syndrome exhibit a greater degree of tissue eosinophilia. These points notwithstanding, Yousem and Lombard[93] have reported several cases of pulmonary vasculitis that bridge the differences just cited. Moreover, the immunologic attributes of these conditions are similar; they lack the presence of immune complex deposition (unlike PAN), and cellular infiltrates in each of them are primarily composed of T cells.[94] Alterations in basement membrane proteins, endothelial antigens, and stromal collagen types parallel those seen in PAN and do not assist in differential diagnosis.

Infectious Vasculitides

Although experienced histopathologists can usually discern the presence of infectious processes that cause vasculitis by conventional morphologic means, such is not always the case. Certain mycobacterial or fungal infections may closely simulate Wegener's

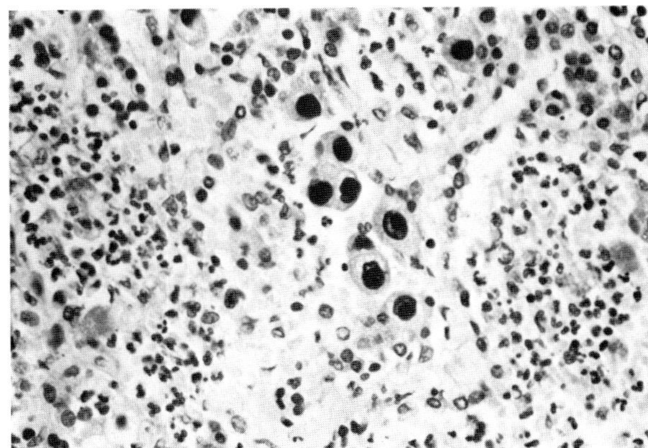

Figure 21-15. Several alveolar macrophages are immunoreactive for a conserved cytomegalovirus antigen (*center of photograph*) in case of viral pneumonitis that had the appearance of diffuse alveolar damage by conventional microscopy.

granulomatosis or allergic angiitis. Therefore, histochemical stains designed to detect such agents must be used in all cases of large-vessel pulmonary vasculitis. Furthermore, Humphrey and Weiner[49] have shown that a certain proportion of mycobacterial pneumonitides are recognizable only with immunohistochemical stains for mycobacterial membrane antigens. Currently, it would appear that approximately 7% of mycobacterioses are immunopositive for these markers in the absence of detectable bacilli on Ziehl-Nielsen or Fite stains[49]; these may be confused diagnostically with the idiopathic vasculitides if arterial involvement is prominent.

SPECIFIC DIFFERENTIAL DIAGNOSTIC CONSIDERATIONS

Several differential diagnoses of interest to pulmonary pathologists have been presented in the context of commentaries on individual disease entities. Others that merit additional emphasis or re-emphasis will be considered here.

Usual Interstitial Pneumonia vs. Viral Pneumonitis

Idiopathic UIP occasionally may be simulated clinically and pathologically by a variety of viral infections, including those due to respiratory syncitial virus, cytomegalovirus, adenovirus, and influenza virus. Antibody reagents that are specific for all these organisms are available and should be applied as indicated by the nuances of the clinical presentation.

Diffuse Alveolar Damage vs. Infectious Processes

Especially in immunosuppressed patients, the diagnosis of idiopathic diffuse alveolar damage is one of exclusion. Cytomegalovirus, herpesvirus, adenovirus, *Pneumocystis,* and *Toxoplasma* all may closely mimic the changes seen in alveolar damage syndromes due to noninfectious causes (Fig. 21-15). Accordingly, immunostains for these microbes are strongly recommended in the context under discussion.

Allograft Rejection vs. Viral Infection

It is well known by transplantation pathologists that tissue changes mediated by allograft rejection in the liver, heart, or kidney may be perfectly recapitulated by viral infection, most commonly with cytomegalovirus. Our preliminary experience would suggest that the lung is no exception to this rule. Hence, immunohistologic or ISH evaluation for occult viral disease is strongly recommended in the assessment of transplant biopsies.

Sarcoidosis vs. Hypersensitivity Pneumonitis vs. Infection

In cases lacking a definitive clinical history for hypersensitivity pneumonitis, its histologic separation from sarcoidosis is challenging. Immunohistologically, one observes a preponderance of CD4+ T cells in the latter condition, but a dominance of CD8+ lymphocytes in the former. Similarly, infection with fungi or mycobacteria can mimic sarcoidosis, and again antibody-enzyme techniques supplement histochemical stains for microorganisms in making this distinction.

Hemorrhagic Pneumonopathies

Goodpasture's syndrome is confused in some cases with idiopathic pulmonary hemosiderosis or with septal capillaritis-pneumonitis of collagen vascular diseases. The characteristic linear staining pattern for IgG and C3 in alveolar septal capillary walls demonstrated in Goodpasture's syndrome contrasts with the granular reactivity seen in lupus erythematosus or rheumatoid arthritis. In contrast, pulmonary hemosiderosis shows no interstitial immunoglobulin binding whatever.

ADJUNCTIVE SEROLOGIC METHODS

No further mention need be made here of the utility of serologic assays for antinuclear antibodies, rheumatoid factor, and circulating immune complexes in the assessment of interstitial pneumonitides. Nevertheless, the recent observation that patients with Wegener's granulomatosis possess antibodies to cytoplasmic neutrophil antigens promises to assist in the definitive diagnosis of this troublesome disorder.[95–97] To date, histologically similar lung diseases have been associated only infrequently with positivity for this assay.

THE FUTURE

This chapter has focused on current knowledge on the specialized tissue immunology of selected pulmonary diseases. However, this field is in its infancy, and the future holds great promise. A more complete understanding of antigenic targets of immunologic lung diseases at a molecular level, together with the development of suitable assays to detect immune derangements involving them, should greatly enhance our abilities to identify and treat these conditions in the years to come.

REFERENCES

1. Coons AH, Creech JH, Jones RN. Immunological properties of an antibody containing a fluorescent group. Proc Soc Exp Biol Med 1941;47:200–202.
2. Sternberger LA, Hardy PH, Cuculis JJ, Meyer HG. The unlabeled antibody enzyme method for immunohistochemistry. Preparation and properties of soluble antigen-antibody complex (horseradish peroxidase–anti-horseradish peroxidase) and its use in the identification of spirochetes. J Histochem Cytochem 1970;18:315–333.
3. Vacca LL, Abrahams SJ, Naftchi NE. A modified peroxidase-antiperoxidase procedure for improved localization of tissue antigens. J Histochem Cytochem 1980;28:297–307.
4. Hsu SM, Raine L, Fanger H. Use of avidin-biotin-peroxidase complex (ABC) in immunoperoxidase techniques: A comparison between ABC and unlabeled antibody (PAP) procedures. J Histochem Cytochem 1981;29:577–580.
5. Swanson PE, Wick MR. Avidin-biotin-peroxidase complex kits. Am J Clin Pathol 1989;91 (suppl 1):S43–S44.
6. Cordell JL, Falini B, Erber W, Gatter KC, Mason DY. Immunoenzymatic labeling of monoclonal antibodies using complexes of alkaline phosphatase and monoclonal anti-alkaline phosphatase (APAAP complexes). J Histochem Cytochem 1984;32:219–229.
7. Suffin SC, Muck KB, Young JC. Improvement of the glucose oxidase immunoenzyme technique. Am J Clin Pathol 1979;71:492–496.
8. Gown AM. Immunoglucose oxidase methods in immunohistochemistry. In: DeLellis RA, ed. Advances in immunohistochemistry. New York: 1988, Raven Press, 31.
9. Swanson PE, Hagen KA, Wick MR. Avidin-biotin-peroxidase-antiperoxidase complex: An immunocytochemical method with enhanced sensitivity. Am J Clin Pathol 1987;88:162–176.
10. Hacker GW, Springall DR, Van Noorden S, Bishop AE, Grimelius L, Polak JM. The immunogold-silver staining method. Virchows Arch (Pathol Anat) 1985;406:449–461.
11. Warhol MJ. Immunoelectron microscopy in diagnostic pathology. In: DeLellis RA, ed. Advances in immunohistochemistry. New York: Raven Press, 1988, 67.
12. Hofler H, DeLellis RA, Wolfe HJ. In situ hybridization and immunohistochemistry. In: DeLellis RA, ed. Advances in immunohistochemistry. New York: Raven Press, 1988, 47.
13. Curran RC, Gregory J. The unmasking of antigens in paraffin sections of tissue by trypsin. Experientia 1977;33:1400–1401.
14. McLean IW. Nakane PK. Periodate-lysine-paraformaldehyde fixative. J Histochem Cytochem 1974;22:1077–1083.
15. Stein H, Gatter KC, Heryet A, Mason DY. Freeze-dried paraffin-embedded human tissue for antigen labeling with monoclonal antibodies. Lancet 1984;ii:71–73.
16. Andrade RE, Hagen KA, Swanson PE, Wick MR. The use of ficin for proteolysis in immunostaining of paraffin sections. Am J Clin Pathol 1988;90:33–39.
17. Warnke R. Alteration of immunoglobulin-bearing lymphoma cells by fixation. J Histochem Cytochem 1979;27:1195–1196.
18. Moll R, Franke WW, Schiller DL, Geiger B, Krepler R. The catalogue of human cytokeratins. Cell 1982;31:11–24.
19. Traub P. Are intermediate filament proteins involved in gene expression? Ann NY Acad Sci 1985;455:68–78.
20. Pinkus GS, Kurtin PJ. Epithelial membrane antigen: A diagnostic discriminant in surgical pathology. Hum Pathol 1985;16:929–940.
21. Momburg F, Moldenhauer G, Hammerling GJ, Moller P. Immunohistochemical study of the expression of a M_r 34,000 human epithelium-specific surface glycoprotein in normal and malignant tissues. Cancer Res 1987;47:2883–2891.

22. Singh G, Singh J, Katyal SL, Brown WE, Kramps JH, Paradis IL, Dauber JH, MacPherson TA, Squeglia N. Identification, cellular localization, isolation, and characterization of human Clara-cell-specific 10 kD protein. J Histochem Cytochem 1988;36:73–80.
23. Kawai T, Torikata C, Suzuki M. Immunohistochemical study of pulmonary adenocarcinoma. Am J Clin Pathol 1988;89:455–462.
24. Finkbeiner WE, Basbaum CB. Monoclonal antibodies directed against human airway secretions: Localization and characterization of antigens. Am J Pathol 1988;131:290–297.
25. Wick MR. Anitbodies to desmin in diagnostic pathology. In: Wick MR, Siegal GP, eds. Monoclonal antibodies in diagnostic immunohistochemistry. New York: Marcel Dekker, 1988, 93.
26. Altmannsberger J, Osborn M, Schauer A, Weber K. Antibodies to different intermediate filament proteins: Cell type-specific markers on paraffin-embedded human tissues. Lab Invest 1981; 45:427–434.
27. Alles JU, Bosslet K. Immunohistochemical and immunochemical characterization of a new endothelial cell-specific antigen. J Histochem Cytochem 1986;34:209–214.
28. Ordonez NG, Batsakis JG. Comparison of *Ulex europaeus* I lectin and factor VIII-related antigen in vascular lesions. Arch Pathol Lab Med 1984;108:129–132.
29. Fleischmajer R, et al. Biology, chemistry, and pathology of collagen. Ann NY Acad Sci 1985;460:1–31.
30. Konomi H, Hayashi T, Nakayasu K, Arima M. Localization of type V collagen and type IV collagen in human cornea, lung, and skin. Am J Pathol 1984;116:417–426.
31. Lee AK. Basement membrane and endothelial antigens. In: DeLellis RA, ed. Advances in immunohistochemistry. New York: Raven Press, 1988, 363.
32. Pusey CD, Dash A, Kershaw MJ, Morgan A, Reilly A, Rees AJ, Lockwood CM. A single autoantigen in Goodpasture's syndrome identified by a monoclonal antibody to human glomerular basement membrane. Lab Invest 1987;56:23–31.
33. Cashman SJ, Pusey CD, Evans DJ. Extraglomerular distribution of immunoreactive Goodpasture antigen. J Pathol 1988;155:61–70.
34. Knapp W, Dorken B, Rieber P, Schmidt RE, Stein H, Von dem Borne AEGK. CD antigens 1989. Am J Pathol 1989;135:420–421.
35. Andrade RE, Wick MR, Frizzera G, Gajl-Peczalska K. Immunophenotyping of hematopoietic malignancies in paraffin sections. Hum Pathol 1988;19:394–403.
36. Cartun RW, Coles FB, Pastuszak WT. Utilization of monoclonal antibody L26 in the identification and confirmation of B-cell lymphomas. Am J Pathol 1987;129:415–421.
37. Pulford KAF, Rigney EM, Micklem KJ, Cordell J, Mason DY. KP1—a new monoclonal antibody that detects a monocyte/macrophage-associated antigen in routinely processed tissue sections. J Clin Pathol 1989;42:414–421.
38. Swerdlow SH, Wright SA. The spectrum of Leu-M1 staining in lymphoid and hematopoietic proliferations. Am J Clin Pathol 1986;85:283–288.
39. Webber D, Tron V, Askin F, Churg A. S-100 staining in the diagnosis of eosinophilic granuloma of lung. Am J Clin Pathol 1985;84:447–453.
40. Kim CK, Swerdlow SH, Ray M, Weiss MA. Immunoperoxidase staining for S-100 protein in the diagnosis of eosinophilic granuloma of lung. Am J Clin Pathol 1986;86:125–126.
41. Flint A, Lloyd RV, Colby TV, Wilson BW. Pulmonary histiocytosis X: Immunoperoxidase staining for HLA-DR antigen and S-100 protein. Arch Pathol Lab Med 1986;110:930–933.
42. Young JD, et al. Mechanisms of membrane damage mediated by human eosinophil cationic protein. Nature 1986;321:613–617.
43. Akiyama JI, Chida K, Sato A, Yamashita A. Four monoclonal antibodies, AMH-1, -2, -3, and -4, give varied reactivities with monocytes, alveolar macrophages, and epithelioid-cell granulomas. J Clin Immunol 1988;8:372–380.

44. Kobzik L, Godleski JJ, Biondi A, O'Hara CJ, Todd RF III. Immunohistologic analysis of a human pulmonary alveolar macrophage antigen. Clin Immunol Immunopathol 1985;37:213–219.

45. Swanson PE. Monoclonal antibodies to monomorphic human histocompatibility antigens: Class I (HLA A,B, C), class II (HLA-DR or Ia-like antigen), and beta-2 microglobulin. In: Wick MR, Siegal GP, eds. Monoclonal antibodies in diagnostic immunohistochemistry. New York: Marcel Dekker, 1988, 309.

46. Crystal RG, Gadek JE, Ferrans VJ, Fulmer JD, Line BR, Hunninghake GW. Interstitial lung disease: Current concepts of pathogenesis, staging, and therapy. Am J Med 1981;70:542–568.

47. Colby TV, Weiss RL. Current concepts in the surgical pathology of pulmonary infections. Am J Surg Pathol 1987;11 (suppl 1):25–37.

48. Kaye VN. Monoclonal antibodies to microbial antigens in diagnostic pathology. In: Wick MR, Siegal GP, eds. Monoclonal antibodies in diagnostic immunohistochemistry. New York: Marcel Dekker, 1988, 623.

49. Humphrey DM, Weiner NH. Mycobacterial antigen detection by immunohistochemistry in pulmonary tuberculosis. Hum Pathol 1987;18:701–708.

50. Eisenberg H, Simmons DH, Barnett EV. Diffuse pulmonary interstitial disease: An immunohistologic study. Chest 1979;75 (suppl):262–264.

51. Dreisin RB, Schwartz MI, Theophilopoulos AM, et al. Circulating immune complexes in the idiopathic interstitial pneumonitides. N Engl J Med 1978;298:354–358.

52. Kallenberg CGM, Schilizzi BM, Beaumont F, De Leij L, Poppema S, The TH. Expression of class II major histocompatibility complex antigens on alveolar epithelium in interstitial lung disease: Relevance to pathogenesis of idiopathic pulmonary fibrosis. J Clin Pathol 1987;40:725–733.

53. Hammar SP, Winterbauer RH, Bockus D, Remington F, Friedman S. Idiopathic fibrosing alveolitis: A review with emphasis on ultrastructural and immunohistochemical features. Ultrastruct Pathol 1985;9:345–372.

54. Kuhn C III, Boldt J, King TE Jr, Crouch E, Vartio T, McDonald JA. An immunohistochemical study of architectural remodeling and connective tissue synthesis in pulmonary fibrosis. Am Rev Respir Dis 1989;140:1693–1703.

55. Saldiva PHN, Delmonte VC, de Carvalho CRR, Kairalla RA, Auler JOC Jr. Histochemical evaluation of lung collagen content in acute and chronic interstitial diseases. Chest 1989;95:953–957.

56. Takiya C, Peyrol S, Cordier JF, Grimaud JA. Connective matrix organization in human pulmonary fibrosis. Virchows Arch (Cell Pathol) 1983;44:223–240.

57. Pines A, Kaplinsky N, Olchovsky D, Rozenman J, Frankl O. Pleuropulmonary manifestations of systemic lupus erythematosus: Clinical features of its subgroups. Chest 1985;88:129–135.

58. Inoue T, Kanayama Y, Ohe A, Kato N, Horiguchi T, Ishii M, Shiota K. Immunopathologic studies of pneumonitis in systemic lupus erythematosus. Ann Intern Med 1979;91:30–34.

59. McCluskey RT, Fienberg R. Vasculitis in primary vasculitides, granulomatoses, and connective tissue diseases. Hum Pathol 1983;14:305–315.

60. Myers JL, Katzenstein A-LA. Microangiitis in lupus-induced pulmonary hemorrhage. Am J Clin Pathol 1986;85:552–556.

61. Warwick MT, Haslam P. Antibodies in some chronic fibrosing lung diseases. Clin Allergy 1971;1:83–95.

62. Braun SR, Flaherty DK, Burrell R, Rankin J. Importance of anti-lung antibody in farmer's lung disease. Am J Med 1983;74:535–539.

63. Eade OE, Hodges JR, Berrill WT, Lang C, Lloyd RS, Wright R. Immunofluorescent antibodies in patients with bird-fancier's lung. Clin Exp Immunol 1978;32:259–262.

64. Ghose T, Landrigan P, Killeen R, Dill J. Immunopathological studies in patients with farmer's lung. Clin Allergy 1974;4:119–128.

65. Smets P, Gari M, Pinon JM, Seguela JP. Diagnosis of pigeon breeder's disease by indirect immunofluorescence on sections of pigeon oviduct. Clin Allergy 1983;13:57–60.

66. Clee MD, Lamb D, Clark RA. Bronchocentric granulomatosis: A review and thoughts on pathogenesis. Br J Dis Chest 1983;77:227–234.

67. Kadison P, Haynes BF. Vasculitis: Mechanisms of vessel damage. In: Gallin J, et al, eds. Inflammation: Basic principles and clinical correlates. New York: Raven Press, 1988, 703.

68. Leatherman JW, Davies SF, Hoidal JR. Alveolar hemorrhage syndromes: Diffuse microvascular lung hemorrhage in immune and idiopathic disorders. Medicine 1984;63:343–361.

69. Beechler CR, Enquist RW, Hunt KK, Ward GW, Knieser MR. Immunofluorescence of transbronchial biopsies in Goodpasture's syndrome. Am Rev Respir Dis 1980;121:869–872.

70. Katzenstein A-LA, Askin FB. Surgical pathology of non-neoplastic lung disease. 2nd ed. Philadelphia: WB Saunders, 1990, 203.

71. Katzenstein A-LA, Askin FB: Surgical pathology of non-neoplastic lung disease. 2nd ed. Philadelphia: WB Saunders, 1990, 11.

72. Last SA, Siefkin AD, Reiser KM. Type I collagen content is increased in lungs of patients with adult respiratory distress syndrome. Thorax 1983;38:364–368.

73. Schmidt JA, et al. Silica-stimulated monocytes release fibroblast proliferation factors identical to interleukin-1. J Clin Invest 1984;73:1462–1468.

74. Katzenstein A-LA, Myers, JL, et al. Bronchiolitis obliterans and usual interstitial pneumonia: A comparative clinicopathologic study. Am J Surg Pathol 1986;10:373–381.

75. Basset F, Ferrans VS, Foler P, Takemura T, Fukuda Y, Crystal RG. Intraluminal fibrosis in interstitial lung disorders. Am J Pathol 1986;122:443–461.

76. Chollet S, Soler P, Dournovo P, et al. Diagnosis of pulmonary histiocytosis X by immunodetection of Langerhans' cells in bronchoalveolar lavage fluid. Am J Pathol 1984;115:225–232.

77. Rosen Y, Athanassiades TJ, Moon S, Lyons H. Nongranulomatous interstitial pneumonitis in sarcoidosis. Chest 1978;74:122–125.

78. Coleman A, Colby TV. Histologic diagnosis of extrinsic allergic alveolitis. Am J Surg Pathol 1988;12:514–518.

79. Rossi GA, Sacco O, Cosulich E, Risso A, Balbi B, Ravazzoni C. Helper T-lymphocytes in pulmonary sarcoidosis. Am Rev Respir Dis 1986;133:1086–1090.

80. Spiteri MA, Clarke SW, Poulter LW. Phenotypic and functional changes in alveolar macrophages contribute to the pathogenesis of pulmonary sarcoidosis. Clin Exp Immunol 1988;74: 359–364.

81. Leatherman JW, Michael AF, Schwartz BA, Hoidal JR. Lung T cells in hypersensitivity pneumonitis. Ann Intern Med 1984;100:390–392.

82. Costabel U, Bross KJ, Ruhle KH, Lohr GW, Matthys H. Ia-like antigens on T-cells and their subpopulations in pulmonary sarcoidosis and in hypersensitivity pneumonitis. Am Rev Respir Dis 1985;131:337–342.

83. Spurzem JR, Saltini C, Kirby M, Konishi K, Crystal RG. Expression of HLA class II genes in alveolar macrophages of patients with sarcoidosis. Am Rev Respir Dis 1989;140:89–94.

84. Glickstein M, Kornstein MJ, Pietra GG, Aronchick JM, Gefter WB, Epstein DM, Miller W. Non-lymphomatous lymphoid disorders of the lung. Am J Roentgenol 1986;147:227–237.

85. Koss MN, Hocholzer L, Langloss JM, et al. Lymphocytic interstitial pneumonia: Clinicopathological and immunopathological findings in 18 cases. Pathology 1987;19:178–185.

86. Addis BJ, Hyjek E, Isaacson P. Primary pulmonary lymphoma: A reappraisal of its histogenesis and its relationship to pseudolymphoma and lymphoid interstitial pneumonia. Histopathology 1988;13:1–17.

87. LeTourneau A, Audouin J, Garbe L, Capron F, Servais B, Monges G, Payan H, Diebold J. Primary pulmonary malignant lymphoma: Clinical and pathological findings, immunocytochemical and ultrastructural studies in 15 cases. Hematol Oncol 1983;1:49–60.

88. Solal-Celigny P, Couderc LJ, Herman D, Herve P, Schaffar-Deshayes L, Brune-Vezinet F, Tricot G, Clauvel JP. Lymphoid interstitial pneumonitis in acquired immunodeficiency syndrome–related complex. Am Rev Respir Dis 1985;131:956–960.

89. Guillon JM, Autran B, Denis M, Fouret P, Plata F, Mayaud CM, Akoun GM. Human immunodeficiency virus–related lymphocytic alveolitis. Chest 1989;94:1264–1270.

90. Rubinstein A, Morecki R, Goldman H. Pulmonary disease in infants and children. Clin Chest Med 1988;9:507–517.

91. Koss MN, Hochholzer L, Langloss JM, Wehunt WD, Lazarus AA, Nichols PW. Lymphomatoid granulomatosis: A clinicopathologic study of 42 patients. Pathology 1986;18:283–288.

92. Lipford EH Jr, Margolick JB, et al. Angiocentric immunoproliferative lesions: A clinicopathologic spectrum of post-thymic T-cell proliferations. Blood 1988;72:1674–1681.

93. Yousem SA, Lombard CM. The eosinophilic variant of Wegener's granulomatosis. Hum Pathol 1988;19:682–688.

94. Gephardt GN, Ahmad M, Tubbs RR. Pulmonary vasculitis (Wegener's granulomatosis): Immunohistochemical study of T and B cell markers. Am J Med 1983;74:700–704.

95. Falk RJ, Jennette JC. Anti-neutrophil cytoplasmic autoantibodies with specificity for myeloperoxidase in patients with systemic vasculitis and idiopathic necrotizing and crescentic glomerulonephritis. N Engl J Med 1988;318:1651–1657.

96. Nolle B, Specks U, Ludemann J, Rohrbach MS, DeRemee RA, Gross WL. Anticytoplasmic autoantibodies: Their immunodiagnostic value in Wegener's granulomatosis. Ann Intern Med 1989;111:28–40.

97. Harrison DJ, Simpson R, Kharbanda R, Abernethy VE, Nimmo G. Antibodies to neutrophil cytoplasmic antigens in Wegener's granulomatosis and other conditions. Thorax 1989;44:373–377.

Index

ISBN 0-397-51051-9